Clinical
BIOCHEMISTRY

Clinical
BIOCHEMISTRY

THIRD EDITION

Nanda Maheshwari MSc BEd
Lecturer
Suburban College of Paramedical Education (SCOPE)
Mumbai, Maharashtra, India

Foreword
SM Arora

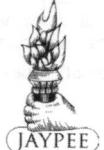

JAYPEE BROTHERS MEDICAL PUBLISHERS
The Health Sciences Publisher
New Delhi | London

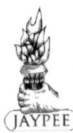 **Jaypee Brothers Medical Publishers (P) Ltd**

Headquarters
Jaypee Brothers Medical Publishers (P) Ltd
EMCA House, 23/23-B
Ansari Road, Daryaganj
New Delhi 110 002, India
Landline: +91-11-23272143, +91-11-23272703
+91-11-23282021, +91-11-23245672
Email: jaypee@jaypeebrothers.com

Corporate Office
Jaypee Brothers Medical Publishers (P) Ltd
4838/24, Ansari Road, Daryaganj
New Delhi 110 002, India
Phone: +91-11-43574357
Fax: +91-11-43574314
Email: jaypee@jaypeebrothers.com

Overseas Office
J.P. Medical Ltd
83 Victoria Street, London
SW1H 0HW (UK)
Phone: +44 20 3170 8910
Fax: +44 (0)20 3008 6180
Email: info@jpmedpub.com

Website: www.jaypeebrothers.com
Website: www.jaypeedigital.com

© 2022, Jaypee Brothers Medical Publishers

The views and opinions expressed in this book are solely those of the original contributor(s)/author(s) and do not necessarily represent those of editor(s) and publisher of the book.

All rights reserved. No part of this publication may be reproduced, stored or transmitted in any form or by any means, electronic, mechanical, photocopying, recording or otherwise, without the prior permission in writing of the publishers.

All brand names and product names used in this book are trade names, service marks, trademarks or registered trademarks of their respective owners. The publisher is not associated with any product or vendor mentioned in this book.

Medical knowledge and practice change constantly. This book is designed to provide accurate, authoritative information about the subject matter in question. However, readers are advised to check the most current information available on procedures included and check information from the manufacturer of each product to be administered, to verify the recommended dose, formula, method and duration of administration, adverse effects and contraindications. It is the responsibility of the practitioner to take all appropriate safety precautions. Neither the publisher nor the author(s)/editor(s) assume any liability for any injury and/or damage to persons or property arising from or related to use of material in this book.

This book is sold on the understanding that the publisher is not engaged in providing professional medical services. If such advice or services are required, the services of a competent medical professional should be sought.

Every effort has been made where necessary to contact holders of copyright to obtain permission to reproduce copyright material. If any have been inadvertently overlooked, the publisher will be pleased to make the necessary arrangements at the first opportunity.

Inquiries for bulk sales may be solicited at: jaypee@jaypeebrothers.com

Clinical Biochemistry

First Edition: 2008
Second Edition: 2017
Third Edition: **2022**
ISBN: 978-93-5465-254-7

Printed at: Sterling Graphics Pvt. Ltd. India.

Dedicated to...

My father Mr Ramesh ji Baheti
and
My mother Mrs Kusumlata Baheti

Mahatma Gandhi said that every home is a university and the parents are the teachers.
I write, as my parents believed in me and have always encouraged and blessed me.

Foreword

It is privilege to present third edition of *Clinical Biochemistry* by Nanda Maheshwari, faculty member of SCOPE. Being associated with the Paramedical Education for a decade, I can acknowledge that this can serve every purpose for Paramedical Students. The contents are divided into three sections: Basic Chemistry, Fundamentals of Biochemistry, and Clinical Biochemistry. This represents perfect blend of her rich practical experience and keen academic interest.

The author has taken tremendous efforts in preparing this book, focusing attention to cover various aspects of the subject. She has maintained simplicity and readability that would help reading and understanding by any beginner and expert alike. The reference diagrams and flowcharts make it easier to relate with tests/practical by students and laboratory professionals. This book has maintained balance between theoretical manual methods and practical world of automation.

I congratulate the author for writing this third edition of *Clinical Biochemistry*. I am sure this book will go a long way in filling the void between academics and industry. May almighty, give her courage and achievements she deserves. I wish her great success in all her endeavors.

SM Arora
Founder
Suburban College of Paramedical Education (SCOPE),
Mumbai, Maharashtra, India

Preface to the Third Edition

"To improve is to change, to be perfect is to be change often."

Journey of this book started in 2008. With continuous adaptation of latest technology, and improved documentation, *Clinical Biochemistry* is ready to launch its third edition in 2022.

Each and every page of the book is presented with thorough revision. Better diagrams, flowcharts, and summary are provided with each chapter for long-term remembrance of the concern topic. From basics to advance, every aspect of the field is discussed in the book.

In this era of Robotics and automation, diagnostic science has made a tremendous progress. With the aim to introduce latest technologies to students, I have updated this edition with topics like Therapeutic Drug Monitoring and Automation in Clinical Biochemistry. Some of the tests which are regular for today's diagnostic world such as tumor markers, details of advanced analytical techniques have been added in this edition. As each topic is covered in a small chapter, it makes it easy for the students to assimilate the concept in totality. I am sure Summary and Practice Questions that are provided for each chapter will prove as additional study support to every student.

The order and style of presentation in this book is similar to the first edition. The orientation of this book is to provide simple yet advanced content such that the book suffices the needs of not only DMLT/MLT/BSc students but also students of diverse backgrounds who require an exposure to this field. This book is successfully serving as a reference book for Laboratory Technician and Paramedical professionals as well. I hope that the simple language and enhanced and illustrative images of this edition will boost your interest in the field of *Clinical Biochemistry*. I welcome constructive criticism and suggestions from teachers, colleagues, students, and interested readers for the next revised edition.

Nanda Maheshwari

Preface to the First Edition

It is a matter of great pleasure to present my third book *Clinical Biochemistry*. In this book, I have tried to explain various concepts using simple language and short sentences. Each topic covered in one small chapter makes it easy for the students to read. The aims and objects of this book are primarily to meet the requirements of CMLT/DMLT and undergraduate courses.

Clinical biochemistry is an important subject of medical laboratory technology courses, but there is non-availability of good books on this subject. The books available are vast and mainly written for MBBS students. I have tried to overcome this problem by writing in easy language and providing exact data. I hope that this book will satisfy the needs of students.

I invite and welcome constructive criticism and suggestions from teachers, colleagues and students for next revised edition.

Nanda Maheshwari

Acknowledgment

It is a feeling of pride for me to introduce the third edition of *Clinical Biochemistry* to my readers. I owe this incredible journey of 13 years to many souls around.

Special thanks to all past and present students and teachers for reading and recommending this book. Feedback from avid readers provided valuable support for me during the course of writing this edition.

In order to learn about the latest technological developments and current laboratory practices in the field, I visited Central Processing Laboratory of Suburban Diagnostics in Mumbai. During my visit, Dr Anupa Dixit, Laboratory Director, and all her staff members were extremely helpful. I would like to express my gratitude toward Dr Pratik Jariwala for allowing me to visit Jariwala Laboratory and Diagnostics, Mumbai.

Dr SM Arora, Founder of Suburban College of Paramedical Education (SCOPE), Mumbai, took great effort to write the foreword of this book. I am sincerely thankful to him. Deep gratitude toward my colleagues for constructive suggestions and discussions while writing this book.

It took me more than a year to finish writing and compiling this work. During this period of research, writing the manuscript, editing, proofreading, etc., my husband Mr Yogendra Maheshwari and my little angels Arushi and Kabir patiently cooperated with me. Thanks a lot to my family for tolerating my incessant disappearances from many family moments. I would like to express my deepest thanks to parents, Mr Ramesh ji Baheti and Mrs Kusumlata Baheti; whatever I am today is because of their blessings and confidence in my abilities. I am fortunate to have good friends and close kin who continuously encouraged me to pursue my work.

Acknowledgment

Thanks to Sukhdev Guruji and Anandvan Yog Kendra for helping me out to be in good state of health so that I can write with more concentration and clarity in mind.

Lastly, my acknowledgment would remain incomplete without mentioning M/s Jaypee Brothers Medical Publishers, New Delhi, India, and their team. My special thanks to them for walking the extra mile and putting in great effort in publishing this book.

Contents

SECTION 1: BASIC CHEMISTRY

Branches of Chemistry 2

1. **Elementary Knowledge of Inorganic Chemistry** 3
   Structure of Atom 4
   Key Terms in Chemistry 5
   Acids, Bases, and Salts 7
   pH 10
   Solutions and Dilutions 19
   Isotope and Radioisotope 25

2. **Elementary Knowledge of Organic Chemistry** 39
   Organic Compounds 39
   Aliphatic and Aromatic Compounds 41
   Functional Groups 42
   Hydrocarbons 44
   Homologous Series 47

3. **Elementary Knowledge of Physical Chemistry** 50
   Osmosis and Diffusion 50
   Colloids 52
   Surface Tension 54

4. **Elementary Knowledge of Analytical Chemistry** 59
   Balances 60
   Centrifuge 67
   pH Meter 69
   Colorimeter 73
   Spectrophotometer 78
   Differences between Colorimeter and Spectrophotometer 81
   Fluorimeter 82
   Flame Photometer 85

Urinometer *88*
Densitometer *89*

5. Elementary Knowledge of Biostatistics 92
Common Statistical Terms *92*
Notations for a Population and Sample Values *94*
Types of Data *95*
Presentation of Data *97*
Measures of Central Tendencies *99*
Measures of Variability *103*
Estimation Statistics *112*
Hypothesis Test *114*
t-Test *117*
Chi-Square Test for Population Standard Deviation *118*

SECTION 2: FUNDAMENTALS OF BIOCHEMISTRY

6. Aim and Scope of Biochemistry 125
History of Biochemistry *125*
Scope of Biochemistry *126*
Aims/Objectives of Clinical Biochemistry *128*

7. Structure of Cell 130
Cell Organelles *131*
Cell Membrane *131*
Cytoplasm *131*
Nucleus *131*
Ribosomes *132*
Endoplasmic Reticulum *132*
Lysosomes *132*
Centrosomes *133*
Vacuoles *133*
Golgi Bodies *133*
Mitochondria *133*
Peroxisomes *134*
Cytoskeleton *134*
Functions of the Animal Cell *134*
Types of Cells *136*

8. Study of Carbohydrates   139
Classification *139*
Detective Tests for Carbohydrate *141*
Metabolism *142*
Carbohydrate Metabolism *144*
Comparisons between Glycolysis and Krebs Cycle *151*
Disorders of Carbohydrate Metabolism *151*
Biochemical Importance of Carbohydrate *155*

9. Study of Proteins   159
Classifications *159*
Detective Tests for Proteins *162*
Metabolism of Protein *162*
Diseases Related to Protein Metabolism *171*
Biochemical Importance of Proteins *175*

10. Study of Lipids   178
Classifications *178*
Detective Tests for Lipids *180*
Lipid Metabolism *180*
Diseases Related to Lipid Metabolism *185*
Disorders of Lipid Metabolism *186*
Biochemical Importance of Lipids *189*

11. Study of Nucleic Acids   192
Components of Nucleic Acids *192*
Structure of DNA *193*
Structure of RNA *195*
Comparisons of DNA and RNA *196*
DNA Replication *197*
Genetic Disorders *204*
Biological Importance of Nucleic Acid *207*

SECTION 3: CLINICAL BIOCHEMISTRY

12. Introduction to Clinical Biochemistry   211
Biochemistry Laboratory *211*
Standard International Units *213*
Laboratory Glassware *220*

Collection of Samples Used in Biochemistry Laboratory 226
Reporting and Interpretation of Results 236

13. Advanced Analytical Techniques–I   242
Chromatography 242
Mass Spectroscopy 255

14. Advanced Analytical Techniques–II   261
Immunoassay 261
Electrophoresis 269
Blotting Techniques 271

15. Enzyme Assay   281
Properties of Enzyme 281
Unit of Enzyme 282
Coenzymes and Cofactors 282
Factors Affecting Enzyme Reaction 287
Importance of Enzymes 288
Amylase 290
Serum Lipase 294
Serum Lactate Dehydrogenase 297
Phosphates 299
Reactions 300
Creatine Phosphokinase Isoenzymes Test 302
Method of Diagnosis for Creatine Kinase Isoenzymes 304
Reagent Composition 305
Procedure 305
Calculations 306

16. Water and Mineral Metabolism   311
Distribution of Water in the Body 311
Water Balance 312
Physiological Functions of Water 313
Regulation of Passage of Water 314
Thirst 314
Minerals 314

17. Inborn Errors of Metabolism   325
Carbohydrate Metabolism 326
Pyruvate Metabolism 331
Protein Metabolism 332

Lipid Metabolism *336*
Nucleic Acid Metabolism *339*
Diagnosis of Inborn Errors of Metabolism *340*

18. Endocrine Glands and Hormones — 344

Functions of Hormones *344*
Chemical Nature of Hormones *345*
Mechanism of Hormone Action *346*
Control of Hormone Secretion *348*
Endocrine Glands *353*
Hormones Secreted by Organs *368*

19. Thyroid Function Tests — 376

Location and Morphology of Thyroid Gland *376*
Synthesis and Release of Thyroid Hormones *377*
Hormones of Thyroid Gland *378*
Parathyroid Gland *379*
Thymus *380*
Thyroid Function Tests *380*
Thyroid-Stimulating Hormone Test *380*
T_3 and T_4 Tests *384*
Clinical Interpretation *387*
Thyroid Function Tests in Pregnancy *387*

20. Diabetic Profile — 391

Types of Diabetes *392*
Diagnosis of Diabetes *396*

21. Liver Function Tests — 418

Morphology and Functions *418*
Serum Bilirubin *420*
Transaminases *426*
Serum Proteins *431*
Alkaline Phosphatase *434*
Urine Analysis: Bile Salt, Bile Pigment, and Urobilinogen *437*

22. Renal Function Tests — 444

Structure and Functions of Kidney *444*
Renal Function Tests *447*

23. Cardiac Function Tests — 469
Structure and Function of Heart *469*
Cardiac Function Tests *471*
Total Lipids *479*

24. Electrolytes — 484
Introduction and Classification *484*
Serum Sodium and Potassium *485*
Urine Sodium and Potassium *491*
Serum and Urine Chloride *492*
Serum and Urine Phosphorus *495*
Serum and Urine Calcium *498*

25. Body Fluids — 502
Seminal Fluid *502*
Amniotic Fluid *507*
Cerebrospinal Fluid *510*
Pericardial Fluid *512*
Pleural Fluid *515*
Peritoneal Fluid *518*
Synovial Fluid *523*

26. Blood pH and Buffer System — 529
Importance of Maintaining Blood pH *529*
Measurement of pH *530*
pH Meter *530*
Procedure and Precaution of Measurement of Blood pH *533*
Need of Buffer System *533*
Buffer Systems in the Body *534*

27. Arterial Blood Gases — 541
Collection of Arterial Blood Specimen *542*
Arterial Blood Gas Analysis *543*
Blood Gas Analyzer *554*
Acid-Base Balance *555*

28. Vitamin Assay — 561
Purpose of Vitamin Deficiency Testing *566*
Essential Vitamins *566*

29. Tumor Markers — 596
Types of Tumor Markers 596
Uses of Tumor Markers 598
List of Tumor Markers 599
Testing of Tumor Markers 607
Limitations of Tumor Markers 609

30. Therapeutic Drug Monitoring — 612
Indications for Drug Level Determination 613
Drugs for Therapeutic Drug Monitoring 613
Information Required for Therapeutic Drug Monitoring 614
Collection of Sample 615
Pharmacokinetic Analysis 616
Target Drug Concentration Range 617

31. Automation in Clinical Biochemistry — 619
Steps in Automated Analysis 620
Classification of Analyzers 623
Care and Maintenance of Analyzers 628
Routine Biochemistry Analyzers 630
Total Laboratory Automation 636
Biosensors 638
Nanotechnology 640

Index 643

Plate 1

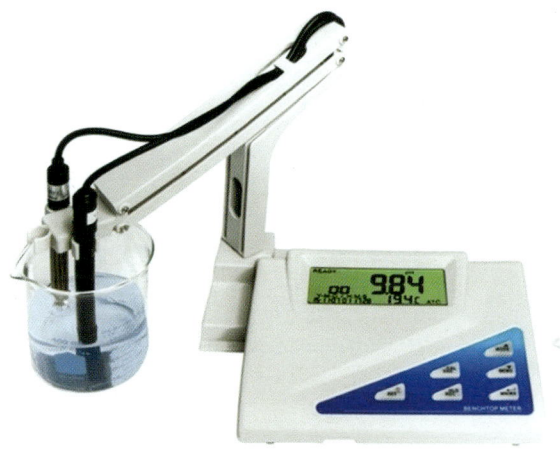

Fig. 1.2: pH meter calibration.

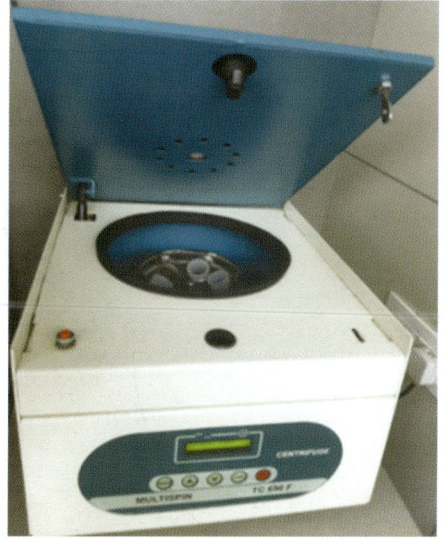

Fig. 4.3: Electric centrifuge.

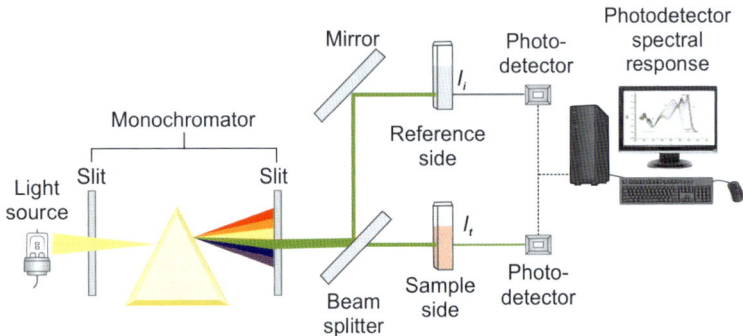

Fig. 4.7: Double-beam spectrophotometer.

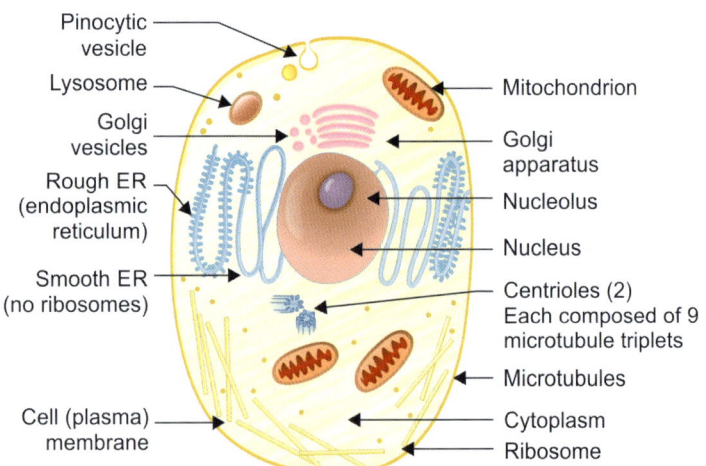

Fig. 7.1: The animal cell.

Plate 3

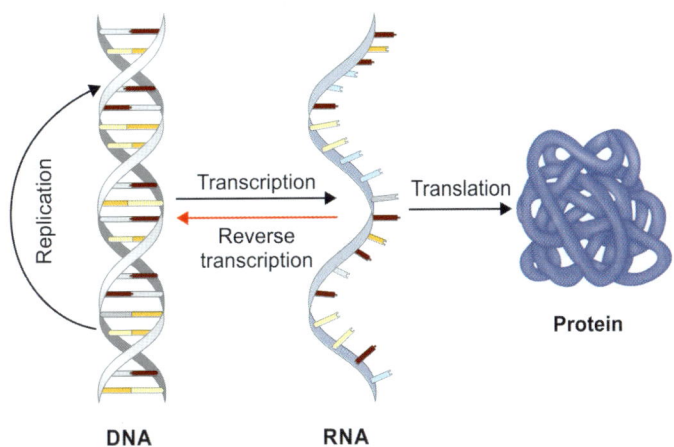

Fig. 9.1: Role of DNA and RNA in protein synthesis.

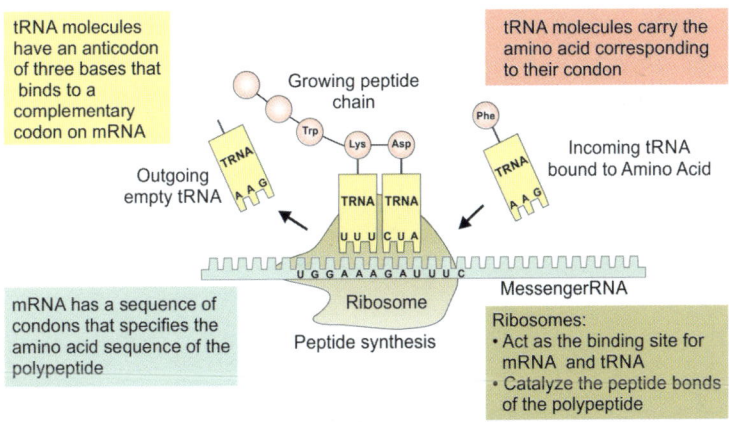

Fig. 9.2: Translation—key components that enable genetic code to synthesize polypeptides.

Plate 4

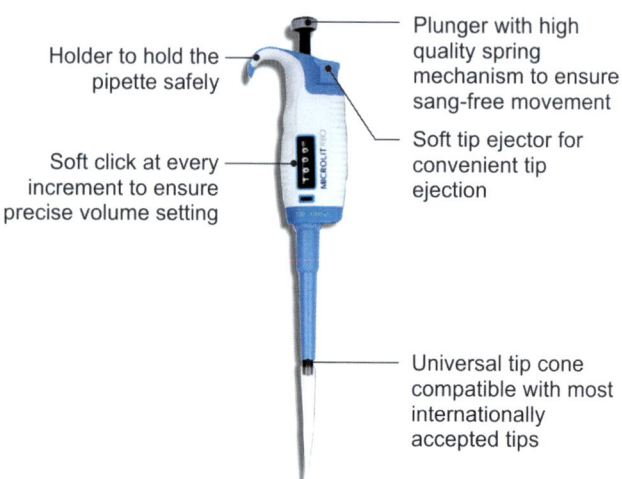

Fig. 12.5: Micropipette.

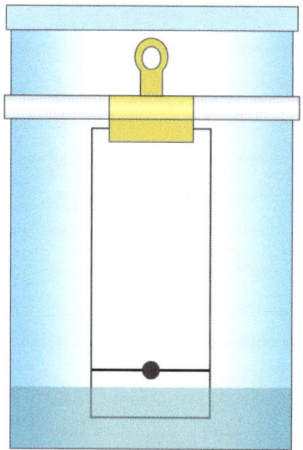

Fig. 13.5B: Paper dipped in a solvent.

Plate 5

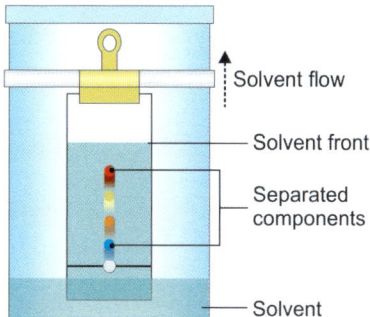

Fig. 13.5C: Components separated.

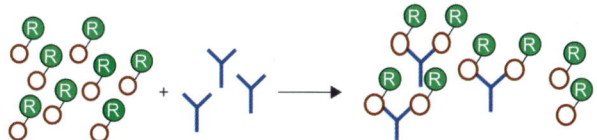

Radiolabeled antigen + antibody gives Ag–Ab complex with radiolabeled Ag

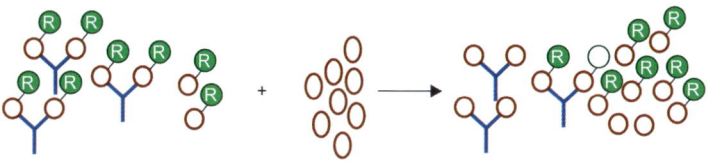

Ag–Ab complex + unlabelled antigen gives Ag–Ab complex attached to unlabelled antigen and radiolabelled antigen becomes free

Fig. 14.1: Principle of radioimmunoassay.

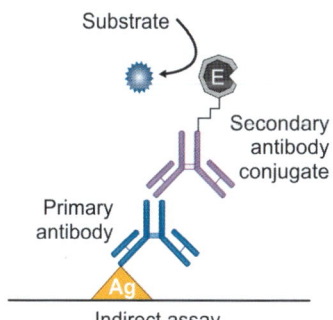

Fig. 14.4: Indirect enzyme-linked immunosorbent assay (ELISA).

Plate 6

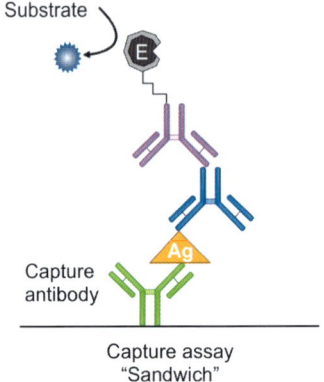

Fig. 14.5: Sandwich enzyme-linked immunosorbent assay (ELISA).

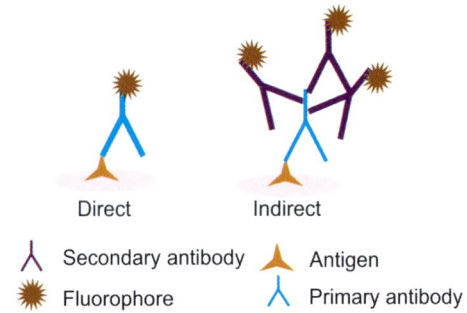

Fig. 14.6: Direct and indirect immunofluorescence.

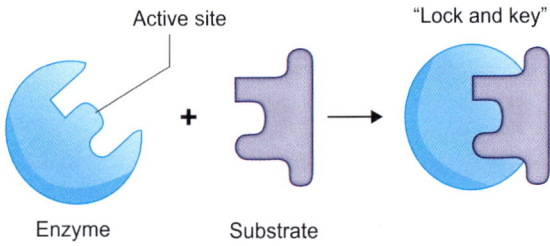

Fig. 15.2: Lock and key model.

Plate 7

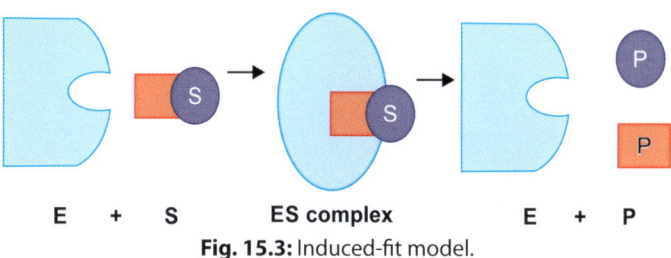

Fig. 15.3: Induced-fit model.

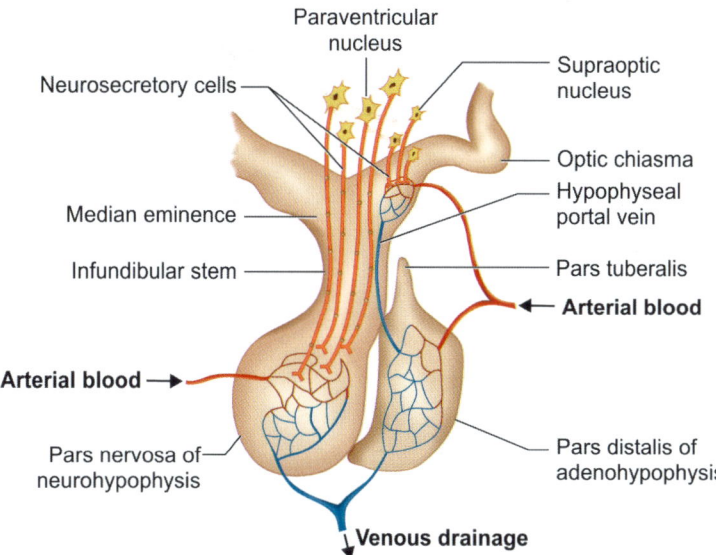

Fig. 18.4: Morphology of pituitary gland.

Plate 8

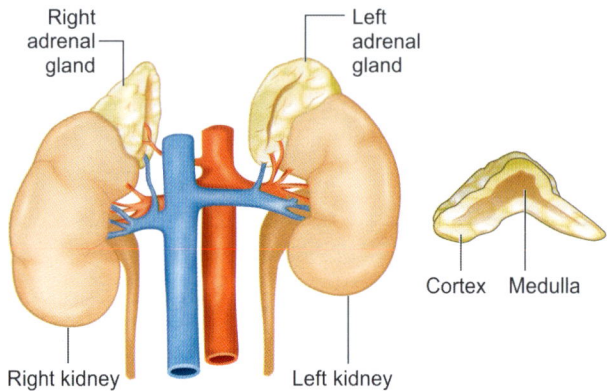

Fig. 18.5: Adrenal gland.

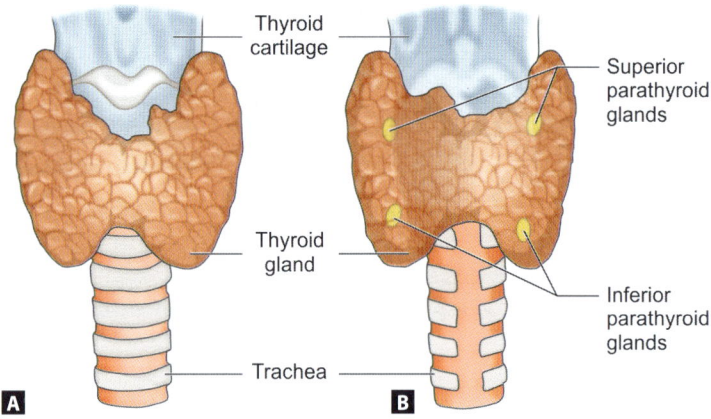

Figs. 19.1A and B: (A) Front view—thyroid gland;
(B) Back view—parathyroid gland.

Plate 9

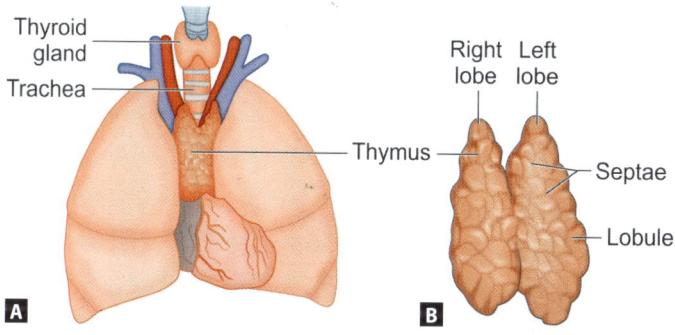

Figs. 19.2A and B: (A) Location of thymus gland; (B) Thymus gland.

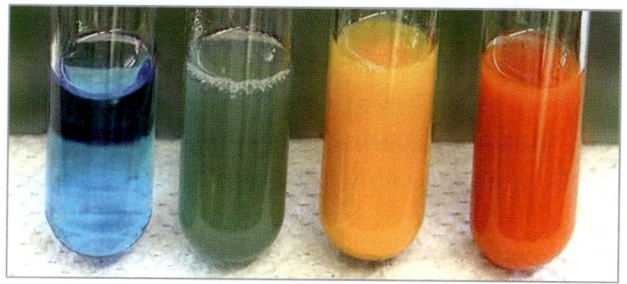

Fig. 20.3: Test tubes showing results of Benedict's test.

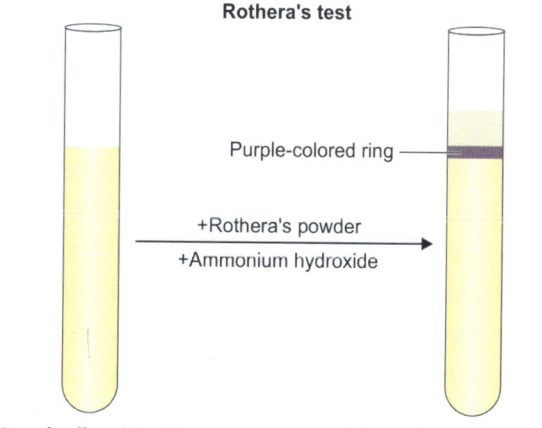

Fig. 20.4: Rothera's test.

Plate 10

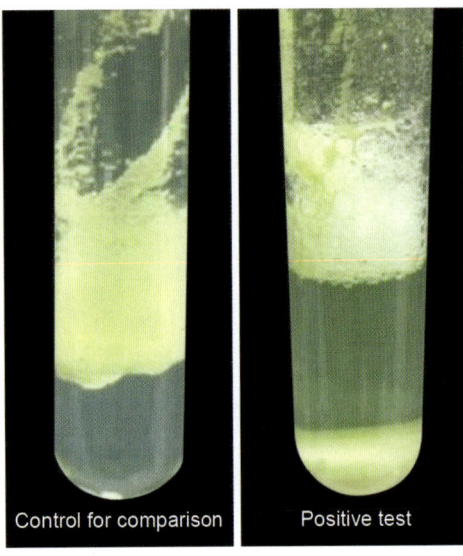

Figs. 21.3A and B: (A) Control for Hay's test: (B) Positive Hay's test.

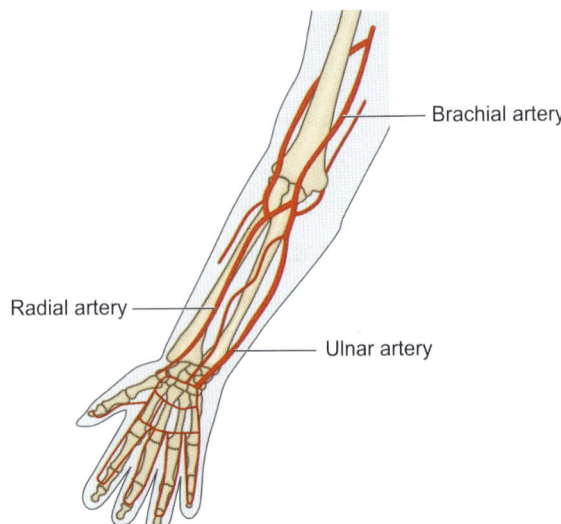

Fig. 27.1: Different arteries for the collection of blood.

Plate 11

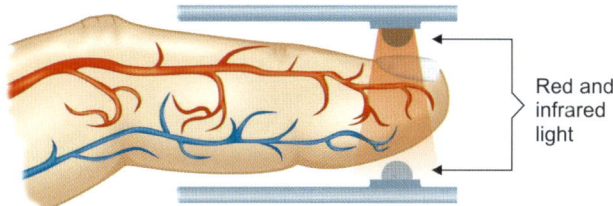

Fig. 27.2: Working of pulse oximeter.

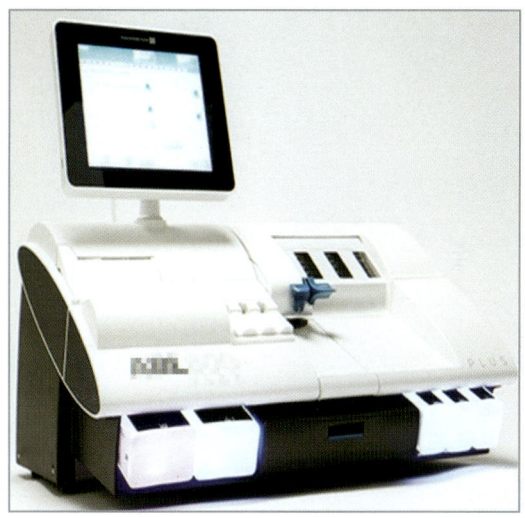

Fig. 27.3: Blood gas analyzer.

SECTION

Basic Chemistry

SECTION OUTLINE

1. Elementary Knowledge of Inorganic Chemistry
2. Elementary Knowledge of Organic Chemistry
3. Elementary Knowledge of Physical Chemistry
4. Elementary Knowledge of Analytical Chemistry
5. Elementary Knowledge of Biostatistics

■ INTRODUCTION

Chemistry is a branch of science which deals with the study of matter composed of atoms and molecules, their properties, composition, structure, behavior, and interactions among constituents of matter.

Everything around us composes of atoms and molecules including our bodies itself. We can see chemistry in our day-to-day activities; right from the production of food in farms to cooking them in a kitchen, from a bicycle to a space rocket, from phones to computers, steel used in buildings, polymers that make plastic bags, cell phone batteries, photosynthesis, detergents, clothes, dyes and colors, beverages, etc., are some of the examples where chemistry is applied. Chemistry helps us to understand the world we see and experience.

■ BRANCHES OF CHEMISTRY

Today, chemistry has become a very diverse subject with large numbers of branches. The five main branches of chemistry are physical chemistry, analytical chemistry, inorganic chemistry, organic chemistry, and biochemistry.

CHAPTER 1

Elementary Knowledge of Inorganic Chemistry

> **Keywords**
> - **Structure of atom:** Atomic structure, ion, element, compound, atomic number, mass number, atomic weight, molecular weight, and equivalent weight
> - **Acids, bases, and salts:** Arrhenius theory, Lowry and Brønsted concept, Lewis concept, and types of salts
> - **pH:** Salt ionization of water, Henderson–Hasselbalch equation, importance of maintaining blood and urine pH, pH indicator, pH meter, and buffer solutions
> - **Solutions and dilutions:** Percent solutions, molarity, normality, dilution factor, stock solution, working solution, diluent, and serial dilutions
> - **Isotope and radioisotope:** Isotope vs nuclide stable isotope and its uses, radioisotope types of radiation, use of radioisotopes in biochemistry, radiation hazard, and radiation safety measures

■ INTRODUCTION

The branch of chemistry that deals with the study of compounds, which does not consist of carbon–hydrogen atoms in it, is called *"Inorganic Chemistry."*

Inorganic substances include all pure elements, salts, many acids and bases, metals and alloys, and minerals. Compounds in which a non-carbon atom forms a chemical bond with hydrogen are inorganic. There are about 100,000 numbers of inorganic compounds in existence. Inorganic chemistry studies the behavior of these compounds along with their properties, their physical and chemical characteristics too. The elements of the periodic table except for carbon and hydrogen come in the lists of inorganic compounds.

Examples of inorganic compounds include:

Sodium chloride (table salt) (NaCl), brass (an alloy), glass and quartz (SiO_2), hydrochloric acid (HCl), sulfuric acid (H_2SO_4), etc.

■ STRUCTURE OF ATOM

All matter is composed of minute discrete particles called as atoms.

Atoms are the foundation of chemistry. They are the basis for everything in the universe. Solids are made of densely packed atoms while gases have atoms that are spread out. Atoms form compounds that help the biological world survive.

An atom is composed of still smaller particles, viz. electrons, protons, and neutrons (**Fig. 1.1**). These are known as atomic or fundamental particles of an atom.

Electrons are the smallest of the three particles that make up atoms. It is a negatively charged particle, found in shells or orbitals that surround the nucleus of an atom.

The proton is a positively charged particle situated in highly dense central part of an atom called nucleus.

The neutron is a neutral particle present in the nucleus of the atom.

As protons and neutrons are found in the nucleus, they are also referred as nucleons.

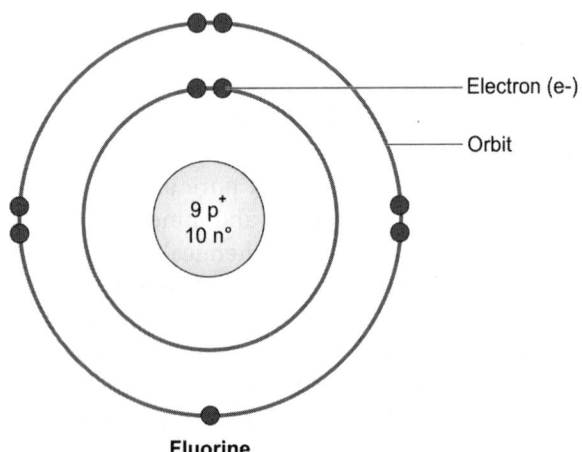

Fluorine
Fig. 1.1: Structure of an atom.

The number of electrons present in the extranuclear part is equal to the number of protons present in the nucleus. Thus, an atom is electrically neutral.

As the electrons have negligible weight, the mass of the atom is concentrated at the nucleus.

■ KEY TERMS IN CHEMISTRY

- **Ion:** An atom or group of atoms that carries a positive or negative electric charge as a result of having lost or gained one or more electrons. Positively charged ions (loss of electron) are called cations; negatively charged ions are (gain of electron) called anions.

  For example, Na^+ (cation of sodium) and Cl^- (anion of chlorine).

- **Element:** An element is a pure substance made up of one kind of atoms only. It can be made up of single atom, two atoms or more than two atoms.

  Elements are classified as metals, non-metals, metalloids, and noble gases.

  For example, Mg (magnesium—metal), O (oxygen—non-metal), B (boron—metalloid), and Ar (argon—noble gas).

- **Compound:** A compound is a pure substance made up of two or more different elements (atoms) combined chemically in a fixed proportion.

  For example, H_2O (water—H and O combines in a fixed proportion—2 atoms of H and 1 atom of O).

- **Atomic number:** The total number of protons in the nucleus of an atom is called the atomic number of that atom. It is represented with the letter "Z." All the atoms of a particular element have the same number of protons, and hence the same atomic number. Atoms of different elements have different atomic numbers.

  For example, all atoms of oxygen have 8 protons in their nucleus. So, the atomic number of oxygen is 8.

- **Mass number:** The number of protons and neutrons combined is called the mass number of an atom. It is represented using the letter "A."

  For example, an atom of carbon has 6 protons and 6 neutrons. Thus, its mass number is 12.

The weight of an electron is almost negligible. Thus, the atomic mass of an atom is almost the same as its mass number.

- **Atomic weight:** Since an atom is very tiny, it is inconvenient to calculate the absolute weight of an atom. Therefore, weight of the atom of an element is compared to the weight of the atom of a standard element like hydrogen or oxygen. Atomic weight of an element is defined as number of times one atom of an element is heavier than the mass of hydrogen atom or number of times one atom of an element is heavier than 1/12th the mass of carbon atom.

  It is measured in atomic mass unit (amu, also known as daltons, D), for example,

Element	Atomic weight (in amu)
Mg	: 24.32
Al	: 26.98
Cu	: 63.54

- **Molecular weight:** Like atoms, molecules are also very small; hence molecular weights such as atomic weights are also relative. Molecular weight of a substance is defined as number of times one molecule of the substance is heavier than the mass of hydrogen atom or number of times one molecule of the substance is heavier than 1/12th the mass of carbon atom.

  Molecular weight of a substance is also the sum of atomic weights of all atoms present in its molecule.

  For example,
  1. Methane (CH_4) = 12 (carbon) + 4 (1 × 4 = 4 hydrogen) = 16
  2. Sulfuric acid (H_2SO_4) = 2 (1 × 2 = 2 hydrogen) + 32 (sulfur) + 64 (16 × 4 oxygen) = 98

- **Equivalent weight:** Whenever an element takes part in a chemical reaction, it must be associated with a definite weight or some multiple of that definite weight.

  Equivalent weight of an element is that weight of it, which can combine with or replace from a chemical combination 8 parts by weight of oxygen or 35.5 parts by weight of chlorine or 1.008 parts by weight of hydrogen.

  It is also defined as the weight of an element, which liberates 11.2 liters of pure and dry hydrogen gas at normal temperature and pressure (NTP) when the equivalent is expressed in grams.

The equivalent weight of an element or radical is equal to its atomic weight or molecular weight divided by the valency as it assumes in compounds.

For example, oxygen has an atomic weight of 16 and always assumes valence 2 in compounds, so its equivalent weight is 8. The sulfate radical (SO_4) has molecular weight 96 and always has valency 2 in compounds, so its equivalent weight is 48. Some elements exhibit more than one valency in forming compounds and thus have more than one equivalent weight. Iron (atomic weight 56) has an equivalent weight of 28 in ferrous compounds (valency 2) and 18.6 in ferric compounds (valency 3).

ACIDS, BASES, AND SALTS

The term acid is derived from a Latin word acidus means sour; while the term alkali is originated from an Arabic word alkali means plant ash.

According to the classical idea, acid is a substance whose water solution:
- Turns blue litmus to red
- Neutralize base
- Reacts with active metals with the evolution of hydrogen gas
- Has sour taste
- Decomposes carbonates into CO_2 and H_2O

According to the classical idea, base is a substance whose water solution:
- Turns red litmus to blue
- Neutralize acid
- Has bitter taste
- Feels soapy
- Absorbs CO_2 to form carbonate

These definitions were applicable to aqueous solution and also do not mention their structures. Therefore, different modern concepts were developed to define acids and bases.

Arrhenius Theory of Acids and Bases (Water-ion-concept)

According to Arrhenius (1887), an acid is a hydrogen compound, which in aqueous solution gives hydrogen ions.

For example, HCl $\rightarrow$ H$^+$ + Cl$^-$

A base is a hydroxide compound, which in aqueous solution produces hydroxyl ions.

For example, NaOH $\rightarrow$ Na$^+$ + OH$^-$

Thus, acidic properties are due to H$^+$ and basic properties are due to OH$^-$ ions.

Lowry and Brønsted Concept of Acids and Bases (Protonic Concept)

According to Lowry and Brønsted (1923), an acid is a substance, which can donate a proton (H$^+$ ion), i.e., acid is a proton donor.

Base is a substance which can accept a proton (H$^+$ ion), i.e., base is a proton acceptor.

For example, HCl + H$_2$O $\rightarrow$ H$_3$O$^+$ + Cl$^-$

Here, since HCl donates a proton to water, it is an acid. Water accepts a proton, hence it is a base.

Lewis Concept of Acids and Bases (Lewis Electronic Theory)

According to Lewis (1923), an acid is a substance which can accept the electron pair to form a coordinate bond. Thus, acid is an electron acceptor.

Base is a substance, which can donate the electron pair to form a coordinate bond. Thus, base is an electron donor.

For example, NH$_3$ + BF$_3$ $\rightarrow$ NH$_3$ BF$_3$

Ammonia + Boron trifluoride. Coordinate complex

In above reaction, BF$_3$ is a Lewis acid and is accepting an electron pair and NH$_3$ is a Lewis base as it is donating an electron pair.

Salts

Salt is a substance of which cation or anion or both the ion reacts with water producing acidity or basicity in the solution.

OR

A salt is a compound formed by the interaction of an acid and a base, placing H$^+$ of the acid by a metal or metal-like radical.

Neutralization is a reaction of acids and base that forms salt and water.

For example, HCl + NaOH → NaCl + H_2O
Acid + Base → Salt + Water

Types of Salts

Depending on the behavior of salts in aqueous solution, there are four types of salts:
1. **Salt of strong acid and strong base:** These salts produce strong acid and strong base when react with water.
   For example, KCl, NaCl, KNO_3, and Na_2SO_4.
2. **Salt of strong acid and weak base:** These salts produce strong acid and weak base when react with water.
   For example, NH_4Cl, $CuSO_4$, and $FeCl_3$.
3. **Salt of weak acid and strong base:** These salts produce weak acid and strong base when react with water.
   For example, KCN, NaCN, and CH_3COONa.
4. **Salt of weak acid and weak base:** These salts produce weak acid and weak base when react with water.
   For example, CH_3COONH_4 and $(NH_4)CO_3$.

The cell contains 1–3% salts.

Sodium chloride is a common salt that is added to prepare food. It regulates plasma volume, acid–base balance and nerve as well as muscle functions. It maintains fluid and electrolyte balance. Chloride of salt is a source of HCl in gastric juice. It also acts as enzyme activator.

The other important mineral salts present in cells and animal body are as follows:

H^+, K^+, Ca^{++}, Mg^{++}, Cl^-, OH^-, HCO_3^-, CO_3^-, SO_4^-, and PO_4^-

The salts serve following functions:
- Salts are essential for construction, survival, and growth of cells.
- The metallic ions function as catalysts of enzymes.
- Ions maintain electrical properties of the cells. For example, Na^+ and K^+ ions are necessary for nerves to conduct impulses.
- Ions act as buffers, e.g., HCO_3 in blood.
- Ions maintain atmospheric pressure.
- Ions are used for synthesis of tissues, e.g., iron is used for synthesis of tissue, calcium is used for synthesis of bones.

■ pH

The pH of an aqueous solution is based on the pH scale which typically ranges from 0 to 14 in water. A pH of 7 is neutral, a pH of less than 7 is acidic and a pH of greater than 7 is basic. Acidic solutions have high hydronium concentrations and lower hydroxide concentrations. Basic solutions have high hydroxide concentrations and lower hydronium concentrations.

Self-ionization of Water

In the self-ionization of water, the amphoteric (capable of functioning either as an acid or as a base) ability of water to act as a proton donor and acceptor allows the formation of hydronium (H_3O^+) and hydroxide ions (OH^-). In pure water, the concentration of hydronium ions equals that of hydroxide ions. At 25° C, the concentrations of both hydronium and hydroxide ions equal 1.0×10^{-7}. The ion product of water K_w, is the equilibrium condition for the self-ionization of water and is expressed as follows:

$$K_w = [H_3O^+][OH^-] = 1.0 \times 10^{-14}$$

- **pH**: The term pH refers to the "potential of hydrogen ion." It was proposed by Danish biochemist Soren Sorensen in 1909 so that there could be a more convenient way to describe hydronium and hydroxide ion concentrations in aqueous solutions since both concentrations tend to be extremely small. It is defined as the negative of the logarithm of the concentration of hydrogen ions. In terms of hydronium ion concentration, the equation to determine the pH of an aqueous solution is:

$$pH = -\log[H_3O^+]$$

- **pOH**: The pOH of an aqueous solution, which is related to the pH, can be determined by the following equation:

$$pOH = -\log[OH^-]$$

This equation uses the hydroxide concentration of an aqueous solution instead of the hydronium concentration.

Henderson-Hasselbalch Equation

Acid dissociation: The Henderson–Hasselbalch equation mathematically connects the measurable pH of a solution with the pK_a

Chapter 1: Elementary Knowledge of Inorganic Chemistry

(which is equal to -log K_a) of the acid. The equation is also useful for estimating the pH of a buffer solution and finding the equilibrium pH in an acid-base reaction. The equation can be derived from the formula of pK_a for a weak acid or buffer. The balanced equation for an acid dissociation is:

$$\underset{\text{Unionized/acid}}{\text{H–A}} \underset{}{\overset{K_a}{\rightleftharpoons}} \underset{\text{Ionized/salt}}{\underset{\text{base}}{\overset{\text{Conjugate}}{H^+ + A^-}}}$$

According to the law of dissociation, the acid dissociation constant K_a can be defined by the equation:

$$K_a = [H^+][A^-]/[HA]$$

where $[H^+]$ and $[A^-]$ are the concentrations of the ionized form of the acid, while $[HA]$ is the concentration of the unionized form.

Taking log on both sides,

$$\log K_a = \log ([H^+][A^-]/[HA])$$

Splitting the log terms, into separate components,

$$\log K_a = \log [H^+] + \log ([A^-]/[HA])$$

Since $pK_a = -\log_{10} K_a$ and $pH = -\log_{10} [H^+]$, therefore:

$$-pK_a = -pH + \log ([A^-]/[HA])$$

Rearranging the terms, we get the Henderson-Hasselbalch equation for acids as:

$$pH = pK_a + \log ([A^-]/[HA])$$

This equation can also be written as:

$$pH = pK_a + \log [(Salt)/(Acid)]$$

or

$$pH = pK_a + \log ([Ionized]/[Unionized])$$

Base dissociation:

$$\underset{\text{Unionized/base}}{\text{B–OH}} \underset{}{\overset{K_b}{\rightleftharpoons}} \underset{\text{Ionized/salt}}{\underset{\text{base}}{\overset{\text{Conjugate}}{B^+ + {}^-OH}}}$$

According to the law of dissociation, the base dissociation constant K_b can be defined by the equation:

$$K_b = [OH^-][B^+]/[BOH]$$

where $[B^+]$ and $[OH^-]$ are the concentrations of the ionized form of the base, while $[BOH]$ is the concentration of the unionized form.

Taking log on both sides,

$$\log K_b = \log([OH^-][B^+]/[BOH])$$

Splitting the log terms into separate components,

$$\log K_b = \log[OH^-] + \log([B^+]/[BOH])$$

Since $pK_b = -\log_{10} K_b$ and $pOH = -\log_{10}[OH^-]$, therefore:

$$-pK_b = -pOH + \log([B^+]/[BOH])$$

Rearranging the terms, we get the Henderson-Hasselbalch equation for bases:

$$pOH = pK_b + \log([B^+]/[BOH])$$

This equation can also be written as:

$$pOH = pK_b + \log[(Salt)/(Base)]$$

or

$$pOH = pK_b + \log([Ionized]/[Unionized])$$

Generally, the term pK_a can be used to measure the strength of an acid and pK_b for bases.

The pK_a of water is 15.7. Any value higher than this pK_a value increases basicity, while values which are lower than this value increases acidity. For example, the pK_a values for strong acids such as HCl can even go into the negative values with a pK_a of −8. While a strong base, such as ammonia (NH_3) has a pK_a of 38.

Applications of Henderson-Hasselbalch Equation:
- The Henderson-Hasselbalch equation calculates the pK_a of a molecule using simple experimental protocols. This in turn gives an idea of the acidity and basicity of molecules.
- The Henderson-Hasselbalch equation gives information of the abundance of ionized and unionized fractions of molecules within a given solution. This is useful for certain reactions as well as important for absorption, distribution and excretion of drugs. Hence, it is very useful in fields of chemistry, biochemistry and pharmacy.
- The Henderson-Hasselbalch equation is useful in estimating the pH of buffer solutions and finding the equilibrium pH in acid-base reactions.

$$\text{Blood pH} = 6.1 + \log(HCO_3^-/(0.03 \times PCO_2))$$

where,
6.1 is dissociation constant
HCO_3^- is plasma bicarbonate (mmol/L)
0.03 is CO_2 solubility constant

p CO_2 is partial pressure CO_2 (mmHg)
Keeping values,
$$pH = 6.1 + \log[24/0.03 \times 40]$$
$$= 7.40$$

Importance of Maintaining Blood pH

In order for the body to function normally, the maintenance of the acidity and alkalinity of the body is vital. The normal pH of blood is 7.35–7.45 with an average of 7.4. This slightly alkaline blood pH must be maintained to avoid detrimental effects on body. This is because, most biochemical reactions essential to life take place in an aqueous environment.

The human body maintains a very delicate pH balance in its fluids, tissues, and systems (within a narrow pH range of 7.35–7.45) so that body's immune system is operating in optimal conditions and is able to fight off illness and disease.

Human body has several self-regulating control mechanisms also called homeostatic systems—that protects us from wide fluctuations in our blood pH levels. The organs involved in the maintenance of blood pH are the lungs and the kidneys. The lungs exhale carbon dioxide to help with pH control while the kidneys excrete hydrogen ions and bicarbonates according to the needs of the body. The formation of carbonic acid and bicarbonate is reversible, so when the body needs more alkalinity, bicarbonate is formed. If the body needs more acidity, carbonic acid is formed.

Mild acidosis can lead to such problems as—if body is not maintained in a state of pH balance, its ability to eliminate the waste products slows down. To protect itself, the body converts acidic waste into solid waste and stores it in less critical areas of the body. The accumulation of solid waste can contribute to many health problems including excess weight, clogged arteries, arthritis, kidney stones, and various other chronic illnesses.

Causes for Acidosis

- Eating food which include meat, fish, poultry, dairy, grains, refined or processed foods, and fast food
- Drinks, such as coffee, soft drinks, alcohol, many types of water (distilled, bottled)

- Stress, worries, anxiety, and negative thoughts
- Pollution and toxins
- Intense physical exercise that produces lactic acid
- Dehydration which slows down the body's ability to cleanse itself through the kidneys
- Tobacco and drug use

Alkalosis can lead to such problems as—alkalosis occurs when body has too many bases. It can occur due to decreased blood levels of carbon dioxide, which is an acid. It can also occur due to increased blood levels of bicarbonate, which is a base. This may lead to:

Confusion (can progress to stupor or coma), hand tremor, lightheadedness, muscle twitching nausea, vomiting, numbness or tingling in the face, hands, or feet, and prolonged muscle spasms.

Causes for Alkalosis

Respiratory alkalosis is caused by low carbon dioxide levels in the blood. This can be due to:
- Fever, being at a high altitude, lack of oxygen, liver disease, lung disease, which is a cause to breathe faster (hyperventilate) and salicylate poisoning.
- Metabolic alkalosis is caused by too much bicarbonate in the blood. It can also occur due to certain kidney diseases.
- Hypochloremic alkalosis is caused by an extreme lack or loss of chloride, such as from prolonged vomiting.
- Hypokalemic alkalosis is caused by the kidneys' response to an extreme lack or loss of potassium. This can occur from taking certain water pills (diuretics).
- Compensated alkalosis occurs when the body returns the acid-base balance to normal in cases of alkalosis, but bicarbonate and carbon dioxide levels remain abnormal.

Importance of Maintaining Urine pH

Urine pH is used to classify urine as either a dilute acid or base solution. The glomerular filtrate of blood is usually acidified by the kidneys from a pH of approximately 7.4 to a pH of about 6 in the

Chapter 1: Elementary Knowledge of Inorganic Chemistry

urine. Depending on the person's acid-base status, the pH of urine may range from 4.5 to 8. The kidneys maintain normal acid-base balance primarily through the re-absorption of sodium and the tubular secretion of hydrogen and ammonium ions. Urine becomes increasingly acidic as the amount of sodium and excess acid retained by the body increases. Alkaline urine, usually containing bicarbonate-carbonic acid buffer, is normally excreted when there is an excess of base or alkali in the body. Secretion of an acid or alkaline urine by the kidneys is one of the most important mechanisms the body uses to maintain a constant body pH. Urine pH is an important screening test for the diagnosis of renal disease, respiratory disease, and certain metabolic disorders.

A highly acidic urine pH occurs in:-
- Acidosis
- Uncontrolled diabetes
- Diarrhea
- Starvation and dehydration
- Respiratory diseases in which carbon dioxide retention occurs and acidosis develops

A highly alkaline urine occurs in:
- Urinary tract obstruction
- Pyloric obstruction
- Salicylate intoxication
- Renal tubular acidosis
- Chronic renal failure
- Respiratory diseases that involve hyperventilation (blowing off carbon dioxide and the development of alkalosis)

pH Indicators

A number of organic substances are known which show distinctly different colours below and above a small pH range.

For example, phenolphthalein is colorless below a pH of 8.3 and distinctly pink above 10. Over the pH range from 8 to 10 it changes color gradually through different shades of pink. Methyl orange shows a distinct red color below pH 3.1 and a yellow color above a pH of 4.4.

Color Change

Indicator	Acid	Alkali	pH range
Thymol blue	Red	Yellow	1.2–2.8
Methyl yellow	Red	Yellow	2.9–4.0
Methyl orange	Red	Yellow	3.1–4.4
Methyl red	Red	Yellow	4.2–6.3
Bromothymol blue	Yellow	Blue	6.0–7.6
Phenol red	Yellow	Red	6.8–8.4
Cresol red	Yellow	Red	7.2–8.8
Phenolphthalein	Colorless	Pink	8.3–10.0

For quickness and convenience, indicator papers are made from universal indicator are available. From the color developed with the universal indicator, one can easily fix the approximate value of the pH of a solution. By comparing the color developed with the already prepared standardized color plates or charts, the pH of a solution under test can be fixed with a remarkable accuracy.

pH Meter

The pH meter is used to measure the pH of a solution.
The pH meter is of two types—digital pH meter and manual pH meter.
pH meter consists of power pack and two electrodes.

The power pack contains an on/off switch, an indicating meter, a temperature compensation knob, a calibrate knob and a wire with a plug pin. The on/off switch is used to supply or cut off electric current. The indicating meter shows pH reading. The temperature compensation knob is used to adjust the temperature. The calibrate knob is used to set pH. The plug pin is connected to the main electric line.

The pH meter contains two electrodes—glass electrode and a calomel electrode. In modern pH meters, the two electrodes are combined into single unit.

The glass electrode has a hard glass tube. At the base, it has a thin bulb. The bulb contains HCl (0.1 mol/L). The bulb is covered by a special membrane of soda glass. It is sensitive to H^+ and it allows H^+

to pass through it. A platinum wire is connected to the HCl through silver-silver chloride electrode. The wire coming out from the glass electrode is connected to the power pack of the pH meter.

The calomel electrode is a reference electrode. It is not sensitive to H^+. It contains a calomel paste. The calomel paste is connected with a platinum wire through mercury. The free end of the calomel electrode has a porous plug. The base of electrode is deposited with KCl crystal. The remaining portion is filled with KCl solution.

The glass electrode in the test solution constitutes a half-cell and the calomel electrode constitutes the other half-cell. The two electrodes complete the circuit.

Principle: If the conductor is immersed into an appropriate electrolyte solution there will be a tendency for its atoms to leave the surface and enter the solution as ions. This is called a half-cell and the conductor is called an electrode. The potential difference between the two half-cell is called the electromotive force (emf). The emf will change if the flow of electrons is changed.

This is what happens in the measurement of pH. The indicator electrode is dipped in a solution whose hydrogen ion concentration is to be measured. H^+ ions are drawn towards the outer surface of the glass membrane. The number of H^+ ions accumulating on the membrane depends on their concentration in the external solution.

The change in the hydrogen ion activity outside the glass bulb changes the potential between the indicator electrode and the calomel electrode. The potential is measured by sensitive voltmeter.

The instrument must be calibrated against buffers of known pH before measuring the pH of unknown specimen.

Most pH measurements today are obtained using a single combination electrode in which both the reference and the pH-dependent electrodes are contained in a single glass or plastic tube. The action of the electrode is based on the fact that certain types of borosilicate glass are permeable to H^+ ions but not to other cations or anions. Therefore, if a thin layer of such glass is interposed between two solutions of different H^+ ion concentrations, H^+ ions will move across the glass from the solution of high to that of low H^+ concentration. Because passage of an H^+ ion through the glass adds a positive ion to the solution of low H^+ concentration and leaves behind a negative ion, an electrical potential develops across the glass. The magnitude of this potential is given by the equation:

$$E = 2.303 \frac{RT}{F} \log \frac{[H^+]_1}{[H^+]_2}$$

where E is the potential, R is the gas constant, T is the absolute temperature, F is the Faraday constant, and $[H^+]_1$ and $[H^+]_2$ are the concentrations inside and outside of the glass, respectively. Clearly if the [H⁺] concentration of one of the solutions is fixed, the potential will be proportional to the pH of the solutions.

pH electrodes are like batteries; they run down with time and use. As an electrode ages, its glass changes resistance. This resistance change alters the electrode potential. For this reason, electrodes need to be calibrated on a regular basis.

Calibration in pH buffer solution corrects for this change (**Fig. 1.2**). Calibration of any pH equipment should always begin with buffer 7.0 as this is the "zero point." The pH scale has an equivalent mV scale. The mV scale ranges from +420 to –420 mV. At a pH of 7.0, the mV value is 0. Each pH change corresponds to a change of ±60 mV. As pH values become more acidic, the mV values become greater. For example, a pH of 4.0 corresponds to a value of 180 mV. As pH values become more basic, the mV values become more negative; pH = 9 corresponds to –120 mV. Dual pH calibration using buffers 4.0 or 10.0 provides greater system accuracy.

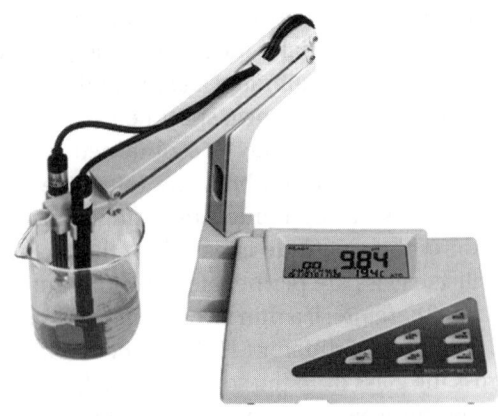

Fig. 1.2: pH meter calibration.
(For color version, see Plate 1)

Buffer Solutions

Buffers are solutions that have constant pH values and the ability to resist changes in that pH level. They are used to calibrate pH measurement systems (electrode and meter). There can be small differences between the output of one electrode and another, as well as changes in the output of electrodes over time. Therefore, the system must be periodically calibrated. Buffers are available with a wide range of pH values, and they come in both premixed liquid form or as convenient dry powder capsules. Most pH testers require calibration at several specific pH values. One calibration is usually performed near the isopotential point (the signal produced by an electrode at pH 7 is 0 mV at 25°C), and a second is typically performed at either pH 4 or pH 10. It is best to select a buffer as close as possible to the actual pH value of the sample to be measured.

Buffer ion plays an important role in restricting pH changes of body fluids.

For example,

Buffers on plasma—
- Bicarbonate—Carbonic acid ($BHCO_3/H_2CO_3$)
- Plasma protein buffer system (B protein/H protein)
- Phosphate buffer system (B_2HPO_4/BH_2PO_4)

Buffers on red blood cells—
- Bicarbonate—Carbonic acid ($BHCO_3/H_2CO_3$)
- Oxyhemoglobinate—Hemoglobin ($BHbO_2/HHbO_2$)
- Hemoglobinate—Hemoglobin (BHb/HHb)

■ SOLUTIONS AND DILUTIONS

Solution

A solution is a homogeneous mixture consisting of a solute dissolved into a solvent. The solute is the substance that is being dissolved, while the solvent is the dissolving medium. When one substance dissolves into another, a solution is formed.

Concentration of solution may be defined as the amount of solute present in the given quantity of the solution. Commonly used units of concentration in biochemistry laboratory are as follows:
1. **Percent Solutions (= parts per hundred):** There are three ways of expressing percentage composition of a solution.

i. *Weight per unit weight (w/w solution):* A 10% w/w solution contains 10 g of solute and 90 g of solvent.
ii. *Weight per unit volume (w/v solution):* A 10% w/v solution contains 10 g of solute dissolved in final volume of 100 mL solution (not the solvent).
iii. *Volume per unit volume (v/v solution):* A 10% v/v solution contains 10 mL of concentrate dissolved in final volume of 100 mL solution (not the solvent).

Sometimes when solutions are too dilute, their percentage concentrations are too low. So, instead of using really low percentage concentrations, such as 0.00001% or 0.000000001%, we choose another way to express the concentrations.

For example, the definition of parts per million: 1 g solute per 1,000,000 g solution (10^6).

Now, divide both values by 1,000 to get a new definition for ppm:
ppm = 0.001 g per 1,000 g solution or
ppm = 1 mg solute per 1 kg solution

For an aqueous solution:
ppm = 1 mg solute per liter of solution

2. **Molarity (M):** This is the most common method for expressing the concentration of a solution in biochemical studies. A mole is defined as exactly $6.023 \times 1,023$ atoms, or molecules, of a substance (this is Avogadro number, N). The mass of one mole of an element is its atomic mass (g).

Therefore,

Mass of solute = Moles × Molecular mass

The molarity of a solution is the number of moles of the solute dissolved per liter of the solution. A solution which contains one mole of the solute in 1 L of the solution is called a molar solution. Molarity of a solution can be calculated as follows:

$$\text{Molarity} = \frac{\text{Weight of a solute in g/L of solution}}{\text{Molecular weight of solute}}$$

It may be noted that in case of molar solutions, the combined total volume of the solute and solvent is 1 L. Thus, for preparing 0.1 M NaOH, one may proceed as follows:

Molecular weight of NaOH = 40
Required molarity of solution = 0.1M

Amount (in g) of NaOH per L of solution = Molecular weight of NaOH × Molarity
= 40 × 0.1
= 4 g

Thus, weigh 4 g of NaOH, dissolve it in a small volume of solvent (water), and make the final volume to 1 L with the solvent.

Sometime, it is desirable to know number of moles of a substance in a reaction mixture. This can be calculated using a simple relationship:

1 M solution = 1 mole of the substance/L of solution
= 1 mmol/mL of solution

Thus,

$$\text{Molarity} = \frac{\text{Moles of solute}}{\text{Volume of solution in L}} \text{ litre}$$

Conversions from % to molarity and from molarity to %:

To convert from % solution to molarity, multiply the % solution by 10 to express the percent solution g/L, then divide by the formula weight.

Note: Formula mass is defined as the sum of atomic masses of the ions present in the formula unit of an ionic compound whereas molecular mass is the sum of the atomic masses of the atoms in a molecule. The units of formula mass "atomic mass unit" (amu).

$$\text{Molarity} = \frac{\% \text{ solution} \times 10}{FW}$$

Example 1: Convert a 6.5 % solution of a chemical with FW = 325.6 to molarity,

$$\text{Molarity} = \frac{6.5 \text{ g}/100 \text{ mL} \times 10}{325.6 \text{ g/mole}}$$

$$= \frac{6.5 \times 10}{325.6}$$

$$= \frac{65}{325.6}$$

$$= 0.1996 \text{ M}$$

To convert from molarity to percent solution, multiply the molarity by the FW and divide by 10:

$$\% \text{ solution} = \frac{\text{Molarity} \times FW}{10}$$

Example 2: Convert a 0.0045 M solution of a chemical having FW 178.7 to percent solution:

$$\% \text{ solution} = \frac{0.0045 \text{ moles/L} \times 178.7 \text{ g/mole}}{10}$$

$$= \frac{0.0045 \times 178.79}{10}$$

$$= 0.08\%$$

3. **Normality (N):** The normality of a solution is the number of gram equivalents of the solute per L of the solution. Therefore, amount of a substance in g/L of solution,

$$\text{Normality} = \frac{\text{Amount of substance in g/L of solution}}{\text{Equivalent wt. of substance}}$$

For example, How many grams of sodium carbonate will be needed to prepare 0.2 N Solution (provided – Eq. wt. of Na_2CO_3 = 53)

$$\text{Normality} = \frac{\text{Amount of substance needed in grams}}{\text{Eq. wt. of substance}}$$

$$0.2 = \frac{\text{Amount of substance needed in grams}}{53}$$

0.2×53 = Amount of substance needed in grams per liter.

∴ 10.6 gm of Na_2CO_3 is needed in a final volume of 1 liter solution to make its normality 0.2 N.

Dilution

Dilution is the process of reducing the concentration of a solute in solution. Usually, it is done simply by mixing with more solvent. It results in increasing volume of solution from V and decrease in concentration of solution.

Terms used in making dilutions:
- **Dilution factor (DF):** Ratio of final volume/Initial volume (final volume = Initial volume + Diluent)
- **Concentration factor (CF):** Ratio of initial volume divided by the final volume (inverse of the dilution factor)

Chapter 1: Elementary Knowledge of Inorganic Chemistry

Simple dilution (dilution factor method based on ratios): A simple dilution is one in which a unit volume of a liquid material of interest is combined with an appropriate volume of a solvent liquid to achieve the desired concentration. The dilution factor is the total number of unit volumes in which your material will be dissolved. The diluted material must then be thoroughly mixed to achieve the true dilution. For example, a 1:5 dilution (read as "1 is to 5" dilution) means combining 1 unit volume of solute (the material to be diluted) + 4 unit volumes of the solvent medium (hence, 1 + 4 = 5 = dilution factor).

To prepare 400 mL of a disinfectant that requires 1:8 dilution from a concentrated stock solution with water. Divide the volume needed by the dilution factor (400 mL/8 = 50 mL) to determine the unit volume. The dilution is then done as 50 mL concentrated disinfectant + 350 mL (400 − 50 = 350 mL) water.

a. **Stock solution:** It is a concentrated solution which is to be diluted to give either the secondary solution or working solution; can be expressed in M or % or even nX concentrate where n is some number greater than 1.

   For example, 10X means that the stock solution is 10 times concentrated than secondary solution or working solution.

b. **Secondary solution:** It is an intermediate solution of the stock solution, to be used to make the working solution.

c. **Working solution:** It is diluted solution that is to be used for the test.

d. **Diluent:** Solution used for diluting stock solution to make the secondary and working solutions, usually water but could be a buffer of some sort or even organic solvents.

Dilutions

Using the algebraic formula below, one can calculate the volume, V_1, of the initial stock solution or C_1 to give the initial working or secondary stock concentration, C_2, final working concentration, and final volume V_2.

The difference of V_2 and V_1 is the volume of water to add to make desired dilution.

If any of the three factors are known, fourth is calculated by using following formula:

$$C_1 \times V_1 = C_2 \times V_2$$

Note that C_1 and C_2 have to be in the same units and V_1 and V_2 have to be in the same units.

For example, if you have 2.5 mL of a 1 M solution of NaCl and you want to make 3 mL of a 0.33 M solution of NaCl, you can use the formula to calculate how much of the 1 M solution you will need.

V_1 of the initial stock solution = ?
C_1 initial working or secondary stock concentration = 1 M
C_2 and final working concentration = 0.33 M
Final volume, = V_2 = 3 mL

$$V_1 \times C_1 = V_2 \times C_2$$
$$(V_1)(1\ M) = (3\ mL)(0.33\ M)$$
$$V_1 = (3\ mL)(0.33\ M)/1\ M$$
$$V_1 = 1\ mL$$

Since the diluted solution is to have a final volume of 3 mL, you can calculate the volume of solvent by subtracting V_1 from V_2: 3 mL – 1 mL = 2 mL. Therefore, adding 2 mL of solvent to 1 mL of a 1 M solution of NaCl will yield 3 mL of a 0.33 M NaCl solution.

Serial Dilutions

Serial dilutions involve the preparation of successive dilutions that vary the concentration of the solute by a constant factor, so that each successive dilution is a multiple of the previous dilution. Usually, the dilution factor at each step is constant, resulting in a geometric progression of the concentration in a logarithmic fashion.

For example, in 10-fold serial dilutions, each successive dilution is one-tenth of the previous dilution yielding dilution ratios of 1/10, 1/100, 1/1,000, and so on. Serial dilutions may be used to prepare a series of standard concentrations for a biochemical assay, or to dilute a very dense culture of microorganisms to a concentration suitable for counting. It is very important to prepare serial dilutions carefully since each successive dilution will magnify the effect of any previous error.

Steps involved in making serial dilution:
- Begin with a stock solution of 1 mg/mL and set up a series of dilutions in which the dilution ratio relative to the stock solution progressively changes by one-half.
- In this instance, the concentrations of the successively diluted solutions would be 1/2, 1/4, 1/8, and 1/16 of the original concentration **(Fig. 1.3)**.

Chapter 1: Elementary Knowledge of Inorganic Chemistry

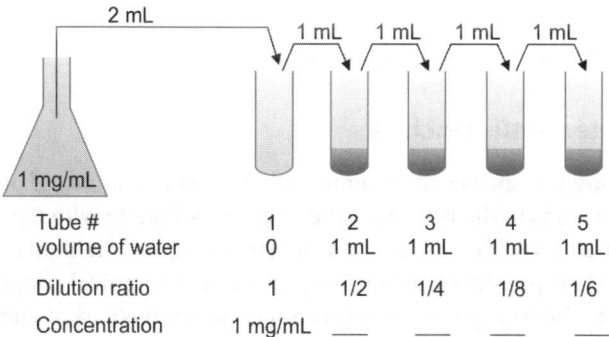

Fill in the concentration of each of the diluted samples

Fig. 1.3: Diagram of two-fold serial dilutions.

- If 1 mL of each dilution is needed, set up a series of five test tubes, with the first one empty and the rest with 1 mL of solvent.
- Pipette out 2 mL (twice the volume needed for your test) into tube 1.
- Then transfer 1 mL of that volume to tube 2, making a 1/2 dilution since there was 1 mL of water in tube 2.
- After mixing the contents of tube 2, half that sample (1 mL) would be transferred to tube 3, making a 1/4 dilution since the 1 mL of water that was already in tube 3 will dilute the incoming 1/2 dilution by 1/2 (1/2 × 1/2 = 1/4).
- This procedure is repeated until the last tube is reached, which will contain 2 mL of a 1/16 dilution of the stock solution.

■ ISOTOPE AND RADIOISOTOPE

Isotopes (from the Greek *iso-*, equal, and *topos*, place; in reference to isotopes of an element having the same position in the periodical table of elements) are forms of a given chemical element that have different atomic masses. The nuclei of isotopes of an element contain identical numbers of protons, and so the isotopes have the same atomic number. Each isotope has a different number of neutrons and thus has a different atomic mass.

For example, carbon-12, carbon-13, and carbon-14 are three isotopes of the element carbon with mass numbers 12, 13, and 14, respectively. The atomic number of carbon is 6, which means that every carbon atom has 6 protons, so that the neutron numbers of these isotopes are 6, 7, and 8, respectively.

Isotope versus Nuclide

A nuclide is a species of an atom with a specific number of protons and neutrons in the nucleus, for example, carbon-13 with 6 protons and 7 neutrons. The nuclide concept (referring to individual nuclear species) emphasizes nuclear properties over chemical properties, whereas the isotope concept (grouping all atoms of each element) emphasizes chemical over nuclear. The neutron number has large effects on nuclear properties, but its effect on chemical properties is negligible for most elements. Even for the lightest elements, whose ratio of neutron number to atomic number varies the most between isotopes, it usually has only a small effect although it matters in some circumstances, for example, hydrogen, the lightest element, the isotope effect is large enough to affect biology strongly.

The term (originally also isotopic elements, now sometimes isotopic nuclides) is intended to imply comparison. For example, the nuclides ^{12}like $^6C_{13}$, and $^6C_{14}$, are isotopes (nuclides with the same atomic number but different mass numbers), but nuclides ^{40}like $^{18}Ar_{40}$, $^{19}K_{40}$ $^{20}Ca_{40}$ are isobars (nuclides with the same mass number).

However, *isotope* is the older term and so is better known than nuclide and is still sometimes used in contexts in which nuclide might be more appropriate, like in nuclear technology and nuclear medicine.

Isotopes are of two types: Stable isotope and radioactive isotope.

Stable Isotope

The discovery of stable "'isotopes" began with JJ Thomson's identification of neon-22 in 1912. More than 90 naturally occurring elements have been identified on the earth; they exist as nearly 270 stable isotopes. Stable isotopes are forms of the elements that do not decay or emit radiation. The various isotopes of a given element differ from one another only in the number of neutrons in their atomic nucleus. Even highly purified samples of an element are generally a mixture of several isotopes. Pure silver, for example, is composed of nearly equal amounts of silver-107 and silver-109. Iron is mostly iron-56 (92%), but it contains small amounts of three other isotopes as well.

Enriched isotope refers to material that consists largely or exclusively of a single isotope. The extra mass made them traceable (usually by mass spectrometry of, for example, blood or urine) as they preceded through various biochemical pathways. Similar labeling of nearly any compound is theoretically possible by synthesizing it with large quantities of an isotope that is relatively rare in nature. In the last two decades, the use of enriched stable isotopes has offered substantial advantages in the rapid growth of research on human body composition, energy balance, protein turnover, and fuel utilization.

Uses of Stable Isotopes

Understanding of the biological processes that control human and animal physiology plays an important role in medical and biochemistry research. These disciplines make use of stable isotope analysis through non-invasive labeling techniques to provide information on biochemical reactions or metabolic pathways within the body, e.g., by breath analysis. Breath analysis using stable isotope analysis allows the non-invasive determination of whole-body CO_2 production. After an isotopically labeled meal is ingested (e.g., ^{13}C-labeled glucose), breath analysis will show that exhaled CO_2 from the patient shows enrichment in ^{13}C levels relative to ^{12}C. The time taken for the ^{13}C isotope to appear in the exhaled breath gives some indication of the metabolic rate of the patient.

The general approach to biomedical studies that use stable isotopes is specialized analytical methods for detection of the specific stable isotopes is used. For example, after ingestion or injection of an isotope of zinc, the absorption of zinc by the human body can be determined by measuring the trace amounts that appear in the blood and urine over a period of days or weeks after ingestion or injection. The dilution of the stable isotope tracer gives information on the distribution of zinc in the body, and the rate of excretion gives information regarding how well a particular mineral is absorbed.

The simultaneous use of two isotopes in two different foodstuffs can be used to determine how absorption of calcium, for example, might vary as a function of mode of intake. A major application is the study of calcium absorption from ingested foodstuffs and its subsequent turnover in bone in relation to osteoporosis. By using simultaneous oral and intravenous administration of two or more stable isotopes (e.g., calcium-42 and calcium-44), the absorption of various calcium supplements and food sources can be investigated. Other uses can be summarized as shown in **Table 1.1**.

Although the introduction of stable isotope tracers revolutionized the understanding of biological processes, the field relies heavily on sophisticated chemical techniques and analytical instrumentation not routinely available. Expensive measurement methods are also limiting applications.

Table 1.1: Selected enriched stable isotopes used in biomedical research.

Stable isotope	Uses
Calcium-42, -44, -46, -48	• Calcium metabolism, bioavailability, and absorption parameters during physical stress, bed rest, and space flight • Osteoporosis research and bone turnover studies • Role of nutritional calcium in pregnancy, growth and development, and lactation • Bone changes associated with diseases, such as diabetes and cystic fibrosis
Carbon-13	• Noninvasive breath tests for metabolic research and diagnosis • Elucidation of metabolic pathways in inborn errors of metabolism
Chromium-53, -54	Adult-onset diabetes mechanisms
Copper-63, -65	Studies of congenital disorders and body kinetics in gastrointestinal diseases
Iron-54, -57, -58	Metabolism, energy expenditure studies
Krypton-78, -80, -82, -84, -86	Diagnosis of pulmonary disease
Lithium-6	• Sodium and renal physiology • Psychiatric diseases
Magnesium-25, -26	Kinetic studies of heart disease and vascular problems
Nitrogen-15	Whole body protein turnover, synthesis, and catabolism
Vanadium-51	• Diabetes, bioavailability, and metabolism • Brain metabolism studies
Xenon-129	Magnetic resonance imaging (MRI)

Radioisotope

The atomic number of an element is the same, but different mass numbers are called isotope of an element. If the nucleus contains either excess of neutrons or protons, the force between these constituents will be unbalanced leading to unstable nucleus. An unstable nucleus will continuously vibrate and will attempt to reach stability by undergoing radioactive decay. The number of neutrons determines whether the nucleus is radioactive or not. The radioactive isotopes of an element are called radioisotopes; they are natural and artificially produced by nuclear reactors and accelerators.

The unstable nuclei of an element can undergo the variety of processes resulting in the emission of radiation in two forms, namely, radioactivity and nuclear reactions. In a radioactive decay, the nucleus spontaneously disintegrates to different species of nuclei or to a lower energy state of the same nucleus with the emission of alpha (α), beta (β), and gamma (γ) radiation is called radioactivity.

In nuclear reaction, the nucleus interacts with another particle or nucleus with subsequently emission of radiation as one of its final products. In some cases, the final product is also radioactive. The radiation emitted in both these processes may be electromagnetic (X-rays and γ-rays) or particle-like α, β, and neutrons. Such isotopes eventually reach stability in the form of nonradioactive isotopes of other chemical elements, their "radiogenic daughters." Decay of a radioisotope to a stable radiogenic daughter is a function of time measured in units of half-lives.

The half-life of a radioactive substance is a characteristic constant. It measures the time it takes for a given amount of the substance to become reduced by half as a consequence of decay, and therefore, the emission of radiation.

The half-life of isotopes from some sample elements are: Oxygen 16—infinite, uranium 238—4,460,000,000 years, carbon 14—5,730 years, and silver 94—0.42 seconds.

Types of Radiation

There are four major types of radiation—alpha, beta, neutrons, and electromagnetic waves such as gamma rays. They differ in mass, energy, and how deeply they penetrate people and objects.

1. **alpha (α) decay:** It results from an excess of mass. In this type of decay, alpha particles are emitted from the nucleus. Alpha particle consists of 2 protons and 2 neutrons. Atomic number and neutron number of the daughter are reduced by two, so the mass number decreases by four.
   An example is the decay of ^{238}U:
   $$^{238}_{92}U \rightarrow ^{234}_{90}Th + ^{4}_{2}He + Y$$

2. **β+ - or "positron decay":** It results from an excess of protons. In this type of decay, a positively charged beta particle and a neutrino are emitted from the nucleus. The atomic number decreases by one and the neutron number is increased by one.
   An example is the decay of radioactive ^{18}F to stable ^{18}O:
   $$^{18}_{9}F \rightarrow ^{18}_{8}O + \beta^{+} + v + Q$$
   where β+ is the positron, v is the neutrino, and Q is the total energy given off.

3. **β- - or "negatron decay":** It results from an excess of neutrons. In this type of decay, a negatively charged beta particle and a neutrino are emitted from the nucleus. The atomic number increases by one and the neutron number is reduced by one.
   An example is the decay of radioactive ^{14}C to stable ^{14}N:
   $$^{14}_{6}C \rightarrow ^{14}_{7}N + \beta^{-} + v^{-} + Q$$
   where β is the beta particle, v is the antineutrino, and Q is the end-point energy (0.156 MeV).

4. **Electron capture:** It results from an excess of protons. In this type of decay, an electron is spontaneously incorporated into the nucleus and a neutrino is emitted from the nucleus. The atomic number decreases by one and the neutron number increases by one. Electron capture may be followed by the emission of a gamma ray. An example is the decay of ^{123}I to ^{123}Te:
   $$^{123}_{53}I + e^{-} \rightarrow ^{123}_{52}Te + v + Y$$

5. **Gamma rays (γ):** Gamma-rays are a form of electromagnetic radiation (photon), emitted from nucleus. Gamma photons are the most energetic photons in the electromagnetic spectrum. The emission of gamma rays is usually the most common mode of nuclear excitation and also occurs through internal conversion.

The three radioisotopes that emit gamma rays and are useful in clinical biochemistry are cobalt-60, caesium-137, technetium-99m, and americium-241.
6. **Neutron radiation:** It is a neutral particle that produces ionization indirectly by emission of γ-rays and charged particles when interacting with matter. These charged particles produce the ionization. It has more penetrating than gamma ray. They are produced by nuclear reaction and spontaneous fission in nuclear reactors.

Use of Radioisotopes in Biochemistry

It is easy to detect the presence or absence of some radioactive material even when it exists in low concentration. Therefore, several radioisotopes-labeled compounds are used to label the molecules of biological samples in vitro **(Table 1.2)**. This way, Radioisotopes help in elucidating the origin and fate of various biomolecules in the body as well as in the understanding of metabolic pathways in radioisotope tracer studies.

A large number of tests have been devised to determine the constituents of blood, serum or urine, hormones, antigens, and many drugs, by means of associated radioisotopes. These procedures are known as radioimmunoassays (RIAs). The RIA kits, manufactured for laboratory use, are very easy to use and give accurate results.

The most common radioactivity isotope used in radioactive tracer is technetium (^{99}Tc). Tumors in the brain are located by injecting intravenously ^{99}Tc and then scanning the head with suitable scanners.

^{131}I and most recently ^{132}I and ^{123}I are used to study malfunctioning thyroid glands. Kidney function is also studied using compound containing ^{131}I. ^{33}P is used in DNA sequencing. Tritium (^{3}H) is frequently used as a tracer in biochemical studies. ^{14}C has been used extensively to trace the progress of organic molecule through metabolic pathways.

A most recent development is positron emission tomography (PET), which is a more precise and accurate technique for locating tumors in the body. A positron emitting radionuclide (e.g., ^{13}N, ^{15}O, and ^{18}F) is injected to the patient, and it accumulates in the target tissue. As it emits positron which promptly combines with nearby

Table 1.2: Use of radioisotopes.

Radioisotope	Applications
Bismuth-213	It is an alpha emitter. Used for cancer treatment, e.g., in the targeted alpha therapy (TAT)
Cesium-131	It emits photon radiation in the X-ray range. Used in brachytherapy of malignant tumors
Chromium-51	Used in diagnosis of gastrointestinal bleeding and to label platelets
Cobalt-605	Used for controlling the cancerous growth of cells
Dysprosium-165	Used for synovectomy treatment of arthritis
Holmium-166	Diagnosis and treatment of liver tumors
Iodine-131	Widely used in treating thyroid cancer and in imaging the thyroid, diagnosis, and renal blood flows
Iron-59	Used in studies of iron metabolism in the spleen
Potassium-42	Used for potassium distribution in bodily fluids and to locate brain tumors
Radium-223	Used to treat prostate cancers that have spread to the bones
Selenium-75	Used to study the production of digestive enzymes
Sodium-24	Used for studies of electrolytes within the body
Ytterbium-169	Used for cerebrospinal fluid studies in the brain

electrons, it results in the simultaneous emission of two γ-rays in opposite directions. These γ-rays are detected by a PET camera and give precise indication of their origin, that is, depth also. This technique is also used in cardiac and brain imaging.

Compound X-ray tomography or computed tomography (CT) scans. The radioactive tracer produces gamma rays or single photons that a gamma camera detects. Emissions come from different angles, and a computer uses them to produce an image. CT scan targets specific area of the body, like the neck or chest, or a specific organ, like the thyroid.

Radiation Hazard

Exposure to any amount of radiation presents a risk of damage to cells or tissue. While our bodies have the ability to repair damage cells, over time if exposure becomes longer and greater, it can result

Chapter 1: Elementary Knowledge of Inorganic Chemistry

in many acute injuries, such as burns, acute radiation syndrome, and long-term health problems, such as cancer and cardiovascular diseases. Collectively it is known as acute radiation syndrome or also known as radiation sickness.

Radiation exposure can be lowered by following the three principles of radiation safety which are mentioned below.

Time

This refers to the amount of time spent near the radioactive source. Time near the radioactive source should be kept at a minimum. Tasks or work activities revolving around the radioactive source should be done quickly as possible, to reduce spending time around the radioactive area more than necessary.

Distance

This refers to the distance between a person and the radioactive source. The greater the distance, the lesser the exposure and dose of radiation workers will be exposed to.

Shielding

Exposure to radiation sources can be minimized through shields. Shielding refers to putting something in between the radiation source and the person involved. The effectiveness of shields will vary depending on the level of radionuclides the radiation source is emitting.

Radiation Safety Measures

Radiation safety measures such as conducting safety inspections help ensure that critical radiation safety precautions are in place to reduce the risk of overexposure. There should be visible warning signs, contamination surveys conducted, and device tests for all radiation-producing equipment. All workers must be trained to limit time of exposure, use radiation shields, and increase the distance of contact with radioactive devices and materials.

Following preventive measures and rules must be strictly followed to avoid critical health conditions:
- Acquire adequate training to better understand the nature of radiation hazards.

Section 1: Basic Chemistry

- Reduce handling time of radioactive materials and equipment.
- Be mindful of your distance from sources of radiation. Increase distance as much as possible. Whenever possible, handle with the help of remote control.
- Use proper shielding for the type of radiation.
- Isolate or contain harmful radioactive materials properly. Store it in thick wall lead containers.
- Armor yourself with appropriate protective clothing and dosimeters. Wear lead aprons.
- Conduct contamination surveys in the work area.
- Do not eat, drink, smoke, or apply cosmetics in an area where unsealed radioactive substances are handled.
- Observe proper radioactive waste disposal.
- Conduct regular radiation safety self-inspections.

SUMMARY

- Study of compounds, which does not consist of carbon–hydrogen atoms in it, is called *"Inorganic Chemistry."*
- All matter is composed of minute discrete particles called as atoms.
- Fundamental particles of an atom are electrons, protons, and neutrons.
- Ion: Atom/group of atoms with charge.
- Element: Pure substance made up of one kind of atoms only.
- Compound: Pure substance made up of two or more different elements.
- Atomic number: Total number of protons in the nucleus.
- Mass number: Total number of protons and neutrons in the nucleus.
- Atomic weight is number of times one atom of an element is heavier than the mass of hydrogen atom.
- Equivalent weight of an element is that weight of it, which can combine with or replace from a chemical combination 8 parts by weight of oxygen or 35.5 parts by weight of chlorine or 1.008 parts by weight of hydrogen.
- Acid has sour taste and turns blue litmus to red.
- Base has bitter taste and turns red litmus to blue.
- Arrhenius theory: An acid in aqueous solution gives hydrogen ions. A base in aqueous solution produces hydroxyl ions.
- Lowry and Brønsted theory: An acid is a proton donor and base is a proton acceptor.
- Lewis theory: Acid is an electron acceptor and base is an electron donor.
- A salt is a compound formed by the interaction of an acid and a base.
- The cell contains 1–3% salts. Sodium chloride is a common salt that is added to food.
- A pH of 7 is neutral, less than 7 is acidic and greater than 7 is basic.

Chapter 1: Elementary Knowledge of Inorganic Chemistry

- The Henderson–Hasselbalch equation gives information of the abundance of ionized and unionized fractions of molecules within a given solution.
- This slightly alkaline blood pH (7.4) must be maintained to avoid detrimental effects on body.
- The pH of urine may range from 4.5 to 8.
- The organic substances which show distinctly different colors below and above a small pH range are pH indicators.
- pH meter measures pH of the solution. Manual pH meter measures potential difference between two electrodes. These electrodes need to be calibrated on a regular basis.
- Buffers are solutions that have constant pH values and the ability to resist changes in that pH level.
- A solution is a homogeneous mixture consisting of a solute dissolved into a solvent.
- Percent solutions can be expressed as—weight per unit, weight per unit volume or volume per unit volume.
- The molarity of a solution is the number of moles of the solute dissolved per liter of the solution.
- The normality of a solution is the number of gram equivalents of the solute per liter of the solution.
- Dilution is the process of reducing the concentration of a solute in solution.
- It is a concentrated solution which is to be diluted to give either the secondary solution or working solution.
- Secondary solution is an intermediate solution of the stock solution, to be used to make the working solution.
- Diluent is a solution used for diluting stock solution to make the secondary and working solutions.
- Serial dilutions involve the preparation of successive dilutions that vary the concentration of the solute by a constant factor.
- A nuclide is a species of an atom with a specific number of protons and neutrons in the nucleus.
- Isotopes have same atomic number but different atomic masses.
- Stable isotopes do not decay or emit radiation.
- Enriched isotope refers to material that consists largely or exclusively of a single isotope.
- Stable isotope analysis provides information on biochemical reactions or metabolic pathways within the body, like breath analysis.
- In a radioactive decay, the nucleus spontaneously disintegrates to different species of nuclei or to a lower energy state of the same nucleus with the emission of alpha (α), beta (β), and gamma (γ) radiation is called radioactivity.
- In nuclear reaction, the nucleus interacts with another particle or nucleus with subsequently emission of radiation as one of its final products.
- Alpha particle consists of two protons and two neutrons.
- β+ - or "positron decay" results from an excess of protons.

- β- or "negatron decay" results from an excess of neutrons.
- In electron capture, an electron is spontaneously incorporated into the nucleus and a neutrino is emitted from the nucleus.
- Gamma-rays are a form of electromagnetic radiation.
- Radioisotopes help in elucidating the origin and fate of various biomolecules in the body as well as in the understanding of metabolic pathways in radioisotope tracer studies.

PRACTICE QUESTIONS

1. What is inorganic chemistry? Name some inorganic compounds.
2. With neat labeled diagram describe the structure of an atom.
3. Define atomic number, mass number, atomic weight, molecular weight, and equivalent weight
4. Differentiate between acid and base.
5. What are salts? Discuss the different types of salts with examples.
6. What is importance of salt in the body?
7. What is Henderson–Hasselbalch equation? Mention its applications.
8. What is the normal pH of blood? Write two causes of acidosis and two causes of alkalosis.
9. What is the normal range of pH for urine? Write two causes of acidic urine and two causes of alkaline urine.
10. What are pH indicators? Give some examples.
11. Discuss the principle of pH meter.
12. Why it is necessary to calibrate pH meter?
13. What are buffer solutions? Discuss its role in body.
14. Define—percent solution, molarity, and normality dilution factor.
15. What are stable isotopes? Mention any four uses.
16. Explain the terms: Nuclide, radioisotope, and half-life.
17. Discuss the types of radiations which emerge from radioisotope.
18. What is radiation syndrome? How it can be lowered?

SOLVED EXAMPLES

Example 1: Consider that 0.8 g of solid NaOH used for the preparation of 500 mL solution. Express the concentration of this solution in terms of g/L, %w/v, mg%. (MW NaOH = 40)
The solution contains 0.8 g/500 mL, or 1.6 g/L.
       %(w/v)………. …1.6 g/L = 0.16 g/100 mL = 0.16%
       mg %………….. 0.16 g/100 mL = 160 mg/100 mL = 160 mg%

Example 2: How many grams of solid NaOH are required to prepare 500 mL of 0.04 M solution? Express the concentration of this solution in terms of %(w/v). (MW NaOH = 40).

Chapter 1: Elementary Knowledge of Inorganic Chemistry

Step 1:

$$\text{Molarity} = \frac{\text{No. of moles required}}{\text{Volume in liter}}$$

Given = Modarity = 0.04 M
Volume = 500 mL = 0.5 lit.

Putting values,

$$0.04 = \frac{\text{No. of moles required}}{0.5}$$

0.04×0.5 = No. of moles required
= 0.02 g of solid NaOH is required to prepare 500 mL of 0.04 M solution

Step 2:

$$\text{\% solution} = \frac{\text{Molarity} \times \text{FW}}{10}$$

$$= \frac{0.04 \times 40}{10}$$

$$= \frac{1.6}{10}$$

= 0.16% (concentration of solution)

Example 3: Dilute 7.0 mL of a 5.0% (w/v) solution to a 3.0% (w/v) solution.

$V1 \times C1 = V2 \times C2$
$7.0 \times 5.0 = V2 \times 3.0$
$V2 = 11.7$ mL

To 7.00 mL of initial solution add 4.7 mL of diluent.

$(11.7 - 7.0 = 4.7$ mL$)$

Describe the preparation of 2 L of a 0.4 M HCl starting with concentrated HCl solution: 28% (w/v) HCl, ρ (s.g.) = 1.15 g/mL. Liters × M = Number of moles.

$V1 \times C1 = V2 \times C2$
$1 \times 0.4 = 0.8$ mole HCl is needed
Wtg = Number of moles × MW
= 0.80 × 36.5
= 29.2 g pure HCl is needed

The stock solution is not pure HCl but only 28% HCl by weight.
Therefore,

$$\frac{29.2}{0.28} = 104.3 \text{ g stock solution is needed.}$$

Instead of weighing out 104.3 g stock solution, we can calculate the volume required.

$$V_{mL} = \frac{Wtg}{\rho \text{ (g/mL)}} = \frac{104.3}{1.15} = 90.7 \text{ mL stock solution is needed.}$$

Therefore, measure out 90.7 mL stock solution and dilute to 2 L with water.

Section 1: Basic Chemistry

PRACTICE NUMERICALS

1. What is the % (w/v) of 1.0 L solution that contains 5.0 g of NaCl?

Ans: 0.5 g/mL (%).

2. Find the percent volume of ethanol in a solution prepared by diluting 30.0 mL of ethanol to 250 mL.

Ans: 12%.

3. (a) How many moles of NaCl (MW = 58.5) are required to prepare 100 mL of a 1.6 M solution?
   (b) How many grams of NaCl are required?

Ans: (a) 0.16 moles
   (b) 9.36 g/100mL.

4. How many moles of HCl are present in 50 mL of 3.0 M HCl solution?

Ans: 0.15 mol.

5. What are the normalities of (a) 0.213 M HCl, and (b) 0.010 M $Ca(OH)_2$?

Ans: (a) 0.213 N
   (b) 0.02 N.

6. A solution contains 15 g of $CaCl_2$ in a total volume of 190 mL. Express the concentration of this solution in terms of (a) g/L, (b) %(w/v), (c) mg%, (d) M (MW of $CaCl_2$ = 110.986 g/mole)

Ans: (a) 78.949/L
   (b) 7.89 w/v
   (c) 7894.736% mg (w/v)
   (d) 0.711 M.

7. What is the molarity of pure ethanol; that is, how many moles are present in 1 L of pure ethanol? The density of ethanol is 0.789 g/mL. The MW of ethanol is 46.07 g/mol.

Ans: 17.12 M.

8. How many grams of NaCl are necessary to prepare 500 mL of a 10% (w/v) solution?

Ans: 50 gm.

Elementary Knowledge of Organic Chemistry

CHAPTER 2

Keywords
Characteristics of organic compounds, covalent bond, aliphatic compounds, aromatic compounds, functional groups, hydrocarbons, alkane, alkene and alkyne, homologous series

■ INTRODUCTION

Organic compounds play an important role in our daily life. The basic structures of life, such as carbohydrates, proteins, and fats, are organic compounds. To understand various biological processes going on in the human body, basic knowledge of organic chemistry is must. They are the basic components of many of the cycles that drive the earth. For example, the carbon cycle that includes the exchange of carbon between plants and animals in photosynthesis and cellular respiration.

■ ORGANIC COMPOUNDS

The term organic chemistry is applied to substances, which were derived from animals or plants, i.e., living organisms.

All organic compounds contain carbon as an essential element, combined with hydrogen, oxygen, nitrogen, sulfur, phosphorus, and/or halogens (chlorine, fluorine, bromine, and iodine).

The general characteristics of organic compounds include the following:
- They can be isolated as well as prepared in laboratory.
- They comprise almost 90% of all known compounds.
- Mostly built up of only three elements—carbon, hydrogen, and oxygen. Other elements like halogen, nitrogen as well as phosphorous are also present but to a lesser extent.

- They possess complex structures and high molecular weights.
- Their properties are decided by certain active atom or group of atoms known as the functional group.
- They are mostly insoluble in water but soluble in organic solvents.
- Organic compounds do not dissociate in solutions, therefore these are poor conductors of electricity.
- They are combustible in nature.
- Chemical reactions involving organic compounds proceed at slower rates.
- Generally, the larger and more complicated the organic substance, the higher its boiling and melting points.

Covalent Bond

Organic compound always form covalent bond **(Fig. 2.1)**.

A covalent bond is a chemical bond that involves the sharing of electron pairs between atoms that in turn results in a balance of attractive and repulsive forces between the atoms. These shared electrons belong to both carbon and hydrogen atoms. The presence

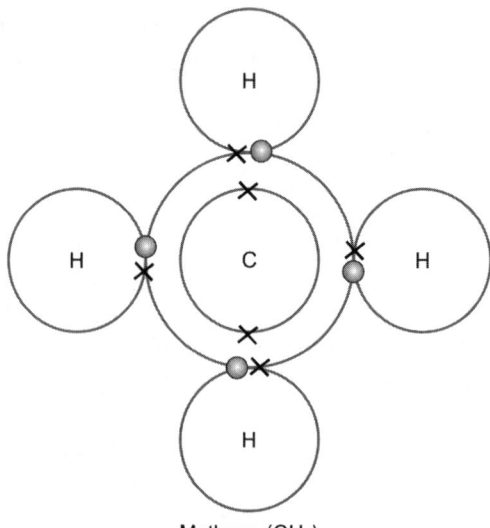

Methane (CH$_4$)

Fig. 2.1: Covalent bond in methane—carbon atom shares one electron with four hydrogen atoms.

of a covalent bond renders certain characteristics to the organic compounds. These include the following:
- Low melting points and boiling points in comparison to the inorganic compounds.
- Organic acids and bases are less strong and thus they have a limited dissociation in an aqueous medium.
- They exhibit the phenomenon of isomerism in which a single molecular formula represents several organic compounds differing in physical and chemical properties.
- They are volatile in nature.

■ ALIPHATIC AND AROMATIC COMPOUNDS

On the basis of structure, organic compounds are classified into the following two groups **(Table 2.1)**:
1. Acyclic/Open chain/Aliphatic compounds
2. Cyclic/Closed chain/Aromatic compounds

Acyclic/Open Chain/Aliphatic Compounds

In aliphatic compounds, the molecules are open-chained or noncyclic. For example,

CH_4 (Methane), $CH_2=CH_2$ (Ethene), H—C—C—H (Ethane)

These compounds may also contain branched chains. For example, isobutene.

$$H_3C—CH(CH_3)—CH_3$$

Table 2.1: Classifications of organic compounds.

Parameter	Aromatic compounds	Aliphatic compounds
Structure	The linking of carbon compounds takes place in the ring structure with the help of conjugated pi electrons	The linking of carbon compounds takes place in a straight line manner
Flame test	A sooty flame is produced when burnt	A sooty flame is not produced when burnt
Odor	Pleasant odor	Unpleasant odor
Example	Benzene and naphthalene	Butane and propane

Cyclic/Closed Chain/Aromatic Compounds

These compounds contain one or more closed chain of carbon atoms and are called cyclic or ring compounds. These compounds possess a pleasant aroma. For example, benzene and naphthalene.

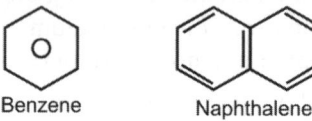

Benzene   Naphthalene

Aromatic compounds are further subdivided as:
- Homocyclic compounds
- Heterocyclic compounds

Homocyclic Compounds

Homocyclic compounds contain a ring or rings of carbon atoms only, e.g., cyclobutane.

$$\begin{array}{c} H_2C \longrightarrow CH_2 \\ | \qquad\qquad | \\ H_2C \longrightarrow CH_2 \end{array}$$

Heterocyclic Compounds

Hetrocyclic compounds contain one or more hetero or noncarbon atoms like oxygen, sulfur, and nitrogen in the rings of the molecules, e.g., furan.

$$\begin{array}{c} HC = CH \\ \| \quad \| \\ H_2C \quad CH_2 \\ \diagdown O \diagup \end{array}$$

■ FUNCTIONAL GROUPS

Classification of Organic Compounds based Upon Functional Group

Functional group is atom or group of atoms that defines the structure of a particular family of organic compounds. The functional group is responsible for determining the properties of a compound. A particular set of properties is characteristic of a particular kind of structure.

Organic compounds have been classified into a number of classes on the basis of their functional group. Organic molecules are built up of two parts:
1. One part represents carbon-hydrogen framework, and
2. Other part represents the functional group.

For example, if an organic compound is represented as R–X, R represents the carbon hydrogen framework and X represents the functional group.

Classes of organic compounds containing C, H, O, N, X, elements are as follows:

- **Aryl halides:** These are monohalogen derivatives of alkanes, represented as R–X where X is a halogen (F, Cl, Br or I) covalently linked to an alkyl group R, e.g. $CH_3-CH_2-CH_2-Br$ (propyl bromide).
- **Alcohol:** These are aliphatic organic hydroxy compounds in which hydroxyl group (–OH) is attached to alkyl group, e.g. CH_3–OH (methyl alcohol).
- **Aldehydes:** They are classified as the first oxidation products of primary alcohols. In aldehydes, the carbonyl group is attached to at least one hydrogen atom (–CHO). It is always present at the beginning of carbonyl chain, e.g. H–CHO (formaldehyde).
- **Ketones:** They are the first oxidation products of secondary alcohols. In ketones, the carbonyl group is attached to two other carbon atoms, i.e. it does not carry hydrogen.

$$-C=O$$
$$|$$
$$C$$

It is always present between the middle of the chain, e.g. CH_3–CO–CH_3 (dimethyl ketone).

- **Carboxylic acids:** They are the first oxidation products of aldehydes and ketones and are defined as the acidic organic compounds containing carboxylic group (–COOH), e.g. CH_3—COOH (acetic acid).
- **Esters:** Esters are the derivatives of carboxylic acids formed by replacing the hydroxyl group of acid (–OH) by a carbonyl group (–OR). These have particular fruit aroma, e.g. CH_3-COO-CH_3 (methyl methanoate).

Section 1: Basic Chemistry

Class	General formula	Functoinal group	Example
Alkyl halides	R – X	– X	CH_3I Methyl iodide
Alcohol	R – OH	– OH	C_2H_5 OH Ethyl alcohol
Aldehydes	$R-C{\lower.5ex\hbox{$<$}}^{H}_{O}$	$-C{\lower.5ex\hbox{$<$}}^{H}_{O}$	HCHO Formaldehyde
Ketones	$R \atop R$ C=O	C=O	CH_3COH_3C Dimethyl ketone
Carboxylic acids	$R \atop R$ C$<^O_{OH}$	$-C<^O_{OH}$	CH_3COOH Acetic acid
Esters	$R-C<^O_{OR}$	$-C<^O_{OR}$	$CH_3COO\ C_2H_5$ Ethyl acetate
Ethers	R – O – R	–C–O–C–	C_2H_5–O–C_2H_5 Diethyl ether
Amines	R–NH_2	–NH_2	C_2H_5–NH_2 Ethyl amine

- **Ethers:** These are alkyl derivatives of alcohols, formed by replacing hydroxyl hydrogen of alcohol (-OH) by carbonyl group (-OR), e.g. C_2H_5-O-C_2H_5 (diethyl ether).
- **Amines:** Amines are the derivatives of ammonia formed by replacing one or more hydrogen atoms by corresponding number of alkyl or aryl group radicals, e.g. H-NH_2 (Ammonia).

■ HYDROCARBONS (TABLE 2.2)

Important classes of organic compounds containing only carbon and hydrogen elements are hydrocarbons. The carbon atoms join together to form the framework of the compound, and the hydrogen atoms attach to them in many different configurations.

Hydrocarbons are the principal constituents of petroleum and natural gas. They serve as fuels and lubricants as well as raw materials for the production of plastics, fibers, rubbers, solvents, explosives, and industrial chemicals. Hydrocarbons are the simplest organic compounds, but they have interesting physiological effects. These effects depend on the size of the hydrocarbon molecules and

Chapter 2: Elementary Knowledge of Organic Chemistry

Table 2.2: Characteristics of hydrocarbons.

Alkanes	Alkenes	Alkynes
Alkanes are hydrocarbons in which all the linkages between the carbon atoms are single covalent bonds	Alkenes are unsaturated aliphatic hydrocarbons which contain one double bond	Alkynes are unsaturated aliphatic hydrocarbons which contain one triple bond
Alkanes are saturated hydrocarbons with general formula C_nH_{2n+2}	Alkenes are unsaturated hydrocarbons with general formula C_nH_{2n}	Alkynes are unsaturated hydrocarbons with general formula C_nH_{2n-2}
They are less reactive because of the non-availability of electrons in the single covalent bond	Alkenes are most reactive than alkanes and alkynes because of the presence of a double bond	Alkynes are more reactive than alkanes because of the present of a triple bond
They undergo substitution reaction	They undergo addition reaction	They undergo addition reaction
Example: Ethane	Example: Ethene	Example: Ethyne
Suffix used for alkane is –ane	Suffix used for alkene is –ene	Suffix used for alkyne is –yne

where on or in the body they are applied. Some gases or light liquid hydrocarbons act as anesthetics. Inhaling these hydrocarbons in gasoline or aerosol propellants for their intoxicating effect is a major health problem that can lead to liver, kidney, or brain damage or to immediate death by asphyxiation by excluding oxygen.

Hydrocarbons are classified into saturated compounds, such as alkanes and unsaturated compounds, such as alkenes and alkynes.

- **Alkane:** A large and structurally simple class of hydrocarbons includes those substances in which all the carbon-carbon bonds are single bonds. These are called saturated hydrocarbons or alkanes. The simplest alkanes are methane (CH_4), ethane (C_2H_6), and propane (C_3H_8). The alkanes are also called as paraffins. In an alkane, all four valencies of the carbon atom are satisfied with other hydrogen atoms. This gives them general formula C_nH_{2n+2} where, $n \geq 1$, e.g., if n = 1, it is CH_4 (methane), if n = 2, it is C_2H_6 (ethane).

Section 1: Basic Chemistry

Class	General formula	Functional group	Example
Saturated hydrocarbons: Alkanes	C_nH_{2n+2}	$-\overset{\mid}{\underset{\mid}{C}}-$	C_2H_6 Ethane
Unsaturated hydrocarbons: Alkenes	C_nH_{2n}	$C=C$	$H_2C=CH_2$ Ethene
Alkynes	C_nH_{2n-2}	$-C\equiv C-$	$H-C\equiv C-H$ Acetylene

- **Alkenes:** Alkenes are the unsaturated hydrocarbons in which there is at least a double bond between two carbon atoms. In these compounds, unsaturation is due to the presence of the double bond.
  Alkenes have the general formula C_nH_{2n}, where n is the number of *carbon atoms* in the molecule (<1). For example,
  - If n = 2, n = 2, the alkene is called as ethene or also as ethylene with the formula C_2H_4.
  - If n = 3, n = 3, the alkene would be called as propene or propylene with the formula C_3H_6.
- **Alkynes:** Alkynes contain one triple bond between two adjacent carbon atoms. They are commonly called as acetylenes. These are also unsaturated compound.
  They have the general formula C_nH_{2n-2}, where n is the number of carbon atoms in the molecule. It is >1.
  For example, if an alkyne has two carbon atoms, then it would be called as *ethyne* with molecular formula C_2H_2. If an alkyne has three carbon atoms, then it would be *propyne* with formula C_3H_4.
  Formula, name, and prefix are based on number of carbon atoms:

  meth—1 carbon
  eth—2 carbons
  prop—3 carbons
  but—4 carbons
  pent—5 carbons
  hex—6 carbons
  hept—7 carbons

oct—8 carbons
non—9 carbons
dec—10 carbons

■ HOMOLOGOUS SERIES

A homologous series (homos is Greek for "the same as") can be defined as the group of compounds in which the various members have similar structural features and similar chemical properties and the successive members differ in their molecular formula by one methylene (CH_2) group.

For example,
C_2H_6 (Ethane) − CH_4 (Methane) = CH_2 unit
C_3H_8 (Propane) − C_2H_6 (Ethane) = CH_2 unit
C_4H_{10} (Butane) − C_3H_8 (Propane) = CH_2 unit
C_5H_{12} (Pentane) − C_4H_{10} (Butane) = CH_2 unit

Carbon chains of varying length have been observed in organic compounds having the same general formula.

The members of the series show a gradual gradation in their physical properties, such as solubility, density, melting, and boiling points. The physical properties generally increase as the molecular mass increases.

There are a number of homologous series in organic compounds. Some important series of aliphatic compounds are listed in **Table 2.3**.

Table 2.3: Homologous series.

S. No.	Name of series	General formula	I-homologue	II-homologue
1.	Alkane	C_nH_{2n+2}	CH_4	CH_3-CH_3
2.	Alkene	C_nH_{2n}	$CH_2=CH_2$	$CH_2=CH-CH_3$
3.	Alkyne	C_nH_{2n-2}	$HC≡CH$	$HC≡C-CH_3$
4.	Halo alkane	$C_nH_{2n+1}X$	CH_3-X	CH_3-CH_2-X
5.	Alcohol	$C_nH_{2n+2}O$	CH_3-OH	CH_3-CH_2-OH
6.	Ether	$C_nH_{2n+2}O$	CH_3-O-CH_3	$CH_3-O-CH_2-CH_3$
7.	Aldehyde	$C_nH_{2n}O$	$H-CHO$	CH_3-CHO

Contd...

Section 1: Basic Chemistry

Contd...

S. No.	Name of series	General formula	I-homologue	II-homologue
8.	Ketone	$C_nH_{2n}O$	$CH_3-\underset{O}{\overset{\|\|}{C}}-CH_3$	$CH_3-\underset{O}{\overset{\|\|}{C}}-CH_2-CH_3$
9.	Carboxylic acid	$C_nH_{2n}O_2$	H–COOH	CH_3–COOH
10.	Ester	$C_nH_{2n}O_2$	$H-\underset{O}{\overset{\|\|}{C}}-O-CH_3$	$H-\underset{O}{\overset{\|\|}{C}}-O-CH_2CH_3$ or $CH_3-\underset{O}{\overset{\|\|}{C}}-O-CH_3$
11.	Amine	$C_nH_{2n+3}N$	CH_3-NH_2	$CH_3-CH_2-NH_2$

SUMMARY

- All organic compounds are derived from animals or plants, i.e., living organisms.
- It contains carbon as an essential element.
- Organic compound always forms covalent bond.
- Aliphatic compounds are open chained while aromatic have one or more closed chain of carbon atoms.
- Functional group is responsible for structure and properties of compound.
- Some of the important functional groups in biological molecules include: Halide (Cl/F/Br/I), hydroxyl (OH), carbonyl (C=O), carboxyl (COOH), amino (NH_2), and phosphate (P) groups.
- Carbon and hydrogen elements are hydrocarbons.
- Hydrocarbons are classified into saturated compounds, such as alkanes and unsaturated compounds, such as alkenes and alkynes.
- Alkanes have suffix ane and general formula C_nH_{2n+2}
- Alkenes have suffix ene and general formula C_nH_{2n}
- Alkynes have suffix yne and general formula C_nH_{2n-2}
- The successive members of homologous series differ in their molecular formula by one methylene (CH_2) group.

PRACTICE QUESTIONS

1. What are organic compounds? Give any four characteristics of it.
2. Discuss the type of bond formed by covalent compounds.
3. Differentiate between aliphatic and aromatic compounds.
4. What are hydrocarbons? Discuss its importance.

Chapter 2: Elementary Knowledge of Organic Chemistry

5. What is meant by functional group? Write down general formula and example for each of the following: (i) Alkyl halides, (ii) Alcohol, (iii) Aldehydes, (iv) Ketones, (v) Carboxylic acids, (vi) Esters, (vii) Ethers, and (viii) Amines.
6. Differentiate between saturated and unsaturated hydrocarbons.
7. Write down molecular formula of the following: (i) Methyl iodide, (ii) Propanol, (iii) Butane, (iv) Ethanoic acid, (v) Diethyl ether, (vi) Butyne, (vii) Chloropropane, (viii) Hexyne, (ix) Pentene, and (x) Benzyne.
8. What is meant by homologous series? Explain with suitable example.

CHAPTER 3

Elementary Knowledge of Physical Chemistry

Keywords
Osmosis, isotonic solution, hypertonic solution, hypotonic solution, interface tension, diffusion, biological significance of diffusion, colloids, sol and gel, Tyndall phenomenon, Brownian movement, surface tension, cohesion, adhesion role of surface tension in physiological processes, significance of surface tension in clinical biochemistry

■ INTRODUCTION

Physical chemistry is the study of macroscopic and particulate phenomena in chemical systems in terms of the principles, practices, and concepts of physics, such as motion, energy, force, time, surface tension, electrochemistry, etc.

It lies at the interface of chemistry and physics, inasmuch as it draws on the principles of physics to account for the phenomena of chemistry. Physical chemistry has an essential role to play in the understanding of the complex processes and molecules characteristic of biological systems and modern materials. It is also an essential component of the interpretation of the techniques of investigation and their findings. This is because these techniques are becoming even more sophisticated and their full potential can be realized only by strong theoretical backing.

■ OSMOSIS AND DIFFUSION

Osmosis
Osmosis is the spontaneous flow of solvent through a semipermeable membrane from a solution of low concentration to one of higher concentration.

Physiological activities, such as absorption from gastrointestinal tract, fluid interchange in various compartments of body [e.g. between plasma and red blood cell (RBC)] follow the principle of osmosis.

Osmotic Pressure

The pressure, which must be applied to prevent passage of water molecules through membrane permeable only for water, is called osmotic pressure. The osmotic pressure of a solution depends solely on the number of particles in the solution.

Importance: Concentration of urine is regulated by osmotic pressure. The osmotic effect of plasma proteins causes water to flow from protein free interstitial fluid into the blood vessels.

Types of Solution

- **Isotonic solution:** Isotonic solutions are a pair of solutions, which produce does not flow through semipermeable membrane. These are the solutions with the same osmotic pressure and are termed as iso-osmotics.
  For example, living red cells if suspended in 0.85% NaCl solution, it neither gain nor loose water.
  Thus, an intracellular fluid of red cells is isotonic with 0.85% NaCl solution.
- **Hypertonic solution:** Hypertonic solution is a solution, which produce flow through semipermeable membrane towards the solution. This results in exosmosis.
  For example, living red cells if suspended in 2% NaCl solution, which is more concentrated than the concentration of solute inside, the cells will shrink due to exosmosis.
- **Hypotonic solution:** Hypotonic solution is a solution, which produce flow through semipermeable membrane towards the cell. This results in endosmosis.
  For example, living red cells if suspended in water, which is less concentrated than the concentration of solute inside the cells, it will result in swelling and hemolysis due to endosmosis.

Diffusion

When a water-soluble substance like sugar or NaCl is added to water it rapidly spreads in the solvent and forms a homogeneous solution. This process is called diffusion.

The uniform spreading over of solute molecules is mainly due to the energy possessed by its molecules.

Diffusion helps in passive transport of substances across the membrane. Substances move in the direction of the physical gradients, which follows the Ficks law. The law is—

$$\frac{ds}{dt} = DA \frac{dc}{dx}$$

where,

$\frac{ds}{dt}$ = Rate of movement of solute

D = Diffusion constant

A = Area of the liquid surface

$\frac{dc}{dx}$ = Difference in concentration between any two planes

Biological Significance of Diffusion

Diffusion is a physiologically important phenomenon of animal life. For example,
1. The mixing of foodstuffs and digestive juices in the gut occurs by diffusion.
2. Absorption of certain foodstuffs in gut occurs by diffusion.
3. Exchange of foodstuffs, oxygen, carbon dioxide between blood and tissue fluid and between tissue fluid and cells occurs by diffusion.
4. Exchange between plasma fluid and RBC occurs by diffusion.
5. Exchange of oxygen and carbon dioxide between lungs and blood is due to diffusion.

■ COLLOIDS

The term colloid is derived from Greek, Koli = glue and eidos = appearance. A colloid is a mixture that has particles ranging between 1 and 1,000 nanometers in diameter, which are able to remain evenly distributed throughout the solution. These are also known as colloidal dispersions, because the substances remain dispersed and do not settle to the bottom of the container. Colloids are suspensions of particles that are larger than these true solutions but still smaller to settle out by gravity. They cannot be filtered by ordinary filters, e.g., white of eggs, milk, and plasma.

A colloidal system consists of the following two components:
1. Dispersed phase
2. Dispersion medium

The phase that is scattered or present in the form of colloidal particles is called the dispersed phase. The dispersed phase consists of macromolecular solids, such as proteins and nucleic acids and liquids, such as oily fats.

The medium in which the colloidal particles are dispersed is called the dispersion medium. It may be solid liquid or gas.

For example, in a starch solution, starch represents the dispersed phase, while water represents the dispersion medium.

Properties of Colloid

1. **Sol and Gel:** A colloid may remain in two states, namely—Sol and Gel. Sol is a liquid and gel is a solid. These two states are reversible.
2. **Brownian movement:** The dispersed particles of colloid constantly move in random zig-zag paths. This haphazard motion of the dispersed particles in dispersion medium is called Brownian movement.
3. **Tyndall phenomenon:** When a beam of light is passed through a colloidal solution, the colloid particles shine due to scattering of light rays. This is called Tyndall phenomenon.
4. Colloid particles carry electric charges, which may be positive or negative.
5. Colloid solution can be precipitated by adding salts, weak acids and weak bases.
6. Colloids exert some osmotic pressure.
7. It shows properties like adsorption and ageing.
8. The colloid particles will not move through semipermeable membrane.

Biological Significance of Colloids

1. Protoplasm exists in colloidal state.
2. Blood plasma, lymph and milk are colloidal emulsions.
3. Blood clotting is a colloidal phenomenon in which sol like plasma is converted into gel like clot.
4. It helps to store water in body.
5. Colloids are dispersed in the form of minute particles. Hence, they provide a very large surface area for various reactions to occur, such as enzyme action, adsorption, surface tension, etc.

■ SURFACE TENSION

The molecules of matter always attract each other. The force of attraction between the molecules of a similar kind is called the force of cohesion. This force is responsible for keeping the molecules of a substance bind together.

The force of attraction between different types of molecules is called the force of adhesion. For example, when a glass filled with water is emptied, some water particles remain sticking to the glass. This is due to the force of attraction between water molecules and glass molecules, i.e. force of adhesion.

Cohesion and Surface Tension

The cohesive forces between liquid molecules are responsible for the phenomenon known as surface tension. The cohesive forces between molecules in a liquid present in any container are shared with all neighboring molecules. Those on the surface have no neighboring molecules above and, thus, exhibit stronger attractive forces upon their nearest neighbors on and below the surface. The stronger cohesion between the water molecules as opposed to adhesion (the attraction of the water molecules to the air). This makes it more difficult to move an object through the surface than to move it when it is completely submerged.

Surface tension could be defined as the property of the surface of a liquid that allows it to resist an external force, due to the cohesive nature of the water molecules.

Surface Tension at a Molecular Level

Water molecules want to cling to each other. At the surface, however, there are fewer water molecules to cling to since there is air above (thus, no water molecules). These results in a stronger bond between those molecules that actually do come in contact with one another, and a layer of strongly bonded water (**Fig. 3.1**). This surface layer (held together by surface tension) creates a considerable barrier between the atmosphere and the water. In fact, other than mercury, water has the greatest surface tension of any liquid.

Within a body of a liquid, a molecule will not experience a net force because the forces by the neighboring molecules all cancel out (**Fig. 3.1**). However for a molecule on the surface of the liquid, there will be a net inward force since there will be no attractive force acting from above. This inward net force causes the molecules on the surface to contract and to resist being stretched or broken. Thus, the surface is under tension, which is probably where the name "surface tension" came from.

Definition: The attractive force exerted upon the surface molecules of a liquid by the molecules beneath that tends to draw the surface molecules into the bulk of the liquid and makes the liquid assume the shape having the least surface area.

Due to the surface tension, small objects will "float" on the surface of a fluid, as long as the object cannot breakthrough and separate the top layer of water molecules. When an object is on the surface of the fluid, the surface under tension will behave like an elastic membrane.

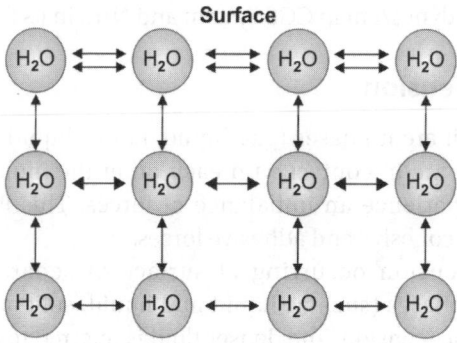

Fig. 3.1: Surface tension—molecules at the surface form stronger bonds.

Role of Surface Tension in Physiological Processes

Substances which lower the surface tension becomes concentrated in the surface layer where as the substances which increase surface tension are distributed in the interior of the liquid. Soaps, oils, proteins and bile salts reduce the surface tension of water while sodium chloride and most inorganic salts increase surface tension. Substances which reduce surface tension are used for emulsification.
1. Bile salts which reduce surface tension bring about stable emulsion of fats and help in the fat absorption.
2. Lipids and proteins which are both surface tension lowering substances are found concentrated in the cell wall. This facilitates adsorption of these substances (taking up of substances from solutions by surface).
3. Surface tension leads to efficient adsorption. This is applied in: (a) enzymatic reactions, (b) formation of complex compounds of proteins and lipids, of proteins and salts, etc. in cytoplasm and (c) in the action of drugs and poisons.

A practical application of lowering surface tension is Hay's test for bile salts in urine. The surface membrane (film) of normal urine is sufficiently dense to prevent fine particles of sulfur sprinkled on the surface from penetrating the skin and sinking to the bottom. The presence of bile salts in the urine of certain types of jaundice lowers the surface tension so much that the surface membrane cannot support sulfur particles, which sink to the bottom of the tube. Thus, bile salts are detected in urine.

Surface tension has the dimension of force per unit length. It is measured in dynes/cm in CGS system and N/m in its SI unit.

Interface Tension

When two different phases (gas/liquid, liquid/liquid, gas/solid or liquid/solid) are in contact with each other the molecules at the interface experience an imbalance of forces. This is because of difference in cohesive and adhesive forces.

Surface tension occurring at surface of separation of two immiscible phases (such as liquid and liquid, solid and liquid) is called interface tension. The denser fluid is referred to as the 'heavy phase' and the lighter fluid is referred to as the 'light phase'.

Significance of Surface Tension in Clinical Biochemistry

Many biological performances and natural processes involve an understanding of wetting and interfacial tension where most biochemical reactions occur not in solution but at the surface and interface. Human biological fluids, such as serum, urine, gastric juice, amniotic fluid, digestive, urinary and reproductive tracts, endocrine glands, middle ear, cerebrospinal and alveolar lining fluid contain numerous surfactants, proteins, and lipids. These low and high-molecular weight surfactants are the common materials in various tissues of the body which control surface tension of human interfaces. The physicochemical processes that take place in these interfaces are of fundamental importance for various tissues and the vital function of body organs.

Pathological features of diseases vary in the nature and the magnitude. Despite this diversity, the common feature of various disorders underlies the physicochemical and biochemical factors, such as surface tension. Changes in the surface tension behavior of human biological fluid are characteristic for some diseases. Studying these interfaces and the changes that occur will provide valuable information relating to various diseases and help to monitor the treatment efficacy. In medicine, surface tension measurement is above all used in connection with various pathological states of lung surfactants, such as adult respiratory distress syndrome, bronchial asthma, and pneumonia. In addition to pneumology, there are other studies which evaluates the surface tension of plasma, urine and other biological fluids.

SUMMARY

- Physical chemistry is the study of macroscopic and particulate phenomena in chemical systems in terms of the principles, practices, and concepts of physics.
- Osmosis is the spontaneous flow of solvent through a semipermeable membrane from a solution of low concentration to one of higher concentration.
- Isotonic solutions are a pair of solutions, with same concentration.
- In hypotonic solution, the solution outside the cell has a higher concentration than inside the cell.

Section 1: Basic Chemistry

- In hypertonic solution, the solution outside the cell has a less concentrated solution than inside the cell.
- The uniform spreading over of solute molecules is diffusion.
- Colloids are mixtures in which microscopically dispersed insoluble particles of one substance are suspended in another substance.
- Colloidal particles make dispersed phase while the medium in which the colloidal particles are dispersed is called the dispersion medium.
- The haphazard motion of the dispersed particles in dispersion medium is called Brownian movement.
- Property of colloidal particles to scatter light is called Tyndall phenomenon.
- The force of attraction between the molecules of a similar kind is cohesion.
- The force of attraction between different types of molecules is adhesion.
- Surface tension is the tendency of fluid surfaces to shrink into the minimum surface area possible.
- Surface tension occurring at surface of separation of two immiscible phases is called interface tension.

PRACTICE QUESTIONS

1. Define: (i) Physical chemistry, (ii) Osmosis, (iii) Diffusion, (iv) Brownian movement, (v) Tyndall phenomenon, and (vi) Interface tension.
2. Differentiate between: (i) Hypotonic and hypertonic solution, and (ii) Diffusion and osmosis.
3. What are colloids? Mention its biological significance.
4. Explain phenomenon of surface tension.
5. Discuss the significance of surface tension in clinical biochemistry.

CHAPTER 4

Elementary Knowledge of Analytical Chemistry

> **Keywords**
>
> Balances—its type, use, and care; centrifuge—principle and types; pH meter working and principle; colorimeter—principle, basic terms, and procedure; Lambert–Beer law spectrophotometer—principle, procedure, and applications; fluorimeter—component and applications; flame photometry—principle, instrumentation, procedure, applications; urinometer—principle and procedure; densitometer

■ INTRODUCTION

Analytical chemistry is a branch of chemistry dealing with the chemical composition of samples and their qualitative and quantitative measurement. It is a comprehensive chemical analysis essential for complete understanding of the chemistry of a substance.

Analytical chemistry studies and uses instruments and methods used to separate, identify, and quantify matter. In practice, separation, identification, or quantification may constitute the entire analysis or may be combined with another method. Separation isolates analytes. Qualitative analysis identifies analytes, while quantitative analysis determines the numerical amount or concentration.

Analytical chemistry consists of classical, wet chemical methods and modern, instrumental methods. Classical qualitative methods use separations, such as precipitation, extraction, and distillation. Identification may be based on differences in color, odor, melting point, boiling point, solubility, radioactivity, or reactivity. Classical quantitative analysis uses mass or volume changes to quantify amount.

Instrumental methods may be used to separate samples using chromatography, electrophoresis, or field-flow fractionation. Then qualitative and quantitative analyses can be performed, often with the same instrument and may use light interaction, heat interaction, electric fields, or magnetic fields. Often the same instrument can separate, identify, and quantify an analyte.

Analytical chemistry is also focused on improvements in experimental design, chemometrics, and the creation of new measurement tools. Analytical chemistry has broad applications to medicine, science, engineering, and diagnostic field. All commonly used laboratory analysis techniques are discussed here.

■ BALANCES

Laboratory balances are used to measure an object's mass to a very high degree of precision. It provides high readability, a broad weighing range, and a high degree of accuracy.

When the instrument balance is discussed scientifically, there is a difference between balance and weighing scale. Balances measure mass, while scales measure weight. A balance does not have effect of specific gravity (SG), whereas the scale will be affected by the gravity.

A balance determines mass by balancing an unknown mass against a known mass. In modern weighing instruments, balances usually use a force restoration mechanism that creates a force to balance the force exerted by the unknown mass.

A scale displays weight by measuring a deflection; the springs are deformed by the load, and the force needed to deform the springs is measured, and converted into weight.

Some Basic Terms Related to Balance

- **Accuracy:** The ability of a scale to provide a result that is as close as possible to the actual value. The best modern balances have an accuracy of better than one part in 100 million when 1kg masses are compared.
- **Calibration:** The comparison between the output of a scale or balance against a standard value. It is usually done with a standard known weight and adjusted so that the instrument gives a reading in agreement.
- **Capacity:** The heaviest load that can be measured on the instrument.

- **Precision:** Amount of agreement between repeated measurements of the same quantity; also known as repeatability. Note: A scale can be extremely precise but not necessarily be accurate.
- **Readability:** This is the smallest division at which the scale can be read. It can vary as much as 0.1–0.0000001 g. Readability designates the number of places after the decimal point that the scale can be read.
- **Tare:** The act of removing a known weight of an object, usually the weighing container, to 0 a scale. This means that the final reading will be of the material to be weighed and will not reflect the weight of the container. Most balances allow taring to 100% of capacity.
- **Rider:** The riders are the sliding pointers positioned on top of the beams to show the pan and beam weight in grams.

Types

There are many types of laboratory balances with wide measuring range. The type of balance can be selected on the basis of its use and availability. Beam balance and analytical balance are discussed in detail.

Beam Balance

The beam balance is a first-order lever with the fulcrum in the middle. It works on the principle of moments. When two equal masses are placed in pans at either ends of a beam supported in the middle, then the beam will be balanced. It is also known as equal arm balance **(Fig. 4.1)**.

Principle

According to the principle of moments, under equilibrium condition, the clockwise moment due to body on one side of the beam equals the anticlockwise moment due to standard weights on the other side of the beam.

Setup

The beam balance consists of light and rigid beam of brass, a metallic pillar, a wooden case, two pans, a metallic pointer, and an ivory scale. The plumb line indicates whether the balance is horizontal. In an ideal condition, the plumb line is aligned with the end of knob fixed

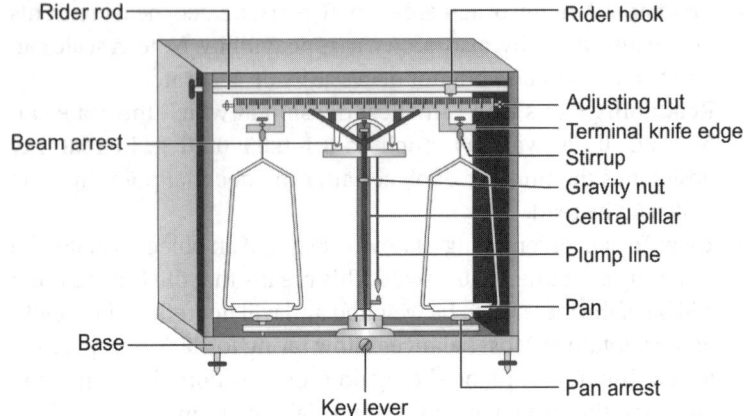

Fig. 4.1: Beam balance.

to the pillar. When the beam is horizontal, the pointer remains on 0 mark on the ivory scale. The device is enclosed in a glass box to avoid effects of air. The box has leveling screws at the bottom to set it horizontal. A lever arrangement is provided at the base board for raising or lowering of the platform.

Working

It is used to find unknown mass by using known standard masses.
- By adjusting leveling screw, the plumb line is brought just above the pointed projection on the balance.
- The beam is raised using the lever and checked that the pointer swings equally on either side of the 0 mark.
- Now, the beam is lowered and an unknown mass is kept in one pan of the common balance.
- The next known masses are put in the second pan such that the pointer lies in the center (0 mark) or the scale swings equally on both sides of the 0 mark.
- The total known mass in the other pan is calculated, which gives mass of the object.

For weighing liquid or gas:
1. First, take the mass of an empty beaker or closed container. Note the mass M_1.
2. Fill the beaker with the liquid or container with the gas, find its mass, and label it as M_2.
3. $M_2 - M_1$ will be the mass of liquid or gas.

Precautions

Do not weigh if the substance is hot.
1. While weighing, only use side doors of the balance.
2. The weights, fractional weights, or rider should not be touched directly with finger.
3. Always use the same balance for weighing different substances to reduce error.
4. Always close the chamber doors before taking final reading.

Electrical Balance

Electrical balance is a significant instrument for the laboratories for precise measurement of chemicals. It is an automated balance based on the principle of generation of current that is proportional to the displacement of the pan. These are designed to measure small masses from around 320 g to submilligram **(Fig. 4.2)**. They are very sensitive pieces of equipment, so they are needed to be treated with care. The main types of laboratory balance are as follows:
- Top-pan balance (200–0.001 g)
- Analytical balance (320–0.0001 g)
- Microbalance (6–0.000001 g)
- Ultramicrobalance (6–0.0000001 g)

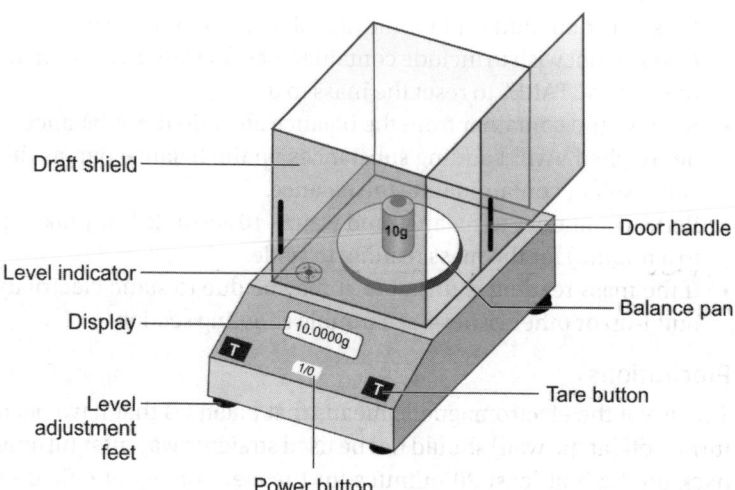

Fig. 4.2: The analytical balance.

Principle

Electrical balances measure weight using an electromagnet. There is an electromagnetic servomotor which generates a force to counter the weight of the mass being measured. The electrical current required to generate this force is proportional to the weight and so can be used, with appropriate calibration, to calculate the mass. This mass is then displayed on the screen. To signal when the weight and electromagnetic forces are equal, many balances have a "null detector" that uses a light source and detector.

Working

The following is a basic procedure for using an analytical balance. Before using a balance, always check the calibration with a check weight.

- Check that the balance is level using the level indicator. If the bubble is not in the center, adjust the level, normally by twisting the feet, until the bubble is in the center of the inner circle.
- Check that the balance is on and that the door is closed. Press the "Tare" button and wait 5-10 seconds for a "*" or similar symbol to appear in the upper left/right hand corner of the display, and the mass to read 0.0000 g.
- Open the door and place a weigh boat, weight paper, or another container on the center of the balance pan (ideally with tweezers or similar).
- Close the door and wait for the digital readout to stabilize ("*").
- If you do not wish to include container mass in your measurement, then press "TARE" to reset the mass to 0.
- Remove the container from the balance and add the substance to be weighed. Avoid adding substances on the balance pan as this can result in contaminating the balance.
- Return container to balance and wait 5-10 seconds (may take up to a minute) for the mass reading to settle.
- If the mass reading is unstable, it may be due to static electricity build-up or other issues—see trouble shooting section.

Precautions

The use of the electromagnetic means that balances that have been turned off (at the wall) should not be used straight away after turning back on. Wait at least 30 minutes for the electromagnetic field to

Chapter 4: Elementary Knowledge of Analytical Chemistry

stabilize (times may vary depending on manufacturer and model). It also means that placing any magnetic materials or magnets near the balance could cause problems for the balance.

Weighing a liquid, powder, or granular substance, these substances must always be weighed using an appropriate weighing container.
1. Place the weighing container on the balance pan and close the doors.
2. Tare the container by briefly pressing the control bar.
3. The readout will read 0 with the container sitting on the pan. This allows the mass of sample to be read directly.

Other balances in use are as follows:
- **Equal-arm balances:** An equal-arm balance is the simplest type of beam balance. This scale incorporates two pans on opposite sides of a lever. It can be used in two different ways. The object to be weighed can be placed on one side and standard weights are added to the other pan until the pans are balanced. The sum of the standard weights equals the mass of the object. Another application for the scale is to place two items on each scale and adjust one side until both pans are leveled. This is convenient in applications, such as balancing tubes or centrifugation where two objects must be of the exact same weight.
- **Unequal-arm balances:** An unequal-arm balance is suspended at a point a very short distance from one of its ends. These are single-pan balances. Only one pan was now visible to the user, and all weights were included in the case and operated by knobs from the outside.
- **Spring balances:** A spring balance consists of a coiled spring fixed to a support at one end, with a hook at the other to which the body to be weighed is applied.
- **Moisture balances:** A moisture balance is used to measure the moisture content in a material sample. They do so by heating the sample, and automatically calculating the percentage of weight lost throughout the heating cycle.
- **Top-loading balances:** A top-loading balance uses a glass or plastic breeze-break atop the scale.
- **Platform balances:** A platform balance is a form of equal-arm balance in which two flat platforms are attached to the top side of the beam, one at each end. On this platform, objects to be weighed

are placed. It allows a heavy object to be placed on a load-bearing platform.

Care and Use and Maintenance of Balance

- Often, the weighing pan is sealed to prevent the ingress of dust or other contaminants. Items to be measured should be at room temperature before weighing. A hot item will give a reading less than the actual weight due to convection currents that make the item more buoyant.
- Another important part of using a balance is cleaning. Scales are exposed to many chemicals that can react with the metal in the pan and corrode the surface. This will affect the accuracy of the scale. Also, keep in mind that a potentially dangerous situation could occur if a dusting of chemicals is left on the balance pan. There is a chance that incompatible chemicals could be brought into contact if left standing or that someone could be exposed to a dangerous chemical that has not been cleaned from the balance. To avoid damaging the scale or putting others in danger, the balance should be kept extremely clean. A hairbrush can be used to remove any dust that can spill over during weighing.
- At the end of the day, the balance can be turned off.
- For most laboratories, an annual service and calibration is sufficient. However, accredited laboratories will often check the calibration every day to ensure that no error has occurred.
- In between calibrations, the key maintenance is to keep the balance clean. Any material that works its way inside a balance can cause major problems, especially if it is a corrosive material. Clean the balance by dusting off the stage and the surrounding area with a paint brush or similar and then gently wipe down the balance, glass panels, and countertop around the balance with a lint-free tissue. Ethanol can sometimes also be used depending on manufacturer and model—always check manufacturer's instructions.
- Other sources of error for laboratory balances include: Buoyancy, friction, improper miscalibration, misalignment, condensation, evaporation, gravitational abnormalities, and seismic disturbances.

■ CENTRIFUGE

A centrifuge is a device that allows the rotation of an object about a single axis, where an outward force is applied perpendicularly to the axis. Centrifugation is a process in which a solution is rotated in circles around a central axis. The centrifugal force and gravitational forces act together on the solution. This results in separation of sediments and supernatant.

Principle

A centrifuge works on the principle of sedimentation, where the high speed of the rotation causes the denser particles to move away from the center while smaller, less dense particles are forced toward the center. Thus, the denser particles settle at the bottom while the lighter particles are collected at the top.

Types of Centrifuges

Centrifuges are of three types:
1. Ordinary centrifuge
2. Electric centrifuge
3. Ultracentrifuge

Ordinary Centrifuge

These are hands-driven centrifuges, which can reach up to 2,000–2,500 rotations per minute (rpm). Hand centrifuges can hold only two to four centrifuge tubes, which are of 15 mL capacity, and usually made of aluminum. Ordinary centrifuge produces heat due to friction with air after long run.

The tubes in the centrifuge must be balanced exactly; otherwise the tubes will be broken due to vibration. Gradually increase or decrease the speed of centrifuge. The tubes must be of the same size and weight.

Electric Centrifuge

These are motor-driven centrifuge, operated through main electric supply. These can reach up to 3,500 rpm and they are usually

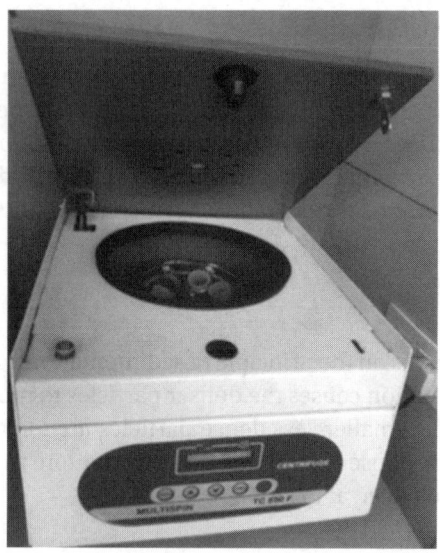

Fig. 4.3: Electric centrifuge.
(For color version, see Plate 1)

provided with a multistage speed regulator to obtain desired speed. The common laboratory centrifuge is used for separation of serum precipitates and sediments of various body fluids, urinary sediments for microscopic examinations, etc **(Fig. 4.3)**.

Ultracentrifuge

This is a high-speed centrifuge. The speed of rotation is more than 60,000 rpm. This centrifugal force permits the cell fractionation of subcellular organelles previously observed only in an electron microscope. This in turn permits assay of their enzymatic constituents providing insight into structure–function relationship. Viruses can be isolated in pure form. DNA, RNA, and proteins can be analyzed completely.

The ultracentrifuge has drive and speed control. The drive assembly has a water-cooled electric motor connected to the rotor by way of a precision gearbox. The speed rotor may be selected by means of rheostat and monitored by a tachometer. If there is overspeed, the instrument is automatically shut down. There is an infrared (IR) radiometric sensor beneath the rotors; it measures and controls the temperature of the rotors continuously and accurately.

Chapter 4: Elementary Knowledge of Analytical Chemistry

To eliminate heating effect, the rotor is sealed and evaluated by two pumping systems. Friction is completely avoided inside the vacuum.

While spinning, the rotors may be kept at an angle of 30° of horizontal.

Application

The primary application of a centrifuge is the separation of particles suspended in a suspension. It can be used for the separation of cell organelles, nucleic acid, blood components, and separation of isotopes.

■ pH METER

pH meter is an electronic instrument used to measure acidity or alkalinity of solutions. It measures the activity of hydrogen ions. It is widely used in different branches of science.

pH indicates the hydrogen ion concentration of any given solution. pH signifies the power of hydrogen. To understand the theory of pH, it is important to know about dissociation of water. The pH scale has been derived from spontaneous dissociation of water. The water spontaneously dissociates into its H^+ and OH^- components. The concentration of H^+ ion found in pure water is 1×10^{-7}. This H^+ ion concentration is neither acidic nor alkaline and hence called neutral.

When the H^+ ion concentration is more than 1×10^{-7}, the solution is acidic; when it is less than 1×10^{-7}, then the solution is alkaline. Low pH indicates high H^+ ion concentration; high pH indicates low H^+ concentration. Hence, the pH scale is inversely related to concentration of H^+ in any given solution and directly related to OH^- ion concentration (**Fig. 4.4**).

$$pH = -\log_{10}[H^+]$$

The pH scale is in the range from 1 to 14. When there is change of pH by unit 1 (e.g., pH changes from 4 to 5), it indicates the change in hydrogen ion concentration by 10 times. When there is change of pH by 2 units, it indicates the change in hydrogen ion concentration by 100 times. Due to this relationship, the pH scale is called logarithmic.

While conducting many laboratory tests, it is important to check the pH of any given solution. For precise noting of pH, an instrument

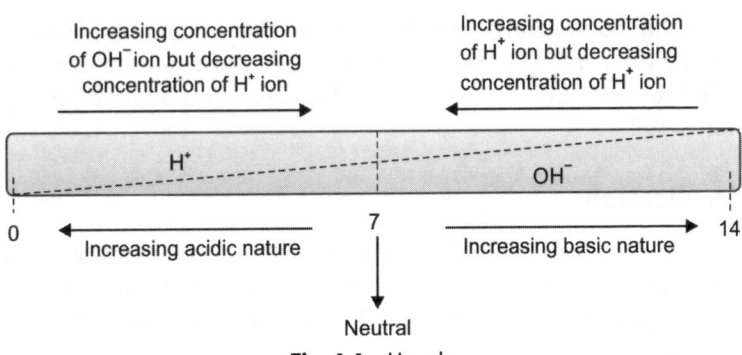

Fig. 4.4: pH scale.

is used and it is called pH meter. The pH meter works on the potentiometric principle.

As the acidic solution has more positive charge (H^+ ion) than alkaline solution, the acidic solution has greater potential to produce current than alkaline solution. The pH meter measures the potential difference (voltage) of test solution and standard or known solution and calculates the pH. Hence, it works like a voltmeter. To complete the circuit, two electrodes are connected which allows the movement of electric current.

Principle

The working of pH meter is based on Nernst equation. The Nernst equation derives the relation between the electric voltage and ion concentration. The Nernst equation derived for H^+ ion concentration is the basis of pH meter. The working principle of pH meter is the potentiometry. The pH meter consists of glass (also called indicator electrode) and reference electrode. The glass electrode consists of glass membrane, which is sensitive to hydrogen ion concentration of test sample solution. The glass electrode potential varies from sample to sample. The reference electrode is standard and has constant potential. The reference electrode does not respond to test sample solution. The pH meter measures and compares the potential difference between both glass and reference electrodes.

Using the Nernst equation, the potential difference is used to measure the hydrogen ion concentration indicating the pH of given solution. Due to the potential difference between two electrodes, the electron flows and generates current. This generated current is measured by a voltmeter. The relationship between the potential difference, generated current, and pH has been derived. The potential difference of 1 pH is 59.16 mV at 25°C and hence when there is a difference of 1 pH unit, there will be change in voltage by 59.16 mV. This relationship is employed in measuring the pH.

Construction of pH meter

The pH probe of a modern pH meter is a combined type, in which glass and reference electrode are placed into a rod-like structure. The combined electrode consists of the following parts:

1. **Glass bulb:** It is a sensor that senses the H^+ ion concentration and it is made from a special type of glass and membrane **(Fig. 4.5)**. The glass bulb consists of 0.1M HCl.
2. **Internal electrode:** It is the silver chloride electrode.
3. **Internal solution:** The silver chloride electrode is dipped in buffer solution of 0.1 mol/L KCl of pH 7.
4. **Reference electrode:** It is also the silver chloride electrode.

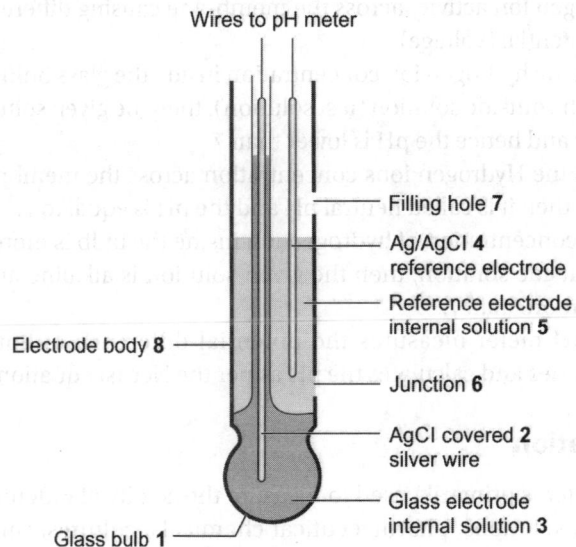

Fig. 4.5: pH meter with combined electrodes.

5. **Internal solution:** The reference electrode is also dipped in buffer solution of 0.1 mol/L KCl of pH 7.
6. **Junction:** It is made from ceramic junction, also called diaphragm, that allows the contact of sample solution and reference electrolyte. It does not disturb the electric connection between the electrodes.
7. **Filling hole:** It is used for refilling the electrolyte.
8. **Electrode body:** The body is from nonconductive glass or plastic.

Working

- The acidic solution is rich in H^+ ion concentration. When the pH probe is dipped in an acidic solution, the H^+ ion moves close to the glass membrane of the sensitive glass bulb (external side of the bulb).
- Similar reaction occurs inside the bulb, which is filled with buffer solution of neutral pH. This neutral buffer solution has a constant number of hydrogen ions.
- The H^+ ions present inside the bulb also move close to glass membrane (internal side of the bulb). Hence, this causes the difference in the concentration of hydrogen ion or degree of hydrogen ion activity across the membrane causing difference in the potential (voltage).
- When the hydrogen ion concentration inside the glass bulb is less than the outside solution (test solution), then the given solution is acidic and hence the pH is lower than 7.
- When the Hydrogen ions concentration across the membrane is same, then it is called neutral pH and the pH is equal to 7.
- If the concentration of hydrogen ion inside the bulb is more than the outside solution, then the given solution is alkaline and the pH is more than 7.
- The pH meter measures the potential difference at both the electrodes and calculates the pH as per the Nernst equation.

Application

A pH meter is primarily used to measure the acidity of different test samples, solutions, pharmaceutical chemicals, cultures, soil, and water treatment plant.

Note: The instrument must be calibrated against buffers of known pH before measuring the pH of an unknown specimen.

■ COLORIMETER

A colorimeter involves the measurement of color and is the widely used method for finding the concentration of biochemical compounds. It measures absorbance and wavelength between 400 and 700 nm (nanometer), i.e., from the visible spectrum of light of the electromagnetic spectrum.

Absorption of Light

Light falling on a colored solution is either absorbed or transmitted. A colored solution absorbs all the colors of white light and selectively transmits only one color. This is its own color.

Principle

A colorimeter is based on the photometric technique which states that when a beam of incident light of intensity I_0 passes through a solution, a part of the incident light is reflected (I_r), a part is absorbed (I_a), and the rest of the light is transmitted (I_t).
Thus,

$$I_0 = I_r + I_a + I_t$$

In a colorimeter, (I_r) is eliminated because of the measurement of (I_0) and it is sufficient to determine the (I_a). For this purpose, the amount of light reflected (I_r) is kept constant by using cells that have identical properties. (I_0) and (I_t) are then measured.

The mathematical relationship between the amount of light absorbed and the concentration of the substance can be shown by the two fundamental laws of photometry on which the colorimeter is based.

Beer's Law

This law states that the amount of light absorbed is directly proportional to the concentration of the solute in the solution.

$$\text{Log}_{10} I_0/I_t = a_s c$$

where,
 a_s = Absorbency index
 c = Concentration of solution

Lambert's Law

The Lambert's law states that the amount of light absorbed is directly proportional to the length and thickness of the solution under analysis.

$$A = \log_{10} I_0/I_t = a_s b$$

Where,
 A = Absorbance of test
 a_s = Absorbance of standard
 b = Length/thickness of the solution

The mathematical representation of the combined form of the Beer–Lambert law is as follows:

$$\log_{10} I_0 / I_t = a_s bc$$

If *b* is kept constant by applying Cuvette or standard cell, then

$$\log_{10} I_0/I_t = a_s c$$

The absorbency index is defined as

$$a_s = A/cl$$

where,
 c = Concentration of the absorbing material (in g/L)
 l = Distance traveled by the light in solution (in cm)

In simplified form, the working principle of the colorimeter is based on the Beer–Lambert law which states that the amount of light absorbed by a color solution is directly proportional to the concentration of the solution and the length of a light path through the solution.

$$A \propto cl$$

where,
 A = Absorbance/optical density of solution
 c = Concentration of solution
 l = Path length

$$A = \epsilon cl$$

ϵ = Absorption coefficient

Parts of Colorimeter

There are five essential parts in a colorimeter **(Fig. 4.6)**.
1. **Light source:** The most common source of light used in a colorimeter is a tungsten filament.
   Condenser lens: The lens makes the beam of light parallel.
2. **Monochromator:** To select the particular wavelength, filter or monochromators are used to split the light from the light source. The filter allows maximum transmission of the color absorbed. The filter is chosen so that Beer's law is obeyed. It is selected according to the color of the solution.
   For example, if a blue solution is under examination, then red color is absorbed and red filter is selected.
   The color of filter should be therefore complementary to the color of the solution under investigation **(Table 4.1)**.
3. **Sample holder:** Test tube or cuvettes are used to hold the color solutions; they are made up of glass at the visible wavelength.

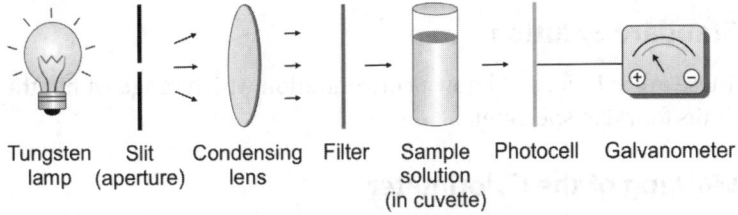

Tungsten   Slit   Condensing   Filter   Sample   Photocell   Galvanometer
lamp   (aperture) lens   solution
                                            (in cuvette)

Fig. 4.6: Colorimeter.

Table 4.1: Range of filters for different colored solution.

Color of solution	Filter
Red-Orange	Blue-Blue Green
Blue	Red
Green	Red
Purple	Green
Yellow	Blue
Yellow-Green	Violate

These are small, test tube-like containers used in a colorimeter. These are filled with the solution of which the optical density is to be measured and kept in the cuvette holder of the colorimeter. The upper end of the cuvette has an arrow mark. The solution is filled up to this mark. The sides of the cuvette facing the beam are cut parallel to each other.

4. **Photodetector system:** When light falls on the detector system, an electric current is generated. This reflects the Galvanometer reading.
5. **Measuring device:** The current from the detector is fed to the measuring device, the Galvanometer, which shows the meter reading that is directly proportional to the intensity of light.

Blank Solution

This is used to set photometer to 0 absorbance (A) or 100% transmittance (% T). This can be distilled water or the reagent solution if colored.

Standard Solution

These are solutions of known concentration which range within the limits found in specimen.

Working of the Colorimeter

When using a colorimeter, it requires being calibrated first which is done by using the standard solutions of the known concentration of the solute that has to be determined in the test solution.

When the monochromatic light (light of one wavelength) reaches the cuvette with test solution, some of the light is reflected, some part of the light is absorbed by the solution, and the remaining part is transmitted through the solution which falls on the photodetector system. The photodetector system measures the intensity of transmitted light and converts it into the electrical signals that are sent to the galvanometer.

The galvanometer measures the electrical signals and displays them in the digital form. That digital representation of the electrical signals is the absorbance or optical density of the solution analyzed.

If the absorption of the solution is higher, then there will be more light absorbed by the solution and if the absorption of the solution is low, then more lights will be transmitted through the solution which affects the galvanometer reading and corresponds to the concentration of the solute in the solution. By putting all the values in the formula given in the below section, one can easily determine the concentration of the solution.

Here is the formula used for determining the concentration of a substance in the test solution.

$$A = \epsilon cl$$

For two solutions, i.e., test and standard,
 ϵ = Constant
 l = Constant (using the same Cuvette or Standard cell)

$$A_T = C_T \ \ldots (i)$$
$$A_S = C_S \ \ldots (ii)$$

From (i) and (ii),

$$A_T \times C_S = A_S \times C_T$$
$$C_T = (A_T/A_S) \times C_S$$

where,
 C_T = Concentration of the test solution
 A_T = Absorbance/optical density of the test solution
 C_S = Concentration of the standard
 A_S = Absorbance/optical density of the standard solution

Procedure

- Set the instrument to 0% transmission setting with the help of 0 setting knob.
- Pour the blank in a cuvette and set the instrument to 100% transmission with the blank setting knob.
- Take the absorbance readings of various standard solutions of different concentrations.
- Each time, the cuvette is rinsed in distilled water and the outer surface of the cuvette is wiped off with soft tissue paper before placing in the cuvette holder.
- Record the readings in a tabular form—absorbance readings against the sequential concentration of standard used.

- Plot the calibration curve on a linear graph paper for absorbance readings (Y-axis) against various concentrations of standard (X-axis). The calibration curve should be at an angle of 45°.

Results

Results are either calculated by optical density (OD) of test and standard or prepared from the calibration curve.

Applications

The colorimeter is commonly used for the determination of the concentration of a colored compound by measuring the optical density or its absorbance.

It can also be used for the determination of the course of the reaction by measuring the rate of formation and disappearance of the light-absorbing compound in the range of the visible spectrum of light like—end-point reaction methods and rate of reaction methods.

In a clinical biochemistry laboratory, the Folin–Wu method, glucose oxidase-peroxidase (GOD-POD) method of glucose, and end-point reaction of enzymes are some examples of tests performed on a colorimeter.

■ SPECTROPHOTOMETER

A spectrophotometer is an instrument used to measure absorbance at various wavelengths. The basic principle of a colorimeter and spectrophotometer is same. It is also based on the Lambert–Beer law.

It is similar to a colorimeter except that it uses prism or diffraction grating to produce monochromatic light. It can be operated in ultraviolet (UV) region, visible spectrum as well as IR region of the electromagnetic spectrum.

Types

The spectrophotometer is of two types:
1. Single-beam spectrophotometer
2. Double-beam spectrophotometer

Chapter 4: Elementary Knowledge of Analytical Chemistry

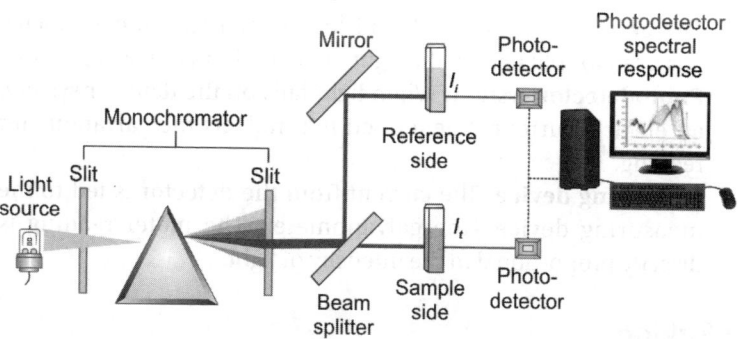

Fig. 4.7: Double-beam spectrophotometer.
(For color version, see Plate 2)

Single-beam spectrophotometer operates between 325- and 1,000-nm wavelength using the single beam of light. The light travels in one direction and the test solution and blank are read in the same.

Double-beam spectrophotometer operates between 185- and 1,000-nm wavelength. It has two photocells. This instrument splits the light from the monochromator into two beams. One beam is used for reference and the other for sample reading. It eliminates the error which occurs due to fluctuations in the light output and the sensitivity of the detector **(Fig. 4.7)**.

Parts

There are seven essential parts of spectrophotometer:

1. **Light source:** In a spectrophotometer, three different sources of light are commonly used to produce light of different wavelengths. For the visible spectrum, it is a tungsten lamp. For UV radiation, the commonly used sources are the hydrogen lamp and the deuterium lamp. The Nernst filament or globar is the most satisfactory source of IR radiation.
2. **Monochromator:** To select the particular wavelength, prism or diffraction grating is used to split the light from the light source.
3. **Sample holder:** Test tube or Cuvettes are used to hold the colored solutions. They are made up of glass at a visible wavelength.
4. **Beam splitter:** It is present only in a double-beam spectrophotometer. It is used to split the single beam of light coming from the light source into two beams.

5. **Mirror:** It is also present only and double beam spectrophotometer. It is used to split light in the right direction from the beam splitter.
6. **Photodetector system:** When light falls on the detector system, an electric current is generated that reflects the galvanometer reading.
7. **Measuring device:** The current from the detector is fed to the measuring device—the galvanometer. The meter reading is directly proportional to the intensity of light.

Working

There is a ray of light with a certain wavelength that is specific for the assay and directed toward the solution. Before reaching the solution, the ray of light passes through a series of diffraction grating, prism, and mirrors. These mirrors are used for navigation of the light in the spectrophotometer and the prism splits the beam of light into different wavelengths and the diffraction grating allows the required wavelength to pass through it and reaches the cuvette containing the standard or test solutions. It analyzes the reflected light and compares with a predetermined standard solution.

When the monochromatic light (light of one wavelength) reaches the cuvette, some of the light is reflected, some part of the light is absorbed by the solution, and the remaining part is transmitted through the solution which falls on the photodetector system. The photodetector system measures the intensity of transmitted light and converts it into the electrical signals that are sent to the galvanometer.

The galvanometer measures the electrical signals and displays it in the digital form. That digital representation of the electrical signals is the absorbance or optical density of the solution analyzed.

In double-beam spectrophotometers, the beam splitters are present which split the monochromatic light into two beams, one for the standard solution and the other for the test solution. In this, the absorbance of standard and the test solution can be measured at the same time and any number of test solutions can be analyzed against one standard. It gives more accurate and precise results and eliminates the errors which occur due to the fluctuations in the light output and the sensitivity of the detector.

Calculation

The formula used for determining the concentration of a substance in the test solution using the absorbance values measured by the spectrophotometer is the same as that of a colorimeter.

$$A_T \times C_S = A_S \times C_T$$
$$C_T = (A_T/A_S) \times C_S$$

where,
- C_T = Concentration of the test solution
- A_T = Absorbance/optical density of the test solution
- C_S = Concentration of the standard
- A_S = Absorbance/optical density of the standard solution

Applications

The spectrophotometer is commonly used for the determination of the concentration of colored as well as colorless compounds by measuring the optical density or its absorbance.

It can also be used for the determination of the course of the reaction by measuring the rate of formation and disappearance of the light absorbing compound in the range of the visible and UV regions of the electromagnetic spectrum. This method is used for serum creatinine, different enzymes, etc.

By a spectrophotometer, a compound can be identified by determining the absorption spectrum in the visible region of the light spectrum as well as the UV region of the electromagnetic spectrum.

DIFFERENCES BETWEEN COLORIMETER AND SPECTROPHOTOMETER (TABLE 4.2)

Table 4.2: Differences between colorimeter and spectrophotometer.

Basis of comparisons	Colorimeter	Spectrophotometer
Basic function	Measuring light absorbance level	Measuring light transmittance level

Contd...

Contd...

Basis of comparisons	Colorimeter	Spectrophotometer
Approach	Psychophysical analysis	Physical analysis
Complexity	It is generally rugged and less complex instrument than a spectrophotometer.	It is generally a more complex instrument than a colorimeter.
Filter	Glass is used.	Prism is used.
Accuracy	Results up to two digits after decimal.	More precise. Results up to four digits after decimal.
Components	It is composed of sensor and simple data processor. It has only a set illuminant and observer combination.	It is composed of sensor and data processor and sometimes includes computer software. It has many available illuminant or observer combinations.
Wavelength	It uses fixed wavelengths in the visible range only.	It uses a wide range of wavelengths in the ultraviolet, visible, and infrared zones.
Data display	Data is displayed on a digital or analog output.	Data is produced and recorded via computer software.
Application	It can be used to determine the concentration of an individual compound based on the amount of absorbance.	It can be used in identification and quantification studies of inorganic and organic biochemical molecules.
Cost	It is cheaper when compared to a spectrophotometer.	It is more costly when compared to a colorimeter.
Nature	It is made up of stationary parts and it is lighter in weight and therefore good for field use.	It is composed of moving parts and it is heavier in weight and only good for bench use.

■ FLUORIMETER

A large number of substances are unknown which can absorb UV or visible light energy. These substances lose some of excess energy through heat and release the remnant energy as electromagnetic radiation of a wavelength longer than that absorbed. The process of emitting radiation is collectively known as luminescence.

Luminescence is of two types:
1. **Fluorescence:** When a beam of light is incident on certain materials, they emit visible light or radiations. This phenomenon is known as fluorescence and the substance showing this phenomenon is known as fluorescent substance. The phenomenon of fluorescence is instantaneous and starts immediately after the absorption of light and stops as soon as the incident light is cut off.
2. **Phosphorescence:** When light radiation is incident on certain materials, they continue to emit light even after the incident light is cut off. This type of delayed fluorescence is called phosphorescence and the substances are called phosphorescent substances.

Principles of Fluorimetry

- When molecules are irradiated with light of the appropriate frequency, it will be absorbed in about 10-15 seconds.
- In the process of absorption, the molecules may move from ground to the first excited singlet electronic state.
- From the excited singlet state, one of the following three phenomena will probably occur, depending on the molecule involved and the conditions.
- The first possibility is that the excited singlet state is relatively unstable; in such a situation, the excited molecules will return to the ground state by collisional deactivation (loosing heat energy) without emitting any radiation.
- The second possibility is that the molecules in the excited singlet state may emit an UV or visible light photon. This process is known as fluorescence.
- The third possibility is that the molecule with a relatively stable excited state may undergo transition and sometime thereafter returns to the ground state, usually by the emission of an UV or visible light photon. This is known as phosphorescence emission.
- Fluorescence spectroscopy analyzes fluorescence from a molecule based on its fluorescent properties. The instruments used for the measurement of fluorescence are known as fluorimeters.

Instrumentation

The components of a fluorimeter are as follows:
1. **Source of light:** This is an excitation source. It is usually in the UV range and emits light of high energy. The use of a xenon lamp is common and gives out radiant energy of discrete wavelength.
2. **Primary filter:** This screens the radiant energy coming out of light source. The filter works like the monochromator that allows selected wavelengths of light in the UV region to pass through. This screened light then hits the specimen and excites the organic compound under study.
3. **Specimen carrier:** This carries the specimen. The test compound present in the specimen is capable of excitation that leads to its fluorescence. The primary filter is absorbed by the specimen and used up in the process of fluorescence. The specimen then emits the light of low energy (wavelength longer than absorbed).
4. **Secondary filter:** This filters the light in the visible range that is emitted by the organic compound present in the specimen. The secondary filter is kept at right angles to the path of exciting light.
5. **Detector:** This measures the amount of light coming through the secondary filter, which is proportional to the concentration of the fluorescing compound. The fluorescence detection system consists of photomultiplier tubes (PMT) that amplify the photon emission and record and display the signal electronically **(Fig. 4.8)**.

As like any other photometric analysis, a calibration curve is made with known concentration of the compound under study. The concentration of unknown is then figured out from the photometric readings of the standard. Fluorescence is directly proportional to the concentration of test analyte.

Applications

Intrinsic fluorophores are molecules with a natural fluorescence whereas extrinsic fluorophores are those that are added to a sample to provide fluorescence or to change the spectral properties. This ability has broadened the scope of fluorometry in biochemical diagnostic to a greater extent.
1. This method is highly sensitive and a valuable tool in the toxicology laboratory.

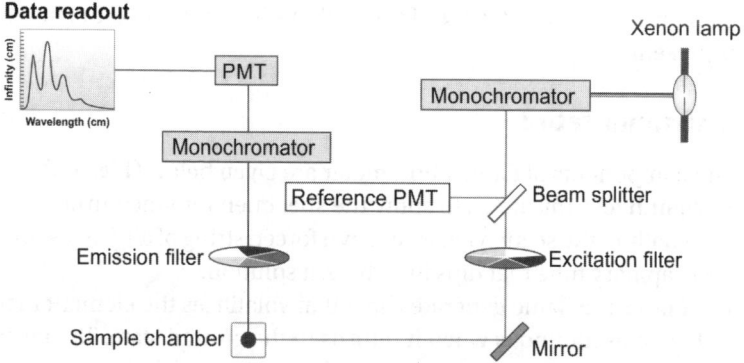

Fig. 4.8: Schematic representation of a fluorimeter.
(PMT: photomultiplier tubes)

2. It is also used in the analysis of various hormones, drugs, specific antibodies, etc.
3. It is used to determine metals, such as calcium, magnesium, and uranium salts in urine.
4. Determination of vitamin B (B1 thiamine and B2 riboflavin) in the food samples, such as meat and cereals

■ FLAME PHOTOMETER

Flame photometry is based on the measurement of intensity of the light emitted when a metal is introduced into a flame.

Principles

When a liquid sample containing a metallic salt solution is introduced into a flame, the processes involved in flame photometry are:
- The solvent is vaporized, leaving particles of the solid salt
- The salt is vaporized or converted into gaseous state
- A part or all of the gaseous molecules are progressively disassociated to give free neutral items or radicals. These neutral items are excited by the thermal energy of the flame. The exited atoms, which are unstable, quickly emit photons and return to lower energy state eventually reaching the unexcited state.

When flame photometry is employed as an analytical tool, the wavelength of the radiation coming from a flame tells us what the element is, and the intensity of color tells us how much of the element is present.

Instrumentation

The components of flame photometer are given below **(Fig. 4.9)**:
- **Nebulizer:** This helps to spray the specimen into the burner. It is usually of the scent type; where by a forced string of air passes over a capillary tube that dips into the test solution.
- **Flame:** The flame generates heat that volatilizes the element that becomes luminous when it returns to the ground state. The most common gas mixture that provides optimum temperature for the routine determination of sodium and potassium is propane-butane or natural gas. The mixture of fuel, gas and air in right proportions is ignited which provides the flame.
- **Monochromators:** These devices increase specificity of the analysis. These are simple filters which screens out all other wavelengths of light except the specific one emitted by the element analyzed, e.g. filters that yield 589 nm for Na and 767 nm for K.

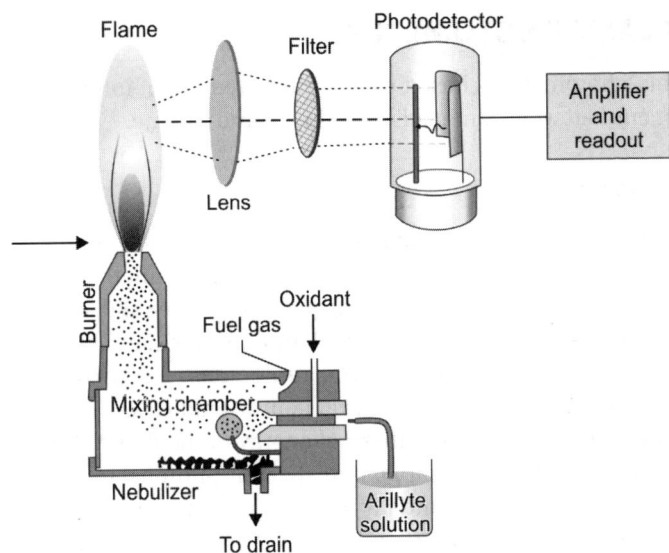

Fig. 4.9: Flame photometer.

Along with the monochromator filters, heat filters are placed between the flame and monochromator filter to stop the passage of heat.
- **Photodetectors:** The photodetector system quantifies the emitted light by converting it into an electrical impulse, which is eventually transmitted to the read out galvanometer.

Procedure

Use of an internal standard like lithium, strontium or cesium can minimize the interference and interaction of other elements present in serum and excited simultaneously. The element used as internal standard is not normally present in serum.
- First of all dilute the specimen and standard (1:200). If the internal standard is to be used, the specimen and the standard are diluted with the internal standard solution.
- Turn on the electrical connections of the flame photometer. Allow it to stabilize for few minutes. Turn on the air compressor and open the fuel valve.
- Ignite the flame by pressing ignition button.
- Put the de-ionized water under the nebulizer inlet tube. Zero the panel reading. Set the internal standard (Lithium) indicator at the required level.
- Replace the water with standard solution and set the levels for sodium and potassium.
- Put into the diluted specimen and take the readings. Most instruments are directly read out and do not require a calibration curve.

Applications

1. Flame photometry is a simple, rapid method for the routine determination of elements that can be easily excited. It provides high sensitivity and high reliability for the determination of elements in the first two columns of the periodic table. Among these elements are sodium, potassium, lithium, calcium, magnesium, strontium and barium. The measurement of these elements is very useful in determining certain transition elements, such as copper, manganese and iron.

2. The main use of flame photometer in clinical biochemistry is to determine level of sodium and potassium from serum.
3. Ion selective electrode is used to determine chloride ion. It is seen more automated instruments in conjunction with the determination of sodium and potassium. It is based on potentiometry (pH meter-principle).

■ URINOMETER

The urinometer is a type of hydrometer for measuring the specific gravity of urine.

Principle

This method is based on the principle of buoyancy (i.e., the ability of a fluid to exert an upward thrust on a body placed in it). The urinometer is placed in a container filled with urine **(Fig. 4.10)**. When solute concentration is high, the upthrust of solution increases and the urinometer is pushed up (high SG). If the solute concentration is low, the urinometer sinks further into the urine (low SG).

Procedure

- Fill a urinometer cylinder to about 1 inch from the top with the urine sample.
- Holding the urinometer float by the stem, slowly insert it into the cylinder. Do not wet the stem above the water line or an inaccurate reading will result.
- Give the float a slight swirl and read the specific gravity from the graduated marks on the stem as it comes to rest.
- Do not accept a reading if the float is against the side of the cylinder.
- Read the specific gravity to the nearest 0.001 according to the scale. Read at the bottom of the meniscus.

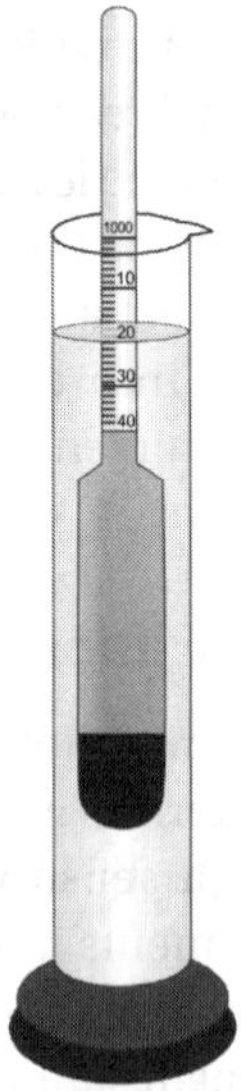

Fig. 4.10: Urinometer.

- Also measure the temperature. The urinometer is calibrated at 15°C. For each 3°C deviation above 15°C, add 0.001 to the reading and subtract 0.001 from the reading for each 3°C below 15°C.
- Rinse and carefully dry the urinometer after use.

Note: If the quantity of urine is not sufficient for measurement of SG, urine can be appropriately diluted and the last two figures of SG are multiplied by the dilution factor.

The normal range for specific gravity of urine is 1.010–1.030.

The specific gravity of urine gives an estimate of the concentration of urinary solids. Long's coefficient (2.66) times the thousands digits (last two digits) of the specific gravity gives the estimate of total solids in grams per liter.

Consider that the specific gravity of urine is 1.018.
So, 18 × 2.66 (last two digits multiplied by Long's coefficient)
= 47.88
This gives an estimate of 47.88 g/L for urinary solids.

The main drawbacks of using a urinometer are—it requires a large volume of urine, it is time consuming, and the specific gravity of a solution is dependent on temperature.

■ DENSITOMETER

A densitometer is essentially a double-filter photometer or spectrophotometer that scans the electrophoretic strip (in the form agarose, cellulose acetate, or polyacrylamide) as it moves past the optical system. One beam scans the dye intensity of the separated bands and the other beam scans the area of the background color of the strip (without the colored bands). The difference between these two signals is presented as a recorder tracing. The area under each graphical peak can be computed by an electronic integrator. The densitometer electrical signal can be converted by an analog to digital converter to print out the percentage of area under each peak. For example, by entering the total protein value in the densitometer keyboard, it is possible to get individual concentrations of separated albumin, α-1, α-2, and β- and γ- globulin. Densitometers have fluorescence capability to measure fluorescence of nicotinamide adenine dinucleotide (NADH) and nicotinamide adenine dinucleotide phosphate (NADPH) coupled enzyme reactions used for the quantitation of separated isoenzymes fractions.

SUMMARY

- Analytical chemistry studies and uses instruments and methods used to separate, identify, and quantify matter.
- A balance determines mass by balancing an unknown mass against a known mass.
- A beam balance works on the principle of moments according to which in equilibrium, the anticlockwise moment due to the weight of an object on the left pan of the beam is equal to the clockwise moment due to the standard weights on the right pan of the beam.
- Electrical analytical balance uses an electromagnet to generate a force to counter the sample and output the result by measuring the force needed to achieve balance.
- A centrifuge is a device that spins liquid samples at high speeds and thus creates a strong centripetal force causing the denser materials to travel toward the bottom of the centrifuge tube and lighter materials remain at the top of it.
- A pH meter measures the hydrogen-ion activity in solutions, indicating its acidity or basicity (alkalinity) expressed as pH value.
- The principle of pH meter is the concentration of hydrogen ions in the solution. It is the negative logarithm of a hydrogen ion.
- The colorimeter is based on the Beer–Lambert law, according to which the absorption of light transmitted through the medium is directly proportional to the medium concentration.
- Spectrophotometry is a method to measure how much a chemical substance absorbs light by measuring the intensity of light as a beam of light passes through sample solution.
- The basic principle is that each compound absorbs or transmits light over a certain range of wavelength.
- A fluorimeter is a device that measures the fluorescence or light emitted by different fluorescing objects. This is a very sensitive and valuable tool in toxicology.
- The principle of a flame photometer is based on the measurement of the emitted light intensity when a metal is introduced into the flame.
- The wavelength of the color gives information about the element and the color of the flame gives information about the amount of the element present in the sample.
- A urinometer is an instrument used to measure the specific gravity of urine. It is based on the principle of buoyancy. Because of increased density of

Chapter 4: Elementary Knowledge of Analytical Chemistry

urine compared to that of water, the urinometer will float higher in urine than in water.
- A densitometer is a device that measures the degree of darkness (the optical density) of a photographic or semitransparent material or of a reflecting surface.
- The densitometer determines the density of a sample placed between the light source and the photoelectric cell from differences in the readings.

PRACTICE QUESTIONS

1. Define analytical chemistry. What role it plays in clinical biochemistry?
2. What is a difference between balance and weighing scale?
3. With a neat-labeled diagram, explain the principle and working of beam balance.
4. What is principle of electric balance? Discuss the precautions to be taken care of while working with it.
5. Mention the principle of centrifuge. Write a note on ultracentrifuge.
6. Discuss the principle of pH meter.
7. With a neat-labeled diagram, discuss the working of pH meter.
8. State and explain Lambert's and Beer's law.
9. With a neat-labeled diagram, explain the principle and working of a colorimeter.
10. Differentiate between colorimeter and spectrophotometer.
11. Mention the principle and applications of a fluorimeter.
12. Mention the principle and components of a flame photometer.
13. What is the use of a urinometer? Discuss the steps to use it.
14. Write a note on densitometer.

Elementary Knowledge of Biostatistics

CHAPTER 5

> **Keywords**
> Common statistical terms, qualitative (discrete) data, quantitative (continuous) data, measures of central tendencies—mean, median, mode, measures of variability—range, standard deviation, variance, and correlation coefficient, standard error of mean (SEM), confidence interval, hypothesis test, Z-test, t-test, Chi-Square test

■ INTRODUCTION

Statistics is the study of the collection, analysis, interpretation, presentation and organization of data. Statistical analysis allows us to use mathematics to reach conclusions about various situations.

Biostatistics (or biometry) is the application of statistics to a wide range of topics in biology. Basic statistical concepts help biologists correctly, prepare experiments, verify conclusions and properly interpret results. Biostatistics covers applications and contributions from health, medicines, nutrition, genetics, biology, epidemiology, and many others.

In nature, blood pressure, pulse rate, amount of hemoglobin or any other measurement or counting varies not only from person to person but also from group to group. The extent of this variability is an attribute or a character, whether it is by chance, i.e. biological or normal, is learnt by studying biostatistics.

Variation more than natural limits may be pathological, i.e. abnormal due to the play of certain external factors. Hence, biostatistics may also be called a science of variation.

■ COMMON STATISTICAL TERMS

Before learning the methods in biostatistics, some terms used, their symbols and notations are the compulsory things to know.

1. **Variable:** A characteristic that takes on different values about different persons, places or things. A quantity that varies within limits, such as height, weight, blood pressure, age, etc. It is denoted as X and notation for orderly series as $X_1, X_2, X_3, \ldots X_n$. The suffix n is symbol for number in the series. Σ (sigma) stands for summation of results or observation.
2. **Constant:** Quantities that do not vary, such as $\pi = 3.141$, $e = 2.718$. They do not require statistical study. In biostatistics, mean, standard deviation, standard error, correlation coefficient and proportion of a particular population are considered as constant.
3. **Observation:** An event and its measurements, such as blood pressure (event) and 120 mm of Hg (measurement).
4. **Observational unit:** The observational unit is the type of subject being sampled.
5. **Data:** A set of values recorded on one or more observational units.
6. **Population:** It is an entire group of people or study elements—persons, things or measurements for which we have an interest at a particular time. Populations are determined by our sphere of interest. It may be infinite or finite. If a population consists of fixed number of values, it is said to be finite, and if population consists of an endless succession of values, the population is an infinite one.

   A statistical population may also be birth weights, hemoglobin levels, readings of a thermometer, number of red blood cells (RBCs) in human body, etc. Such a population mostly gives quantitative data. It is finite or small in number or infinite or unlimited in number that cannot be easily counted.
7. **Sampling unit:** Each member of a population.
8. **Sample:** It may be defined as a part of a population. It is a group of sampling units that form part of a population, generally selected so as to be representative of the population whose variables are under study. There are many kinds of sample that can be selected from a population.
9. **Parameter:** It is a summary value or constant of a variable that describes the population, such as mean, variance, correlation coefficient, proportion, etc. Familiar examples are mean height, mean birth rate, mean morbidity and mean mortality rates, etc.

10. **Statistic:** It is a summary value that describes the sample, such as its mean, standard deviation, standard error, correlation coefficient, proportion, etc. This value is calculated from the sample and is often applied to population but may or may not be a valid estimate of population. Though not desirable, parameter and statistic are often used as synonyms.
11. **Parametric test:** It is one in which population constants as described above are used, such as mean, variances, etc. and data tend to follow one assumed or established distribution, such as normal, binomial, poisson, etc.
12. **Nonparametric tests :** Tests, such as χ^2 test, in which no constant of a population is used. Data do not follow any specific distribution and no assumptions are made in nonparametric tests, e.g. to classify good, better and best you allocate arbitrary numbers or marks to each category.

NOTATIONS FOR A POPULATION AND SAMPLE VALUES

Roman letters are used for statistics of samples and Greek for parameters of population.

Common notations are:

Summary value	Sample statistics	Population parameters
Mean	$\bar{X}$	μ
Standard deviation	s	σ
Variance	s^2	σ^2
Proportion	p	P
Complement of proportion	q	Q

Other symbols commonly used are:
    = : Equal to
    > : Greater than
    < : Less than
    Z : The number of standard deviation from the mean or standard normal deviate/variate
    % : Percent
    γ : Pearson's correlation coefficient
    ρ : Spearman's correlation coefficient

O : Observed number
E : Expected number
d.f. or f : Degrees of freedom
K : Number of groups or classes
P : Probability

■ TYPES OF DATA

Statistical methods for analysis mainly depend on type of data. The statistical data obtained from above sources can be divided into two broad categories:
1. Qualitative or discrete data
2. Quantitative or continuous data

Qualitative or Discrete Data

In such data, there is no notion of magnitude or size of the characteristic (or attribute) as it cannot be measured. They are classified by counting individuals having the same characteristic. There is only one variable, i.e. the number of persons and not the characteristic.

For example, number of deaths due to bacterial/viral/ protozoan diseases, persons with different blood groups in a population, etc.

The results thus obtained are expressed as a ratio, proportion, percentage or a rate.

Qualitative data is of following types:
- **Nominal data:** This is also called as categorical data where data is simply assigned "names" (nominal) or categories based on the presence or absence of certain attributes/characteristics without any ranking between the categories. Thus, nominal data have no order and thus only gives names or labels to various categories.
  For example, persons classified on the basis of their nationality like Indian, Sri Lankan, Italian, American, etc.
- **Dichotomous data:** It is also referred as binominal data, which refers to two possible outcomes.
  For example, patients are categorized by gender as males or females, outcome of cancer may be death or survival, or drug therapy with drug 'X' will show improvement or no improvement at all.
- **Ordinal data:** It is also called as ordered, categorical, or graded data. The variables may have two or more categories. Generally,

this type of data is expressed as scores or ranks. There is a natural order among categories and they can be ranked or arranged in order. However, the interval between two measurements is not meaningful.

For example, pain may be classified as mild, moderate and severe. Since, there is an order between the three grades of pain, this type of data is called as ordinal. To indicate the intensity of pain, it may also be expressed as scores (mild = 1, moderate = 2, severe = 3). Hence, data can be arranged in an order and rank.

Quantitative or Continuous Data

The qualitative data have a magnitude. The characteristic is measured either on an interval or on a ratio scale. In this type, there are two variables—the characteristic (such as height) and the frequency, i.e. the number of persons with the same characteristic and with the same range.

Height varies from person-to-person; it may be 150 cm in one and 160 cm in another person of the same age and sex. Number of persons with 150 cm or in the range of 150–152 cm, may be 10 while those with height 160 cm or in the range of 160–162 cm, may be 20. Thus, we find the characteristic as well as the frequency both vary from person-to-person as well as from group-to-group.

The quantitative data obtained from characteristic variable are also called continuous data as each individual has one measurement from a continuous range.

- **Interval variable:** This type of data is characterized by an equal and definite interval between two measurements.

  For example, the difference between a temperature of 100° and 90° is the same difference as between 90° and 80°. This kind of data may have fractional values.

- **Ratio variable:** It has all the properties of an interval variable and also has a clear definition of 0.0. When the variable equals 0.0, there is none of that variable. Variables like height, weight, enzyme activity are ratio variables.

  Temperature, expressed in F or C, is not a ratio variable. A temperature of 0.0 on either of those scales does not mean 'no heat'. However, temperature in Kelvin is a ratio variable, as 0.0 Kelvin really does mean 'no heat'. Another counter example is pH.

It is not a ratio variable, as pH = 0 does not mean 'no acidity' (quite the opposite!).

In case of ratio variables (but not interval variables), if the ratio of two measurements is taken, it gives a constant value. A weight of 4 grams is twice a weight of 2 grams, because weight is a ratio variable. A temperature of 100° C is not twice as hot as 50° C, because temperature C is not a ratio variable. A pH of 3 is not twice as acidic as a pH of 6, because pH is not a ratio variable.

Sometimes, certain data may be converted from one form to another form to reduce asymmetrical distribution and make it to follow the normal distribution. Data can be transformed by taking the logarithm, square root, reciprocal, or in the form of ratios between measurements as well as intervals.

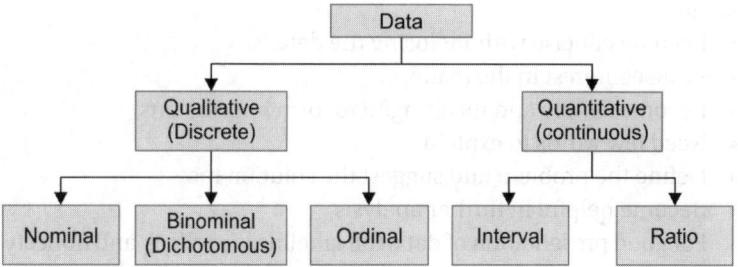

■ PRESENTATION OF DATA

The quantitative data obtained from characteristic variable are also called continuous data as each individual has one measurement from a continuous spectrum or range, such as body temperature from 35°C to 42°C, height 150-180 cm, pulse rate 68-84 per minute and so on. The observations ascend or descend from 0 or any starting point in the range of spectrum, such as systolic blood pressure of 100 individuals rising from lowest 90 mm Hg to highest 150 mm Hg. There can be infinite values between any given range.

The characteristic may be measurable in whole numbers and fractions, such as chest circumference—33 cm, 34.5 cm, 35.2 cm, 36 cm, 37.3 cm and so on or it may be measurable or countable in discrete whole numbers only, such as pulse rate; cholesterol; blood pressure; EST; blood sugar; etc. In medical studies, such statistics are mostly collected in anatomy and physiology, i.e. in health, to define the normal or to find the limits of deviation from the normal in healthy persons. When the measurement or counting crosses the normal limits, it becomes unusual and may indicate pathology. Some of the statistical methods employed in analysis of such data are mean, range, standard deviation, coefficient of variation and correlation coefficient.

Data collected and compiled from experimental work, records and surveys should be accurate and complete. They must be checked for accuracy and adequacy before processing further. So far they lie in masses or are scattered in the records, in other words they are mixed and unsorted. Next step, therefore is sorting or classification of the data into characteristic groups or classes as per age, sex, social class, attacks, etc. They should be presented in such a way that data should:
- Become concise without losing the details
- Arouse interest in the reader
- Become simple and meaningful to form impressions
- Need few words to explain
- Define the problem and suggest the solution too
- Become helpful in further analysis

For good presentation of data, full labeling, simplicity and honesty are essential requirements.

Depending upon its types, data can be presented by various ways like tabulation, histogram, bar diagram, pie chart, line graph, frequency curve, etc.

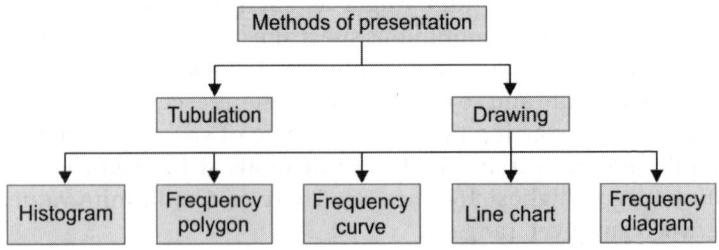

Statistical method has two major branches mainly descriptive and inferential. Descriptive statistics explain the distribution of population measurements by providing types of data, estimates of central tendency (mean, mode and median), and measures of variability (standard deviation, correlation coefficient), whereas inferential statistics is used to express the level of certainty about estimates and includes hypothesis testing, standard error of mean, and confidence interval.

Descriptive statistics are used to describe the basic features of the data in a study. They provide simple summaries about the sample and the measures. Together with simple graphics analysis, they form the basis of virtually every quantitative analysis of data.

Descriptive statistics describes what the data shows. Descriptive statistics are used to present quantitative descriptions in a manageable form. In a research study, we may have lots of measures. Or we may measure a large number of people on any measure. Descriptive statistics help us to simplify large amounts of data in a sensible way.

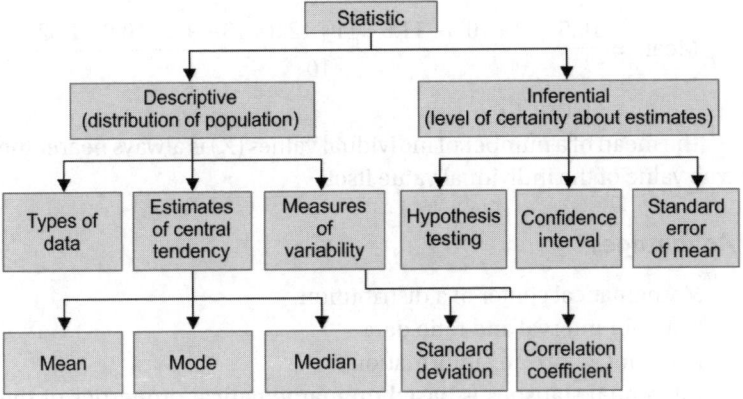

■ MEASURES OF CENTRAL TENDENCIES

A measure of central tendency is a single value that attempts to describe a set of data by identifying the central position within that set of data. These also mean measures of central location or summary statistics. These are of three types (i) mean, (ii) median, and (iii) mode.

Mean (Arithmetic)

The mean (or average) is the most popular and well-known measure of central tendency. The mean is equal to the sum of all the values in the data set divided by the number of values in the data set. So, if we have n values in a data set and they have values $x_1, x_2, ..., x_n$, the sample

(A sample is a portion of a population selected for further analysis) mean, usually denoted by $\bar{x}$ (pronounced x bar), is:

$$\bar{x} = \frac{(x_1 + x_2 + \ldots + x_n)}{n}$$

This formula is usually written in a slightly different manner using the Greek capital letter, Σ, pronounced "sigma", which means "sum of...":

$$\bar{x} = \frac{\Sigma x}{n}$$

For example, value of hemoglobin (in g/dL) of females in a society are—10.5, 11, 10.9, 11.5, 11, 12.3, 13, 9.5, 10.9, 11.2.

$$\text{Mean} = \frac{10.5 + 11 + 10.9 + 11.5 + 11 + 12.3 + 13 + 9.5 + 10.9 + 11.2}{10}$$

= 11.18 g/dL

The mean of a number of individual values (X) is always nearer the true value of the individual value itself.

Advantages

- Mathematical center of a distribution
- Good for interval and ratio data
- Does not ignore any information
- Inferential statistics is based on mathematical properties of the mean

Disadvantages

- Influenced by extreme scores and skewed distributions
- May not exist in the data
- Not suitable for qualitative data

Median

The median is the middle score for a set of data that has been arranged in order of magnitude. Median is a better indicator of central value when one or more of the lowest or the highest observations are wide apart or are not evenly distributed. The median is less affected by outliers and distorted data.

Chapter 5: Elementary Knowledge of Biostatistics

In order to calculate the median, suppose we have the data of age of patients coming to laboratory are as below:

65	55	89	56	35	14	56	55	87	45	92

We first need to rearrange that data into order of magnitude (smallest first):

14	35	45	55	55	**56**	56	65	87	89	92

Our median mark is the middle mark - in this case, 56 (highlighted in bold). It is the middle mark because there are 5 scores before it and 5 scores after it. This works fine when for an odd number (as 11 here) of score but for an even number of scores (as 10 here) take the middle two scores and average the result. So, if we look at the example below:

65	55	89	56	35	14	56	55	87	45

We again rearrange that data into order of magnitude (smallest first):

14	35	45	55	**55**	**56**	56	65	87	89

Only now we have to take the 5th and 6th score in our data set and average them to get a median of 55.5.

Thus, median is an average, which is obtained by getting middle values of a set of data arranged or ordered from lowest to the highest (or *vice versa*). In this process, 50% of the population has the value smaller than and 50% of samples have the value larger than median.

Advantages

- Not influenced by extreme scores or skewed distribution
- Good with ordinal data
- Easier to compute than the mean
- Considered as the typical observation

Disadvantages

- May not exist in the data
- Does not take actual values into account

Mode

The mode is the most frequent score in data set or it is the point of maximum concentration. The number, which occurred repeatedly, contributes mode in a distribution of quantitative data. It represents the highest bar in a bar chart. Therefore, mode is considered as the most popular parameter/characteristic.

An example of a mode is presented below:

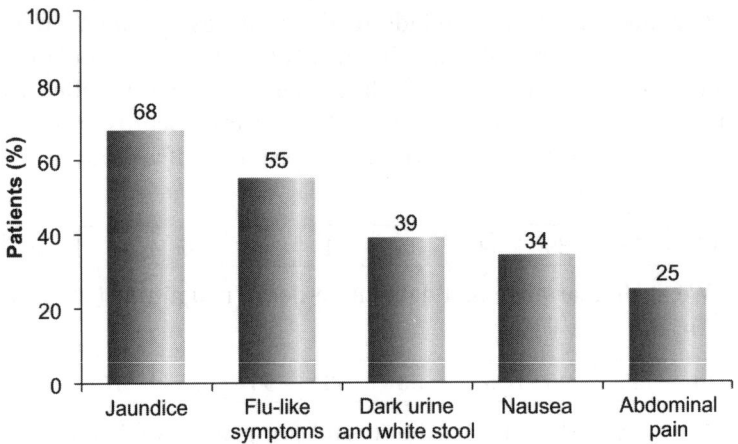

Normally, the mode is used for categorical data where we wish to know the most common category, as illustrated above. Here it indicated that jaundice is most common form of disease from given samples at a particular time.

Advantages

- Good with nominal data
- Bimodal distribution might verify clinical observations (pre and postmenopausal breast cancer)
- Easy to compute and understand
- The score exists in the data set

Disadvantages

- Ignore most of the information in a distribution
- Small samples may not have a mode
- More than one mode might exist

■ MEASURES OF VARIABILITY

Variability within populations is most common part of statistics. Measures of variability are statistical procedures to describe how spread out (variable) the data is.
- The indices used to measure variation or dispersion among scores are as follows:
  - Range
  - Standard deviation
  - Variance
  - Correlation coefficient

Range

Range is the simplest method of examining variation among scores. It refers to the difference between the highest and lowest values produced.

For example, range of:

Systolic blood pressure	: 100–140 mm
Diastolic blood pressure	: 80–90 mm
Fasting blood sugar	: 70–100 mg/dL

Range is not a satisfactory measure as it is based only on two extreme values, ignoring the distribution of all other observations within extremes. These extreme values vary from study-to-study. The normal range covers the observations falling in 95% confidence limits.

For example, a person cannot be labeled as normal or pathologic on single observation whether it is within the range or outside it. One should go by total picture of a clinical case.

Percentile is one of the methods to express range of variables.

Percentiles (or Quartiles)

- Percentiles are values in a series of observations arranged in ascending order of magnitude which divide the distribution into 100 equal parts. Thus, the median is 50th percentile. The 50th percentile will have 50% observations on either side.
- A percentile is a value at or below which a given percentage or fraction of the variable values lie.
- The p-th percentile is the value that has p% of the measurements below it and (100-p)% above it.

- For example, if you are in the 80th percentile on a real GMAT result, you scored better on that section than 80% of the students taking the GMAT and 20% students scored more than you.
- If children at age 4 years form 10th percentile, if means 10% of entire population is below 4 years of age and 90% is above that.

Thus, percentiles are used to divide a distribution into convenient groups.

Standard Deviation

The standard deviation is the most widely applied measure of variability. Standard deviation is how much variation is there from the average (mean). If all of the scores are grouped around the average, then standard deviation will be lower. If scores are all over the map and not grouped together at all, then standard deviation will be huge.

It is important to distinguish between the standard deviation of a population and the standard deviation of a sample.

Standard Deviation of a Population

A population is defined as the complete collection of data to be studied.

They have different notation, and they are computed differently.
The steps for calculating standard deviation of a population are as follows:
- Calculate the average (mean)
- Calculate the deviations, which are the scores minus the average (mean)
- Square the deviations
- Sum up (Σ) the squared deviations
- Divide this by the number of scores in your data set (or multiply by 1/N, same thing)
- Take the square root

The standard deviation of a population is defined by the following formula:

$$\sigma = \text{sqrt(square root)} \left[\Sigma (X_i - X)^2 / N \right]$$

Where,

σ is the population standard deviation,
X_i is the ith element from the population,

X is the population mean, and
N is the number of elements in the population.

Example: Consider a population consisting of the following values:
2, 4, 4, 4, 5, 5, 7, 9
- There are eight data points in total, with a mean (or average) value of 5:

$$\frac{2+4+4+4+5+5+7+9}{8} = 5$$

- To calculate the population standard deviation, first compute the difference of each data point from the mean, and square the result:

$$(2-5)^2 = (-3)^2 = 9 \quad (5-5)^2 = 0^2 = 0$$
$$(4-5)^2 = (-1)^2 = 1 \quad (5-5)^2 = 0^2 = 0$$
$$(4-5)^2 = (-1)^2 = 1 \quad (7-5)^2 = 2^2 = 4$$
$$(4-5)^2 = (-1)^2 = 1 \quad (9-5)^2 = 4^2 = 16$$

- Next divide the sum of these values by the number of values and take the square root to give the standard deviation:

$$\sqrt{\frac{9+1+1+1+0+0+4+16}{8}} = 2$$

- Therefore, the above population has a standard deviation of 2. This indicates the variability of the observation about the mean.

Standard Deviation of a Sample

A sample is defined as a section of the population understudy. This can be anywhere from 1% to 99% of them. The standard deviation of a sample is defined by slightly different formula:

$$s = \text{sqrt}\left[\frac{\sum(x_i - x)^2}{(n-1)}\right]$$

Where,
s is the sample standard deviation,
x_i is the i th element from the sample,
x is the sample mean, and n is the number of elements in the sample.

Find SD of the erythrocyte sedimentation rate (ESR), In normal 5 members it found to be
4, 2, 5, 8, 6

1. Calculate the mean:

$$\bar{x} = \frac{\sum x}{N}$$

$$= \frac{x_1 + x_2 + \ldots + x_N}{N} = \frac{4+2+5+8+6}{5} = 5$$

2. Calculate $x - \bar{x}$ for each value in the sample:

$$x_1 - \bar{x} = 4 - 5 = -1$$
$$x_2 - \bar{x} = 2 - 5 = -3$$
$$x_3 - \bar{x} = 5 - 5 = 0$$
$$x_4 - \bar{x} = 8 - 5 = 3$$
$$x_5 - \bar{x} = 6 - 5 = 1$$

3. Calculate $\sum(x - \bar{x})^2$:

$$\sum(x - \bar{x})^2 = (x_1 - \bar{x})^2 + (x_2 - \bar{x})^2 + \ldots + (x_N - \bar{x})^2$$
$$= (-1)^2 + (-3)^2 + 0^2 + 3^2 + 1^2 = 20$$

4. Calculate the standard deviation:

$$s = \sqrt{\frac{\sum(x - \bar{x})^2}{N - 1}}$$

$$= \sqrt{\frac{20}{5 - 1}} = 2.24$$

Therefore, standard deviation for given data is 2.24.

Variance

The variance is a numerical value used to indicate how widely individuals in a group vary. If individual observations vary greatly from the group mean, the variance is big; and vice versa.

It is important to distinguish between the variance of a population and the variance of a sample. They have different notation, and they are computed differently. The variance of a population is denoted by σ^2; and the variance of a sample, by s^2.

The variance of a population is defined by the following formula:

$$\sigma^2 = \sum (X_i - X)^2 / N$$

where σ^2 is the population variance, X is the population mean, X_i is the ith element from the population, and N is the number of elements in the population.

The variance of a sample is defined by slightly different formula:

$$s^2 = \Sigma (x_i - x)^2 / (n - 1)$$

where s^2 is the sample variance, x is the sample mean, x_i is the i th element from the sample, and n is the number of elements in the sample. Using this formula, the variance of the sample is an unbiased estimate of the variance of the population.

This concludes that, the variance is equal to the square of the standard deviation.

Correlation Coefficient

Correlation is relationship between two variables. It is used to measure the degree of linear relationship between two continuous variables. Correlation may be due to some direct relationship between two variables. This also may be due to some inherent factors common to both variables. The correlation is expressed in terms of coefficient.

The sign describe the direction and the absolute value indicates the magnitude of the relationship between two variables of a correlation coefficient.

- The value of a correlation coefficient ranges between -1 and 1.
- The greater the absolute value of a correlation coefficient, the stronger the *linear* relationship.
- The strongest linear relationship is indicated by a correlation coefficient of -1 or 1.
- The weakest linear relationship is indicated by a correlation coefficient equal to 0.
- A positive correlation means that if one variable gets bigger, the other variable tends to get bigger.
- A negative correlation means that if one variable gets bigger, the other variable tends to get smaller.

Larger the correlation coefficient, stronger is the association.

Correlation between the two variables does not necessarily suggest the cause and effect relationship. It indicates the strength of association for any data in comparable terms as for example, correlation between height and weight, age and height, weight loss and poverty, parity and birth weight, socioeconomic status and hemoglobin. While performing these tests, it requires x and y variables to be normally distributed. It is, generally, used to form hypothesis and to suggest areas of future research.

Correlation coefficient only measures linear relationships. Therefore, a correlation of 0 does not mean zero relationship between two variables; rather, it means zero *linear* relationship. (It is possible for two variables to have zero linear relationship and a strong curvilinear relationship at the same time.)

Scatter Plots and Correlation Coefficients

The scatter plots below show how different patterns of data produce different degrees of correlation.

Several points are evident from the scatter plots.
- When the slope of the line in the plot is negative, the correlation is negative; and vice versa.
- The strongest correlations (r = 1.0 and r = −1.0) occur when data points fall *exactly* on a straight line.
- The correlation becomes weaker as the data points become more scattered.
- If the data points fall in a random pattern, the correlation is equal to zero.
- Correlation is affected by outliers. Compare the first scatter plot with the last scatter plot. The single outlier in the last plot greatly reduces the correlation (from 1.00 to 0.71).

Calculation of Correlation Coefficient

Correlation coefficient for sample data is denoted by "r". The formula for Pearson correlation coefficient r is given by:

$$r = \frac{n(\Sigma xy) - (\Sigma x)(\Sigma y)}{\sqrt{\left[n\Sigma x^2 - (\Sigma x)^2\right]\left[n\Sigma y^2 - (\Sigma y)^2\right]}}$$

Where,
  r = Correlation coefficient
  x = Values in first set of data
  y = Values in second set of data
  n = Total number of values

Example: The two given sets of data are....
  X = Value of hemoglobin of people living in slum
  Y = Value of hemoglobin of people living in high society

X	15	16	12	10	8
Y	12	11	10	14	16

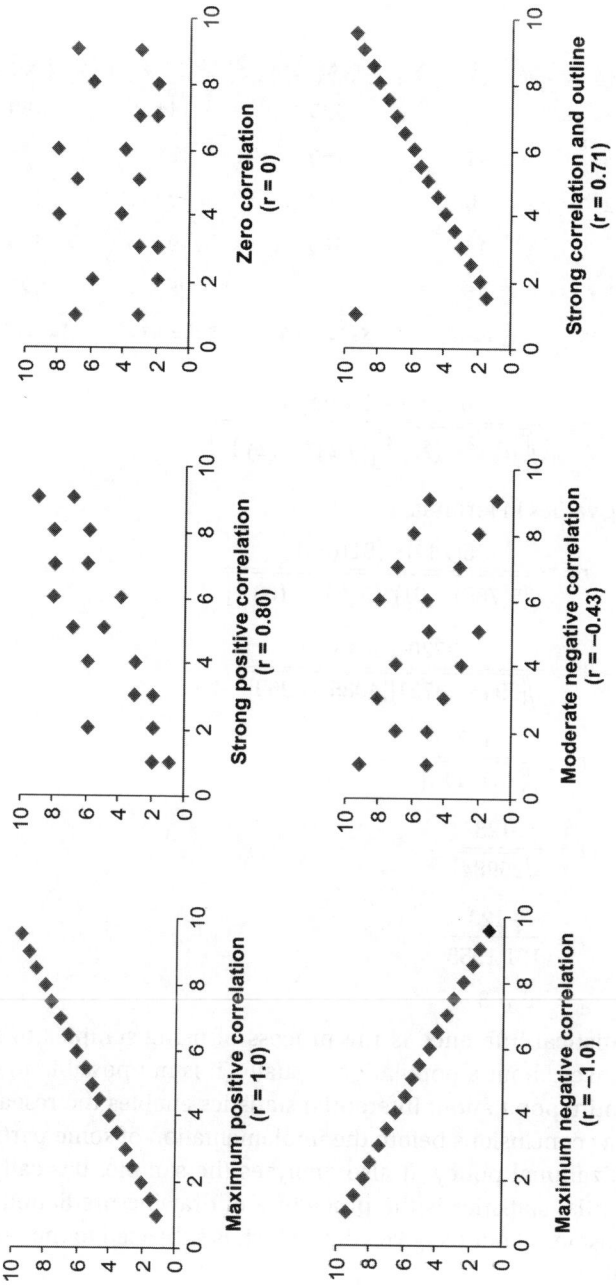

Construct the following table:

x	y	x^2	y^2	xy
15	12	225	144	180
16	11	256	121	176
12	10	144	100	120
10	14	100	196	140
8	16	64	256	128
$\Sigma x = 61$	$\Sigma y = 63$	$\Sigma x^2 = 789$	$\Sigma y^2 = 817$	$\Sigma xy = 744$

$$r = \frac{n(\Sigma xy)-(\Sigma x)(\Sigma y)}{\sqrt{\left[n\Sigma x^2 - (\Sigma x)^2\right]\left[n\Sigma y^2 - (\Sigma y)^2\right]}}$$

Putting values in formula,

$$r = \frac{5(744)-(61)(63)}{\sqrt{[5(789)-(61)^2\,[5(817-(63)^2]}}$$

$$r = \frac{3720-3843}{\sqrt{[3945-3721][4085-3969]}}$$

$$r = \frac{-123}{\sqrt{[224][116]}}$$

$$r = \frac{-123}{\sqrt{25984}}$$

$$r = \frac{-123}{161.1955}$$

$$r = -0.763$$

Statistical inference is the process of using samples to make inferences about a population. Usually, it is not possible to study the entire population. Inferential statistics enables the researcher to draw conclusions before the implementation of some particular organizational policy. It also analyzes the sample. Basically, the inferential statistics is the procedure of drawing predictions and conclusions about the given data which is subjected to the random variations.

Differences between Descriptive and Inferential Statistics

Although, descriptive and inferential statistics both are used for purpose of analysis of the data, still both of them are different in various ways. Let us learn about this differences below:
1. The descriptive statistics gives a description about a sample, while the inferential statistics predicts and infers about a much larger data or population.
2. Descriptive statistics just describes the certain characteristics about a data. Whereas, inferential statistics deeply analyzes the statistical data and observations.
3. Descriptive statistics deals with central tendency and spread of the frequency distribution. While in inferential statistics, more details, such as hypothesis tests and confidence interval are studied.
4. The measures of descriptive statistics (mean, median, mode) are numbers. On the other hand, the measures in inferential statistics are not always exact numbers.
5. Descriptive statistics deals with small samples which enables us to produce results without errors. But inferential statistics takes whole population for drawing conclusions which may not have the extent of required accuracy.
6. In descriptive statistics, the conclusions cannot be made beyond the given data. In inferential statistics, the educated predictions and guesses can be made on the basis of the parameters of the given population, it does not matter how big the population is.

Examples

Examples of descriptive statistics:
- Estimation of number of students (boys and girls separately) in a school
- Population of particular country or city
- Frequency of the variables
- Estimation of number of damaged or cavity teeth by a dentist

Examples of inferential statistics:
- Average marks obtained by all the students
- Grades or percentile of the scores
- Average score in cricket

- Prediction by a dentist about the teeth those are susceptible to have cavity or damage in future

Inferential statistics includes detection and prediction of observational and sampling errors. This type of statistics is being utilized in order to make estimates and test the hypotheses using given data.

There are two main areas of statistical inference, estimation and hypothesis testing.

■ ESTIMATION STATISTICS

"Estimation statistics" is estimating population values based on sample data. This can be done by two types—standard error of mean (SEM) and confidence interval (CI).

Standard Error of Mean

The sample mean is called a point estimate, and it is used to estimate the corresponding population mean. If repeated samples are taken from the same population there is no reason to assume that the population mean will be exactly equal to the sample mean. The degree of variation between means from repeated samples can be measured by the *standard error of the mean (SEM)*.

$$SEM = \frac{s}{\sqrt{n}}$$

Where **S** = Standard deviation and **n** = Sample size

Greater the SD, greater will be SE as will happen in small sample. Sampling error can be minimized by reducing the standard deviation which can be done only by taking large sample.

Confidence Interval

Since, statistics uses a sample space and predicts the trends for the whole population, it is quite natural to expect a certain degree of error and uncertainty. This is captured through the confidence interval.

Suppose the survey shows that 34% of the blood sample found positive for malaria. The confidence that these results are accurate for the whole group can never be 100%; for this the survey would need to be taken for the entire group. Therefore, if it is assumed to be 95% confidence interval in the results, it could mean that the final result would be 30–38%. If confidence interval is higher, 99%, then the uncertainty in the result would increase to 28–40%.

The confidence interval depends on a variety of parameters, like the number of people taking the survey and the way they represent the whole group.

For most practical surveys, the results are reported based on a 95% confidence interval. The inverse relationship between the confidence interval width and the certainty of prediction should be noted.

The confidence interval is represented in the form of an interval that provides a range for the parameter of given population.

The CI gives a range around the mean where we expect the "true" (population) mean to lie, using the formula:

The formula for a confidence interval for a mean is:

$$\bar{x} \pm (z \text{ critical value}) \frac{s}{\sqrt{n}}$$

Confidence limits are two extremes of measurements within which 95% of observations would lie.

Lower confidence limit = $\bar{x} - (Z \text{ critical value}) \frac{s}{\sqrt{n}}$

Upper confidence limit = $\bar{x} + (Z \text{ critical value}) \frac{s}{\sqrt{n}}$

Where,
- Z = Critical value from a two-tail test
- $\bar{x}$ = Sample mean
- s = Standard deviation
- and n = Sample size

Z-values for various confidence levels

Confidence level	z-value
80%	1.28
90%	1.645 (by convention)
95%	1.96
98%	2.33
99%	2.58

Note: The width of the CI depends on the sample size and on the variation of data values. A very wide interval may indicate that more data should be collected before anything very definite can be said about the population mean.

■ HYPOTHESIS TEST

Hypothesis testing is simply another way of drawing conclusions about a population parameter. Hypothesis testing is the most common kind of statistical inference. Statistical data analysis allows us to use mathematical principles to decide how likely it is that our sample results match our hypothesis about a population.

Two hypotheses or presumptions are made to draw the inference from the sample value.

1. **Null hypothesis:** It is a hypothesis of no difference [H_0] between statistic of a sample and a parameter of population or between statistic of two samples. This hypothesis nullifies the claim that the experimental result is different from or better than the one observed already.
2. **Alternative hypothesis:** It is a hypothesis of significant difference [H_1] stating that the sample result is different—greater or smaller than the hypothetical value of the population.

Next step is to choose between null hypothesis [H_0] and alternate hypothesis [H_1] by applying relevant statistical technique.

One and Two-Sided Tests:
Hypothesis tests can be one or two-sided (tailed)
- One tailed tests are directional
  - $H_0 : \mu_1 - \mu_2 \leq 0$
  - $H_A : \mu_1 - \mu_2 > 0$
- Two tailed tests are not directional
  - $H_0 : \mu_1 - \mu_2 = 0$
  - $H_A : \mu_1 - \mu_2 \neq 0$

Z test: To make minimum error in choice of hypothesis, the sampling distribution or area under the normal curve into two zones:
1. **A zone of acceptance:** If the sample falls in the plain area, i.e, within mean ± 1.96 SE the null hypothesis accepted.
2. **A zone of rejection:** If the sample falls in the shaded area, i.e. beyond mean ± 1.96 SE the null hypothesis rejected and alternate hypothesis is accepted.

Level of significance (α): The value of α represents the boundary between results that are statistically significant (where we reject H_0) and results those are not statistically significant (where we do not reject H_0). Thus, α is called the level of significance of the hypothesis test.

This form of acceptance or rejection interprets estimated difference from the universe parameters at 5% level of significance.

Type I error: In certain circumstances, the null hypothesis is rejected even when the estimate falls in the zone of acceptance at 5% level say at point A, it means level of significance is changed from 5 to 6, 8, or 10%. It is also called as alpha (α) error. It can be minimized by taking large random sample.

Type II error: In certain circumstances, the null hypothesis is accepted even when the estimate falls in the zone of rejection. Say at point B. It means level of significance is changed from 5 to 4, 3, 2 or 1%. It is also called as beta (β) error.

***p*-value:** The *p*-value is the probability of observing a sample statistic (such as $\bar{x}$ or Z data) at least as extreme as the statistic actually observed if we assume that the null hypothesis is true. Roughly speaking, the *p*-value represents the probability of observing the sample statistic if the null hypothesis is true. Since, the term "*p*-value" means "probability value," its value must always lie between 0 and 1.

A small *p*-value indicates a conflict between your sample data and the null hypothesis. Therefore, since the data are real and the hypothesis is a conjecture, this *small p-value will lead us to reject H_0*.

The rejection rule for performing a hypothesis test using the *p*-value method is,

Reject H_0 when the p-value is less than α

Strength of evidence against the null hypothesis for various levels of *p*-value

p-Value	Strength of evidence against H_0
p-value ≤ 0.001	Extremely strong evidence
0.001 <p-value ≤ 0.01	Very strong evidence
0.01, <p-value ≤ 0.05	Solid evidence
0.05, <p-value ≤ 0.10	Mild evidence
0.10, <p-value ≤ 0.15	Slight evidence
0.15, <p-value	No evidence

Z test for the Population Mean μ: p-Value Method
When a random sample of size n is taken from a population where the population standard deviation σ is known, Z test can be used if either of the following conditions is satisfied:
Case 1: The population is normal, or
Case 2: The sample size is large ($n \geq 30$).

Step 1: State the hypotheses and the rejection rule.
Use one of the forms to write H_0 and H_a. Define σ (that is, "σ represents the population mean "). The rejection rule is "Reject H_0 if the p-value is less than α".

Step 2: Find Z data.
Either use technology to find the value of the test statistic Z data, or calculate the value of Z data as follows:

$$Z \text{ data} = \frac{\overline{X} - \mu_0}{\sigma \overline{x}} = \frac{\overline{X} - \mu_0}{\sigma/\sqrt{n}}$$

Step 3: Find the p-value.
Either use technology to find the p-value, or calculate it using the p distribution table that corresponds to hypotheses.

Step 4: State the conclusion and interpretation.
If the p-value is less than α, then reject H_0. Otherwise, do not reject H_0.

Z test: Critical Value Method
The critical region consists of the range of values of the test statistic Z data for which we reject the null hypothesis.

The noncritical region consists of the range of values of the test statistic Z data for which we do not reject the null hypothesis.

The value of Z that separates the critical region from the noncritical region. Table of critical values Z_{crit} for common values of the level of significance α.

Form of Hypothesis Test

	$H_0: \mu \leq \mu_0$	$H_0: \mu \geq \mu_0$	$H_0: \mu = \mu_0$
Level of significance α	$H_a: \mu > \mu_0$	$H_a: \mu < \mu_0$	$H_a: \mu \neq \mu_0$
0.10	$Z_{crit} = 1.28$	$Z_{crit} = -1.28$	$Z_{crit} = 1.645$
0.05	$Z_{crit} = 1.645$	$Z_{crit} = -1.645$	$Z_{crit} = 1.96$
0.01	$Z_{crit} = 2.33$	$Z_{crit} = -2.33$	$Z_{crit} = 2.58$

Chapter 5: Elementary Knowledge of Biostatistics

Test for the Population Mean: Critical Value Method

When a random sample of size n is taken from a population where the population standard deviation σ is known, Z test can be used if either of the following conditions is satisfied:
- Case 1: The population is normal, or
- Case 2: The sample size is large ($n \geq 30$).

Step 1: State the hypotheses

Step 2: Find Z_{crit} and state the rejection rule. Use Z distribution table

Step 3: Find Z_{data}. Either use technology to find the value of the test statistic Z data or calculate the value of Z data as follows:

$$Z_{data} = \frac{\overline{X} - \mu_0}{\sigma_{\overline{x}}} = \frac{\overline{X} - \mu_0}{\sigma/\sqrt{n}}$$

Step 4: State the conclusion and the interpretation. If Z_{data} falls in the critical region, then reject H_0. Otherwise, do not reject H_0.

■ t-TEST

t statistic(**t-data**) is a t distribution with $n-1$ degrees of freedom (if either the population is normal or the sample size is large).

Test for the Population Mean μ: p-Value Method

When a random sample of size n is taken from a population, t test is used if either of the following conditions is satisfied:
Case 1: The population is normal, or
Case 2: The sample size is large ($n \geq 30$).

Step 1: State the hypotheses and the rejection rule. Define μ. The rejection rule is "Reject H_0 if the p-value is less than α."

Step 2: Find t-data. Either use technology to find the value of the test statistic t data or calculate the value of t data as follows:

$$t \text{ data} = \frac{\overline{X} - \mu_0}{s/\sqrt{n}}$$

Step 3: Find the p-value. Either use technology to find the p-value or estimate the p-value using t-distribution table.

Step 4: State the conclusion and the interpretation. If the *p*-value is less than α, then reject H_0. Otherwise, do not reject H_0.

CHI-SQUARE TEST FOR POPULATION STANDARD DEVIATION (σ)

χ^2 (Chi (pronounced as kye)-Square) Distribution

If a random sample of size *n is taken* from a normal population with mean σ and standard deviation *s*, then the statistic follows a χ^2 distribution with *n*–1 degrees of freedom, where σ^2 represents the sample variance.

$$\chi^2 = \frac{(n-1)s^2}{\sigma}$$

When the observed value of χ^2 data is unusual or extreme on the assumption that H_0 is true, it should be rejected. If, there is insufficient evidence against H_0, it should be accepted.

Chi- square Test for σ: p-Value Method

This hypothesis test is valid only if we have a random sample from a normal population.

Step 1: State the hypotheses and the rejection rule. State the rejection rule as "Reject H_0 when the *p*-value is less than α." Clearly define σ.

Step 2: Find χ^2 data. Either use technology to find the value of the test statistic χ^2 data or calculate the value of χ^2 data as follows:

$$\chi^2 = \frac{(n-1)s^2}{\sigma_0^2}$$

Which follows a χ^2 distribution with *n*–1 degrees of freedom, and where s^2 represents the sample variance.

Step 3: Find the *p*-value. Either use technology to find the *p*-value or estimate the *p*-value using probability table for chi-square (χ^2) distribution.

Step 4: State the conclusion and the interpretation. If the *p*-value is less than α, then reject H_0. Otherwise, do not reject H_0.

tTable

t- distribution table

cum. prob	$t_{.50}$	$t_{.75}$	$t_{.80}$	$t_{.85}$	$t_{.90}$	$t_{.95}$	$t_{.975}$	$t_{.99}$	$t_{.995}$	$t_{.999}$	$t_{.9995}$
one-tail	0.50	0.25	0.20	0.15	0.10	0.05	0.025	0.01	0.005	0.001	0.0005
two-tails	1.00	0.50	0.40	0.30	0.20	0.10	0.05	0.02	0.01	0.002	0.001
df											
1	0.000	1.000	1.376	1.963	3.078	6.314	12.71	31.82	63.66	318.31	636.62
2	0.000	0.816	1.061	1.386	1.886	2.920	4.303	6.965	9.925	22.327	31.599
3	0.000	0.765	0.978	1.250	1.638	2.353	3.182	4.541	5.841	10.215	12.924
4	0.000	0.741	0.941	1.190	1.533	2.132	2.776	3.747	4.604	7.173	8.610
5	0.000	0.727	0.920	1.156	1.476	2.015	2.571	3.365	4.032	5.893	6.869
6	0.000	0.718	0.906	1.134	1.440	1.943	2.447	3.143	3.707	5.208	5.959
7	0.000	0.711	0.896	1.119	1.415	1.895	2.365	2.998	3.499	4.785	5.408
8	0.000	0.706	0.889	1.108	1.397	1.860	2.306	2.896	3.355	4.501	5.041
9	0.000	0.703	0.883	1.100	1.383	1.833	2.262	2.821	3.250	4.297	4.781
10	0.000	0.700	0.879	1.093	1.372	1.812	2.228	2.764	3.169	4.144	4.587
11	0.000	0.697	0.876	1.088	1.363	1.796	2.201	2.718	3.106	4.025	4.437
12	0.000	0.695	0.873	1.083	1.356	1.782	2.179	2.681	3.055	3.930	4.318
13	0.000	0.694	0.870	1.079	1.350	1.771	2.160	2.650	3.012	3.852	4.221
14	0.000	0.692	0.868	1.076	1.345	1.761	2.145	2.624	2.977	3.787	4.140
15	0.000	0.691	0.866	1.074	1.341	1.753	2.131	2.602	2.947	3.733	4.073

Contd...

Contd...

cum. prob	t_{50}	t_{75}	t_{80}	t_{85}	t_{90}	t_{95}	t_{975}	t_{99}	t_{995}	t_{999}	t_{9995}
one-tail	0.50	0.25	0.20	0.15	0.10	0.05	0.025	0.01	0.005	0.001	0.0005
two-tails	1.00	0.50	0.40	0.30	0.20	0.10	0.05	0.02	0.01	0.002	0.001
21	0.000	0.686	0.859	1.063	1.323	1.721	2.080	2.518	2.831	3.527	3.819
22	0.000	0.686	0.858	1.061	1.321	1.717	2.074	2.508	2.819	3.505	3.792
23	0.000	0.685	0.858	1.060	1.319	1.714	2.069	2.500	2.807	3.485	3.768
24	0.000	0.685	0.857	1.059	1.318	1.711	2.064	2.492	2.797	3.467	3.745
25	0.000	0.684	0.856	1.058	1.316	1.708	2.060	2.485	2.787	3.450	3.725
26	0.000	0.684	0.856	1.058	1.315	1.706	2.056	2.479	2.779	3.435	3.707
27	0.000	0.684	0.855	1.057	1.314	1.703	2.052	2.473	2.771	3.421	3.690
28	0.000	0.683	0.855	1.056	1.313	1.701	2.048	2.467	2.763	3.408	3.674
29	0.000	0.683	0.854	1.055	1.311	1.699	2.045	2.462	2.756	3.396	3.659
30	0.000	0.683	0.854	1.055	1.310	1.697	2.042	2.457	2.750	3.385	3.646
40	0.000	0.681	0.851	1.050	1.303	1.684	2.021	2.423	2.704	3.307	3.551
60	0.000	0.679	0.848	1.045	1.296	1.671	2.000	2.390	2.660	3.232	3.460
80	0.000	0.678	0.846	1.043	1.292	1.664	1.990	2.374	2.639	3.195	3.416
100	0.000	0.677	0.845	1.042	1.290	1.660	1.984	2.364	2.626	3.174	3.390
1000	0.000	0.675	0.842	1.037	1.282	1.646	1.962	2.330	2.581	3.098	3.300
z	0.000	0.674	0.842	1.036	1.282	1.645	1.960	2.326	2.576	3.090	3.291
	0%	50%	60%	70%	80%	90%	95%	98%	99%	99.8%	99.9%

Confidence Level

Table of χ^2 Probability (p)

DF	0.995	0.2	0.1	0.05	0.02	0.01	0.005	0.002	0.001
1	3.9E-05	1.642	2.706	3.841	5.412	6.635	7.879	9.55	10.828
2	0.01	3.219	4.605	5.991	7.824	9.21	10.597	12.429	13.816
3	0.0717	4.642	6.251	7.815	9.837	11.345	12.838	14.796	16.266
4	0.207	5.989	7.779	9.488	11.668	13.277	14.86	16.924	18.467
5	0.412	7.289	9.236	11.07	13.388	15.086	16.75	18.907	20.515
6	0.676	8.558	10.645	12.592	15.033	16.812	18.548	20.791	22.458
7	0.989	9.803	12.017	14.067	16.622	18.475	20.278	22.601	24.322
8	1.344	11.03	13.362	15.507	18.168	20.09	21.955	24.352	26.124
9	1.735	12.242	14.684	16.919	19.679	21.666	23.589	26.056	27.877
10	2.156	13.442	15.987	18.307	21.161	23.209	25.188	27.722	29.588
11	2.603	14.631	17.275	19.675	22.618	24.725	26.757	29.354	31.264

Other hypothesis testing methods includes ANOVA test. This is Analysis of Variance Test. It can compare more than two samples drawn from corresponding normal population.

SUMMARY

- Biostatistics is "the science of collecting and analyzing biologic or health data using statistical methods.
- Qualitative or discrete data are classified by counting individuals having the same characteristic. It has only one variable i.e., the number of persons and not the characteristic.
- Quantitative or continuous data have a magnitude. The characteristic is measured either on an interval or on a ratio scale. There are two variables—the characteristic and the frequency.
- Depending upon its types, data can be presented by various ways, such as tabulation, histogram, bar diagram, pie chart, line graph, and frequency curve.
- The mean is equal to the sum of all the values in the data set divided by the number of values in the data set.
- The median is the middle score for a set of data that has been arranged in order of magnitude.
- The mode is the most frequent score in our data set or it is the point of maximum concentration.

Section 1: Basic Chemistry

- Measures of variability are statistical procedures to describe how spread out (variable) the data is.
- Range is the difference between the highest and lowest values produced.
- Percentiles are values in a series of observations arranged in ascending order of magnitude which divide the distribution into 100 equal parts.
- Standard deviation is how much variation is there from the average (mean).
- The variance is a numerical value used to indicate how widely individuals in a group vary.
- Correlation is used to measure the degree of linear relationship between two continuous variables, it is expressed in terms of coefficient.
- The descriptive statistics gives a description about a sample, while the inferential statistics predicts and infers about a much larger data or population.
- "Estimation statistics" is estimating population values based on sample data. This can be done by two types—standard error of mean (SEM) and confidence interval (CI).
- The degree of variation between means from repeated samples can be measured by the standard error of the mean (SEM).
- Since statistics uses a sample space and predicts the trends for the whole population, a certain degree of error and uncertainty is expected. This is captured through the confidence interval.
- Hypothesis testing is simply another way of drawing conclusions about a population parameter. Z test, t-test, and Chi-Square test are tests used for hypothesis testing.
- Z test is when a random sample of size n is taken from a population where the population standard deviation σ is known.
- t statistic (**t data**) is a t distribution with $n - 1$ degrees of freedom (if either the population is normal or the sample size is large).
- Chi-Square test is when a random sample of size n is taken from a normal population with mean σ and standard deviation s.

PRACTICE QUESTIONS

1. What is biostatistics? Discuss its applications.
2. Discuss the different types of statistical data.
3. Why is there a need of presentation of data?
4. What are measures of central tendencies? Discuss its types.
5. Write a short note on—range, standard deviation, variance, and correlation coefficient.
6. Differentiate between descriptive and inferential statistics.
7. What is estimation statistics? How it can be performed?
8. What are two hypotheses or presumptions made to draw the inference from the sample value?
9. Write a note on—Z Test, t-test, and Chi-Square test.

SECTION 2

Fundamentals of Biochemistry

SECTION OUTLINE

6. Aim and Scope of Biochemistry
7. Structure of Cell
8. Study of Carbohydrates
9. Study of Proteins
10. Study of Lipids
11. Study of Nucleic Acids

CHAPTER 6

Aim and Scope of Biochemistry

> **Keywords**
> **Carl Neuberg, Claude Bernard,** enzymology, endocrinology, molecular biochemistry, clinical biochemistry, genetic engineering, biomolecules

■ INTRODUCTION

The most conspicuous attribute of living organisms is that they are complicated and highly organized. All living organisms are made of cells which possess intricate internal structure containing many kinds of complex molecule and chemical reactions. The term "biochemistry" is derived from a combination of biology and chemistry.

The term "biochemistry" was first introduced by a German chemist, Carl Neuberg, in 1903. Biochemistry is defined as a science concerned with the chemical nature and chemical behavior of the living matter. It takes into account the studies related to the nature of the chemical constituents of living matter, their transformations in biological systems, and the energy changes associated with these transformations.

■ HISTORY OF BIOCHEMISTRY

Modern biochemistry developed out of and largely came to replace what in the 19th and early 20th centuries was called physiological chemistry, which dealt more with extracellular chemistry, such as the chemistry of digestion and of body fluids. However, work in this very living, aspect of chemistry had started in early 19th century. Claude Bernard is accredited with the sirehood (father) of biochemistry. He was the first to conceive and present to the scientific community the idea of a "fixed internal milieu." His most important contribution was his concept of the internal environment of the organism, which led to the present understanding of homeostasis—the self-regulation of vital processes.

During the later part of the 19th century, eminent scientists contributed a great deal to the elucidation of the chemistry of fats, proteins, and carbohydrates. At this period, some very fundamental aspects of enzymology were under close scrutiny. Study of nucleic acid is central to the knowledge of life but its fusion with biochemistry started with works of Fredrick Sanger and Har Gobind Khurana. Their experiments involved a subtle bland of enzymology and chemistry. In 1990s, research turned to finding the structural details of cell.

■ SCOPE OF BIOCHEMISTRY

Biochemistry has advanced more since mid-20th century with the development of new techniques, such as chromatography, X-ray diffraction, nuclear magnetic resonance (NMR) spectroscopy, radio-isotopic labeling, electron microscopy, and molecular dynamics simulations.

The knowledge of biochemistry is growing speedily; newer disciplines are emerging from biochemistry, such as enzymology (study of enzymes), endocrinology (study of hormones), clinical biochemistry (study of diseases), and molecular biochemistry (study of biomolecules and their functions). Along with these branches, certain other specialties have also come up, such as agricultural biochemistry and pharmacological biochemistry.

The field of molecular biochemistry has also expanded its horizons beyond human imagination with the introduction of polymerase chain reaction (PCR). It created waves of appreciation from every field of medicine and now coming out of the laboratory to help establish better therapies for various diseases by introduction of gene therapy. Biochemistry has promises to the world of science in development of new path-breaking research and coming times would surely prove these promises to be fulfilled.

Advances in biochemistry have found large-scale applications in various areas, such as industry, agriculture, medicine, and pharmacy.

1. **Genetic engineering:** By applying biochemical techniques, improved strains of domestic animals and cultivated plants are

produced through genetic engineering, nitrogen fixing genes of bacteria are transferred to higher plants (wheat and maize).
2. **Feed proteins:** New strains of microorganisms are being employed in the production of low-cost feed protein and essential amino acids for domestic animals.
3. **Biological control:** To protect cultivated plants from the pests, biological preparations of superior quality that are not harmful to human or animals are currently being manufactured.
4. **Control of pollution:** Biological methods for the disposal of industrial and domestic wastes and for the cleaning up oil spills, common contaminants of the seas (using specially cultivated bacterial mutants) have proved to be of substantial value.
5. **Industrial development:** Biochemical processes are widely used in the food industry (in the preparation of bread, cheese, wine, etc.) and in the leather industry. Detergents with enzyme additions are also commonly available.
6. **Medical field:** Biochemical methods are increasing by gaining acceptance in pharmaceutical practice. Enzymes are used in technology for the synthesis of drugs such as steroid hormones.
7. **Diagnostic field:** Clinical biochemistry is an important tool in the diagnostic world. It is analytical and interpretative science. The analytical part involves the determination of the level of chemical components in body fluids and tissues. The interpretative part examines these results and uses them in the diagnosis of disease, the screening for susceptibility to specific diseases, and monitoring of progress of treatment. The clinical biochemistry may aid in:
   - Discovering occult disease
   - Preventing irreparable damage
   - Early diagnosis after onset of signs or symptoms

Based on the symptoms described by the patient, physician can get clue on the biochemical change and the associated disorder. For example, if a patient complains about stiffness in small joints, then physician may predict it to be gout and get confirmed by evaluating uric acid levels in the blood, as uric acid accumulation in blood results in gout. Almost all the diseases or disorders have some biochemical involvement. So, the diagnosis of any clinical condition is easily possible by biochemical estimations.
- Differential diagnosis of various possible diseases
- Determining the stage of the disease

- Estimating the activity of the disease
- Detecting the recurrence of the disease
- Monitoring the effect of therapy
- Genetic consulting in familial problems
- Medicolegal problems, such as paternity suits
- Isolation, structural elucidation, and the determination of mode of action of biomolecules
- Study of oncogenes in cancer cells
- The relationship of biochemistry with genetics, physiology, immunology, pharmacology, and toxicology
- Physiology: Biochemistry helps one understand the biochemical changes and related physiological alteration in the body.
- The application of bacterial techniques has enabled scientists to develop convenient and economical methods for the commercial synthesis of pharmaceuticals, such as insulin, vitamins, antibiotics, antibodies, amino acids, nucleotides, and nucleosides.

AIMS/OBJECTIVES OF CLINICAL BIOCHEMISTRY

The objective of biochemistry is complete understanding of all the chemical processes associated with living cells at the molecular level. To achieve this objective, biochemists have attempted to isolate numerous molecules (biomolecules) found in cells, to determine their structures and to analyze how they function.

Thus, principal objective of biochemist is to fill the wide gap between the highly intricate functions of the living cell and the various properties of its individual chemical constituents. A biochemist, therefore, has to perform an important arduous task carrying the research work with utmost sincerity, patience, and honesty.

The American Society of Biological Chemists has defined biochemist as "A biochemist is an investigator who utilizes chemical, physical or biological techniques to study chemical nature and behavior of living matter."

Biochemical studies have illuminated many aspects of disease and the study of certain diseases has opened up new therapeutic approaches.

Chapter 6: Aim and Scope of Biochemistry

SUMMARY

- The term "biochemistry" was first introduced by a German chemist, Carl Neuberg, in 1903.
- Biochemistry is a science concerned with the chemical nature and chemical behavior of the living matter.
- Claude Bernard is accredited with the sirehood of biochemistry.
- Advances in biochemistry have found large-scale applications in various areas, such as industry, agriculture, medicine, and pharmacy.
- Principal objective of biochemist is to fill the wide gap between the highly intricate functions of the living cell and the various properties of its individual chemical constituents.
- A biochemist is an investigator who utilizes chemical, physical, or biological techniques to study chemical nature and behavior of living matter.
- Clinical biochemistry is helpful in diagnosis of disease, the screening for susceptibility to specific diseases, and monitoring of progress of treatment.

PRACTICE QUESTIONS

1. Define biochemistry and biochemist.
2. What are the emerging disciplines of biochemistry?
3. Discuss the applications of biochemistry in the field of diagnosis.
4. What is the principle and objective of biochemistry?
5. Discuss the role of a biochemist in a diagnostic laboratory.
6. Discuss the importance of biochemistry in the field other than clinical biochemistry.

CHAPTER 7

Structure of Cell

> **Keywords**
> Cell organelles, cell membrane, cytoplasm, centrioles, endoplasmic reticulum, Golgi apparatus, lysosomes, microfilaments, microtubules, mitochondria, nucleus, DNA, chromosomes, peroxisomes, plasma membrane, ribosomes

■ INTRODUCTION

All living organisms are made up of cells. Cells are building blocks of life. A cell is the smallest unit of life. It helps in carrying out functions, such as respiration, nutrition, digestion, and excretion, so it is called the structural and functional unit of life. A cell is a microscopic structure which consists of cytoplasm and nucleus enclosed in a membrane.

Animal cells consist of different kinds of shapes and sizes. The size of animal cells range from a few millimeters to micrometers. The largest animal cell is the ostrich egg which has a 5-inch diameter, weighing about 1.2–1.4 kg and the smallest animal cells are the neurons of about 100 microns in diameter.

Animal cells are smaller than the plant cells and they are generally irregular in shape taking various forms of shapes, due to lack of the cell wall. Some cells are round, oval, flattened or rod-shaped, spherical, concave, and rectangular. This is due to the lack of a cell wall.

Animal cells are eukaryotic. Animal cells have an outer boundary known as the plasma membrane. The nucleus and the organelles of the cell are bound by a membrane. The genetic material (DNA) in animal cells is within the nucleus that is bound by a double membrane.

■ CELL ORGANELLES

Animal cell contains membrane bound nucleus, it also contains other membrane bound structure, called cellular organelles. These cellular organelles carry out specific functions that are necessary for the normal functioning of the cell. Animal cells lack cell wall, a large vacuole and plastids. Due to the lack of the cell wall, the shape and size of the animal cells are mostly irregular.

The cell organelles are centrioles, endoplasmic reticulum (ER), Golgi apparatus, lysosomes, microfilaments, microtubules, mitochondria, nucleus, peroxisomes, plasma membrane, and ribosomes.

■ CELL MEMBRANE

- A typical cell membrane is 75 Å in thickness.
- It is a semipermeable barrier, allowing only a few molecules to move across it.
- An electron microscopic study of cell membrane shows the lipid bi-layer model of the plasma membrane, it is also known as the fluid mosaic model.
- The cell membrane is made up of phospholipids, which have polar (hydrophilic) heads and nonpolar (hydrophobic) tails.
- It encloses cytoplasm in which various cell organelles are present.

■ CYTOPLASM

- The fluid matrix that fills the cell is the cytoplasm.
- The cellular organelles are suspended in this matrix of the cytoplasm.
- This matrix maintains the pressure of the cell, ensures the cell does not shrink or burst.

■ NUCLEUS

- It is a dense spherical structure present in the center of the cell. It is covered with a double-layered membrane called nuclear envelope.
- A fluid present within nuclear envelope is called nucleoplasm.

- Nucleus is the house for most of the cells genetic material—the DNA and RNA.
- DNA is divided into 46 individual molecules, one for each chromosome. In order for the functioning of DNA, it is combined with proteins and organized into a compact and dense string such as fiber, called chromatin or chromosomes.
- The RNA moves in/out of the nucleus through these pores.
- Proteins needed by the nucleus enter through the nuclear pores.
- The RNA helps in protein synthesis through transcription process.
- The nucleus controls the activity of the cell and is known as the control center.
- The nucleolus is the dark spot in the nucleus, and it is the location for ribosome formation.

■ RIBOSOMES

- Ribosome is the site for protein synthesis where the translation of the RNA takes place.
- As protein synthesis is very important to the cell, ribosomes are found in large number in all cells.
- Ribosomes are found freely suspended in the cytoplasm and also are attached to the ER.

■ ENDOPLASMIC RETICULUM

- Within cytoplasm of the cell is an extensive network of membrane arranged in plates and tubules, collectively called as endoplasmic reticulum (ER).
- ER is the transport system of the cell. It transports molecules that need certain changes and also molecules to their destination.
- ER is of two types—rough and smooth.
- ER bound to the ribosomes appears rough and is called the rough endoplasmic reticulum; while the smooth ER does not have the ribosomes.

■ LYSOSOMES

- It is the digestive system of the cell.
- They have digestive enzymes, which help in breaking down the waste molecules and also help in detoxification of the cell.

- If the lysosomes were not membrane bound, the cell could not have used the destructive enzymes.
- They are referred to as the suicide bags of the cell. They have digestive enzymes and are involved in clearing the unwanted waste materials from the cell. They also engulf damaged materials like the damaged cells, and invading microorganisms, and digest food particles.

■ CENTROSOMES

- It is located near the nucleus of the cell and is known as the "microtubule organizing center" of the cell.
- Microtubules are made in the centrosome.
- During mitosis, the centrosome aids in dividing of the cell and moving of the chromosome to the opposite sides of the cell.

■ VACUOLES

- They are bound by single membrane and small organelles.
- In many organisms, vacuoles are storage organelles.
- Vesicles are smaller vacuoles which function for transport in/out of the cell.

■ GOLGI BODIES

- Golgi bodies are compact and consist of parallel membrane plates and tubule.
- It is the site for enzyme secretion. It participates in the formation of lysosomes.
- The Golgi bodies modify the molecules from the rough ER by dividing them into smaller units with membrane known as vesicles.
- It is involved with processing and packaging of the molecules that are synthesized by the cells. The crude proteins that are passed on by the ER to the apparatus are developed by the Golgi apparatus into primary, secondary, and tertiary proteins.

■ MITOCHONDRIA

- Mitochondrion is the main energy source of the cell.
- They are called the power house of the cell because energy [adenosine triphosphate (ATP)] is created here.

- All enzymes which are present in Krebs cycle are present in mitochondria.
- Mitochondria consist of inner and outer membrane. It is composed of largely proteins and lipids.
- Each mitochondrion is composed of tubular or paired lamellae called cristae.
- Its main function is to produce energy for cell by the process of cellular respiration.
- It is spherical or rod-shaped organelle.
- It is an organelle which is independent as it has its own hereditary material.

■ PEROXISOMES

- Peroxisomes are single membrane-bound organelle that contain oxidative enzymes that are digestive in function.
- They help in digesting long chains of fatty acids and amino acids and help in the synthesis of cholesterol.

■ CYTOSKELETON

- It is the network of microtubules and microfilament fibers.
- They give structural support and maintain the shape of the cell.

■ FUNCTIONS OF THE ANIMAL CELL

The animal cells perform variety of activities by the aid of the cellular organelles. These cells function as a unit and the cells together form tissues. A group of tissues with similar function form an organ and a group of organs of specific function to perform become an organ system. Thus, the microscopic cells form the basic unit for the activities and coordination and help survival of the organism (**Fig. 7.1**).

Some significant functions of animal cells include obtaining food and oxygen, keeping internal conditions stable, moving, and reproducing.

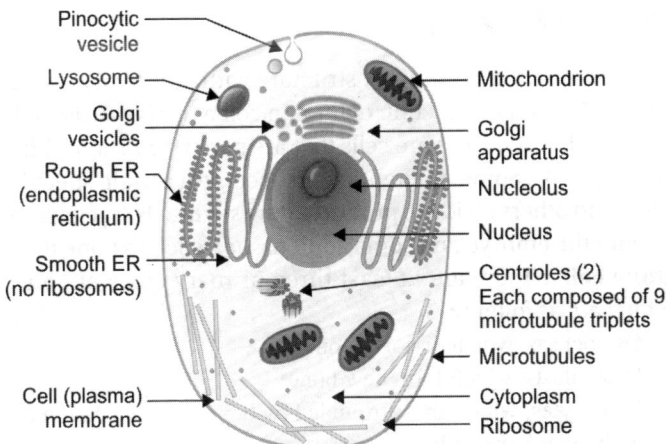

Fig. 7.1: The animal cell.
(For color version, see Plate 2)

Furthermore, animal cells are highly specialized to carry out specific tasks. Also, each cell type has the organelles suited to its particular task.

Some examples of this may include the cardiac muscles of the heart that beat in unison or the digestive tract cells that have cilia which are finger-like projections that increase surface area for nutrients absorption.

There are four primary functions which are certainly common to all cells:

1. **Growth:** Cells carry the primary function of physical growth in living being.
2. **Respiration:** Cells help in breaking down or oxidizing food substances to release energy for other vital life processes.
3. **Metabolism:** Cells help in converting food into energy, thereby promoting the performance of various regular activities. This process is called as metabolism.
4. **Reproduction:** Cells produce an exact copy of its genetic material before splitting into two genetically identical cells. This process of cell reproduction is mitosis. Cellular reproduction in animals enables their body to replace dying, diseased, or damaged cells and in cases of pregnancy to perpetuate the specific species.

TYPES OF CELLS

Human body is a very complex structure with hundreds of different types of cell. A small selection of human cell types is discussed here.

- **Stem cells:** Stem cells are cells that are parent to various different types of cells. Some differentiate to become a certain specific cell type, and others divide to produce more stem cells. They are found in both the embryo and some adult tissues, such as bone marrow.
- **Bone cells:** There are at least three primary types of bone cell which are as follows:
  a. Osteoclasts, which dissolve bone
  b. Osteoblasts, which form new bone
  c. Osteocytes, which are surrounded by bone and help communicate with other bone cells
- **Blood cells:** There are three major types of blood cell, which are as follows:
  a. Red blood cells, which carry oxygen around the body
  b. White blood cells, which are part of the immune system
  c. Platelets, which help blood clot to prevent blood loss after injury
- **Muscle cells:** These are also known as myocytes, muscle cells are long, tubular cells. Muscle cells are important for a huge range of functions, including movement, support, and internal functions, such as peristalsis—the movement of food along the gut.

  Sperm cells: These tadpole-shaped cells are the smallest in the human body.

  They are motile, meaning that they can move. They achieve this movement by using their tail (flagellum), which is packed with energy-giving mitochondria.
- Sperm cells cannot divide; they only carry one copy of each chromosome (haploid), unlike the majority of cells, which carry two copies (diploid).
- **Female egg cell:** Compared with the sperm cell, the female egg cell is a giant; it is the largest human cell. The egg cell is also haploid (with half number of chromosomes) so that the DNA from the sperm and egg can combine to create a diploid cell.

- **Fat cells:** Fat cells are also called adipocytes and are the main constituent in adipose tissue. They contain stored fats called triglycerides that can be used as energy when needed. Once the triglycerides are used up, the fat cells shrink. Adipocytes also produce some hormones.
- **Nerve cells:** Nerves cells are the communication system of the body. Also called neurons, they consist of two major parts—the cell body and nerve processes. The central body contains the nucleus and other organelles, and the nerve processes (axons or dendrites) run like long fingers, carrying messages far and wide. Some of these axons can be over 1 meter long.

SUMMARY

- Cells are basic structural and functional unit of life.
- Cells can be of different shapes and sizes.
- Animal cells are eukaryotic cells—they contain a nucleus and numerous organelles.
- The plasma membrane surrounds an animal cell.
- Almost all of a cell's DNA is kept inside its nucleus.
- ER is a network of membranes connected to the nucleus—it includes the smooth ER and the rough ER.
- Cell membrane is a semipermeable membrane that controls passage of materials into and out of the cell.
- Centriole takes part in cell production.
- Cytoplasm is fluid matrix that consists of various cell organelles.
- Lysosome digests materials in the cell.
- Mitochondrion is composed of tubular or paired lamellae called cristae. It produces energy for the cell.
- ER transports substances within the cell.
- Smooth ER is without ribosomes; it assembles lipids.
- Rough ER is closest to the nucleus; it assembles proteins out of amino acid.
- Golgi apparatus transports substances to the surface of the cell and proteins get finishing touches; modify, pack, and sorts.
- Nuclear envelope surrounds nucleus and controls passage of materials into and out of nucleus.
- Nucleolus takes part in production of ribosomes.
- Nucleus controls all cell functions. It contains chromosomes.
- Ribosome makes protein for the cell.
- Cytoskeleton gives structural support and maintains the shape of the cell.

- Different types of specialized cells are found in different tissues according to its function. It includes—stem cells, blood cells, nerve cells, bone cells, sperm cells, egg cells, fat cells, etc.

PRACTICE QUESTIONS

1. Why cells are called structural and functional unit of life?
2. Explain four primary functions of the cell.
3. Write a short note on:
    i. Stem cells
    ii. Bone cell
    iii. Blood cell
    iv. Muscle cells
    v. Sperm cells
    vi. Egg cell
    vii. Fat cells
    viii. Nerves cells
4. Draw a neat labeled diagram of an animal cell.
5. Complete the following table:

Cell organelles	Structure	Function
Cell membrane		
	Matrix that fill the cell	
Nucleus		
		Site for protein synthesis
Endoplasmic reticulum		
		Suicide bags of cells
Centrosome		
Golgi bodies		
		Power house of the cell
Cytoskeleton		

CHAPTER 8

Study of Carbohydrates

> **Keywords**
> Monosaccharides, oligosaccharide, polysaccharide, iodine test, Benedict's test, Fehling's test, mucic acid test, basal metabolic rate, glycogenesis, glycolysis, citric acid cycle, hexose monophosphate shunt (HMP pathway), galactosemia, fructose intolerance, disorders of pyruvate metabolism, biochemical importance of carbohydrate

■ INTRODUCTION

Carbohydrates constitute the greatest proportion of organic material on earth. They are the main components of the food. Carbohydrates are the important components of our clothing, housing furniture, etc.

Carbohydrates are defined as polyhydroxy aldehydes or ketones and their derivatives.

■ CLASSIFICATION

Carbohydrates are classified as **(Flowchart 8.1)**:
1. **Monosaccharides:** These are the simplest members of carbohydrate, which are represented by the general formula $C_nH_{2n}O_n$. Monosaccharides are grouped according to the number of carbon atoms present in a sugar molecule, such as trioses (3), tetroses (4), pentoses (5), and hexoses (6). Each of these can be further named as aldoses or ketoses depending on the presence of aldehyde or ketone group, respectively.
   For example, glucose—it is a hexose carbohydrate. It is an aldose sugar.
2. **Oligosaccharide:** These are condensation products of two to ten simple sugars or monosaccharide. They are represented by general formula $C_n(H_2O)_{n-1}$. Oligosaccharides are grouped according to number of monosaccharide units present in a molecule.

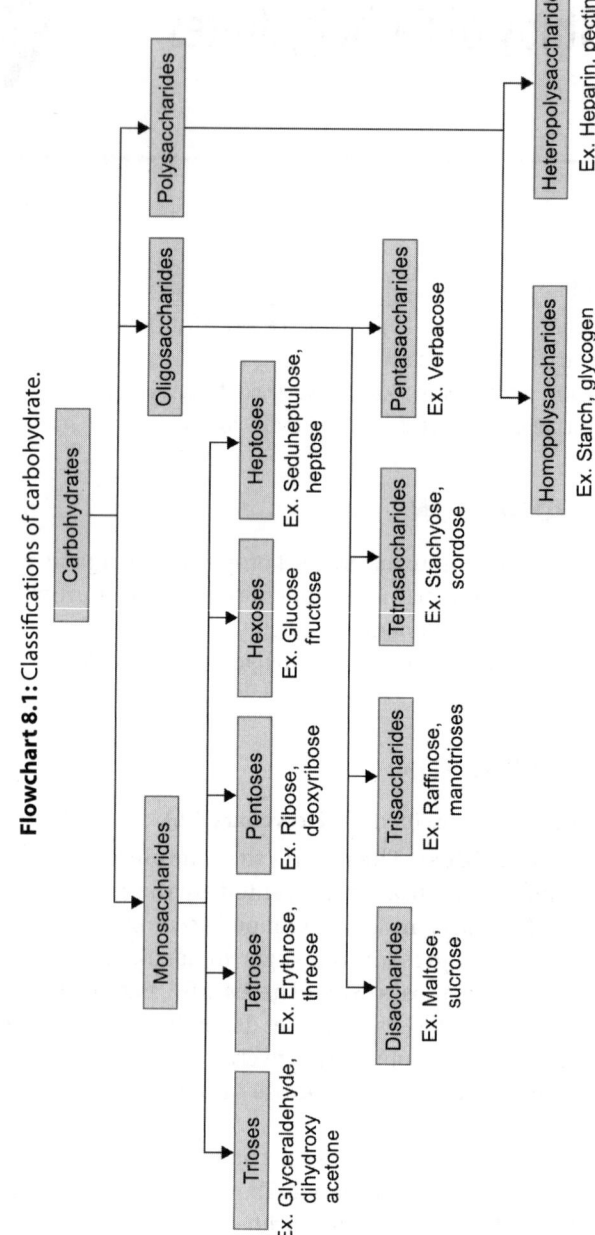

Flowchart 8.1: Classifications of carbohydrate.

For example, maltose, lactose and sucrose are disaccharides and raffinose is trisaccharide.

3. **Polysaccharide:** These are the majority of carbohydrates found in natural sources. These are high molecular weight polymers of monosaccharides represented by general formula $(C_6H_{10}O_5)n$. They are classified as homopolysaccharide and heteropolysaccharide depending on the presence of either the same monosaccharide or more than one simple sugar.

For example, cellulose and glycogen are homopolysaccharides while glucuronic acid is a heteropolysaccharide.

■ DETECTIVE TESTS FOR CARBOHYDRATE

1. **Dehydration:** Carbohydrates on dehydration give furfural or its derivatives. Concentrated sulfuric acid is used as dehydrating agent e.g., Moilsch test. It is general test for carbohydrate identification. Furfural or its derivatives formed during dehydration react with α-naphthol to give violet color.

$$\text{Ribose} \xrightarrow{\text{conc. } H_2SO_4} \text{Furfural}$$

2. **Reducing properties:** Carbohydrates having free carbonyl group acts as reducing agent. It reduces certain metal ions like copper, mercury, etc. based on this property following tests detect reducing sugars.
   - *Benedict's test:* Carbohydrates are heated with alkaline copper sulfate, copper ions get reduced and give red precipitate of Cu_2O.
   - *Fehling's test:* Reducing sugar reduces copper ions present in Fehling's solution so as to give red precipitates of Cu_2O.
   - *Formation of osazone:* When reducing sugar is heated with phenylhydrazine, yellow crystalline compounds called osazones are formed. Definite crystalline forms of osazone are obtained from different reducing sugars. For example, glucose phenylhydrazone react with two molecules of phenylhydrazine to give glucosazone, aniline and ammonia.

3. **Reduction:** The carbonyl group of sugar can be reduced by variety of reagents such as H_2 and Pt to an alcohol. Such carbohydrate derivatives are called alditols. For example,

$$\text{Glucose} \xrightarrow{H_2 - Pt} \text{Sorbitol}$$

4. **Oxidation:** Sugar on oxidation gives acid. The oxidation product depends upon oxidizing agent used in the reaction. For example,

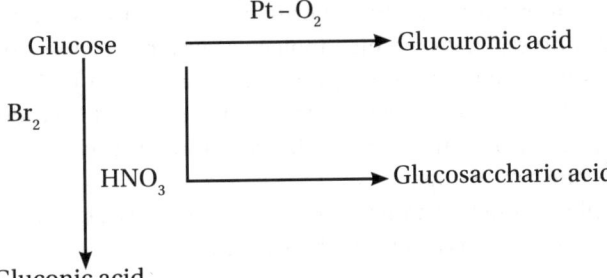

5. **Mucic acid test:** This test is used for identification of galactose and lactose. Galactose/lactose on oxidation in presence of concentrated nitric acid gives galactosaccharic acid (mucic acid). The mucic acid is insoluble and gets crystallized. The crystals are colorless and broken glass type.
6. **Iodine test:** Iodine reacts with different sugars to form different colors. For example,

Types of polysaccharide	Color with iodine
Starch	Blue
Dextrin	Brown
Glycogen	Pink
Amylase	Deep blue
Amylopectin	Purple

■ METABOLISM

Metabolism of a substance is defined as series of biochemical reactions occurring within the living organism from the time of incorporation until its excretion. Metabolism consists of anabolism and catabolism.

Anabolism: Anabolism or synthesis is defined as series of biochemical reactions involved in the process of synthesis of larger molecules from smaller ones.

Catabolism: Catabolism or analysis is defined as series of reactions involved in the process of breakdown of larger molecules into smaller ones for supply of energy.

Energy metabolism: There will be continuous exchange of energy between living body and its surrounding environment. This energy exchange is based on first law of thermodynamics which states that energy is neither gained nor lost when it is converted from one form to another form. These forms are chemical, electrical, mechanical, thermal, etc.

Basal metabolism: Energy produced as by-product of cellular metabolism is essential for sustenance of life. Although, there is variation in requirement of amount of energy, rate of production of energy in body remains more or less constant under some standard conditions known as basal metabolism.

Basal metabolic rate: The rate of production of energy at basal conditions per hour per meter square of body surface area is called basal metabolic rate. Its normal value in adult male is 40 calories per hour per meter square and 37 calories per hour per meter square in adult female.

Unit of energy: It is mainly calorie. It is defined as amount of heat energy which can raise the temperature of 1 g of water from 15°C to 16°C. Amount of heat can also be expressed as joule.

$$1 \text{ kilocalorie} = 4.19 \text{ kilojoules}$$

Uses of energy in body: Energy obtained from food sources is used in body for several purposes such as:
- Synthesis of protoplasmic constituents like DNA, RNA, phospholipids, etc.
- Functioning of different organs like heart, kidneys, etc.
- Maintenance of body temperature.
- Generation of electrical potentials in central nervous system (CNS), autonomic nervous system (ANS), heart, etc.
- Transport of substances against concentration gradient.
- Growth and maintenance.

Food sources that give us energy are mainly carbohydrate, protein and fat.

■ CARBOHYDRATE METABOLISM

Carbohydrates are converted to monosaccharides in the process of digestion in the digestive system. Mainly they are glucose, fructose and galactose. They are absorbed from the small intestines into portal circulation. Major function of carbohydrates is release of energy by undergoing oxidation. Carbohydrates are mainly used by cells in the form of glucose. Especially brain cells use glucose only. Fructose and galactose are also converted to glucose in liver. Different metabolic processes undergone by carbohydrates in the body are given below:

- **Glycogenesis:** It is the synthesis of glycogen from glucose.

    Glucose ⟶ glycogen

- **Gluconeogenesis:** It is formation of glucose from non-carbohydrates as glycerol.

    Glycerol ⟶ glucose

- **Glycogenolysis:** It is the conversion of glycogen to glucose.

    Glycogen ⟶ glucose

- **Glycolysis:** It is the oxidative pathway of glycogen or glucose.
- **Citric acid cycle:** It is also oxidative pathway of glucose.
- Hexose monophosphate shunt is alternative to glycolysis and citric acid cycle for oxidation of glucose.

Glycolysis

Glycolysis is also known as Embden Meyerhoff pathway. Anaerobic glycolysis is anaerobic degradation of glucose to yield lactic acid.

Stages of glycolysis: There are two stages in glycolysis **(Flowchart 8.2)**. In the first stage, glucose is converted to glyceraldehyde 3-phosphate, a three carbon compound. In the second stage, glyceraldehyde 3-phosphate is converted into pyruvate. It is regarded as the preparatory (or investment) phase, since they consume energy to convert the glucose into two three-carbon sugar phosphates. This pyruvate enters citric acid cycle in aerobic conditions. The second half of glycolysis is known as oxidative (or the pay-off phase) it is characterized by oxidation of glucose to pyruvate, with a net gain of the energy-rich molecules ATP and NADH. In anaerobic conditions, pyruvate is converted to lactate.

Flowchart 8.2: Glycolysis.

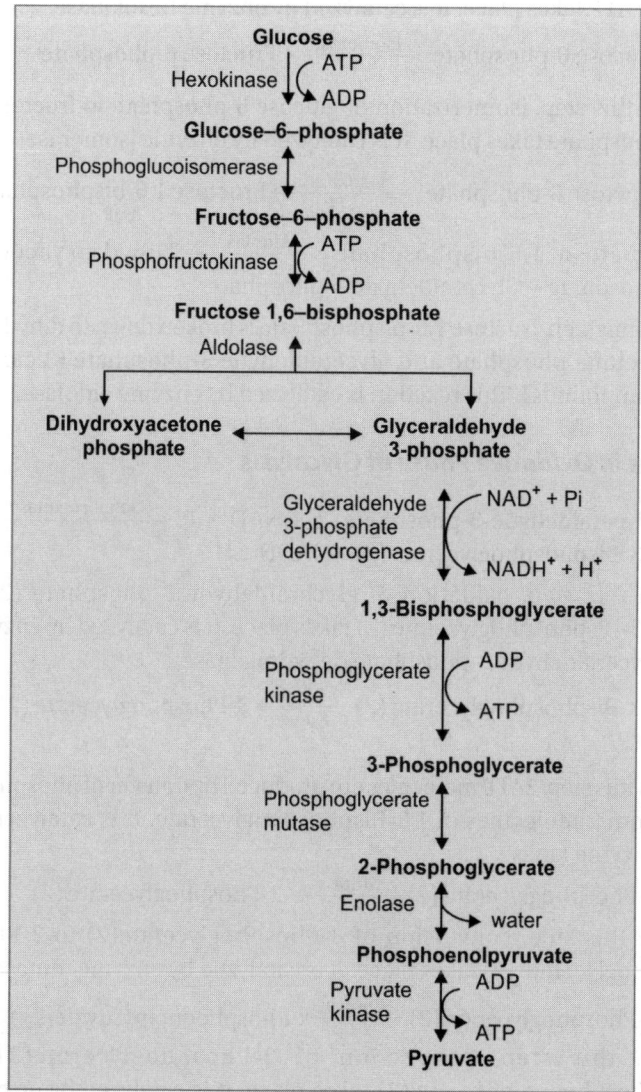

Steps in Preparatory Phase of Glycolysis

1. Glucose $\xrightarrow[\text{ATP} \quad \text{ADP}]{\text{Hexokinase}}$ Glucose 6-phosphate

In this step, phosphorylation of D-Glucose to glucose 6-phosphate by ATP takes place. It is catalyzed by enzyme hexokinase.

2. Glucose 6-phosphate $\xrightarrow{\text{Isomerase}}$ Fructose 6-phosphate

   In this step, isomerization of glucose 6-phosphate to fructose 6-phosphate takes place. It is catalyzed by enzyme isomerase.

3. Fructose 6-phosphate $\xrightarrow[\text{ATP}]{\text{Hexokinase}}$ Fructose 1,6-bisphosphate ADP

4. Fructose 1,6-bisphosphate $\xrightarrow{\text{Aldolase}}$ Dihydroxyacetone phosphate + Glyceraldehyde 3-phosphate

   In this step, fructose 1,6-bisphosphate is broken down to dihydroxy acetone phosphate and glyceraldehyde 3-phosphate (3 carbon compounds). This reaction is catalyzed by enzyme aldolase.

Steps in Oxidative Phase of Glycolysis

1. Glyceraldehyde-3-phosphate (2) + NAD^+ + Pi $\xrightarrow{\text{Dehydrogenase}}$ 1,3-Bisphosphoglycerate (2) + NADH + H^+

   In this step, oxidation of glyceraldehyde 3-phosphate (2) to 1,3-Bisphosphoglycerate (2) takes place. It is catalyzed by enzyme glyceraldehyde 3-phosphate dehydrogenase.

2. 1,3-Bisphosphoglycerate (2) $\xrightarrow[\text{Kinase}]{\text{2ADP}}$ 3-Phosphoglycerate (2) + 2 ATP

   In this step, 2ATP molecules are produced by transfer of phosphates from 2 molecules of 1,3-Bisphosphoglycerate. It is catalyzed by enzyme kinase.

3. 3-Phosphoglycerate (2) $\xrightarrow{\text{Mutase}}$ 2-Phosphoglycerate (2)

   In this step, conversion of 3-Phosphoglycerate(2) to 2-Phosphoglycerate (2) takes place. It is catalyzed by enzyme mutase.

4. 2-Phosphoglycerate (2) $\xrightarrow{\text{Enolase}}$ Phosphoenolpyruvate(2) + H_2O

   In this step, conversion of 2-Phosphoglycerate(2) to phosphoenolpyruvate (2) takes place. It is catalyzed by enzyme enolase.

5. Phosphoenolpyruvate (2) + 2ADP $\xrightarrow{\text{Kinase}}$ Pyruvate (2) + 2 ATP

   In this step, conversion of phosphoenolpyruvate (2) to pyruvate (2) takes place. It is catalyzed by enzyme kinase.

2 ATP molecules are produced by transfer of phosphates from phosphoenolpyruvate.

6. Pyruvate + NADH + H$^+$ $\xrightarrow{\text{LDH}}$ Lactate + NAD$^+$

In anaerobic conditions, pyruvate is converted to lactate by enzyme lactate dehydrogenase (LDH). In aerobic conditions, pyruvate enters citric acid cycle.

Glycolysis yields two molecules of ATP (4 ATPs are produced, 2 ATPs are consumed. Net yield of ATP is 2), two molecules of pyruvic acid and two "high energy" electron carrying molecules of NADH.

Tricarboxylic Acid Cycle

Tricarboxylic acid cycle (TCA) cycle is a cyclic sequence of reactions in which pyruvate formed in glycolysis is completely oxidized to CO_2 and H_2O.

It was postulated by HA Krebs in 1937. Its original name is citric acid cycle.

TCA cycle is the common pathway for degradation of two carbon acetyl residues derived not only from carbohydrates but also from fatty acids and, which is amino acids. TCA cycle actually takes place in intact cells. It accounts quantitatively for oxidation of carbohydrates, fatty acids and amino acids.

TCA cycle is both catabolic and anabolic pathway. It also generates precursors for anabolic pathways. α-ketoglutarate and oxaloacetate serve as precursors of amino acids. α-ketoglutarate and oxaloacetate are intermediates of this cycle. Citrate can be removed from this cycle and can be used as precursor of extramitochondrial acetyl-CoA for fatty acid biosynthesis. Succinyl-CoA can also be removed from the cycle for biosynthesis of heme.

The Net Equation

Acetyl-CoA + 3 NAD$^+$ + FAD + GDP + HPO$_4^{-2}$ ⟶ 2CO$_2$ + 3 NADH + FADH$_2$ + GTP + CoA

Reaction 1: Formation of Citrate

The first reaction of the cycle is the condensation of acetyl-CoA with oxaloacetate to form citrate, catalyzed by citrate synthase.

Once oxaloacetate is joined with acetyl-CoA, a water molecule attacks the acetyl leading to the release of coenzyme A from the complex. It is catalyzed by citrate synthatase forming citrate.

$$\text{Acetyl-CoA} + \text{Oxaloacetate} + H_2O \xrightarrow{\text{Citrate synthase}} \text{Citrate} + \text{CoA}$$

Reaction 2: Formation of Isocitrate

The citrate is rearranged to form an isomeric form, isocitrate by an enzyme aconitase.

The effect of this conversion is that the –OH group is moved from the 3' to the 4' position on the molecule.

$$\text{Citrate} \xrightarrow{\text{Aconitase}} \textit{Cis}\text{-Aconitate} \xrightarrow{\text{Aconitase}} \text{Isocitrate}$$

Reaction 3: Oxidation of Isocitrate to α-Ketoglutarate

In this step, isocitrate dehydrogenase catalyzes oxidative decarboxylation of isocitrate to form α-ketoglutarate.

In the reaction, generation of NADH from NAD is seen. The enzyme isocitrate dehydrogenase catalyzes the oxidation of isocitrate to yield an intermediate which then has a carbon dioxide molecule removed from it to yield α-ketoglutarate.

$$\text{Isocitrate} + NAD^+(NADP^+) \longrightarrow \text{α-Ketoglutarate} + CO_2 + NADH (NADPH) + H^+$$

Reaction 4: Oxidation of α-Ketoglutarate to Succinyl-CoA

Alpha-ketoglutarate is oxidized, carbon dioxide is removed, and coenzyme A is added to form the 4-carbon compound succinyl-CoA. During this oxidation, NAD^+ is reduced to NADH and H^+. The enzyme that catalyzes this reaction is α-ketoglutarate dehydrogenase.

$$\text{α-ketoglutarate} + NAD^+ + \text{CoA} \longrightarrow \text{Succinyl-CoA} + CO_2 + NADH + H^+$$

Reaction 5: Conversion of Succinyl-CoA to Succinate

Coenzymes A is removed from succinyl-CoA to produce succinate. The energy released is used to make guanosine triphosphate (GTP) from guanosine diphosphate (GDP) and Pi by substrate-level phosphorylation. GTP can then be used to make ATP. The enzyme succinyl-coA synthase catalyzes this reaction of the citric acid cycle.

$$\text{Succinyl-CoA} + \text{Pi} + \text{GDP} \xrightarrow{\text{Succinyl-CoA synthetase}} \text{Succinate} + \text{GTP} + \text{CoA-SH}$$

Reaction 6: Oxidation of Succinate to Fumarate

Succinate is oxidized to fumarate. During this oxidation, FAD is reduced to $FADH_2$. The enzyme succinate dehydrogenase catalyzes the removal of two hydrogens from succinate.

$$\text{Succinate} + \text{E-FAD} \xrightarrow{\text{Succinate dehydrogenase}} \text{Fumarate} + \text{E-FADH}_2$$

Reaction 7: Hydration of Fumarate to Malate

The reversible hydration of fumarate to L-malate is catalyzed by fumarase (fumarate hydratase).

Fumarase continues the rearrangement process by adding hydrogen and oxygen back into the substrate that had been previously removed.

$$\text{Fumarate} + H_2O \xrightarrow{\text{Fumarase}} \text{L-malate}$$

Reaction 8: Oxidation of Malate to Oxaloacetate

Malate is oxidized to produce oxaloacetate, the starting compound of the citric acid cycle by malate dehydrogenase. During this oxidation, NAD^+ is reduced to NADH and H^+.

Significance of Krebs Cycle

1. Amino acids are formed from α-ketoglutaric acid, pyruvic acids and oxaloacetic acid.
2. Krebs cycle (citric acid cycle) releases plenty of energy (ATP) required for various metabolic activities of cell **(Fig. 8.1)**.
3. By this cycle, carbon skeleton are got, which are used in process of growth and for maintaining the cells.
4. The potential of NADH and $FADH_2$ is converted to more ATP through an electron transport chain with oxygen as the "terminal electron acceptor".*

---

*Number of adenosine triphosphate (ATP) formed from a molecule of glucose.

Section 2: Fundamentals of Biochemistry

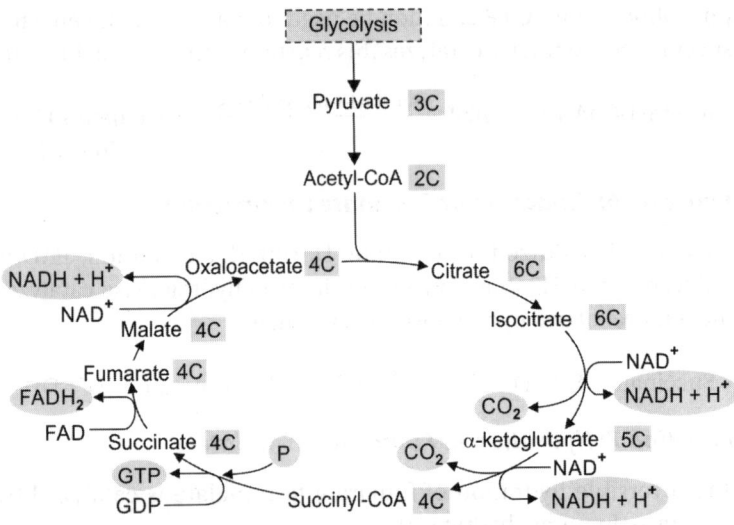

Fig. 8.1: Cyclic representation of TCA cycle.

The stoichiometry of coenzyme reduction and ATP formation in the aerobic oxidation of a molecule of glucose via glycolysis, the pyruvate dehydrogenase reaction, and the citric acid cycle

Reaction	Number of ATP or reduced coenzymes directly formed	Number of ATP ultimately formed*
Glucose to glucose-6-phosphate	−1 ATP	−1
Fructose-6-phosphate to fructose-1,6-bisphosphate	−1 ATP	−1
2 glyceraldehyde-3-phosphate to 2 1,3-bisphosphoglycerate	2 NADH *	6
2 1,3-bisphosphoglycerate to 2 3-phosphoglycerate	2 ATP	2
Phosphoenolpyruvate to 2 pyruvate	2 ATP	2
2 pyruvate to 2 acetyl-CoA	2 NADH *	6
2 isocitrate to α-ketoglutarate	2 NADH*	6
2 α-Ketoglutarate to 2 succinyl-CoA	2 NADH *	6
2 succinyl-CoA to 2 succinate	2 ATP (or 2 GTP)	2
2 succinate to 2 fumarate	2 FADH$_2$ *	4
2 malate to 2 oxaloacetate	2 NADH *	6
Total		38

*One molecule of glucose metabolizes to give 38 ATPs.

COMPARISONS BETWEEN GLYCOLYSIS AND KREBS CYCLE

Glycolysis	Krebs Cycle
It is the first step of respiration yielding two molecules of pyruvic acids after the partial breakdown of a glucose molecule in a set of enzymatic processes	Krebs cycle is the second step of aerobic respiration in which pyruvate is oxidized completely into inorganic substances forming carbon dioxide
Occurs in all the living organisms	Occurs in aerobes
Occurs inside the cytoplasm	Occurs inside the mitochondria
No carbon dioxide evolved	Carbon dioxide evolved
Oxygen not required for glycolysis	Oxygen is required for Krebs cycle
Four adenosine triphosphate (ATP) molecules are produced in the glycolysis for each glucose molecule	One ATP or guanosine triphosphate (GTP) molecule is produced by substrate-level phosphorylation in each turn of the Krebs cycle
Consumes two molecules of ATP for initial phosphorylation of substance molecules	Does not consume ATP
Net gain of two molecules of ATP and two molecules of nicotinamide adenine dinucleotide (NADH) gained for every molecule of glucose broken down	Each turn of the Krebs cycle yields three molecules of NADH and two molecules of flavin adenine dinucleotide ($FADH_2$)
Occurs as a linear sequence	Occurs as a cyclic sequence

Both glycolysis and the Krebs cycle are enzyme-mediated and are under constant regulation based on the energy requirement of the cell/organism. The rates of these processes vary under various conditions, such as the well-fed state, fasting state, exercised state, and starvation state.

DISORDERS OF CARBOHYDRATE METABOLISM

As discussed above, carbohydrates must be broken down by the body into simpler constituents. This process needs many enzymes. If an enzyme needed to process a certain sugar is missing, the sugar can accumulate in the body, causing problems.

- **Glycogen storage diseases:** Glycogen is made of many glucose molecules linked together. The sugar glucose is the body's main source of energy for the muscles (including the heart) and brain. Any glucose that is not used immediately for energy is held in reserve in the liver, muscles, and kidneys in the form of glycogen and is released when needed by the body.

  There are many different glycogen storage diseases (also called glycogenoses), each identified by a roman numeral. These diseases are caused by a hereditary lack of one of the enzymes that is essential to the process of forming glucose into glycogen and breaking down glycogen into glucose. About 1 in 20,000 infants has some form of glycogen storage disease **(Table 8.1)**.
    - *Symptoms:* Some of these diseases cause few symptoms. Others are fatal. The specific symptoms, age at which symptoms start, and their severity vary considerably among these diseases. For types II, V, and VII, the main symptom is usually weakness. For types I, III, and VI, symptoms are low levels of sugar in the blood and protrusion of the abdomen (because excess or abnormal glycogen may enlarge the liver). Low levels of sugar in the blood cause weakness, sweating, confusion, and sometimes seizures and coma. Other consequences for children may include stunted growth, frequent infections, and sores in the mouth and intestines.

      Glycogen storage diseases tend to cause uric acid (a waste product) to accumulate in the joints, which can cause gout, and in the kidneys, which can cause kidney stones). In type I glycogen storage disease, kidney failure is common.
    - *Diagnosis and treatment:* The specific type of glycogen storage disease is diagnosed by examining a piece of muscle or liver tissue under a microscope (biopsy).

      Treatment depends on the type of glycogen storage disease. For most types, eating many small carbohydrate-rich meals everyday helps prevent blood sugar levels from dropping.
- **Galactosemia:** Galactose is a sugar that is present in milk and in some fruits and vegetables. A deficient enzyme or liver dysfunction can alter the metabolism, which can lead to high levels of galactose in the blood (galactosemia). There are different forms of galactosemia, but the most common and the most severe form is referred to as classic galactosemia.

Table 8.1: Types and characteristics of glycogen storage diseases.

Name	Affected organs, tissues, or cells	Symptoms
Type O	Liver or muscle	Episodes of low blood sugar levels (hypoglycemia) during fasting if the liver is affected
von Gierke's disease (type IA)	Liver and kidney	Enlarged liver and kidney, slowed growth, very low blood sugar levels, and abnormally high levels of acid, fats, and uric acid in blood
Type IB	Liver and white blood cells	Same as in von Gierke's disease but may be less severe Low white blood cell count, recurring infections, and inflammatory bowel disease
Pompe's disease (type II)	All organs	Enlarged liver and heart and muscle weakness
Forbes' disease (type III)	Liver, muscle, and heart	Enlarged liver or cirrhosis, low blood sugar levels, muscle damage, heart damage, and weak bones in some people
Andersen's disease (type IV)	Liver, muscle, and most tissues	Cirrhosis, muscle damage, and delayed growth and development
McArdle disease (type V)	Muscle	Muscle cramps or weakness during physical activity
Hers' disease (type VI)	Liver	Enlarged liver Episodes of low blood sugar during fasting Often no symptoms
Tarui's disease (type VII)	Skeletal muscle and red blood cells	Muscle cramps during physical activity and red blood cell destruction (hemolysis)

- *Symptoms:* Newborns with galactosemia seem normal at first but, within a few days or weeks, lose their appetite, vomit, become jaundiced, have diarrhea, and stop growing normally. White blood cell function is affected, and serious infections can

develop. If treatment is delayed, affected children remain short and become intellectually disabled or may die.
  - *Diagnosis:* Galactosemia is detectable with a blood test which detects presence of enzymes needed for metabolism of galactose.
- **Hereditary fructose intolerance:** Hereditary fructose intolerance is caused by lack of the enzyme needed to metabolize fructose. Very small amounts of fructose cause low blood sugar levels and can lead to kidney and liver damage.

  In this disorder, the body is missing an enzyme that allows it to use fructose, a sugar present in table sugar (sucrose) and many fruits. As a result, a by-product of fructose accumulates in the body, blocking the formation of glycogen and its conversion to glucose for use as energy. Ingesting more than tiny amounts of fructose or sucrose causes low blood sugar levels (hypoglycemia), with sweating, confusion, and sometimes seizures and coma. Children who continue to eat foods containing fructose develop kidney and liver damage, resulting in jaundice, vomiting, mental deterioration, seizures, and death.

  For most types of this disorder, early diagnosis and dietary restrictions started early in infancy can help prevent these more serious problems.

  The diagnosis is made when a chemical examination of a sample of liver tissue determines that the enzyme is missing.
- **Mucopolysaccharidoses:** Complex sugar molecules called mucopolysaccharides are essential parts of many body tissues. In mucopolysaccharidoses, the body lacks enzymes needed to break down and store mucopolysaccharides. As a result, excess mucopolysaccharides enter the blood and are deposited in abnormal locations throughout the body.

  During infancy and childhood, short stature, hairiness, and abnormal development become noticeable. The face may appear coarse. Some types of mucopolysaccharidoses cause intellectual disability to develop over several years. In some types, vision or hearing may become impaired. The arteries or heart valves can be affected. Finger joints are often stiff.

  A doctor usually bases the diagnosis on the symptoms and a physical examination. The presence of a mucopolysaccharidosis in other family members also suggests the diagnosis. Urine tests may help but are sometimes inaccurate. X-rays may show characteristic bone abnormalities.

- **Disorders of pyruvate metabolism:** Pyruvate is a substance that is formed in the processing of carbohydrates and proteins and that serves as an energy source for cells. Problems with pyruvate metabolism can limit a cell's ability to produce energy and allow a buildup of lactic acid, a waste product. Many enzymes are involved in pyruvate metabolism. A hereditary deficiency in any one of these enzymes results in one of a variety of disorders, depending on which enzyme is missing. Symptoms may develop any time between early infancy and late adulthood. Exercise and infections can worsen symptoms, leading to severe lactic acidosis. These disorders are diagnosed by measuring enzyme activity in cells from the liver or skin.
- **Pyruvate dehydrogenase complex deficiency:** This disorder is caused by a lack of a group of enzymes needed to process pyruvate. This deficiency results in a variety of symptoms, ranging from mild to severe. Some newborns with this deficiency have brain malformations. Other children appear normal at birth but develop symptoms, including weak muscles, seizures, poor coordination, and a severe balance problem, later in infancy or childhood. Intellectual disability is common.

  This disorder cannot be cured, but some children are helped by a diet that is high in fat and low in carbohydrates.
- **Absence of pyruvate carboxylase:** Pyruvate carboxylase is an enzyme. A lack of this enzyme causes a very rare condition that interferes with or blocks the production of glucose from pyruvate in the body. Lactic acid and ketones build up in the blood. Often, this disease is fatal. Children who survive have seizures and severe intellectual disability, although there are recent reports of children with milder symptoms. There is no cure, but some children are helped by eating frequent carbohydrate-rich meals and restricting dietary protein.

BIOCHEMICAL IMPORTANCE OF CARBOHYDRATE

1. Carbohydrates are important constituents of the cell structure in the form of glycolipid, glycoproteins, heparin, cellulose, starch and glycogen.

2. Carbohydrates serve as an important source and store of energy.
3. Carbohydrates play important role in metabolism of amino acids and fatty acids.
4. Lactose promotes the growth of desirable bacteria in the small intestine. It also increases calcium absorption.
5. They protect friction surfaces, such as blood vessels, trachea, etc. against mechanical damage.
6. It plays an important role in maintaining osmotic and ionic regulation of body.
7. It works as an intracellular cementing material.
8. It spares protein.
9. Heparin is a carbohydrate, which works as an anticoagulant in body.

SUMMARY

- Carbohydrates are defined as polyhydroxy aldehydes and ketones and their derivatives.
- These are the simplest members of carbohydrate, grouped according to the number of carbon atoms present.
- Oligosaccharides are compound sugars that yield 2–10 molecules of the same or different monosaccharides on hydrolysis.
- Polysaccharides contain >10 monosaccharide units and can be hundreds of sugar units in length.
- Carbohydrates on dehydration give furfural or its derivatives.
- Carbohydrates having free carbonyl group act as reducing agent.
- Metabolism of a substance is a series of biochemical reactions occurring within the living organism.
- The rate of production of energy at basal conditions per hour per meter square of body surface area is called basal metabolic rate.
- Calorie is the unit of energy.
- In the process of digestion, carbohydrates are converted to monosaccharides, mainly as glucose, fructose, and galactose.
- Glycogenesis is the synthesis of glycogen from glucose.
- Gluconeogenesis is the formation of glucose from noncarbohydrates as glycerol.
- Glycolysis is the oxidative pathway of glycogen or glucose. It turns glucose into pyruvate, so it can enter into the Krebs cycle to produce more energy and generate ATP (energy) in the process.
- Overall, the process of glycolysis produces a net gain of two pyruvate molecules, two ATP molecules, and two NADH molecules for the cell to use for energy.

Chapter 8: Study of Carbohydrates

- Tricarboxylic acid cycle (TCA) cycle is a cyclic sequence of reactions in which pyruvate formed in glycolysis is completely oxidized to CO_2 and H_2O.
- Each turn of the cycle forms three NADH molecules and one $FADH_2$ molecule, one ATP and three H^+.
- Hexose monophosphate shunt is alternative to glycolysis and citric acid cycle for oxidation of glucose.
- Any glucose that is not used immediately for energy is held in reserve in the liver, muscles, and kidneys in the form of glycogen.
- There are many different glycogen storage diseases each identified by a roman numeral (also called glycogeneses).
- These diseases are caused by a hereditary lack of one of the enzymes that is essential to the process of forming glucose into glycogen and breaking down glycogen into glucose.
- A deficient enzyme or liver dysfunction can alter the metabolism of galactose, which can lead to high levels of galactose in the blood (galactosemia).
- Hereditary fructose intolerance is caused by lack of the enzyme needed to metabolize fructose.
- In mucopolysaccharidoses, the body lacks enzymes needed to break down and store mucopolysaccharides.
- Problems with pyruvate metabolism can limit a cell's ability to produce energy and allow a buildup of lactic acid.
- Carbohydrates serve as an important source and store of energy.
- These are important constituents of the cell structure.
- Carbohydrates play an important role in maintaining osmotic and ionic regulation of body.

PRACTICE QUESTIONS

1. What are carbohydrates? Write a note on its classification.
2. What are the chemical properties of carbohydrates? Discuss any three detection tests based on it.
3. Define Metabolism, Basal metabolic rate, Calorie, Anabolism, and Catabolism.
4. With the help of a flowchart, discuss the various steps involved in glycolysis.
5. Give an account of glycolysis. Where does it occur? What is the end product? Trace the fate of these products in both aerobic and anaerobic respiration.
6. With the help of a flowchart, discuss the cyclic events involved in Krebs cycle.
7. Mention the significance of Krebs cycle.
8. Compare the process of glycolysis and Krebs cycle.
9. What is glycogen? Write a note on glycogen storage diseases.

10. What is hereditary fructose intolerance? Discuss the cause, symptom, diagnosis, and treatment of the disorder.
11. What are mucopolysaccharides? Discuss the condition associated with mucopolysaccharidoses.
12. Why pyruvate metabolism is important? Discuss the disorders associated with it.
13. Enlist the biochemical importance of carbohydrates.

Study of Proteins

CHAPTER 9

Keywords
Simple protein, conjugated proteins, derived proteins, Biuret test, trichloroacetic acid (TCA) test, importance of NADPH, urea cycle, kwashiorkor, marasmus, phenylketonuria (PKU), maple syrup urine disease, homocystinuria, deficiency of G6PD, thiamine deficiency, biochemical importance of proteins codons, transcription, translation transamination, deamination, urea cycle

Proteins are one of the chief constituents of all living organisms. Proteins are defined as high molecular weight mixed polymers of α-amino acids joined together with peptide linkage (CO-NH).

The total numbers of amino acids, the sequence in which amino acids are arranged and the overall three-dimensional structure of the molecule is characteristic of each protein and is responsible for its biological activity.

■ CLASSIFICATIONS

Proteins can be classified on the basis of their solubility and composition as follows **(Flowchart 9.1)**:
1. **Simple protein:** These proteins on hydrolysis yield α-amino acids and their derivatives. They are subdivided on the basis of solubility into following groups:
    a. *Albumins:* These are water-soluble proteins, which coagulates on heating, e.g. egg albumin, serum albumin.
    b. *Globulin:* These proteins are insoluble in water and soluble in dilute salt solution.
    c. *Glutelins:* These proteins are insoluble in water and soluble in dilute acids and alkalies. These are mostly found in plants, e.g. glutenin (wheat) and oryzenin (rice).

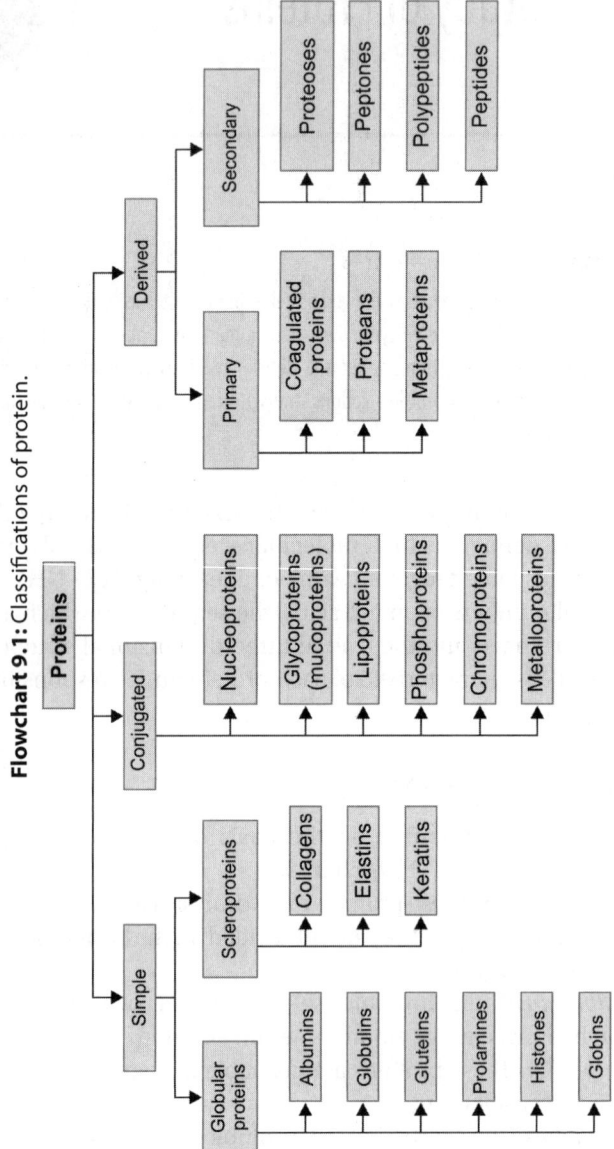

Flowchart 9.1: Classifications of protein.

d. *Prolamins:* These proteins are insoluble in water and soluble in 70 percent alcohol, e.g. zein (corn) and gliadin (wheat).
e. *Scleroproteins:* These proteins are structural and protective in function. These are insoluble in all solvents, e.g. keratin (horn, nail, hoof and feathers), collagen (bone and skin).

2. **Conjugated proteins:** Conjugated proteins are those which on hydrolysis yield a non-protein substance called as prosthetic group. These are subdivided on the basis of prosthetic group attached to proteins.
   a. *Nucleoproteins:* These proteins occur in combination with nucleic acids, e.g. deoxyribonucleoproteins and nucleohistones.
   b. *Phosphoproteins:* These proteins contain phosphorus radical as a prosthetic group, e.g. casein (milk) and vitellin (egg yolk).
   c. *Glycoproteins:* These contain carbohydrate as a prosthetic group, e.g. mucin (saliva) and ovomucoid (egg white).
   d. *Porphyrinoproteins:* These are proteins which have porphyrin (with a metal ion) as their prosthetic group, e.g. hemoglobin (Fe— iron is prosthetic group).
   e. *Lipoproteins:* Lipoproteins are combination of proteins with lipids, such as fatty acids, cholesterol, etc. (e.g. α and β lipoproteins of blood).
   f. *Flavoproteins:* These are the proteins which have riboflavin as their prosthetic group.
   g. *Metalloproteins:* These are the proteins which have metal ions as their prosthetic group, e.g. ceruloplasmin (Cu).

3. **Derived proteins:** These are the proteins which arise as a result of partial hydrolysis of proteins or due to removal of prosthetic group or due to other changes in the molecule.
   These proteins have been subclassified as follows:
   a. *Primary derived proteins:* These are denatured forms of various proteins formed by action of dilute acids/enzymes/or water. For example, metaproteins are formed by the action of slightly stronger acids and alkalies, e.g. myosan. Coagulated proteins are formed by the action of heat, X-rays, UV-rays and alcohol (e.g. coagulated albumin).
   b. *Secondary derived proteins:* These proteins are formed due to the hydrolytic cleavage of peptide bonds in proteins, e.g. peptones, peptides.

■ DETECTIVE TESTS FOR PROTEINS

1. **Heat test:** When a protein solution is heated in a boiling water bath, the proteins get coagulated and loose their biological activity, e.g. boiling of eggs.
2. **Test with trichloroacetic acid (TCA):** TCA denatures the protein. It is normally used to precipitate proteins from their solution.
3. **Biuret test:** Biuret reagent consists of copper sulfate in an alkaline medium. When proteins are treated with biuret reagent, it shows violet color.
4. **Hydrolysis test:** Protein on hydrolysis gives free amino acids. Hydrolysis can be carried out by acids like HCl, H_2SO_4, etc. or alkalies like NaOH, KOH, etc.
5. **Xanthoproteic test:** Nitration of aromatic amino acids of proteins gives yellow color. Concentrated nitric acid can be used for nitration.
6. **Millon's test:** Phenolic group of tyrosine of proteins react with mercuric sulfate in the presence of sodium nitrite and sulfuric acid to give red color.
7. **Precipitation test:** Proteins are precipitated by using different agents, e.g. salts like sodium chloride, ammonium sulphate, organic solvents like acetone, alcohol, heavy metals like Cu, mercury salts acids like TCA, HCl, CH_3COOH.

■ METABOLISM OF PROTEIN

During digestion, proteins are converted into their constituent amino acids by the action of various proteolytic enzymes. Amino acids are then absorbed into blood and transported to the liver. They are used in the body to synthesize new proteins for growth and repair.

Protein Synthesis

Protein synthesis is process of synthesis of proteins within the cells. The process involves two major steps—Transcription and Translation. This process involves important role of DNA and RNA (**Fig. 9.1**).

The Genetic Code

DNA provides instruction for making amino acids or forms a polypeptide chain (proteins-enzymes). The sequence of the bases

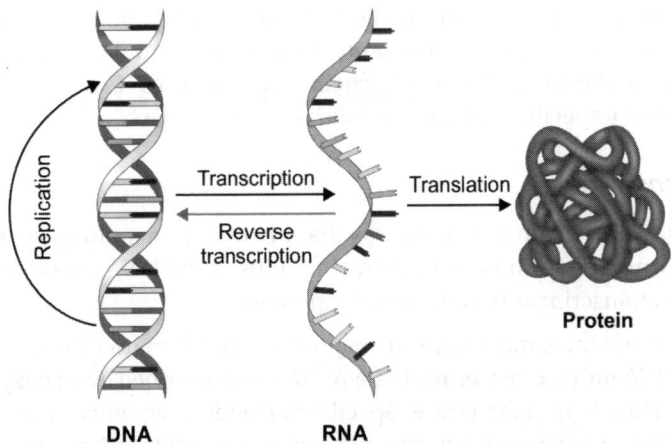

Fig. 9.1: Role of DNA and RNA in protein synthesis.
(For color version, see Plate 3)

A, C, G and T, in DNA determines unique genetic code and provides the instructions needed to make the proteins and molecules essential for our growth, development, and health. The cell reads the DNA code in groups of three bases. Each triplet of bases, also called a codon, specifies which amino acid will be added next during protein synthesis.

For example:
- Triplets on DNA e.g. CAC TCA
- Codons on mRNA e.g. GUG AGU
- Anticodons on tRNA e.g. CAC UCA
  (must be complementary to the codon of mRNA)

Each triplet codes for one amino acid. Single amino acid may have up to 6 different triplets for it due to the redundancy of the code (code is degenerate). Some amino acids are coded by more than one codon. The code is universal. That is, same triplet code will give the same amino acid in virtually all organisms. The codes are nonoverlapping. That is, no base of one triplet contributes to part of the code next to it.

We have 64 possible combinations of the 4 bases in triplets. There are 20 different amino acids, which are the building blocks of proteins. Different proteins are made up of different combinations of amino acids. This gives them their own unique 3D structure and function in the body. Out of 64 of 61 codons are used to specify the 20 amino acids. For example, ATG = methionine.

There are three codons that do not code for an amino acid. These codons mark the end of the protein and stop the addition of amino acids to the end of the protein chain. These are UAA UAG UGA. Also there is a specific codon to start the process e.g. AUG.

Transcription

DNA transcription is a process that involves transcribing genetic information from DNA to RNA. The transcribed DNA message, or RNA transcript, is used to produce proteins.

There are three main steps to the process of DNA transcription:
1. **RNA polymerase binds to DNA:** DNA is transcribed by an enzyme called RNA polymerase. Specific nucleotide sequences indicate RNA polymerase where to begin and where to end. RNA polymerase attaches to the DNA at a specific area called the promoter region. The DNA in the promoter region contains specific sequences that allow RNA polymerase to bind to the DNA.
2. **Elongation:** Certain enzymes called transcription factors unwind a section of the double stranded DNA helix and break the bonds between the complementary base-pairs in the unwinded section. This allows RNA polymerase to transcribe only a single strand of DNA into a single stranded RNA polymer called messenger RNA (mRNA). The strand that serves as the template is called the antisense strand. The strand that is not transcribed is called the sense strand.

   Like DNA, RNA is composed of nucleotide bases. RNA, however, contains the nucleotides adenine, guanine, cytosine and uracil (U). When RNA polymerase transcribes the DNA, guanine pairs with cytosine (G-C) and adenine pairs with uracil (A-U). For example, if part of one strand of the unravelled DNA reads GATCAT, the complementary mRNA sequence will read CUAGUA.
3. **Termination:** RNA polymerase moves along the DNA until it reaches a terminator sequence. At that point, RNA polymerase releases the mRNA polymer and detaches from the DNA.

   Finally, after the complementary mRNA is made, the section of DNA is rewound into its original double helix conformation.

Translation

Since proteins are constructed in the cytoplasm of the cell, mRNA must cross the nuclear membrane to reach the cytoplasm cells. Once in the cytoplasm, ribosomes and another RNA molecule called transfer RNA work together to translate mRNA into a protein. This process is called translation **(Fig. 9.2)**.

Ribosomes, carry out protein synthesis, attach themselves to the mRNA strand and move down, reading the sequence of nucleotides and putting together the appropriate protein as they move. The first set of 3 nucleotides the ribosome will read is always AUG. This is because the AUG sequence serves start codon, telling the ribosome to "start reading here."

As the ribosome proceeds along the mRNA, it adds the appropriate amino acid to the growing chain correspond each set of three nucleotides that code for a specific amino acid is called a codon. All 20 amino acids used to make biological proteins have at least one corresponding codon. For example, the codon GCA codes for an amino acid called alanine. And the codon AAU codes for an amino acid called asparagine. Therefore, a portion of an mRNA sequence that reads: AUG GCA AAU will result in the following string of amino acids: methionine-alanine-asparagine.

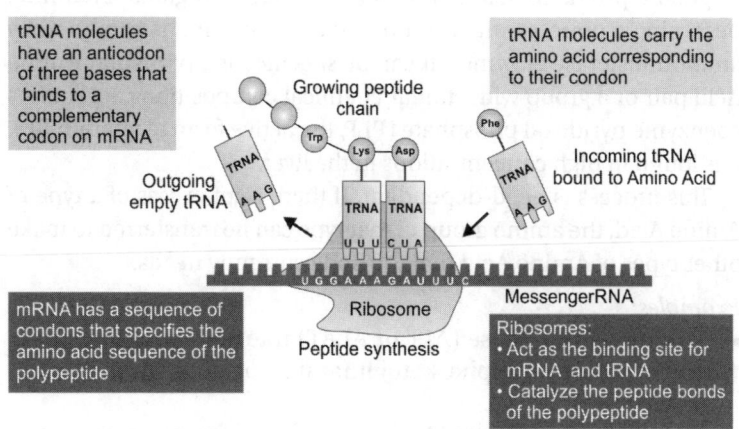

Fig. 9.2: Translation—key components that enable genetic code to synthesize polypeptides.
(For color version, see Plate 3)

By reading the entire mRNA sequence, the ribosome constructs a long chain of amino acids, which make up the protein.

Proteins can be manufactured in large quantities because a single DNA sequence can be transcribed by many RNA polymerase molecules at once.

Catabolism of Proteins

Unlike carbohydrates and triglycerides, which are stored, proteins cannot be stored for later use. In fact, any amino acid which is not needed for immediate biosynthetic needs is deaminated and the carbon skeleton is used as a metabolic fuel.

The amino acids undergo certain common reactions like transamination followed by deamination for the liberation of ammonia. Ammonia then enters in urea cycle for complete degradation of proteins with non toxic product, which is urea.

Transamination

Transamination is the transfer of an amino group from an alpha-Amino Acid to an alpha-keto acid, which is an Amino Acid with an alpha-keto group (=O). The original Amino Acid loses an amino group and gains a keto group, becoming an alpha-keto acid. The original alpha-keto acid loses its keto group and gains an amino, becoming a nonessential Amino Acid. The reaction is catalyzed by aminotransferase enzymes. It can be specific for a particular Amino Acid pair or a group with similar chemical compositions. It requires coenzyme pyridoxal phosphate (PLP, the active form of vitamin B6). It is found in high concentrations in the liver.

This process is need-dependent. If there is an excess of a type of Amino Acid, the amino group of that type can be transferred to make other types of Amino Acid that the body currently needs.

Examples:
- Alanine transaminase (ALT or ALAT) transfers an amino group from alanine to alpha-ketoglutarate, forming pyruvate and glutamate.
- Aspartate transaminase (AST or ASAT) transfers an amino group from aspartate to alpha-ketoglutarate, forming oxaloacetate and glutamate.

Both are reversible reactions.

Deamination

The removal of amino group from the amino acids as NH_3 is deamination. It results in the liberation of ammonia for urea synthesis. Simultaneously, the carbon skeleton of amino acids is converted to keto acids.

Deamination may be either oxidative or non-oxidative.

Oxidative Deamination

Oxidative deamination is the liberation of free ammonia from the amino group of amino acids coupled with oxidation. This takes place mostly in liver and kidney.

Role of glutamate dehydrogenase : In the process of transamination as well as deamination, glutamate acts as the central molecule.

Glutamate rapidly undergoes oxidative deamination, catalysed by glutamate dehydrogenase (GDH) to liberate ammonia. This enzyme is unique in that it can utilize either NAD+ or NADP+ as a coenzyme. Conversion of glutamate to α-ketoglutarate occurs through the formation of an intermediate, α-iminoglutarate.

After ingestion of a protein-rich meal, liver glutamate level is elevated. It is converted to α-ketoglutarate with liberation of NH_3. Further, when the cellular energy levels are low, the degradation of glutamate is increased to provide α-ketoglutarate which enters TCA cycle to liberate energy.

Example: Oxidative deamination by amino acid oxidases.

L-Amino acid oxidase and D-amino acid oxidase are flavoproteins, possessing FMN and FAD, respectively. They act on the corresponding amino acids (L or D) to produce α-keto acids and NH_3. In this reaction, oxygen is reduced to H_2O_2, which is later decomposed by catalase **(Fig. 9.3)**.

Non-oxidative Deamination

Some of the amino acids can be deaminated to liberate NH_3 without undergoing oxidation.

a. **Amino acid dehydrases:** Serine, threonine and homoserine are the hydroxy amino acids. They undergo non-oxidative deamination catalysed by PLP-dependent dehydrases (dehydratases).

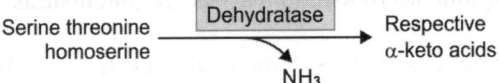

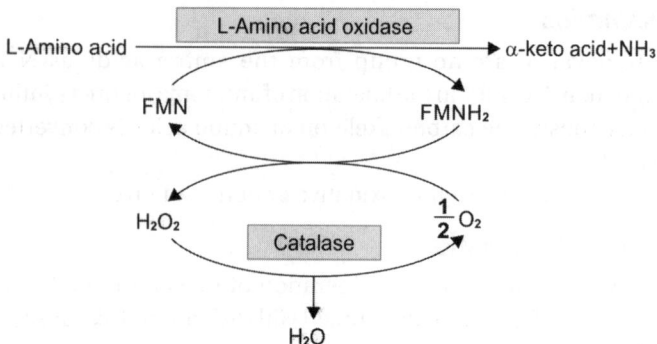

Fig. 9.3: Oxidative deamination of amino acids.

b. **Amino acid desulfhydrases:** The sulfur amino acids, namely cysteine and homocysteine, undergo deamination coupled with desulfhydration to give keto acids.

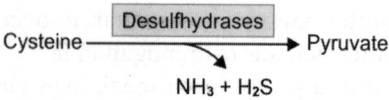

c. **Deamination of histidine:** The enzyme histidase acts on histidine to liberate NH_3 by non-oxidative deamination process.

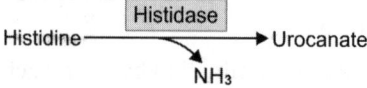

Urea Cycle

Ammonia (NH_3), the product of deamination reaction, is toxic even in small amount and must be removed from the body. Urea cycle is the conversion reactions of ammonia to urea **(Fig. 9.4)**. This reaction occur in liver (certain occur in cytosol and mitochondria). The urea is then transferred to kidney where it is then excreted. Urea cycle involves following reactions:

Step 1: Formation of carbamoyl phosphate from ammonia (NH_3) and bicarbonates (HCO^{-3})/Carbon dioxide (CO_2) using ATP as energy source. It occurs in the mitochondria, catalyzed by carbamoyl phosphate synthetase, and requires N-acetylglutamate as an activator and 2 ATP.

$$HCO^{-3} + NH_3 + 2ATP \rightarrow \text{Carbamoyl phosphate} + 2ADP + P_i$$

Chapter 9: Study of Proteins

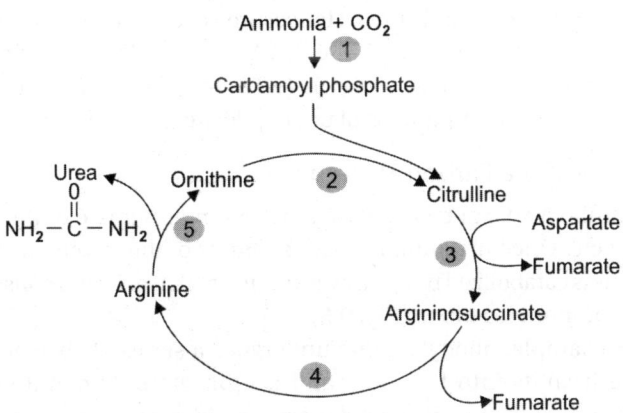

Fig. 9.4: Urea cycle.

Step 2: Transfer of carbamoyl group (O=C–NH$_2$) to ornithine to produce citrulline. It occurs in the mitochondria, catalyzed by ornithine carbamoyltransferase

Carbamoyl phosphate + Ornithine → Citrulline + P$_i$

Step 3: Removal of second urea nitrogen from ASP.
It occurs in the cytosol, catalyzed by argininosuccinate synthetase, requires 1 ATP

Citrulline + Aspartate → Argininosuccinate

Step 4: Elimination of arginine from the aspartate carbon skeleton to form fumarate.

Argininosuccinate → Arginine + Fumarate

It occurs in the cytosol, catalyzed by argininosuccinate lyase. Fumarate either enters the CAC (TCA) or transforms into oxaloacetate, which can be turned into aspartate and re-enter the urea cycle.

Step 5: Hydrolysis of arginine to yield urea and regenerate ornithine. It occurs in cytosol, catalyzed by arginase. End product urea enters the bloodstream. Ornithine is transported back into the mitochondrial matrix for step 2.

Net Reaction Per Cycle

NH$_4$ + CO$_2$ + Asparate + 3ATP → Urea + Fumarate + 2ADP + 2P$_i$ + AMP + PP$_i$

The urea cycle brings two amino groups and HCO$_3$ together to form urea. Thus toxic, insoluble ammonia is converted into non-toxic, water soluble, excretable urea. Hence, urea cycle disposes two waste products i.e. NH_4 and HCO_3^-. Though 3 ATPs are utilized, the ultimate cost of making a molecule of urea is 4 ATPs (one ATP is converted into AMP). The rate limiting steps of urea cycle are 1, 2, and 5

The Fate of the Carbon Skeleton

Any amino acid can be converted into an intermediate of the citric acid cycle. Once the amino group is removed, the α-keto acid that remains is catabolized by a pathway unique to that acid and consisting of one or more reactions **(Fig. 9.5)**.

For example, phenylalanine undergoes a series of six reactions before it splits into fumarate and acetoacetate. Fumarate is an intermediate in the citric acid cycle, while acetoacetate must be converted to acetoacetyl-coenzyme A (CoA) and then to acetyl-CoA before it enters the citric acid cycle.

Those amino acids that can form any of the intermediates of carbohydrate metabolism can subsequently be converted to glucose via a metabolic pathway known as gluconeogenesis. Gluconeogenesis is the synthesis of glucose from non-carbohydrate sources. These amino acids are called glucogenic amino acids.

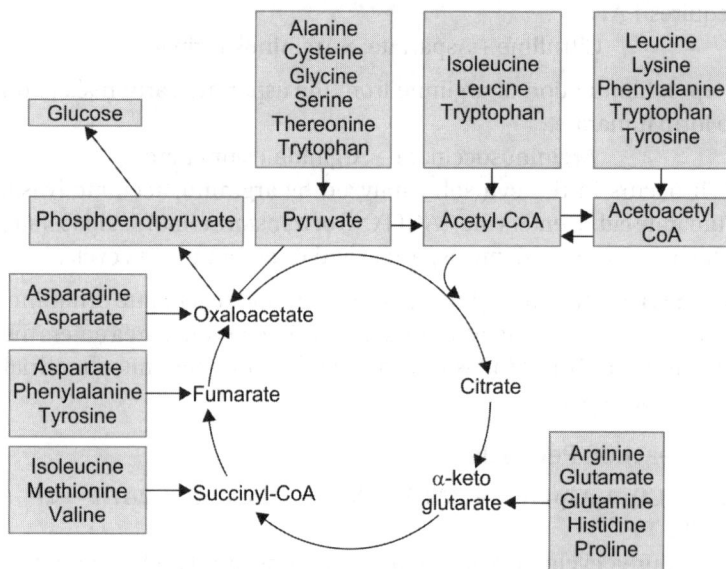

Fig. 9.5: Fates of the carbon skeletons of amino acids.

Amino acids that are converted to acetoacetyl-CoA or acetyl-CoA, which can be used for the synthesis of ketone bodies but not glucose, are called ketogenic amino acids.

Some amino acids fall into both categories. Leucine and lysine are the only amino acids that are exclusively ketogenic. Figure summarizes the ultimate fates of the carbon skeletons of the 20 amino acids.

■ DISEASES RELATED TO PROTEIN METABOLISM

Deficiency Diseases of Protein

Deficiency diseases of protein are caused by inadequate intake of proteins. Protein energy malnutrition (PEM) is generally reported in children of growing age. This causes two types of diseases:

i. **Kwashiorkor:** It is a protein deficiency disease. It is the most widely spread kind of malnutrition. It commonly affects infants and children between 1 to 3 years of age.

   The common symptoms of kwashiorkor are underweight, stunted growth, poor brain development, loss of appetite, anemia, protruding belly, slender legs and bulging eyes. Edema of lower legs and face and change in skin and hair color may also occur in kwashiorkor.

   The basic causes of disease are protein deficient or inadequate diet due to ignorance and poverty and infectious diseases, such as diarrhea, measles, respiratory infections, intestinal worms, which weaken the child. Other contributory factors include ill spacing of children, large family, poor mental health, early termination of breastfeeding, late introduction of supplementary diet, etc.

ii. **Marasmus:** This form of a disease affects infants under one year of age. Marasmus is caused by simultaneous deficiency of protein and total caloric value, which is deficiency of all nutrients. This is the case when mother's milk is replaced too early or mother conceives before her infant is ready.

   Due to protein deficient diet, stored fats and tissue proteins are used as sources of energy. This impairs physical growth and retards mental development. Subcutaneous fat disappears, ribs became very prominent, limbs become thin and skin becomes dry, thin and wrinkled. There is emaciation (extreme leanness) and loss of weight. Digestion and absorption of food stop due to atrophy of digestive glands and intestinal mucosa. This leads to diarrhea.

Hereditary Disorders

Amino acids are the building blocks of proteins and have many functions in the body. Hereditary disorders of amino acid processing can result from defects either in the breakdown of amino acids or in the body's ability to get amino acids into cells. Because these disorders cause symptoms early in life, newborns are routinely screened for several common ones like phenylketonuria, maple syrup urine disease, homocystinuria, tyrosinemia and a number of other inherited disorders.

Phenylketonuria (PKU)

Phenylketonuria (PKU) is a disorder that causes a buildup of the amino acid phenylalanine, which is an essential amino acid that cannot be synthesized in the body but is present in food. Excess phenylalanine is normally converted to tyrosine, another amino acid and eliminated from the body. Without the enzyme that converts it to tyrosine, phenylalanine builds up in the blood and is toxic to the brain, causing intellectual disability.

Symptoms: Newborns with PKU rarely have symptoms right away, although sometimes they are sleepy or eat poorly. If not treated, affected infants progressively develop intellectual disability over the first few years of life, eventually becoming severe. Other symptoms include seizures, nausea and vomiting, an eczema-like rash, lighter skin and hair than their family members, aggressive or self-injurious behavior, hyperactivity and sometimes psychiatric symptoms. Untreated children often give off a mousy body and urine odor as a result of a by-product of phenylalanine (phenylacetic acid) in their urine and sweat.

Diagnosis: PKU is usually diagnosed with a routine screening test.

PKU occurs in most ethnic groups. If PKU runs in the family and DNA is available from an affected family member, amniocentesis or chorionic villus sampling with DNA analysis can be done to determine whether a fetus has the disorder.

Maple Syrup Urine Disease

Maple syrup urine disease is caused by lack of the enzyme needed to metabolize amino acids. By-products of these amino acids cause the urine to smell like maple syrup.

Children with maple syrup urine disease are unable to metabolize certain amino acids. By-products of these amino acids build up, causing neurologic changes, including seizures and intellectual disability. These by-products also cause body fluids, such as urine and sweat, to smell like maple syrup.

There are many forms of maple syrup urine disease. In the most severe form, infants develop neurologic abnormalities, including seizures and coma, during the first week of life and can die within days to weeks. In the milder forms, children initially appear normal but during infection, surgery, or other physical stress, they can develop vomiting, staggering, confusion and coma.

Infants with severe disease are treated with dialysis. Some children with mild disease benefit from injections of vitamin B_1 (thiamine). After the disease has been brought under control, children must always consume a special artificial diet that is low in three amino acids (leucine, isoleucine, and valine). During times of physical stress or flare-ups, it may be necessary to monitor blood tests and give fluids by vein.

Homocystinuria

Homocystinuria is caused by lack of the enzyme needed to metabolize homocysteine. This disorder can cause a number of symptoms, including decreased vision and skeletal abnormalities.

Children with homocystinuria are unable to metabolize the amino acid homocysteine, which along with certain toxic by-products, builds up to cause a variety of symptoms. Symptoms may be mild or severe, depending on the particular enzyme defect.

Infants with this disorder are normal at birth. The first symptoms, including dislocation of the lens of the eye, causing severely decreased vision, usually begin after 3 years of age. Most children have skeletal abnormalities, including osteoporosis. Children are usually tall and thin with a curved spine, chest deformities, elongated limbs, and long, spider-like fingers. Without early diagnosis and treatment, mental (psychiatric) and behavioral disorders and intellectual disability are common. Homocystinuria makes the blood more likely to clot spontaneously, resulting in strokes, high blood pressure, and many other serious problems.

A test measuring enzyme function in liver or skin cells confirms the diagnosis.

Tyrosinemia

Tyrosinemia is caused by lack of the enzyme needed to metabolize tyrosine. The most common form of this disorder mostly affects the liver and the kidneys.

There are two main types of tyrosinemia: Type I and type II.
1. **Type I tyrosinemia:** Children with this disorder typically become ill sometime within the first year of life with dysfunction of the liver, kidneys, and nerves, resulting in irritability, rickets, or even liver failure and death. Restriction of tyrosine in the diet is of little help. Often, children with type I tyrosinemia require a liver transplant.
2. **Type II tyrosinemia** is less common. Affected children sometimes have intellectual disability and frequently develop sores on the skin and eyes.

Deficiency of G6PD

It is an inherited sex-linked trait. It is more severe in RBC. Decreased activity of G6PD impairs the synthesis of NADPH in RBC. This results in the accumulation of methemoglobin and peroxides in erythrocytes leading to hemolysis.

The deficiency is manifested only when exposed to certain drugs or toxins, e.g. intake of antimalarial drug like primaquine and ingestion of fava beans (favism) and sulpha drugs also precipitate the hemolysis.

Some patients developed severe symptoms like—jaundice, decrease in Hb, and destruction of RBCs. In deficiency of G6PD, Hb can no longer be maintained in the reduced form. Hb molecules then cross-link with one another to form aggregates called Heinz bodies on membranes. Membranes damaged by the Heinz bodies and ROS become deformed and the cell undergo lysis, hemolytic anemia.

G6PD deficiency is associated with resistance to malaria (caused by plasmodium infection).

Thiamine Deficiency

The transketolase activity is measured in RBCs is an index of the thiamine status of an individual. The occurrence and manifestation of Wernicke-Korsakoff syndrome (encephalopathy) which is seen in alcoholics and those with thiamine deficiency is due to a genetic defect in the enzyme transketolase. The symptoms include mental disorder, loss of memory and partial paralysis.

■ BIOCHEMICAL IMPORTANCE OF PROTEINS

1. Protein is one of the important components of diet. It is required to maintain growth and healthy function of the body.
2. Proteins are structural component of protoplasm, cells and tissues.
3. Enzymes and few hormones are proteinous in nature.
4. Antibodies, hemoglobin are also protein. Protein play important role in cell-mediated immunity mechanism.
5. Blood clotting is formed by protein-fibrinogen.
6. Protein may serve as mechanical support to biological structures, e.g. keratin, collagen.
7. The nerve impulses are transmitted through synapse, with the help of receptor proteins.
8. Many hormones are protein, e.g. insulin.

SUMMARY

- Proteins are defined as high molecular weight mixed polymers of α amino acids joined together with peptide (CO-NH) linkage.
- Proteins are classified on the basis of their solubility and composition.
- Simple proteins on hydrolysis yield α amino acids and their derivatives.
- Conjugated proteins on hydrolysis yield a nonprotein substance called as prosthetic group.
- Derived proteins are the proteins which arise as a result of partial hydrolysis of proteins or due to removal of prosthetic group or due to other changes in the molecule.
- On the basis of hydrolysis and denaturation properties, proteins can be detected by different tests, such as Biuret test, xanthoproteic test, and Millon's test.

- Intermediate products of glycolysis, the citric acid cycle, and the pentose phosphate pathway can be used to make all 20 amino acids.
- Urea cycle that occurs in liver is the conversion reactions of ammonia to urea at the cost of four adenosine triphosphates (ATPs).
- Kwashiorkor is a protein-deficiency disease, affecting children between 1 and 3 years of age, it is the most widely spread kind of malnutrition.
- Marasmus affects infants under 1 year of age. It is caused by simultaneous deficiency of protein and all nutrients.
- Phenylketonuria (PKU) is a disorder that causes a buildup of the amino acid phenylalanine. It is toxic to the brain, causing intellectual disability.
- Maple syrup urine disease is caused by lack of the enzyme needed to metabolize amino acids.
- Homocystinuria is caused by lack of the enzyme needed to metabolize homocysteine. This disorder can cause decreased vision and skeletal abnormalities.
- Tyrosinemia is caused by lack of the enzyme needed to metabolize tyrosine. It mostly affects the liver and the kidneys.
- Deficiency of glucose-6-phosphate dehydrogenase (G6PD) is an inherited sex-linked trait. It impairs the synthesis of NADPH in red blood cells (RBCs).
- Thiamine deficiency is due to a genetic defect in the enzyme, transketolase. The symptoms include mental disorder, loss of memory, and partial paralysis.
- Proteins perform important functions like to maintain growth, blood clotting, structural component of protoplasm, etc.
- Enzymes and few hormones are proteinous in nature.
- mRNA provides a template for gene coding during protein synthesis, tRNA carries the amino acids to the ribosomes, which has to be added to the polypeptide chain and rRNA forms ribosomes along with proteins.
- DNA transcription is a process that involves transcribing genetic information from DNA to RNA.
- Ribosomes and transfer RNA work together to translate mRNA into a protein. This process is called translation
- Transamination is the transfer of an amino group from an alpha-Amino Acid to an alpha-keto acid, which is an Amino Acid with an alpha-keto group (=O).
- The removal of amino group from the amino acids as NH_3 is deamination.
- Urea cycle is the conversion reactions of ammonia to urea.

PRACTICE QUESTIONS

1. What are proteins? Discuss its classification in detail.
2. Write any four detective tests for proteins.
3. With the help of a flowchart, explain HMP shunt pathway.
4. Discuss the role of NADPH in the body.

5. What is the importance of urea cycle? With the help of a cyclic representation, discuss its steps.
6. Compare between kwashiorkor and marasmus.
7. Write a note on:
    i. Phenylketonuria
    ii. Maple syrup urine disease
    iii. Homocystinuria
    iv. Tyrosinemia
    vi. Deficiency of G6PD
    vii. Thiamine deficiency
8. Justify—biochemically, proteins are very important molecule.
9. What is meant by a codon? Describe its role in protein synthesis.
10. Discuss the process of DNA transcription in detail.
11. Discuss the process of translation in detail.
12. What is transamination? Explain with example.
13. What is deamination? Discuss its type.
14. With a cyclic representation, explain urea cycle.
15. What happens to carbon skeleton during catabolism of protein?

Study of Lipids

Keywords
Fatty acids, waxes, phospholipids, glycolipid, lipoproteins steroid, rancidity emulsification, beta-oxidation, lipogenesis, steatorrhea, Gaucher disease, Tay–Sachs disease, Niemann–Pick disease, Fabry disease, MCAD deficiency, Wolman disease, sitosterolemia, Refsum disease, biochemical importance of lipids

■ INTRODUCTION

Lipids include a diverse group of compounds which include fats, oils, steroids, waxes, and related compounds. These are largely nonpolar in nature. Nonpolar molecules are hydrophobic (water fearing), or insoluble in water. This is because they are hydrocarbons that include mostly nonpolar carbon–carbon or carbon–hydrogen bonds. These are soluble in organic solvents.

■ CLASSIFICATIONS

Lipids can be classified according to their hydrolysis products and according to similarities in their molecular structures. Three major subclasses are as follows:
1. Simple lipids
2. Compound lipids
3. Derived lipids

Simple Lipids

These lipids are esters of fatty acids with certain alcohols. These are subclassified according to the nature of alcohol.
- **Fats and oils:** The fats and oils are similar chemically but difference is on the basis of their physical states at room temperature. It is

customary to call a lipid a fat if it is solid at 25°C, and oil if it is a liquid at the same temperature. These yield fatty acids and glycerol upon hydrolysis. Fats and oils are called triacylglycerols because they are esters composed of three fatty acids joined to glycerol and trihydroxy alcohol. The three fatty acids may be same, like palmitic acids forming tripalmetine, or may be different forming triglycerides with three different fatty acids. The differences in melting points reflect differences in the degree of unsaturation of the constituent fatty acids.

- **Waxes:** These yield fatty acids and long-chain alcohols (12–34 carbon atoms in length) upon hydrolysis. Wax is an ester of long-chain alcohol (usually monohydroxy) and a fatty acid. These are solid at room temperature.

  For example, spermaceti, a wax, liquid at body temperature, obtained from the head of a sperm whale.

Compound Lipids

These are esters of fatty acids with alcohols, containing additional groups. These are subclassified as follows:
- **Phospholipids:** These lipids contain phosphorus as additional group, e.g., plasmalogen.
- **Glycolipid:** Combination of carbohydrate and lipids are glycolipids. These are found in chloroplast membranes.
- **Lipoproteins:** Combination of lipid and protein is lipoprotein, e.g., cholesterol and glycerol. They may be glycerophospholipids or sphingophospholipid depending upon the alcohol group present (glycerol or sphingosine).

Derived Lipids

These are the lipids, which arise as a result of partial hydrolysis of lipid.
- **Fatty acids:** These are hydrolysis products of fats and other lipids. Naturally occurring fats generally contain an even number of carbon atoms. These may be saturated (without double or triple bond) or unsaturated (with double or triple bond), e.g., linoleic acid.
- **Steroids:** Steroids are naturally occurring cyclic compounds having a common structural base of cyclopentanoperhydro-

phenanthrene ring. These have different physiological properties, e.g., testosterone.

■ DETECTIVE TESTS FOR LIPIDS

1. **Iodine absorption test:** This test is for unsaturated fatty acids. A drop of iodine is added to fat solution (fat solution is prepared from chloroform) and shaken. The solution will decolorize if unsaturated fatty acid is present.
2. **Rancidity:** When fat is allowed to stand for a sufficient length of time in contact with air and moisture in presence of light, it gets oxidized and becomes rancid.
3. **Emulsification:** When oil/fat is shaken with water; it is finally divided and dispersed in the water to form emulsion.
4. **Formation of acrolein:** Glycerol from fats dehydrated with the help of solid potassium bisulfate and acrylic aldehyde or acrolein is produced. It is noted by irritating odor.

$$\text{Glycerol} \xrightarrow{KHSO_4} \text{Acrolein}$$

5. **Sudan III test procedure:** 0.5 mL ether or chloroform is taken in a test tube. 0.5 mL of sample is added drop by drop till the sample is fully dissolves. Add one drop of Sudan III reagent. If red color appears, fat is present in the sample.
6. **Huble's test:** This test is used to know the degree of unsaturation in the given sample. Oils on reaction with Huble's reagent fades the violet color of iodine, then it is unsaturated and if the color persists, then the given fat or oil is saturated.

■ LIPID METABOLISM

About 40% of the calorie intake is derived from lipids and almost all of these calories come from fats, the triglycerols.

Fatty acid metabolism is predominantly performed in liver. The liver may play a modifying part in fat storage and retrieval. The major source of lipids entering the liver in free fatty acid form released from adipose tissue and transported in the systemic blood plasma complexed with albumin. Fatty acid oxidation yields twice the usable chemical energy that carbohydrates can deliver. As an example, 130 moles of adenosine triphosphate (ATP) result from the oxidation of one mole of palmitic acid, as compared to 38 moles of ATP from one mole of glucose. On a weight basis, the calorie yield from fatty acids is about double that from carbohydrates; 9 kcal/g from fat vs. 4 kcal/g from carbohydrate or protein).

The major aspects of lipid metabolism are involved with *fatty acid oxidation* to produce energy or the synthesis of lipids, which is called lipogenesis.

The sequence of reactions involved in the formation of lipids is known as lipogenesis. Lipogenesis is not simply the reverse of the fatty acid spiral, but does start with acetyl-CoA and does build up by the addition of two carbons units. The synthesis occurs in the cytoplasm in contrast to the degradation (oxidation), which occurs in the mitochondria. Many of the enzymes for the fatty acid synthesis are organized into a multienzyme complex called fatty acid synthetase.

The major points in the overall lipogenesis reactions are:
1. ATP is required.
2. The reactions are reductions (addition of H^+ and use of NADPH) which are the reverse of the oxidations in the fatty acid spiral.

Biosynthesis of fatty acids requires acetyl-CoA as a key intermediate. It gets decarboxylated to malonyl CoA. The acetyl-CoA is first converted to citrate within mitochondrion by condensation with oxaloacetate. The citrate then passes out to cytoplasm and cleaved back to oxaloacetate and acetyl-CoA with the consumption of ATP.

Acetyl groups are then used for fatty acid synthesis and oxaloacetate is converted to pyruvate. Pyruvate then passes back to mitochondria and used for either regeneration of oxaloacetate or conversion of acetyl-CoA.

The hydrogens required for reductive reactions are all supplied by NADPH. The overall reaction is:
1 acetyl-CoA + 7 malonyl-CoA + 14 $NADPH_2$ are catalyzed by fatty acid synthetase to yield = palmitate* + 7 CO_2 + 14 NADP + 8 CoA

Beta-oxidation of Fatty Acids

Most fats are stored as triglycerides. In order to enter into beta-oxidation bonds must be broken usually with the use of a lipase.

---

*Palmitate is most common form of fatty acid

Section 2: Fundamentals of Biochemistry

The end results of these broken bonds are a glycerol molecule and three fatty acids in the case of triglycerides. Other lipids are capable of being degraded as well. This process is known as beta-oxidation because the oxidation and splitting of two carbon units occur at the beta carbon atom. The oxidation of the hydrocarbon chains occur by a sequential cleavage of two carbon atoms **(Fig. 10.1)**.

Steps of Beta-oxidation

Activation
- Once the triglycerides are broken down into glycerol and fatty acids they must be activated before they can enter into the mitochondria and proceed on with beta-oxidation. This is done by acyl-CoA synthetase to yield fatty acyl-CoA.
- After the fatty acid has been acylated it is now ready to enter into the mitochondria.
- There are two carrier proteins (carnitine acyltransferase I and II), one located on the outer membrane and one on the inner membrane of the mitochondria. Both are required for entry of the Acyl-CoA into the mitochondria.
- Once inside the mitochondria the fatty acyl-CoA can enter into beta-oxidation.

Oxidation
1. A fatty acyl-CoA is oxidized by acyl-CoA dehydrogenase to yield a trans alkene. This is done with the aid of an [FAD] prosthetic group. As a result of this process, a trans double bond is introduced into the acyl chain.

$$\text{Acyl-CoA} \xrightarrow[\text{Dehydrogenase}]{\text{Acyl-CoA-}} \text{trans-}\Delta^2\text{-Enoyl-CoA}$$
(FAD → FADH$_2$)

Hydration
2. The trans alkene is then hydrated with the help of enoyl-CoA hydratase. As a result, double bond introduced in the previous step, yielding an alcohol (-C-OH).

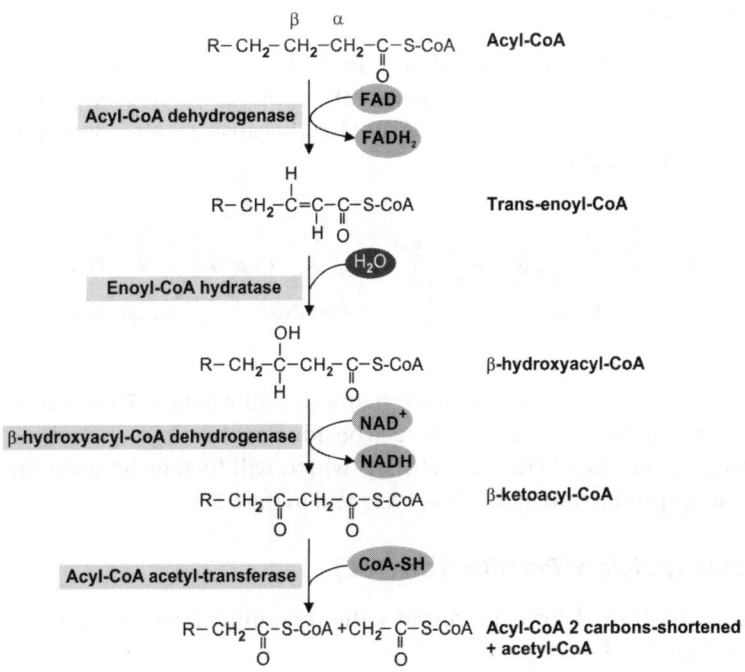

Fig. 10.1: Cyclic representation of beta-oxidation.

Oxidation

The alcohol of the hydroxyacly-CoA is then oxidized by NAD⁺ to a carbonyl with the help of hydroxyacyl-CoA dehydrogenase. NAD⁺ is used to oxidize the alcohol.

Cleavage

Finally acetyl-CoA is cleaved off with the help of thiolase to yield an acyl-CoA that is two carbons shorter than before. The cleaved acetyl-CoA can then enter into the TCA and ETC because it is already within the mitochondria.

$$R-\text{CO-CH}_2\text{-CO-S-CoA} \xrightarrow{+ \text{CoA-SH}}_{\text{Thiolase}} R\text{-CO-S-CoA} + H_3C\text{-CO-S-CoA}$$

3-Ketoacyl-CoA → Acyl-CoA + Acetyl-CoA

In the case of our 16 carbon palmitic acid we have 7 rounds of beta-oxidation. As you can see, besides acetyl-CoA, the whole process yields $FADH_2$ and NADH, which will further be used for energy production in the TCA cycle and in the ETC.

Energy Yield of Palmitic Acid (16C)

8 acetyl-CoA (1 for each round + the remaining from the last two carbons).

7 $FADH_2$, 7 NADH

Each acetyl-CoA yields 12 ATPs, thus 8 acetyl-CoA will yield 96 ATPs. Each $FADH_2$ yields 2 ATPs while each NADH yields 3 ATPs So:

8 acetyl-CoA × 12 = 96 ATPs

7 $FADH_2$ × 2 = 14 ATPs

7 NADH × 3 = 21 ATPs

The total energy yield is 131 (96 + 14 + 21 = 131) ATPs, but the activation of the fatty acid (step 1) requires 2 ATPs so the net yield of energy is 129 ATPs for a molecule of palmitic acid (16 carbon).

Besides, longer chain fatty acids yield even more energy. For example, an 18 carbon fatty acid (stearic acid) yields 146 ATPs, while a 20 carbon fatty acid will yield 163 ATPs-oxidation can be broken down into a series of discrete steps.

This cycle repeats until the fatty acid has been completely reduced to acetyl-CoA, which is fed through the TCA cycle to ultimately yield cellular energy in the form of ATP.

The metabolism of fatty acids and glycogenesis is coordinated in response to dietary sugars. The increase in cellular G-6-P levels

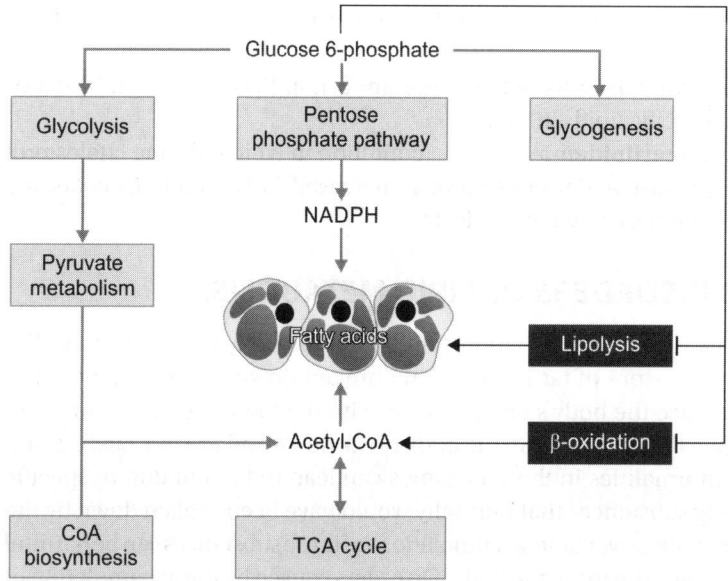

Fig. 10.2: Interconnection between various cycles of lipid and carbohydrate metabolism.

leads to the regulation of several metabolic processes important in the metabolism of lipids. The majority of G-6-P is channeled through glycolysis, resulting in elevated pyruvate and the production of acetyl-CoA. The process is coordinated with increased levels of CoA biosynthesis. Acetyl-CoA is utilized by the TCA cycle to produce intermediates of amino acid metabolism, ATP, NADH, and citrate. Citrate is further channeled to the fatty acid biosynthesis. The process of lipid metabolism is accompanied with the activity of the pentose phosphate pathway yielding the necessary reductive power in the form of NADPH. Parallel to the fatty acid synthesis, elevated levels of G-6-P shut down the process of lipid catabolism through lipolysis and generation of acetyl-CoA through b-oxidation **(Fig. 10.2)**

■ DISEASES RELATED TO LIPID METABOLISM

1. **Steatorrhea:** Maldigestion of fats due to inadequate secretion of pancreatic lipase or bile salts or even may be defective absorption due to intestinal diseases like celiac disease results in excessive excretion of fat in feces. This is called as steatorrhea.

2. Obesity is another disorder due to accumulation of excess of body fat.
3. **Lipidosis:** This denotes the abnormal lipoproteins in blood or specific lipids in tissues.
4. **Hyperlipidemia:** This is a condition in which plasma cholesterol or plasma triglyceride level is increased. This condition occurs due to inherent genetic defects.

■ DISORDERS OF LIPID METABOLISM

Fats (lipids) are an important source of energy for the body. The body's store of fat is constantly broken down and reassembled to balance the body's energy needs with the food available. Groups of specific enzymes help the body break down and process fats. Certain abnormalities in these enzymes can lead to the buildup of specific fatty substances that normally would have been broken down by the enzymes. Over time, accumulations of these substances can be harmful to many organs of the body. Disorders caused by the accumulation of lipids are called lipidoses. Other enzyme abnormalities prevent the body from converting fats into energy normally. These abnormalities are called fatty acid oxidation disorders.

- **Gaucher's disease:** Gaucher's disease is caused by a buildup of glucocerebrosidase, (which are a product of fat metabolism) in tissues. Children who have the infantile form usually die within a year, but children and adults who develop the disease later in life may survive for many years.

  Gaucher's disease leads to an enlarged liver and spleen and a brownish pigmentation of the skin. Accumulations of glucocerebrosidase in the eyes cause yellow spots called pinguecula to appear. Accumulations in the bone marrow can cause pain and destroy bone.

  - *Type 1:* The chronic form of Gaucher's disease, is the most common. It results in an enlarged liver and spleen and bone abnormalities. Most commonly diagnosed during adulthood, type 1 Gaucher's disease may lead to severe liver disease, including increased risk of bleeding from the stomach and esophagus and liver cancer. Neurologic problems can also occur.

- *Type 2:* The infantile form, usually causes death in the first year of life. Affected infants have an enlarged spleen and severe neurologic problems.
- *Type 3:* The juvenile form, can begin at any time during childhood. Children with type 3 disease have an enlarged liver and spleen, bone abnormalities, and slowly progressive neurologic problems. Children who survive to adolescence may live for many years.

Many people with Gaucher's disease can be treated with enzyme replacement therapy, in which enzymes are given by vein, usually every 2 weeks. Enzyme replacement therapy is most effective for people who do not have nervous system complications.

- **Tay-Sachs disease:** Tay-Sachs disease is caused by a buildup of gangliosides in the tissues. This disease results in early death.

In Tay-Sachs disease, gangliosides, which are products of fat metabolism, accumulate in tissues. At a very early age, children with this disease become progressively intellectually disabled and appear to have floppy muscle tone. Spasticity develops and is followed by paralysis, dementia, and blindness. These children usually die by age 3 or 4. The disease cannot be treated or cured.

Before conception, parents can find out whether they carry the gene that causes the disease. During pregnancy, Tay-Sachs disease can be identified in the fetus by chorionic villus sampling or amniocentesis.

- **Niemann-Pick disease:** Niemann-Pick disease is caused by a buildup of sphingomyelin or cholesterol in the tissues. This disease causes many neurologic problems.

In Niemann-Pick disease, the deficiency of a specific enzyme results in the accumulation of sphingomyelin (a product of fat metabolism) or cholesterol. Niemann-Pick disease has several forms, depending on the severity of the enzyme deficiency, which determines how much sphingomyelin or cholesterol accumulates. In the most severe form (type A), children fail to grow normally and have several neurologic problems. These children usually die by age 3. Children with type B disease develop fatty growths in the skin, areas of dark pigmentation, and an enlarged liver, spleen, and lymph nodes. They may be intellectually disabled. Children with type C disease develop symptoms during childhood, with seizures and neurologic deterioration.

Some forms of Niemann-Pick disease can be diagnosed in the fetus by chorionic villus sampling or amniocentesis. After birth, the diagnosis can be made by a liver biopsy (removal of a tissue specimen for examination under a microscope). None of the types of Niemann-Pick disease can be cured, and children tend to die of infection or progressive dysfunction of the central nervous system. Currently, some therapies that may slow or halt the progression of symptoms in types B and C are being studied.

- **Fabry's disease:** In Fabry's disease, glycolipid, which is a product of fat metabolism, accumulates in tissues. Because the defective gene for this rare disorder is carried on the X chromosome, the full-blown disease occurs only in males. The accumulation of glycolipid causes noncancerous (benign) skin growths (angiokeratomas) to form on the lower part of the trunk. The corneas become cloudy, resulting in poor vision. A burning pain may develop in the arms and legs, and children may have episodes of fever. Children with Fabry's disease eventually develop kidney failure and heart disease, although most often, they live into adulthood. Kidney failure may lead to high blood pressure, which may result in stroke. Fabry's disease can be diagnosed in the fetus by chorionic villus sampling or amniocentesis. The disease cannot be cured or even treated directly, but researchers are investigating a treatment in which the deficient enzyme is replaced by transfusion. Treatment consists of taking analgesics to help relieve pain and fever or anticonvulsants. People with kidney failure may need a kidney transplant.

- **Fatty acid oxidation disorders:** Several enzymes help break down fats so that they may be turned into energy. An inherited defect or deficiency of one of these enzymes leaves the body short of energy and allows breakdown products, such as acyl-CoA, to accumulate. The enzyme most commonly deficient is medium chain acyl-CoA dehydrogenase (MCAD). Other enzyme deficiencies include short chain acyl-CoA-dehydrogenase deficiency (SCAD), long chain-3-hydroxyacyl-CoA-deficiency (LCHAD), and trifunctional protein deficiency (TFP). This, results in delayed mental and physical development.

- **MCAD deficiency:** Medium-chain acyl-CoA dehydrogenase (MCAD) deficiency is a condition that prevents the body from converting certain fats to energy. This disorder is one of the most common inherited disorders of metabolism.

Symptoms usually develop between birth and age 3. Children are most likely to develop symptoms if they go without food for a period of time (which depletes other sources of energy) or have an increased need for calories because of exercise or illness. The level of sugar in the blood drops significantly, causing confusion or coma. Children become weak and may have vomiting or seizures. Over the long-term, children have delayed mental and physical development, an enlarged liver, heart muscle weakness, and an irregular heartbeat. Sudden death may occur.

Other Rare Hereditary Disorders of Lipid Metabolism

- **Wolman's disease** results when specific types of cholesterol and glycerides accumulate in tissues. This disease causes enlargement of the spleen and liver. Calcium deposits in the adrenal glands cause them to harden, and fatty diarrhea (steatorrhea) also occurs. Infants with Wolman's disease usually die by 6 months of age.
- **Cerebrotendinous xanthomatosis** occurs when cholestanol, a product of cholesterol metabolism, accumulates in tissues. This disease eventually leads to uncoordinated movements, dementia, cataracts, and fatty growths (xanthomas) on tendons. The disabling symptoms often appear after age 30. If started early, the drug chenodiol helps prevent progression of the disease, but it cannot undo any damage already done.
- **Sitosterolemia**, fats from fruits and vegetables accumulate in blood and tissues. The buildup of fats leads to atherosclerosis, abnormal red blood cells, and xanthomas on tendons.
- **Refsum's disease**, phytanic acid, which is a product of fat metabolism, accumulates in tissues. A buildup of phytanic acid leads to nerve and retinal damage, spastic movements, and changes in the bone and skin.

■ BIOCHEMICAL IMPORTANCE OF LIPIDS

1. Lipids are source of energy. They are superior to carbohydrate and protein since they yield twice the energy produced by carbohydrates or proteins.

Section 2: Fundamentals of Biochemistry

2. In addition to provide flavors and satiety to diet, fats serve as natural solvents for fat soluble vitamins, such as vitamin A, D, E, and K.
3. They contain essential fatty acids, which are not synthesized by human body.
4. Lipids in adipose tissue serve as energy store.
5. Lipids have a role in protection and fixation of internal organs such as kidneys.
6. Lipids in myelin sheath of nerve fibers serve as electrical insulator.
7. Lipids under the skin serve as thermal insulator.
8. Lipoproteins are essential components in the structure of cell membrane and mitochondria. They also play important role in lipid transport in blood.

SUMMARY

- Lipids are heterogeneous group of oily/greasy organic compounds, which are relatively insoluble in water but soluble in organic solvents.
- Simple lipids are esters of fatty acids with certain alcohols.
- Lipid is a fat if it is solid at 25°C, and oil if it is a liquid at the same temperature.
- Waxes yield fatty acids and long-chain alcohols upon hydrolysis.
- Compound lipids are esters of fatty acids with alcohols, containing additional groups.
- Derived lipids are the lipids, which arise as a result of partial hydrolysis of lipid.
- Detective tests for lipids are based on important characteristics of lipids such as rancidity and emulsification.
- Huble's test is used to know the degree of unsaturation in the given sample.
- The sequence of reactions involved in the formation of lipids is known as lipogenesis.
- Lipid metabolism involves β-oxidation. It is named because the oxidation a tes in tissues.
- Wolman disease results when specific types of cholesterol and glycerides accumulate in tissues.
- Sitosterolemia results when fats from fruits and vegetables accumulate in blood and tissues.
- Lipids are source of energy and they also dissolves fat-soluble vitamins.
- Lipids serve as thermal insulator. These are important constituent of cell membrane and mitochondria.

Chapter 10: Study of Lipids

PRACTICE QUESTIONS

1. What are lipids? Write a note on derived lipids.
2. Differentiate between simple and compound lipids.
3. Discuss the test that identifies saturated and unsaturated fats.
4. What is acrolein? How does it help to confirm presence of lipid in sample?
5. Explain lipogenesis.
6. What is β-oxidation? Why it is called so?
7. Discuss the various steps involved in β-oxidation.
8. Explain the following terms:
    i. Steatorrhea
    ii. MCAD deficiency
    iii. Sitosterolemia
    iv. Refsum disease
9. Write cause and symptoms of:
    i. Fabry disease
    ii. Niemann–Pick disease
    iii. Tay–Sachs disease
    iv. Gaucher disease

CHAPTER 11

Study of Nucleic Acids

> **Keywords**
> Nucleotides, purine, pyrimidine, cytosine, adenine, guanine, thymine, uracil, nucleoside, nucleotide, deoxyribonucleic acid (DNA), ribonucleic acid (RNA), mRNA, rRNA, tRNA, hemophilia, Turner syndrome, Huntington disease, thalassemias, karyotype, DNA replication, replication fork, leading strand, lagging strand, termination, de novo synthesis pathway, salvage pathway, purine catabolism, gouts, hyperuricemia, catabolism

■ INTRODUCTION

Nucleic acid is an important class of macromolecules found in all cells. Nucleic acids were so named because they were first found in the nucleus of cells, and have acid property. It is made up of carbon, hydrogen, oxygen, nitrogen, and phosphorus.

Nucleic acids are the most important macromolecules for the continuity of life. They carry the genetic blueprint of a cell and carry instructions for the functioning of the cell.

The two main types of nucleic acids are deoxyribonucleic acid (DNA) and ribonucleic acid (RNA). DNA is the genetic material found in all living organisms, ranging from single-celled bacteria to multicellular mammals. And also in viruses which are on border of living and nonliving. It is found in the nucleus of eukaryotes and in the organelles, chloroplasts, and mitochondria. In prokaryotes, the DNA is not enclosed in a membranous envelope.

■ COMPONENTS OF NUCLEIC ACIDS

Nucleic acid molecule is a long-chain polymer. It is composed of monomeric units, called nucleotides. Each nucleotide consists of nucleoside and a phosphate group. Each nucleoside consists of a pentose sugar and a nitrogenous base. The sugar is ribose in case of RNA and deoxyribose in case of DNA.

Nitrogenous bases are of two types namely—purine and pyrimidine.

There are two main purine bases—adenine and guanine.

Similarly, there are three main pyrimidine bases. These are—cytosine, thymine, and uracil. Cytosine and thymine are commonly found in DNA. Cytosine and uracil are found in RNA.

Nucleoside: A base combined with a sugar molecule is called nucleoside. In DNA, four different nucleosides are present. These are adenosine, guanosine, cytosine, and thymine. In RNA, deoxyribose sugar is replaced by ribose sugar and the base thymine is replaced by uracil.

Nucleotides: A nucleotide is derived from nucleoside by the addition of a molecule of phosphoric acid. A number of nucleotide units link with one another to form a polynucleotide chain.

■ STRUCTURE OF DNA

DNA molecules consists of two polynucleotide chains running in opposite directions and coiled in such a way that adenine of one strand is always in front of thymine of other strand. Guanine of one chain always faces cytosine in complementary strand. These pairs of bases (A:T, G:C) are bonded by weak hydrogen bonds. This

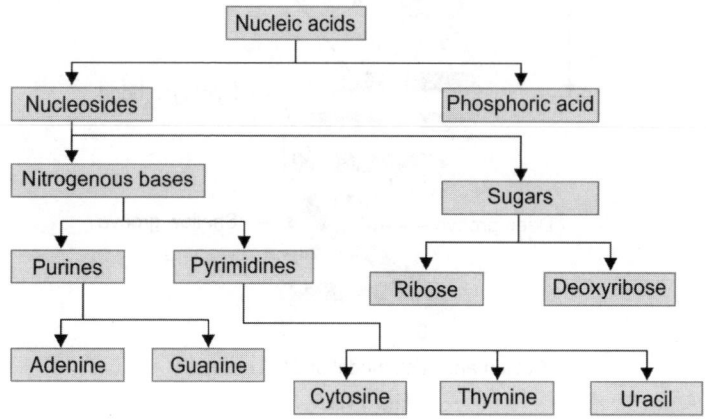

arrangement of bases is called base pairing rules and the overall structure is called as double helical structure **(Fig. 11.1A)**.

The sugar present in DNA is called deoxyribose. It is a pentose sugar, which contains five carbon atoms ($C_5H_{10}O_4$). It contains one oxygen atom less than the ribose sugar.

In each DNA molecule, the deoxyribose sugar is attached to a phosphoric acid at one side and a nitrogenous base at other side. The phosphoric acid molecule is linked to sugar at carbon atom no. 3 or 5. The nitrogen base molecule is joined to the sugar by a glycosidic bond. This is formed between carbon atom no. 1 of deoxyribose and nitrogen atom 3 or 9 of nitrogen base. A phosphodiester bond joins two nucleotides. It is formed between the carbon atom no. 3 of sugar of one nucleotide and phosphate component at the 5th position of another nucleotide **(Fig. 11.1B)**.

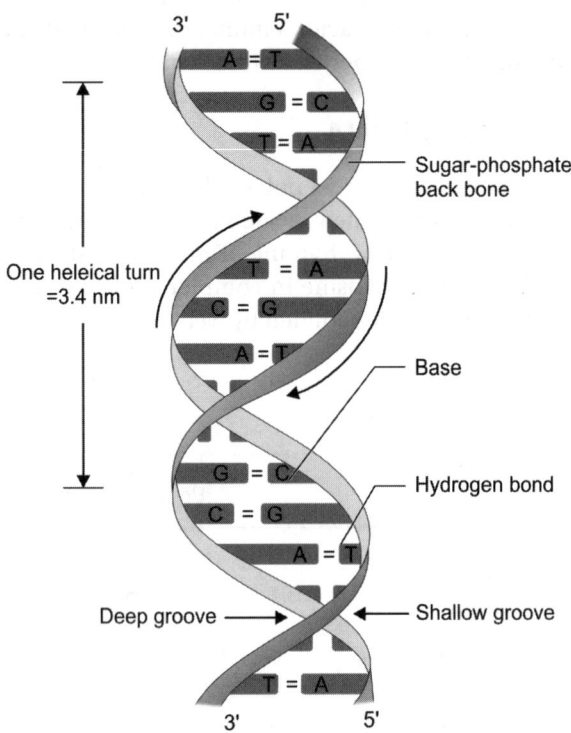

Watson and crick model of DNA molecule

Fig. 11.1A

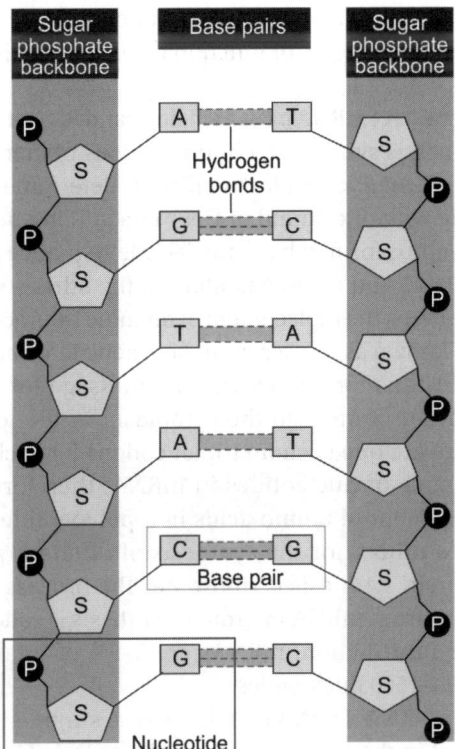

Fig. 11.1B
Figs. 11.1A and B: Structure of DNA.

At one end of polynucleotide chain, 3rd carbon of sugar is free called as 3' end and at the other end 5th carbon of sugar is free, called as 5' end. The 3' end of one chain lies close to 5' end of other chain. Hence, two strands of DNA are antiparallel. The polynucleotide chains of DNA molecule are linked by nucleotides of adjacent chain.

In mammalian cells, DNA is always formed in nucleus where it exists in combination with basic proteins (histones) giving rise to structures, which are called chromosomes.

■ STRUCTURE OF RNA

These are single-stranded polynucleotides involved in the translation of genetic information contained in DNA. The pyrimidines present in

RNA are cytosine and uracil. The number of purine and pyrimidine are not equal. Three types of functionally different RNAs are found in living cells.

1. **Messenger RNA (mRNA):** It is a single strand RNA of low molecular weight which is synthesized in the nucleus of mammalian cells. The sequence of nucleotides in mRNA is determined by the base-paring rule with one strand of DNA as a guiding polynucleotide. The mRNA thus formed has a nucleotide sequence similar to one strand of DNA and complementary to the other strand, the only difference being the replacement of thymine by uracil in RNA. This process is known as transcription of genetic information.

   The mRNA thus formed carries the message for the synthesis of appropriate protein to the cytoplasm in the form of triplet code. There are one or more triplet codons for each amino acid. The sequence of nucleotides in mRNA, therefore determines the arrangement of amino acids in a polypeptide chain. There is separate mRNA for the synthesis of different proteins. The site of protein synthesis is ribosome. The process of transfer of information from mRNA in protein synthesis is called translation of genetic information. mRNAs are 3–5% of total RNA. These contain 500–1500 nucleotides.

2. **Ribosomal RNA (rRNA):** It is also a single-stranded RNA synthesized in the same manner as the mRNA. However, it does not contain any genetic information. It is associated with the ribosome where it is found in combination with proteins. The main function of rRNA is to maintain the structural integrity of ribosome and to bind the mRNA, the tRNA and enzymes required in the protein synthesis. rRNAs are 80% of total RNA. These contain many nucleotides.

3. **Transfer RNA (tRNA):** It is low molecular weight RNA which is involved in the transfer of amino acids pool to the site of protein synthesis, i.e. ribosomes. For each amino acid, there is a specific tRNA. tRNAs are 10–15% of total RNA. The molecule of tRNA is folded to attain a shape of cloverleaf. It contains 73–95% nucleotide.

■ COMPARISONS OF DNA AND RNA

For comparison *see* **Table 11.1**.

Table 11.1: Comparisons of DNA and RNA.

Criteria	DNA	RNA
Acid name	Deoxyribonucleic acid	Ribonucleic acid
Stability	Very stable, long life	Less stable, short life
Location	Nucleus and mitochondria	Nucleus and cytoplasm
Copier enzyme	DNA polymerase	RNA polymerase
Structure	Long nucleotide chain Two complementary strands A, B, or C form helix	Short nucleotide chain One complementary strands Only A form helix
Pentose sugar	Deoxyribose	Ribose
Nucleobases	Cytosine, adenine, guanine, and thymine	Cytosine, adenine, guanine, and uracil
Base pairing	Adenine–Thymine Cytosine–Guanine	Adenine–Uracil Cytosine–Guanine
Function	Repository of genetic information	Involved in protein synthesis and gene regulation; carrier of genetic information in some viruses
Types	———	mRNA, tRNA, and rRNA

■ DNA REPLICATION

DNA replication is the process by which DNA makes a copy of itself during cell division. It involves the following steps **(Fig. 11.2)**:

Step 1: Replication Fork Formation
Step 2: Primer Binding and Elongation
Step 3: Termination

Step 1: Replication Fork Formation

- The first step in DNA replication is to 'unzip/uncoil' the double helix structure of the DNA molecule.
- This is carried out by an enzyme called helicase which breaks the hydrogen bonds between the complementary bases of DNA together (A with T, C with G).
- The separation of the two single strands of DNA creates a 'Y' shape called a replication 'fork'. The two separated strands will act as templates for making the new strands of DNA.

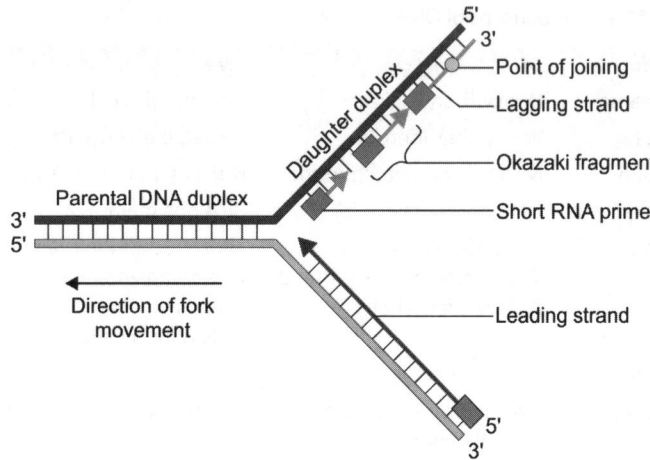

Fig. 11.2: DNA replication.

Step 2: Primer Binding and Elongation

One of the strands is oriented in the 3' to 5' direction (towards the replication fork), this is the leading strand. The other strand is oriented in the 5' to 3' direction (away from the replication fork), this is the lagging strand. As a result of their different orientations, the two strands are replicated differently:

Elongation of Leading Strand

- A short piece of RNA called a primer (produced by an enzyme called primase) comes along and binds to the end of the leading strand. The primer acts as the starting point for DNA synthesis.
- DNA polymerase III binds to the strand at the site of the primer and begins adding new base pairs complementary to the strand of DNA in the 5' to 3' direction. This is called elongation.
- This sort of replication is called continuous.

Elongation of Lagging Strand

- Numerous RNA primers are made by the primase enzyme and bind at various points along the lagging strand.
- Pieces of DNA, called Okazaki fragments, are then added to the lagging strand also in the 5' to 3' direction.

- This type of replication is called discontinuous as the Okazaki fragments will need to be joined up later.

Step 3: Termination
- Once both the continuous and discontinuous strands are formed, an enzyme called exonuclease removes all RNA primers from the original strands.
- These primers are then replaced with appropriate bases. Another exonuclease "proof reads" the newly formed DNA to check, remove and replace any errors.
- Another enzyme called DNA ligase joins Okazaki fragments together forming a single unified strand.
- The ends of the parent strands consist of repeated DNA sequences called telomeres. Telomeres act as protective caps at the end of chromosomes to prevent nearby chromosomes from fusing.
- Once completed, the parent strand and its complementary DNA strand coils into the familiar double helix shape.
- In the end, replication produces two DNA molecules, each with one strand from the parent molecule and one new strand.
- The result of DNA replication is two DNA molecules consisting of one new and one old chain of nucleotides. This is why DNA replication is described as semi-conservative, half of the chain is part of the original DNA molecule, half is brand new.

Purine and Pyrimidine Metabolism

There are two kinds of nitrogen-containing bases - purines and pyrimidines. Purines consist of a six-membered and a five-membered nitrogen-containing ring, fused together. Pyridmidines have only a six-membered nitrogen-containing ring. Two purines and three pyrimidines are of prime importance.
- **Purines:**
    - Adenine = 6-amino purine, Guanine = 2-amino-6-oxy purine

Adenine

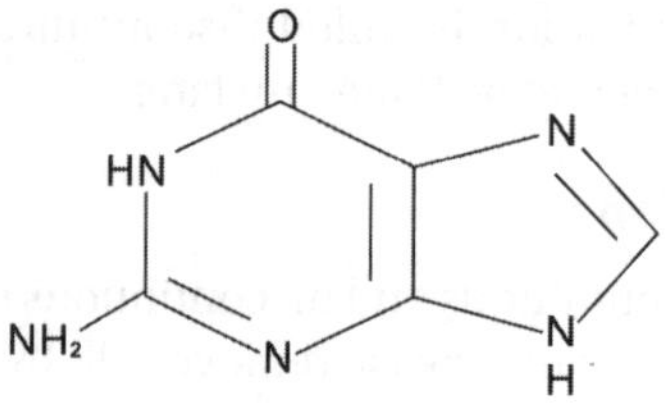

Guanine

- Adenine and guanine are found in both DNA and RNA.s.
- **Pyrimidines:**
    - Uracil = 2,4-dioxy pyrimidine, Thymine = 2,4-dioxy-5-methyl pyrimidine

Cytosine = 2-oxy-4-amino pyrimidine,

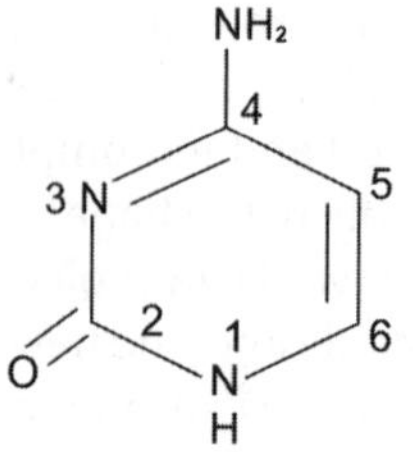

Cytosine 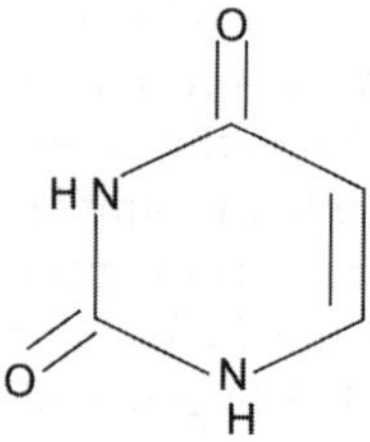   **Uracil**

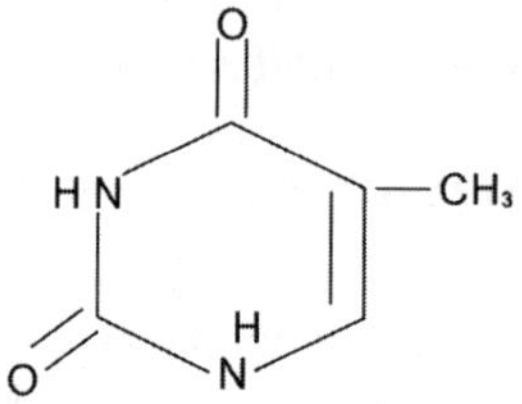

Thymine

- Cytosine is found in both DNA and RNA. Uracil is found only in RNA. Thymine is normally found in DNA. Sometimes tRNA will contain some thymine as well as uracil.

Hydrolysis of Polynucleotides

Nucleotides joined together by 3'-5' phosphodiester bonds are called as Polynucleotides.

The nucleic acids are hydrolyzed by nucleases to give a mixture of polynucleotides. These are further cleaved by phosphodiesterases (exonucleases) to a mixture of the mononucleotides. The mononucleotides are hydrolyzed by nucleotidases to give the nucleosides and P_i. The sugar phosphate can either be reincorporated into nucleotides or metabolized via the Hexose Monophosphate Pathway. Nitrogenous bases are catabolised as follows:

- **Purine catabolism:**
    - The end product of purine catabolism in is uric acid. Uric acid is formed primarily in the liver and excreted by the kidney into the urine.
    - If the methyl is on an $-NH_2$, it is removed along with the $-NH_2$ and the core is metabolized in the usual fashion. If the methyl is on a ring nitrogen, the compound is excreted unchanged in the urine.
    - Both adenine and guanine nucleotides forms a common intermediate xanthine. Adenine, is oxidized to xanthine by the enzyme xanthine oxidase. Guanine is deaminated, with the amino group released as ammonia, to xanthine. Most of the ammonia will be transported to the liver as glutamine for ultimate excretion as urea.
    - Xanthine, is oxidized by oxygen and xanthine oxidase with the production of hydrogen peroxide. In man, the urate is excreted and the hydrogen peroxide is degraded by catalase.
    - Urate salts coprecipitate with calcium salts and can form stones in kidney or bladder. A very high concentration of urate in the blood leads to a group of diseases called to as gout.
- **Pyrimidine catabolism:** In contrast to purines, pyrimidines undergo ring cleavage and the usual end products of catabolism are beta-amino acids plus ammonia and carbon dioxide. Pyrimidines from nucleic acids are acted upon by nucleotidases and pyrimidine nucleoside phosphorylase to yield the free bases. The 4-amino group of both cytosine and 5-methyl cytosine is released as ammonia.
- **Purine and pyrimidine anabolism:** There are two pathways of synthesis of nucleotides: *De novo* synthesis pathway, and Salvage pathway.
    - *De novo synthesis of purine nucleotides:*
        + The de novo synthesis of purine nucleotide is the main synthesis pathway of nucleotides. Phosphoribose, amino

acids, one carbon units and CO_2 are used as raw materials to synthesize purine nucleotide from the beginning.
- Purine synthesis occurs in all tissues. The major site of purine synthesis is in the liver and, to a limited extent, in the brain.
- Substrates: Ribose-5-phosphate; glycine; glutamine; H_2O; ATP; CO_2; aspartate.
- Products: GMP; AMP; glutamate; fumarate; H_2O.
- Reactions: Ribose-5-phosphate (as provided by the pentose-phosphate pathway) is converted into PRPP (Phosphoribosyl pyrophosphate) by PRPP synthetase, in a step requiring one ATP.
- An α-amino group is then added to PRPP from glutamine to form 5-phosphoribosylamine. This reaction is catalyzed by glutamine PRPP amidinotransferase.
- A series of nine reactions results in the formation of IMP (Inosine 5′-monophosphate).
- IMP can then be transformed either to GMP by IMP dehydrogenase, or to AMP by adenylosuccinate synthetase
  - *De novo synthesis of pyrimidine nucleotides:*
    - The pyrimidine synthesis is a similar process than that of purines. In the de novo synthesis of pyrimidines, the ring is synthesized first and then it is attached to a ribose-phosphate to for a pyrimidine nucleotide. It occurs in the cytosol of cells in all tissues.
    - Substrates: CO_2; glutamine; ATP; Aspartate; H_2O; NAD^+; Phosphoribosyl pyrophosphate (PRPP).
    - Products: UTP; CTP; glutamate; NADH; CO_2
    - Glutamine's amide nitrogen and carbon dioxide provide atoms 2 and 3 or the pyrimidine ring. They do so, however, after first being converted to carbamoyl phosphate. The other four atoms of the ring are supplied by aspartate. The sugar phosphate portion of the molecule is supplied by PRPP.
- **Purine salvage pathway:**
  - A salvage pathway is a pathway in which nucleotides are synthesized from intermediates in the degradative pathway for nucleotides. Purine synthesis via the salvage pathways occurs in all tissues. It is especially important in the brain and the bone marrow.
  - *Substrates:* Hypoxanthine; PRPP; guanine; adenine.

- *Products:* GMP; AMP; IMP
- Bases from degraded nucleic acids can be converted back into purine nucleotides via the salvage pathways.
- Base + PRPP = Base-ribose-phosphate (BMP) + PPi
- Hypoxanthine can be combined with PRPP (which acts as the donor of ribose-5 phosphate) to form IMP in a reaction catalyzed by Hypoxanthine-guanine phosphoribosyltransferase (HGPRT).
- IMP can subsequently be transformed into AMP or GMP via the last few steps of the pathway of de novo purine synthesis.
- HGPRT also catalyzes the reaction which combines PRPP with guanine to form GMP. Adenine phosphoribosyltransferase converts adenine and PRPP to form AMP.
- **Pyrimidine synthesis via salvage pathways:**
  - Pyrimidines can be salvaged from orotic acid, uracil, and thymine but not from cytosine. Salvage is accomplished by the enzyme pyrimidine phosphoribosyl transferase. It involves two steps
  - Base + Ribose 1-phosphate = Nucleoside + Pi (nucleoside phosphorylase)
  - Nucleoside + ATP = Nucleotide + ADP (nucleoside kinase - irreversible)
  - There is a uridine phosphorylase and kinase and a deoxythymidine phosphorylase and a thymidine kinase which can salvage some thymine in the presence of dR 1-P.
- **Interconversion of nucleotides:**
  - The monophosphates are the forms synthesized *de novo* although the triphosphates are the most commonly used forms. But, of course, the three forms are in equilibrium. There are several enzymes classified as nucleoside monophosphate kinases which catalyze the general reaction: (= represents a reversible reaction)
  - Base-monophosphate + ATP = Base-diphosphate + ADP, e.g. enzyme adenylate kinase: AMP + ATP = 2 ADP
  - There is a different enzyme for GMP, one for pyrimidines and also enzymes that recognize the deoxy forms.
  - Similarly, the diphosphates are converted to the triphosphates by nucleoside diphosphate kinase:
  BDP + ATP = BTP + ADP

- **Formation of deoxyribonucleotides:** *De novo* synthesis and most of the salvage pathways involve the ribonucleotides (Exception is the small amount of salvage of thymine indicated above). Deoxyribonucleotides for DNA synthesis are formed from the ribonucleotide diphosphates.

■ GENETIC DISORDERS

Genes are the building blocks of heredity. They are passed from parent to child. They hold DNA, the instructions for making proteins. Proteins do most of the functions in cells. They move molecules from one place to another, build structures, break down toxins and do many other maintenance jobs.

Sometimes there is a mutation, a change in a gene or genes. The mutation changes the gene's instructions for making a protein, so the protein does not work properly or is missing entirely. This can cause a medical condition called a genetic disorder.

A gene mutation can be inherited from one or both parents. A mutation can also happen during lifetime of an individual.

There are three types of genetic disorders:
1. Single-gene disorders, where a mutation affects one gene. Sickle cell anemia is an example.
2. Chromosomal disorders, where chromosomes (or parts of chromosomes) are missing or changed. Chromosomes are the structures that hold our genes. Down syndrome is a chromosomal disorder.
3. Complex disorders, where there are mutations in two or more genes. Often your lifestyle and environment also play a role. Colon cancer is an example.

There are many genetic disorder diseases. Some of them are discussed as follows:
- **Sickle cell anemia:** It is caused due to point mutation (base substitution) in gene for hemoglobin.

  As a result, blood cells have a deformed, sickle shape. They get caught in blood vessels and restrict blood flow to tissue causing damage, pain and possibly death. They break leading to a lower red blood cell count.

  Symptoms are fatigue, headaches, muscle cramps, kidney and heart damage.

- **Cystic fibrosis:** It is caused due to mutation in gene for the transport protein (plasma/cell membrane) responsible for transporting chloride ions.
  This results in misshapen transport protein in cells of digestive tract and respiratory system, mucus accumulation in lungs and pancreas.
  Symptoms are difficulty breathing and digesting food, many lung infections.
- **Hemophilia:** This is X-linked recessive gene disorder. It causes mutation in gene, builds defective form of a protein needed to clot blood. As a result, blood does not clot.
  Symptoms are difficulty in healing, bleeding without stopping, internal bleeding, lots of bruising, arthritis (long-term).
- **Turner's syndrome:** Turner's syndrome is a sex-linked (non-disjunction) disorder of missing of an X chromosome. In this case, female is XO.
  Symptoms are short stature, (swelling) of the hands and feet, broad chest (*shield chest*) and widely-spaced nipples, low hairline, low-set ears, reproductive sterility, crude ovaries, absence of menstrual period, increased weight, obesity, shield-shaped thorax of heart, small fingernails, webbing of the neck, poor breast development.
- **Huntington's disease:** This is an inherited disease which causes certain nerve cells in the brain and central nervous system to degenerate. Loss of these nerve cells causes symptoms, such as behavior changes, unusual, snake-like movements (chorea), uncontrolled movement, difficulty walking, loss of memory, speech and cognitive functions and difficulty in swallowing.
- **Duchenne muscular dystrophy:** Symptoms of Duchenne muscular dystrophy typically show themselves before the age of 6. The condition causes fatigue and weakness of the muscles, which starts in the legs and then gradually progresses to the upper body, leaving individuals wheelchair bound by the age of 12. It affects mostly boys with symptoms, such as heart and respiratory difficulties, deformity of the chest and back and potential mental retardation.
- **Celiac disease:** This digestive, genetic disorder inflicts patients with gluten intolerance—basically those afflicted with celiac

disease are unable to digest any products or food containing gluten (i.e. foods processed from wheat and related grain). If left undiagnosed, the disease will often lead to malnutrition and dehydration due to severe diarrhea. Additional signs of the condition include abdominal bloating and digestive pain.
- **Thalassemias:** Thalassemias refer to a collection of genetic blood disorders. It occurs when hemoglobin cannot be synthesized by red blood cells. A thalassemias often leads to anemia (which typically occurs with decreased hemoglobin in the blood) and causes similar symptoms to occur—like fatigue, an engorged spleen, bone pain, a propensity to broken bones, shortness of breath, lack of appetite, dark urine, jaundice (a yellowing of the skin and whites of the eyes) and liver dysfunction.
- **Transient neonatal diabetes:** Transient neonatal diabetes mellitus is an insulin-requiring hyperglycemia within the first month of life. The disease can be transient and resolve within first few months of life, or can persist as a permanent form of diabetes. Many cases can also develop type II diabetes later in life. A form of transient neonatal diabetes (TNDM3) is caused by mutations in the gene.
- **Down syndrome:** It results from an extra chromosome 21. Each body cell has 47 chromosomes.

  This severely alters the individual's phenotype, like facial features, short stature, heart defects, susceptibility to respiratory infections and mental retardation.

  It is caused by non-disjunction during gamete formation.

Detection of Genetic Disorders

Karyotypes

Chromosomal mutations can be detected by making a karyotype (a chart of chromosome pairs). There are two techniques used to detect karyotype of a fetus during pregnancy.
1. **Amniocentesis:** Needle is inserted into the uterus and 10 mL of amniotic fluid is extracted. Tests can be done on the cells that are in the fluid extracted.
2. **Chorionic villi sampling:** Small amount of fetal tissue is taken from the placenta. Tests are done on the cells in this tissue.

Gene mutations can sometimes be detected by using the DNA fingerprinting. In this test, DNA is cut with restriction enzymes and then the fragments are separated using gel electrophoresis. Every individual has a unique band pattern.

■ BIOLOGICAL IMPORTANCE OF NUCLEIC ACID

- The nucleic acids play an important role in preserving and transmitting the genetic properties of an organism.
- The DNA stores the hereditary character of a cell in the form of sequence of nucleotides and transfers this information to daughter cells by replication.
- Nucleic acids synthesize the various proteins of the protoplasm.
- RNA is associated with memory storage functions in brain.
- DNA produces mutations resulting in new characters.

SUMMARY

- Nucleic acid is an important class of macromolecules found in all living organisms and viruses.
- The two main types of nucleic acids are DNA and RNA.
- Both DNA and RNA are made from nucleotides, each containing a five-carbon sugar backbone, a phosphate group, and a nitrogen base.
- Purine and pyrimidine are two types of nitrogenous bases. Two main purine bases are adenine and guanine. Three main pyrimidine bases are—cytosine, thymine, and uracil.
- A base combined with a sugar molecule is called nucleoside.
- A nucleotide is addition of a molecule of phosphoric acid to nucleoside.
- *DNA is a double helix:* Two complementary strands of polynucleotides that run in opposite directions and are held together by hydrogen bonds between them.
- RNA is single-stranded polynucleotides. The pyrimidines present in RNA are cytosine and uracil.
- Mutation in genes can be inherited and results in genetic disorders. Thalassemia, Huntington disease, hemophilia, and sickle cell anemia are some important genetic disorders.
- Chromosomal mutations can be detected by making a karyotype.
- The nucleic acids play an important role in preserving and transmitting the genetic properties of an organism.
- DNA provides the code for the cell's activities, while RNA converts that code into proteins to carry out cellular functions.
- DNA Replication involves the production of identical helices of DNA from one double-stranded molecule of DNA.

- DNA replication is semi-conservative, invoving process of Replication Fork Formation, Primer Binding, Elongation, and Termination.
- Purines have double carbon ring while pyrimidine have single carbon ring structure.
- The nucleic acids are hydrolyzed randomly by nucleases to yield a mixture of polynucleotides. These are further cleaved by phosphodiesterases (exonucleases) to a mixture of the mononucleotides.
- Except ring-methylated, purines are deaminated, the amino group contribute to the general ammonia pool and rings oxidized to uric acid for excretion.
- Pyrimidines are acted upon by nucleotidases and pyrimidine nucleoside phosphorylase to yield the free bases.
- There are two pathways of synthesis of nucleotides: De Novo synthesis pathway, and Salvage pathway.
- The nucleotides are interconvertable.

PRACTICE QUESTIONS

1. Explain the following terms:
    i. Nucleoside
    ii. Nucleotide
    iii. Nitrogenous bases
2. Discuss the structure of DNA, mRNA, tRNA, and rRNA.
3. Compare between DNA and RNA.
4. What are genes? Which condition can lead to genetic disorders?
5. Write a note on:
    i. Thalassemia
    ii. Hemophilia
    iii. Sickle cell anemia
    iv. Turner syndrome
    v. Transient neonatal diabetes
6. What is meant by a karyotype? Discuss its applications.
7. Justify: "Nucleic acids are the most important macromolecules for the continuity of life".
8. With a neat labelled diagram, explain process of DNA replication.
9. Give reason—DNA replication is semi-conservative.
10. Differentaite between purine and pyrimidine.
11. Write a note on:
    i. Hydrolysis of polunuvleotides
    ii. Purine catabolism
    iii. Pyrimidine catabolism
    iv. De novo synthesis pathway
    v. Salvage pathway
12. What is gout? How it is related to nucleic acid metabolism?

SECTION 3

Clinical Biochemistry

SECTION OUTLINE

12. Introduction to Clinical Biochemistry
13. Advanced Analytical Techniques–I
14. Advanced Analytical Techniques–II
15. Enzyme Assay
16. Water and Mineral Metabolism
17. Inborn Errors of Metabolism
18. Endocrine Glands and Hormones
19. Thyroid Function Tests
20. Diabetic Profile
21. Liver Function Tests
22. Renal Function Tests
23. Cardiac Function Tests
24. Electrolytes
25. Body Fluids
26. Blood pH and Buffer System
27. Arterial Blood Gases
28. Vitamin Assay
29. Tumor Markers
30. Therapeutic Drug Monitoring
31. Automation in Clinical Biochemistry

CHAPTER 12

Introduction to Clinical Biochemistry

Keywords

Diagnosis, treatment, prognosis, screening, biochemical profiling, SI base units, SI derived units, ampere—elementary charge, kilogram—Planck constant, second—cesium frequency, meter—speed of light in vacuum, Kelvin—Boltzmann constant, Mole—Avogadro constant, Candela—luminous efficacy, metric conversions, borosilicate glass, quartz glass, fritted glass, silanized glass, amber glass, volumetric glassware, micropipettes, alconox, chromic acid, ultrasonic cleaners, phlebotomy, specimen labeling, blood collection tubes, additives, order of draw, sampling errors, testes that require fasting, 24-hour entire urine sample, timed sample, fecal collection, cerebrospinal fluid, pleural fluid, ascitic fluids, synovial fluids, semen, sputum, batch analyzer, random access auto analyzers, precision and accuracy, sensitivity and specificity, reference ranges

■ BIOCHEMISTRY LABORATORY

Introduction

Clinical biochemistry tests comprise over one-third of all hospital laboratory investigation. Clinical biochemistry is a branch of laboratory medicine which applies chemical and biochemical methods to the study of disease. In theory, clinical biochemistry embraces all non-morphological studies, while in practice, it is usually, though not exclusively, confined to studies on blood and urine because of the relative ease in obtaining such specimens. Although analysis is made on other body fluids such as gastric aspirate, cerebrospinal fluid (CSF), etc. as well.

Use of Biochemical Tests

The biochemical tests are performed for four main reasons—diagnosis, treatment, prognosis, and screening.

1. **Diagnosis:** Clinical diagnosis is usually based on history, physical examination, and results of investigations. Up to 80% of cases can be diagnosed from history and clinical findings alone.
2. **Treatment:** Biochemical tests are most often used in the managing treatment of patients. These are used for monitoring treatment or to follow the progress of the disease. Serial measurements are valuable in management, e.g., in patients with diabetic ketoacidosis, frequent measurements of blood glucose help to access the response to insulin and to adjust dosage.

    Biochemical tests are also useful in assessing the severity of the disease (**Fig. 12.1**). For example, in renal failure, the greater plasma urea and creatinine, the more severe is reduction in renal function.
3. **Prognosis:** Prognosis is a forecast of the likely outcome of a situation. Biochemical tests, either individually or in combination, can give an indication of the prognosis. For example, in patients with malignant tumors, serial measurements of tumor markers are of value in assessing the response to treatment and possibility of recurrence.
4. **Screening:** When tests are done to detect the presence of a disease before clinical features are evident, it is described as screening. These tests are done on apparently healthy population to identify those who may have subclinical disease (asymptomatic form) or those who are at risk of developing a disease. It can detect the disease before irreversible damage has occurred.

    It can be performed on different groups:
    - *Population screening:* The population at risk can be defined and screened, like phenylketonuria and hypothyroidism in a newborn and cervical screening for detection of cervical carcinoma.

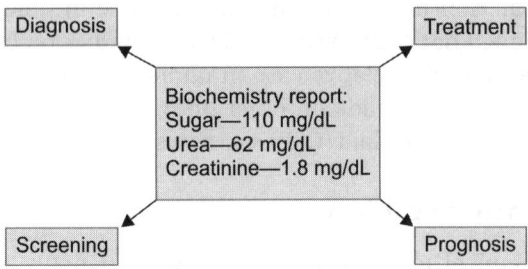

Fig. 12.1: How biochemical tests are used.

- *Selective screening:* It can be applied to a subgroup of the population known to be at risk of developing that disease, like family members of a patient with hypercholesterolemia or premature coronary heart disease could be screened for high cholesterol.
- *Individual screening:* An individual is screened for a particular disease based on individual's history. For example, antenatal screening of a fetus for inherited disease when a previous child of the parents has been found to have that disease or when there is a strong family history of that disease.
- *Opportunistic screening:* When a patient is screened for certain diseases when he presents to the doctor with an unrelated condition. For example, detection of hypertension.

Biochemical Profiling

With availability of multichannel analyzers, it is now possible to analyze a small blood sample for a large number of biochemical tests. When a group of test is applied to otherwise healthy individuals or to all admitted to hospitals, it is termed biochemical profiling.

■ STANDARD INTERNATIONAL UNITS

Every field of science involves taking measurements, understanding them, and communicating them to others. Unit is a chosen reference quantity, which may be used for comparison of quantities of the same dimension.

For example, kilometer, meter, and centimeter all are units of length.

Globally, laboratories are producing, communicating, and exchanging millions of laboratory examination values to multiple parties every day. For most values, "measurement units" are required to make the numerical values comparable and meaningful. However, a nonsystematic use of "measurement units" can create errors in communication between healthcare providers and becomes a risk to patient safety. Therefore, the Committee of Nomenclature for Properties and Units (C-NPU) recommends using an unambiguous terminology of "measurement units," for daily patient care and scientific publications.

The International System of Units, universally abbreviated SI (from the French Le Système International d'Unités), is the modern metric system of measurement. The SI was established in 1960 by the 11th General Conference on Weights and Measures (CGPM, Conférence Générale des Poids et Mesures).

The worldwide scientific laboratory societies have accepted and, to a large extent, implemented the SI units for presentation of laboratory reports in health care and research. This modern form of the metric system is based around the number 10 for convenience. Set units of prefixes have been established and are known as the SI prefixes or the metric prefixes (or units). The prefixes indicate whether the unit is a multiple or a fraction of the base 10. Multiple and fractional SI units are defined by prefix multipliers according to powers of 10 ranging from 10^{-24} to 10^{24}. It allows the reduction of zeros of a very small number or a very larger number.

For example, 0.000000001 meter is 1 nanometer and 7,500,000 Joules into 7.5 Megajoules.

These SI prefixes also have a set of symbols that precede unit symbol.

The commonly used prefixes are shown in Table 12.1.

Table 12.1: SI prefixes list.

Prefix	Symbol	10^n	Scale
yotta (gr. *okto*—eight)	Y	10^{24}	Septillion
zetta (lat. *septem*—seven)	Z	10^{21}	Sextillion
eksa (gr. *ex*—six)	E	10^{18}	Quintillion
peta (gr. *penta*—five)	P	10^{15}	Quadrillion
tera (gr. *teras*—monster)	T	10^{12}	Trillion
giga (gr. *gigas*—giant)	G	10^9	Billion
mega (gr. *megas*—great)	M	10^6	Million
kilo (gr. *khilioi*—thousand)	k	10^3	Thousand
hecto (gr. *hekaton*—hundred)	h	10^2	Hundred
deca (gr. *deka*—ten)	da	10^1	Ten
		10^0	One/Unit
decy (lat. *decimus*—tenth)	d	10^{-1}	Tenth
centy (lac. *centum*—hundredth)	c	10^{-2}	Hundredth

Contd...

Contd...

Prefix	Symbol	10^n	Scale
milli (lac. *mille*—thousand)	m	10^{-3}	Thousandth
mikro (gr. *mikros*—small)	μ	10^{-6}	Millionth
nano (gr. *nanos*—dwarf)	n	10^{-9}	Billionth
pico (it. *piccolo*—small)	p	10^{-12}	Trillionth
femto (den. *femten*—fifteen)	f	10^{-15}	Quadrillionth
atto (den. *atten*—eighteen)	a	10^{-18}	Quintillionth
zepto (lat. *septem*—seven)	z	10^{-21}	Sextillionth
yokto (gr. *okto*—eight)	y	10^{-24}	Septillionth

SI units are divided into two classes: Base units and Derived units.

SI Base Units

These definitions are modified from time to time as techniques of measurement evolve in order to allow more accurate realizations of the base units. There are seven dimensionally independent, base units (or fundamental units). These are—time, length, mass, electric current, thermodynamic temperature, amount of substance, and luminous intensity. In 2019, the SI base units were redefined in agreement with the International System of Quantities, effective on the 144th anniversary of the Metre Convention, 20 May 2019. In the redefinition, four of the seven SI base units—the kilogram, ampere, Kelvin, and mole—were redefined by setting exact numerical values. The second, meter, and candela were already defined by physical constant **(Fig. 12.2)**.

1. **Ampere (A):** Defining constant—elementary charge (e).
   Definition: The ampere, symbol A, is the SI unit of electric current. It is defined by taking the fixed numerical value of the elementary charge e to be $1.602176634 \times 10^{-19}$ when expressed in the unit C, which is equal to A s, where the second is defined in terms of Δv_{Cs}.
2. **Kilogram (kg):** Defining constant—Planck constant.
   The kilogram, symbol kg, is the SI unit of mass. It is defined by taking the fixed numerical value of the Planck constant h to be $6.62607015 \times 10^{-34}$ when expressed in the unit J s, which is equal to kg m²s⁻¹, where the meter and the second are defined in terms of c and Δv_{Cs}.

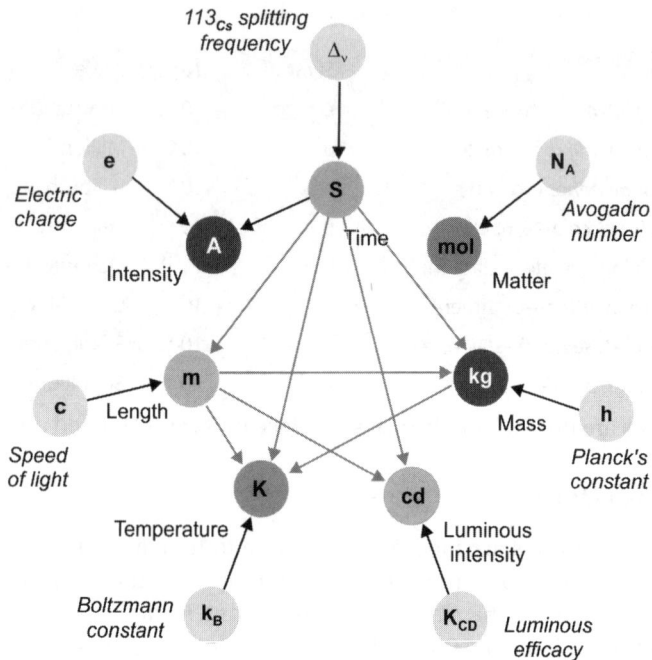

Fig. 12.2: Seven SI units and their constants.

3. **Second (s):** Defining constant—Cesium frequency.
   The second, symbol s, is the SI unit of time. It is defined by taking the fixed numerical value of the cesium frequency Δv_{Cs}, the unperturbed ground-state hyperfine transition frequency of the cesium 133 atom, to be 9,192,631,770 when expressed in the unit Hz, which is equal to s^{-1}.

4. **Meter (m):** Defining constant—speed of light in vacuum.
   The meter, symbol m, is the SI unit of length. It is defined by taking the fixed numerical value of the speed of light in vacuum c to be 299,792,458 when expressed in the unit m/s, where the second is defined in terms of Δv_{Cs}.

5. **Kelvin (K):** Defining constant—Boltzmann constant.
   The Kelvin, symbol K, is the SI unit of thermodynamic temperature. It is defined by taking the fixed numerical value of the Boltzmann constant k to be 1.380649×10^{-23} when expressed in the unit J K^{-1}, which is equal to kg $m^2 s^{-2} K^{-1}$, where the kilogram, meter, and second are defined in terms of h, c, and Δv_{Cs}.

Table 12.2: The seven defining constants of the International system.

Symbols	Value	Descriptions
Δ_{vCs}	9,192,631,770 Hz	The unperturbed ground state hyperfine transition frequency of the cesium 133 atom
c	299,792,458 m/s	The speed of light in vacuum
h	$6.62607015 \times 10^{-34}$ J s	Planck's constant
e	$1.602176634 \times 10^{-19}$ C	The elementary charge
k	1.380649×10^{-23} J/K	Boltzmann's constant
N_A	$6.02214076 \times 10^{23}$/mol	Avogadro's constant
K_{cd}	683 lm/W	The luminous efficacy of monochromatic radiation of frequency 540×10^{12} Hz

6. **Mole (mol):** Defining constant—Avogadro constant, N_A.
   The mole, symbol mol, is the SI unit of amount of substance. One mole contains exactly $6.022140769 \times 10^{23}$ elementary entities. This number is the fixed numerical value of the Avogadro constant, N_A, when expressed in the unit mol^{-1} and is called the Avogadro number. The amount of substance, symbol n, of a system is a measure of the number of specified elementary entities. An elementary entity may be an atom, a molecule, an ion, an electron, any other particle, or specified group of particles.
7. **Candela (cd):** Defining constant—luminous efficacy.
   The candela, symbol cd, is the SI unit of luminous intensity in a given direction. It is defined by taking the fixed numerical value of the luminous efficacy of monochromatic radiation of frequency 540×10^{12} Hz, K_{cd}, to be 683 when expressed in the unit lm W^{-1}, which is equal to cd sr W^{-1}, or cd sr kg^{-1}m^{-2}s^{3}, where the kilogram, meter, and second are defined in terms of h, c, and Δv_{Cs}.

The seven defining constants of the International System are shown in **Table 12.2**.

SI Derived Units

A large number of derived units formed by combining base units according to the algebraic relations of the corresponding quantities, some of which are assigned special names and symbols and which themselves can be further combined to form even more derived units **(Table 12.3)**.

Table 12.3: Derived quantities and their units.

Quantity	Equation	Unit name	Unit symbol	
Area	Area = Length × Width	square meter		m^2
Volume	Volume = Length × Width × Time	cubic meter		m^3
Frequency	Frequency = $\dfrac{1}{\text{Period}}$	hertz	Hz	s^{-1}
Density	Density = $\dfrac{\text{Mass}}{\text{Volume}}$	kilogram per cubic meter		$mg \cdot m^{-3}$
Volocity, speed	Velocity = $\dfrac{\text{Displacement}}{\text{Time}}$	meter per second		$m \cdot s^{-1}$
Acceleration	Acceleration = $\dfrac{\text{Velocity change}}{\text{Time}}$	meters per second squared		$m \cdot s^{-2}$
Force	Force = Mass × Acceleration	Newton	N	$kg \cdot m \cdot s^{-2}$
Pressure, stress	Pressure = $\dfrac{\text{Force}}{\text{Area}}$	Pascal	Pa	$N \cdot m^{-2}$
Energy, work	Work = Force × Displacement	Joule	J	$N \cdot m$
Power	Power = $\dfrac{\text{Work}}{\text{Time}}$	watt	W	$J \cdot s^{-1}$
Quantity of electricity	Quantity of charge = Current × Time	Coulomb	C	$A \cdot s$
Potential difference, electromotive force	Potential difference = $\dfrac{\text{Energy}}{\text{Charge}}$	Volt	V	$W \cdot A^{-1}$
Electric resistance	Resistance = $\dfrac{\text{Potential difference}}{\text{Current}}$	Ohm	Ω	$V \cdot A^{-1}$

- The derived units are coherent in the sense that they are all mutually related only by the rules of multiplication and division with no numerical factor other than 1 needed.
- The derived units are also complete in the sense that one and only one unit exists for every defined physical quantity. Some derived units are used for more than one physical quantity.
- The SI has special names for 22 of these derived units (for example, hertz, the SI unit of measurement of frequency), but the rest merely reflect their derivation. For example, the square meter (m^2), the SI derived unit of area; and the kilogram per cubic meter (kg/m^3 or $kg \cdot m^{-3}$), the SI derived unit of density.

Basic Units in Biochemistry

Unit of quantity: Basic unit of mass or quantity is grams. Following are its conversions commonly used in biochemistry laboratory (**Fig. 12.3**).

The milligram (mg) = 0.001 gram (1/1,000 as milli = 1,000 and equals 1/1,000 of a gram).

The centigram (cg) = 0.01 gram (1/100 as centi = 100 and equals 1/100 of a gram).

The decigram (dg) = 0.1 gram (1/10 as deci = 10 and equals 1/10 of a gram).

Unit of volume: Basic unit of volume is liter. Following are its conversions commonly used in biochemistry laboratory.

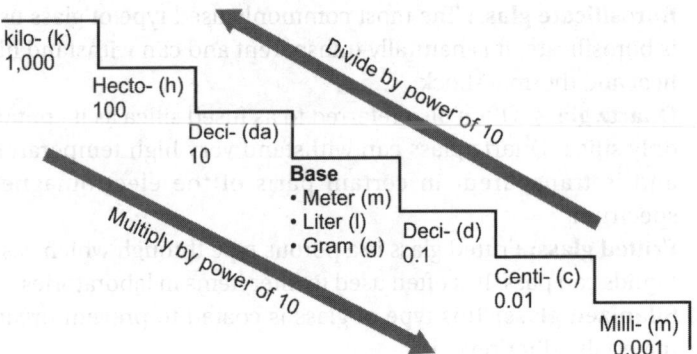

Fig. 12.3: Metric conversion.

The milliliter (mL) = 0.001 liter (1/1,000 as milli = 1,000 and equals 1/1,000 of a liter).

The centiliter (cL) = 0.01 liter (1/100 as centi = 100 and equals 1/100 of a liter).

The deciliter (dL) = 0.1 liter (1/10 as deci = 10 and equals 1/10 of a liter).

■ LABORATORY GLASSWARE

Laboratory glassware refers to a variety of equipment made of glass used for scientific experiments and other work in science. It is found in abundance in laboratories and comes in all shapes and sizes. Though it has become preferable in recent years to substitute glass vessels for cheaper, more durable and less fragile plastic materials, some substances and experiments or applications still require the use of glassware.

The reasons for these are manifold. Firstly, glass is relatively inert, meaning it will not react with the chemicals or substances placed inside and thereby upset or skew the results. It is also transparent, allowing for easy monitoring, and heat-resistant, allowing for high temperatures. Furthermore, it is easy to shape and mold into any form required.

Types of Glass Used

Different types of glass are used to produce laboratory glassware. Each glass variety has specific properties that make it suited to different applications.

- **Borosilicate glass:** The most commonly used type of glass used is borosilicate. It is naturally transparent and can withstand high heat and thermal shock.
- **Quartz glass:** Often also referred to as fused silica as it contains only silica. Quartz glass can withstand very high temperatures and is transparent in certain parts of the electromagnetic spectrum.
- **Fritted glass:** Fritted glass is a porous type through which gas or liquids can pass. It is often used to filter items in laboratories.
- **Silanized glass:** This type of glass is coated to prevent organic materials adhering to it.

- **Amber glass:** Amber glass is darkened to block out ultraviolet (UV) and infrared radiation, thereby making it ideal for storing fluids.

Types of Glasswares

Volumetric glassware is the most commonly used in biochemistry laboratories. Volumetric glasswares are specialized pieces of glassware which are used to measure volumes of liquids very precisely in quantitative laboratory work **(Fig. 12.4)**.

Here are some of the different types of glass instruments used in laboratories:

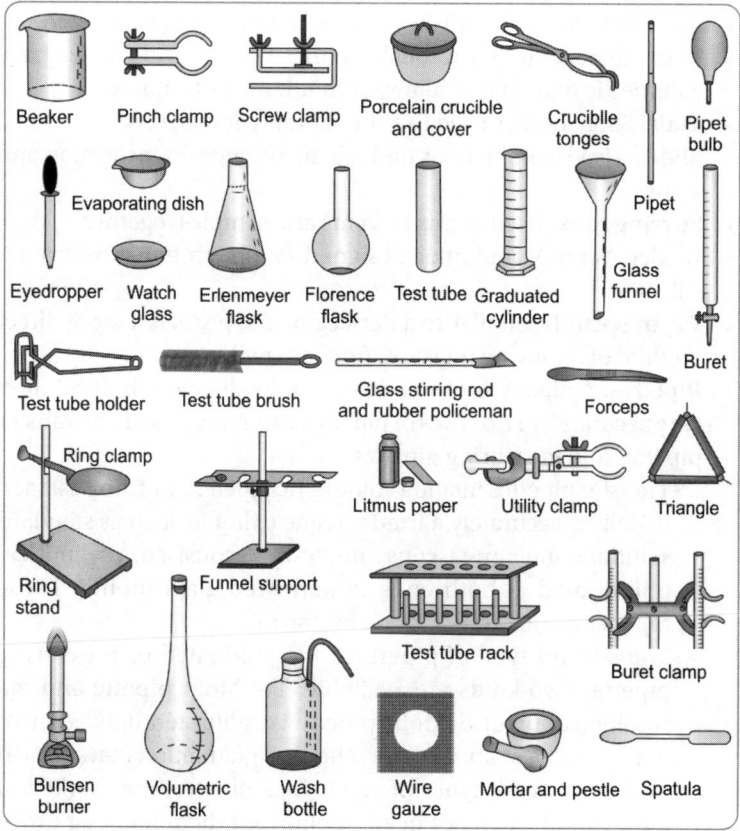

Fig. 12.4: Glassware in biochemistry laboratory.

- **Bulb and graduated pipettes:** These are used to transport specific amounts of fluids from one place to another.
- **Burettes:** These are used to dispense exact quantities of liquid into another vessel.
- **Beakers:** Simple containers used to hold samples and reagents.
- **Volumetric flasks:** Similar to beakers, these are used to hold samples, but usually come in a conical or spherical shape with a tapering neck.
- **Condensers:** Specifically used to cool heated liquid or gas.
- **Retorts:** These are used for distillation purposes.
- **Funnels:** The tapered neck of a funnel allows easy pouring of a liquid into a narrow orifice.
- **Petri dishes:** Shallow dishes used to culture living cells.
- **Petri dishes:** Similar to beakers, these cylindrical vessels have volumetric markings to allow for monitoring of volume.
- **Vials:** Small bottles used to store samples or reagents.
- **Slides:** Used to hold items under a microscope for inspection and study.
- **Stirring rods:** Used to mix solvents and samples together.
- **Desiccators:** A container designed to absorb moisture from a substance.
- **Drying pistols:** Similar to a desiccator, the pistol is a more direct method of removing moisture from a sample.
- **Pipettes:** A pipette is used to measure small amounts of solution very accurately. Two types of pipettes commonly used are transfer pipettes and measuring pipettes.
  - Transfer pipettes include volumetric pipettes and are designed to deliver accurately a fixed volume of liquid such as standard solutions and non-viscous samples, and consist of a cylindrical bulb joined at both ends to narrowed glass tubing. These pipettes are allowed to drain by gravity.
  - The second type of pipette is the graduated or measuring pipette. Two kinds are available: The Mohr pipette and the serological pipette. Mohr pipette is calibrated between two marks on the stem, and the other has graduation marks down to the tip. Some types of serological pipettes are marked of blow-out, these types need to blow-out the remaining drops of liquid in the tip. Mohr pipette delivers between their calibration marks.

Measuring pipettes are principally used for the transfer of reagents and are not generally considered accurate enough to pipette samples and standards. Volumetric pipettes are more accurate than measuring pipettes.

Aqueous solutions form a curved surface when placed in a container. This surface is called a meniscus. To accurately read the level of liquid in a piece of glassware, it is important that eye be on the same level as the surface of the liquid in order to avoid parallax errors. The level of the liquid is then read at the bottom of the meniscus.

- *Automatic pipetting systems:* For the delivery of especially small volumes (0.5 μL to 5 mL) of solutions, automatic pipettors and fitted polypropylene tips can be used. Set the digital micrometer to the desired volume using the adjustment knob. Attach a disposable tip to the shaft of the pipette.

Using Micropipettes

Micropipettes are utilized in the laboratory to transfer small quantities of liquid, usually down to 0.1 μL **(Fig. 12.5)**.

Following steps should be followed for exact measurement of a substance using micropipette.

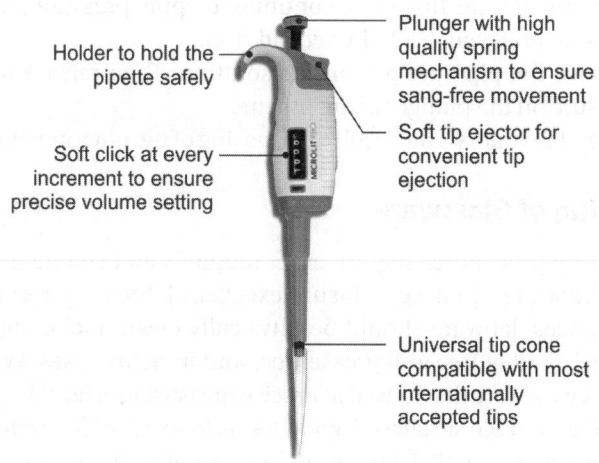

Fig. 12.5: Micropipette.
(For color version, see Plate 4)

- **Examine micropipette.** At the top, it has a plunger that can be pushed into empty the micropipette; next to the plunger is an ejector one can use to eject the plastic tip from the end of the micropipette. Along the side, it has a volume adjustment wheel use to adjust the volume the pipette will take up or contain.
  Look at the volume dial along the side of the micropipette. Micropipettes measure volumes in microliters. Determine what the volume is set to at present and adjust that volume with the volume adjustment wheel to reach the appropriate or desired volume
- Insert the end of the micropipette shaft into one of the plastic tips in plastic tip box. Do not handle the plastic tip with fingers.
- Depress the plunger with thumb until you reach the first stop.
- Insert the plastic tip of the pipette just below the surface of the fluid or water in your beaker.
- Release thumb pressure on the plunger, slowly and gently, drawing fluid into the plastic tip of the micropipette. Once the plunger has traveled all the way out, remove the pipette tip from the solution.
- Transfer the pipette to the receiving vessel/beaker/microfuge tube and place the tip just below the surface of the fluid in the receiving vessel. Do not submerge it completely.
- Depress the plunger slowly and gently to expel all the fluid in the micropipette tip. This time, continue to apply pressure past the first stop until you reach the second stop.
- Remove the pipette tip from the solution. Then release thumb pressure on the plunger of the pipette.
- Follow laboratory's protocol for disposing of the micropipette tips.

Cleaning of Glassware

Laboratory procedures require exact methods and should include good glassware cleaning to insure excellent laboratory results. In all instances, labware should be physically clean, including both chemical residue free and grease free, and in many cases, even be sterile. A glassware that is used in precise measuring of liquids should have fully wettable surfaces. A good test is to use distilled water and see if the water wets all the inner surfaces equally. Grease or residues will not only contaminate the reaction and test results but will also alter the measurement of the liquids.

Good cleaning practices should also be accompanied by good inspection of the glass surfaces for chips, cracks, or abrasions which will cause mechanical failure.

- Always wash glass labware immediately after use. If a thorough cleaning is not immediately possible, always allow the glassware to soak. If not cleaned immediately, some residues may be difficult to remove.
- Most new glasswares are slightly alkaline and should be washed upon receipt and generally can be soaked in a 1% HCl or HNO_3 solution before wash and distill water rinse.
- Never soak for long periods in strong alkaline solutions as it will damage the glass.
- Always follow up a soap or acid wash with a good distill water rinse.
- Always use soft brushes with a wooden or soft plastic handle to avoid abrasion. Do not use wire brushes or brushes with a wire core as it can abrade the glass.

Glass Cleaners

A detergent such as a non-abrasive dishwasher soap will also work well. Always use soft brushes. Always rinse glass well and do a final distill water rinse. If you need to do an acid wash, always rinse the soap off the glass completely or it may cause a reaction and leave a film on the glass.

- **Alconox** is the best as it is not abrasive: It is anionic detergent which consists primarily of a homogeneous blend of sodium linear alkyl aryl sulfonate, alcohol sulfate, phosphates, and carbonates.
- **Chromic acid or chromerge:** It is a great cleaner and also removes organic residues. Use gloves and well ventilate the area when using chromic acid as it is a carcinogen and very corrosive. Make sure metal clamps or flanges are removed. It is best to fill the vessel or soak the item in the solution for a short time in a plastic tub so that the wash material can be added, then rinse immediately several times before proceeding to a detergent wash.

Occasionally stronger acid washes are necessary for certain types of precipitates or residues: This method should only be used when absolutely necessary. Always remember that disposal

of seriously stained glass maybe a less troublesome and less expensive course of action than using strong acid washes. One other caution is that strong acid or chromerge type washes may damage the graduation markings.
- **Removal of grease:** Grease is best removed by boiling the glass in a weak solution of sodium carbonate. Acetone or any other organic solvent can be used also, followed by several water and distill water rinses.
  - For permanganate stains, use a mixture of equal 3% sulfuric acid and 3% hydrogen peroxide.
  - For iron stains, use a solution containing one part hydrochloric acid and one part water.
  - For blood stains, use 3% solution of hydrogen peroxide.
- **Ultrasonic cleaners:** Ultrasonics is a good method of cleaning glassware. Ultrasonic cleaners that are heated will be the best and generally with a mild detergent, they will clean most residues off of glassware.
- **Rinsing:** Glassware should always have a water rinse after any cleaning procedure followed by a distill water rinse. It is best to give smaller pieces such as test tubes a soaking rinse followed by a distill water soaking rinse.
- **Drying:** Oven drying at 100°C is best for all glassware. If not convenient, rack drying will work.
- **Steam autoclaving or sterilizing:** Proper protocol for steam autoclaving of borosilicate glassware is 15–20 minutes at 100–120°C. Always leave closures off or loose during autoclaving.
- **Inspection after cleaning:** Always inspect all glasswares before steam autoclaving for cracks, chips, or damage. The autoclave procedure will cause glassware to break if already damaged.

COLLECTION OF SAMPLES USED IN BIOCHEMISTRY LABORATORY

Today's technologies allow testing on an impressively wide variety of samples collected from the human body. Most often, sample required is a blood and urine sample. However, samples of sputum, feces, semen, and other bodily fluids and tissues are also tested.

Blood

The first step in acquiring a quality laboratory test result for any patient is the specimen collection procedure. Blood has to be tested in most of the blood-related disorders, metabolic disorders, and various infections. The act of drawing or removing blood from the circulatory system through a cut (incision) or puncture in order to obtain a sample for analysis and diagnosis is called as phlebotomy. Phlebotomist is a person who draws blood for diagnostic tests or to remove blood for treatment purposes.

Depending upon the site of collection, there are three popular methods of blood collection:
1. **Arterial blood collection:** This form of blood collection takes place within a hospital environment. It is done mainly for respiratory gases.
2. **Capillary blood collection:** Capillary blood is obtained by pricking the tip of finger, lobe of ear, from the toe, and in infants, it is obtained from the heel. This method can be used when few drops of blood sample is required like test for hemoglobin.
3. **Venous blood collection:** This is the most common site of blood collection required for biochemistry laboratory. For venipuncture large veins of arm are used, these are the median cubital, cephalic, or basilic veins.

Procedure for Collection of Blood

1. First of all decide the amount of blood required and select the container according to the test to be done.
2. Now ensure the patient what is to be done.
3. Lay the arm of the patient on the table.
4. Apply the tourniquet and select the prominent vein of the patient.
5. With cotton swab, disinfect the puncture site.
6. The cotton swab should be previously soaked in the disinfectant.
7. Assemble needle and syringe, check that, it is sharp and unblocked, and it is moving smoothly. Passing air through the syringe can do this. But there should not be any air present in the syringe at the time of blood collection.
8. With the left hand, hold patient's arm, so that skin over vein is tightened. Ask the patient to open and close the wrist.

9. Take the syringe in right hand, holding index finger against the base of the needle, keep the point of needle to upper side and push firmly and steadily without any hesitation into the center of vein.
10. The angle between skin and needle should not be more than 30°. The moment needle enters in vein, blood flows back into the syringe.
11. With your left hand, slightly pull back the piston till required amount of blood is obtained in the syringe.
12. Now, remove the tourniquet, place cotton swab over the needle and wound. Withdraw the needle slowly, and ask the patient to place a cotton swab over the wound. This stops bleeding from wound.
13. Remove the needle from the syringe and gently expel the blood into appropriate container.
14. If anticoagulant is used, gently shake the bottle for proper mixing. Or gently invert at least five times to ensure proper mixing of additive.
15. Discard the needle and syringe properly. If reusable syringe is used immediately, wash it with water using water tray.

Specimen Labeling

Each blood sample must be labeled immediately following collection in the presence of the patient. The minimum amount of information required is:
- Patient's full name (last name first, first name second)
- Identification number (may be the patient's Date of Birth or mobile no. or other unique number)
- Date and time of collection. Many laboratories require the use of military time.
- Phlebotomist's initials.

Note: Never label tubes before collecting the sample, never take the tubes to another location to label them.

Blood collection tubes are available with different colors of cap. These colors of cap represent additives present in tube. The additives can be anticoagulant, when plasma is to be obtained and it is clot activator if serum is desired. Different types of anticoagulants are selected according to the test to be done and method applied. The order of draw is recommended when drawing multiple specimens for

Table 12.4: Order of draw (increasing order of 1 to 10), additives as per cap color of collection bottle.

Cap color	Use	Additive	Special directions
Special sterile tube or bottle	Blood culture	Culture media	Must draw first: Use sterile technique
Clear (discard tube)	Fill before filling blue—top tube when using butterfly set	None	Discard tube
Light blue	Coagulation studies	Sodium citrate	Invert 3–4 times
Red	Chemistry	No anticoagulant (glass), silicon Coating (plastic)	Do not invert (glass) invert 5 times (plastic)
Red\gray	Chemistry	Clot activator, gel separator	Invert 5 times
Gold (SST)	Chemistry	Gel separator, clot activator	Invert 5 times
Green	Chemistry	Heparin	Invert 8 times
Lavender	Hematology Hemoglobin A1c	EDTA	Invert 8 times
Gray	Blood alcohol	Potassium oxalate, Sodium fluoride	Do not clean site with alcohol, Invert 8–10 times
Gray	Glucose	Potassium oxalate, Sodium fluoride	Invert 8–10 times

(EDTA: ethylenediaminetetraacetic acid)

medical laboratory testing during a single venipuncture. The purpose is to avoid possible test result error due to additive carryover. Order of draw, additives as per cap color of collection bottle is fixed. It can be summarized in **Table 12.4**.

Sampling Errors

There are a number of potential errors which may contribute to the success or failure of the laboratory to provide the correct answers to the clinician's question. These can be summarized as:

- **Blood sampling technique:** Difficulty in obtaining a blood specimen may lead to hemolysis with consequent release of potassium and other red cells constituents. Results for these will be falsely elevated.
- **Prolonged stasis:** During venipuncture, Plasma water diffuses into the interstitial space and the serum or plasma sample obtained will be concentrated. Proteins and protein-bound components of plasma such as calcium or thyroxine will be falsely elevated.
- **Insufficient specimen:** Each biochemical analysis requires a certain volume of specimen to enable the test to be carried out it may prove to the impossible for the laboratory to measure everything requested on a small volume specimen.
- **Errors in timing:** The biggest source of error in the measurement of any analyte in a 24-hour urine specimen is in the collection of an accurately timed volume of urine.
- **Incorrect specimen container:** For many analyses, the blood must be collected into a container with anticoagulant and preservative. For example, samples for glucose should be collected into a special container containing fluoride which inhibits glycolysis; otherwise the time taken to deliver the sample to the laboratory can affect the result. If a sample is collected into the wrong container, it should never be decanted into another type of tube. For example, blood which has been exposed even briefly to ethylenediaminetetraacetic acid (EDTA) (an anticoagulant used in sample containers for lipids) will have a markedly reduced calcium concentration, approaching zero.
- **Inappropriate sampling site:** Blood samples should not be taken "down-stream" from an intravenous drip. Laboratory often receives a blood glucose request on a specimen taken from an intravenous drip.
- **Incorrect specimen storage:** A blood sample stored overnight before being sent to the laboratory will show falsely.

Delivery and Storage of Samples

Samples should be kept cold during transport and delivered to the laboratories as soon as possible (within 2 hours). When this is not possible, blood samples for tests utilizing serum or plasma should be centrifuged and separated before storage either in the refrigerator or freezer. Some tests require additional precautions such as protection from light. Details of specific storage and precautions are given with the relevant tests.

For biochemistry laboratory, sample for certain blood tests require to be withdrawn in fasting condition. This is because nutrients in food and drinks go into bloodstream and can change things measured by the tests, skewing the results.

This may need 8–12 hours of fasting. So, if appointment for sample collection is at 8 AM, patient should be instructed to fast for 8 hours, only water is okay after midnight. Patient shouldn't smoke, chew gum (even sugarless), drink alcohol, or exercise. These things can rev up your digestion, and that can affect your results. Patient is allowed to take prescription medications unless your doctor tells to skip them.

These tests typically require fasting:
- Fasting blood glucose measures the amount of glucose in blood to test or diabetes or prediabetes.
  Typical fasting time: At least 8 hours.
- Lipid profile is used to check the level of cholesterol and other blood fats. High levels indicate risk for developing heart disease.
  Typical fasting time: 9–12 hours.
- Basic or comprehensive metabolic panel is often part of a routine physical. The tests check blood sugar, electrolyte, fluid balance, and kidney and liver function.
  Typical fasting time: 10–12 hours.
- Vitamin B12 test measures amount of vitamin in blood. It can help diagnose a specific type of anemia and other problems.
  Typical fasting time: 6–8 hours.
- Iron tests are used to see if iron levels are too low or too high.
  Typical fasting time: 12 hours

Urine Collection

Urine is another fluid commonly used for testing in clinical chemistry laboratories. It is especially suitable for tests that evaluate kidney functions, waste products that are excreted by the kidneys, and for metabolites that are cleared quickly from the bloodstream and accumulate in the urine, such as drugs of abuse. Sometimes both serum and urine concentrations of a substance are useful to know in order to evaluate how well the analyte is being excreted—either to ensure that expected excretion is taking place or to determine if unexpected leakage is occurring.

Different types of urine samples, representing collection at different times of day and for different durations of time, are used for laboratory analyses.

- **Mid-stream sample:** For bacteriological examinations, the first 10 mL of voided urine is discarded then urine is collected. External genitalia must be cleaned properly before for such collection.
- **First morning sample:** Provides a concentrated sample of urine that contains the overnight accumulation of metabolites. Useful for detection of proteins or compounds like HCG (pregnancy test) or unusual analytes. The patient should be instructed to collect the specimen immediately upon rising from a night's sleep.
- **Random sample:** Convenient sample that can be collected at any time. Most often used for routine screening tests. A randomly collected specimen may be collected at unspecified times and is often more convenient for the patient.
- **Timed sample:** Typically 2–6 hours of urine output is collected to give a representative sample; duration of collection depends on the analytes.
- **24-hour entire urine sample:** A 24-hour urinalysis is a timed urine collection used in the metabolic evaluation of urinary stone disease, proteinuria evaluation, and estimation of renal function via creatinine clearance, estimating residual renal function in end-stage renal disease with urea and creatinine clearance.

Instructions for collecting a 24-hour urine sample vary by the laboratory and the test to be performed. Typically, the patient's first voided morning urine is discarded. Note the exact time (e.g., 6:15 AM) when urine collection begins. Subsequent urine produced for next 24 hours, including the next morning's first voided specimen, is collected in containers that are provided by the laboratory. Collect every drop of urine during the day and night. Store the container at room temperature or in the refrigerator. Finish by collecting the first urine passed the next morning, adding it to the collection bottle. This should be within 10 minutes before or after the time of the first morning void on the first day (which was flushed). In this example, it would be between 6:05 and 6:25 on the second day.

Once a full 24 hours of urine is collected, the total volume is recorded. Label the container with full name of patient, date of birth, and the date and time of start and finish of the collection.

A preservative solution is added to the urine collection to stabilize the sample for later analysis. Most preservatives are added to reduce bacterial metabolism or to prevent chemical decomposition of the analyte(s) of interest. This is typically done by adjusting the pH to an acidic or basic range. Some of the common urine preservatives include potassium phosphate, benzoic acid, sodium bicarbonate, acetic acid, hydrochloric acid (6 mol/L—30 mL per 24 hour collection) and boric acid.

Urine specimens should be delivered within 2 hours of collection or refrigerated and transported to the laboratory as soon as possible.

Fecal Collection

A stool analysis is a series of tests done on a stool (feces) sample to help diagnose certain conditions affecting the digestive tract. These conditions can include infection, poor nutrient absorption, or cancer, hidden (occult) blood, fat, meat fibers, bile, and sugars called reducing substances.

Label the container and give instructions to patient.

Instructions given to patient: Collect stool into a clean, dry container or a container provided by laboratory. Specimens must not be contaminated with urine or water. Deliver the specimen to the laboratory immediately. Refrigerate it if there is a delay in delivery.

Cerebrospinal Fluid

A sample of CSF is obtained by lumbar puncture, often called a spinal tap. It is a special but relatively routine procedure. It is performed while the person is lying on their side in a curled up, fetal position or sometimes in a sitting position. The back is cleaned with an antiseptic and a local anesthetic is injected under the skin. A special needle is inserted through the skin, between two vertebrae, and into the spinal canal. The health practitioner collects a small amount of CSF in multiple sterile vials; the needle is withdrawn and a sterile dressing and pressure are applied to the puncture site. The patient will then be asked to lie quietly in a flat position, without lifting their head, for one or more hours to avoid a potential post-test spinal headache.

Other body fluids are collected using procedures similar to that used for CSF in that they require aspiration of a sample of the fluid through a needle into a collection vessel, use of a local anesthetic, and a resting period following sample collection.

Pleural Fluid

This fluid is present in the pleural space. This is taken out by the needle and the procedure is called cerebrospinal fluid. This fluid is analyzed for the diagnosis of malignancy and may be used for culture and some biochemical tests.

Ascitic Fluids

This fluid is collected from the abdominal cavity in case of ascites. This ascitic fluid may be analyzed to diagnose benign or malignancy. Also, some biochemical tests are done. The procedure is known as paracentesis.

Synovial Fluids

This is the joint fluid aspirated aseptically and its analysis gives the diagnosis for its formation. The procedure is known as arthrocentesis.

Semen

Male patients ejaculate into a specimen container, avoiding lubricants, condoms, or any other potentially contaminating materials. Usually, men need to refrain from ejaculating for at least 2 days prior but <7 days before collecting the specimen. The specimen must not be refrigerated but kept as close to body temperature as possible by placing the container in a pocket and delivering it to the laboratory within 60 minutes.

Sputum

Patients are instructed to cough up sputum from as far down in the lungs as possible. (A health practitioner may assist the patient in some situations.) This is best accomplished first thing in the morning before eating or drinking, by taking several deep breaths before expectorating into the collection cup. Sputum should be relatively thick and not as watery as seen when producing saliva.

All samples must be labeled and transported properly.

Methods in Clinical Laboratory

1. **Manual procedures:** Few laboratories are using these procedures. Manual methods are good for small-sized laboratories. Work is tedious and time-consuming. **Table 12.5** shows comparisons between small and large size laboratory
2. **Semi-automated procedures or full automated procedures:** Many laboratories are using these procedures. It saves time and manpower. It requires stringent quality control. However, these are expensive.
   - The early forms of automation were semiauto analyzers.
   - Then came auto analyzer based on continuous flow system.
   - Later discrete analyzers were introduced.
   - Batch analyzer—semiautomated and fully automated.
   - Stat or random access analyzers.

Batch analyzer: The reagent mixture is mixed and fed automatically. One reagent is stored in the machine at a time, enabling one batch of a specific test to be automatically conducted, e.g., RA 100 and ASCA.

Random access auto analyzers: These analyzers can store more than one reagent. Samples are placed in the machine and the computer

Table 12.5: General comparisons between small and large laboratory.

Small laboratories	Large laboratories
Multistep manual methods are used	Monostep methods replaced multistep methods
Reagents prepared manually	Reagents are commercially available
Mouth pipetting is done	Dispensers and diluters are used
Workload is less	Workload has increased tremendously
Methods and procedures are lengthy and time-consuming	Test procedure is short and fast
More manpower is needed	Less manpower is needed due to automation

is programmed to carry out any number of selected tests on each sample, e.g., Hitachi series, RxL series, AU 400,640,2700, etc.

For many laboratories, volume of work increased, and need for simplification arose. This increasing workload led to automation. It saves time and effort as:
- Monostep methods replaced multistep methods
- No manual pipetting
- Efficiency increased by the use of dispensers and diluters
- The automated instruments not only save the labor and time, but allow reliable quality control, reduce the subjective errors, and work economically by using smaller quantities of sample and reagents.

Big laboratories and hospital-based laboratories may have laboratory information system.

Laboratories today are held together by a system of software programs and computers that exchange data about patients, test requests, and test results known as a Laboratory Information System or LIS. The LIS may be interfaced with the hospital information system.*

REPORTING AND INTERPRETATION OF RESULTS

Following criteria should be kept in mind while reporting/reading laboratory test results.
- **Error:** There is a certain error in all results. Usually laboratory will claim 95% confidence in its result, i.e., ±2 standard deviation (SD). Thus a blood sugar report of 100 mg/100 mL with a SD of 1 mg/100 mL would really be 100 + 2 mg/100 mL. For simplicity, the variation is not usually reported with the individual result. The SD for the method should be indicated and the result given with the understanding that the variation is understood.
- **Significant figures:** From mathematical calculations results may be obtained to many decimal places but these will not usually be significant. When reporting a result then each figure given should have a meaning. Thus result should be rounded off to the nearest significant figure before reporting. What is or is not significant must be established for each test.

---

*More about automation is given in separate chapter.

Like in a blood sugar report, 100.2 mg/100 mL is not written as 0.2 mg is not a significant part of the result for most blood sugar methods.

Use of zeros after a decimal point can give misleading information if they are not significant.

For example, 7.0 g means between 6.95 and 7.05 g, while 7 g means between 6.5 and 7.5 g.

- **Precision and accuracy:** Precision is the reproducibility of an analytical method. Accuracy defines how close the measured value is to the actual value. It is the objective in all biochemical method to have good precision and accuracy.
- **Sensitivity and specificity:** Sensitivity of an assay is a measure of how little of the analyte the method can detect. As new methods are developed, they may offer improved detection limits which may help in the discrimination between normal results and those in patients with the suspected disease. Specificity of an assay is related to how good the assay is at discriminating between the requested analyte and potentially interfering substances.
- **Reference ranges:** Biochemical test results are usually compared to a reference range considered to represent the normal healthy state. A reference range for a particular measurement is defined as the prediction interval between which 95% of values of a reference group fall into, in such a way that 2.5% of the time a sample value will be less than the lower limit of this interval, and 2.5% of the time it will be larger than the upper limit of this interval, whatever the distribution of these values.

Reference ranges are sometimes termed normal ranges/normal values. However, using the term normal may not be appropriate as not everyone outside the interval is abnormal (false positive), and people who have a particular condition may still not fall within this interval (false positive). In practice, there are no rigid limits demarcating the diseased population from the healthy; however, the further a result is from the limits of the range, the more likely it is to represent pathology.

Reference ranges are either population based or risk based. Population-based reference ranges are determined by taking samples from a defined population and reference range is calculated as mean ±2 SD. For cholesterol, reference range is given as risk based, 4.0 mmol/L or lower carries a low risk of coronary heart disease.

Biological Factors Affecting the Interpretation of Results

The discrimination between normal and abnormal results is affected by various physiological factors which must be considered when interpreting any given result. These include:

- **Sex of the patient:** Reference ranges for some analytes such as serum creatinine are different for men and women.
- **Age of the patient:** There may be different reference range for neonates, children, adults, and the elderly.
- **Effect of diet:** The sample may be inappropriate if taken when the patient is fasting or after a meal.
- **Time of sample collection:** There may be variations during the day and night.
- **Stress and anxiety:** It may affect the analyte of interest.
- **Posture of the patient:** Redistribution of fluid may affect the result.
- **Effects of exercise:** Strenuous exercise can release enzymes from tissues.
- **Medical history:** Infection and/or tissue injury can affect biochemical values independently of the disease process being investigated.
- **Pregnancy:** It alters some reference ranges.
- **Menstrual cycle:** Hormone measurements will vary through the menstrual cycle.
- **Drug history:** Drugs may have specific effects on the plasma concentration of some analytes.

SUMMARY

- Clinical biochemistry is a branch of laboratory medicine which applies chemical and biochemical methods to the study of disease.
- The biochemical tests are performed for four main reasons—diagnosis, treatment, prognosis, and screening.
- When a group of test is applied to otherwise healthy individuals or to all admitted to hospitals, it is termed biochemical profiling.
- The International System of Units (SI) is the modern form of the metric system, with an official status in nearly every country in the world.
- The seven SI base units are: Length—meter (m), time—second (s), amount of substance—mole (mol).

- Electric current—ampere (A), temperature—kelvin (K), luminous intensity—candela (cd), and mass—kilogram (kg).
- Magnitudes of all SI units have been defined by declaring exact numerical values for seven defining constants when expressed in terms of their SI units. These defining constants are the speed of light in vacuum, c, the hyperfine transition frequency of cesium Δv_{Cs}, the Planck constant h, the elementary charge e, the Boltzmann constant k, the Avogadro constant N_A, and the luminous efficacy K_{cd}.
- A derived unit is a SI unit of measurement comprised of a combination of the seven base units.
- Laboratory glassware refers to a variety of equipment made of glass used for scientific experiments and other work in science.
- Different types of glasses used to make labwares are: Borosilicate glass, quartz glass, fritted glass, silanized glass, and amber glass.
- Volumetric glasswares are specialized pieces of glassware which are used to measure volumes of liquids very precisely in quantitative laboratory work.
- A pipette is used to measure small amounts of solution very accurately. It can be transfer pipette or measuring pipette.
- Washing immediately after use, use of ultrasonic cleaners, hot water, chromic acid, and acetone are some methods to clean glasswares.
- Blood and urine are most common samples used in biochemistry laboratory. Other samples tested are sputum, feces, semen, and other bodily fluids and tissues.
- Blood can be collected from capillary, artery, or vein depending upon tests to be done.
- Specimen labeling, choice of collection tube according to additives, and order of draw are few things to be kept in mind while handling blood collection.
- Avoid sampling errors of time, technique, transportation, site, or storage.
- Some tests that require 8–12 hours of fasting are: Fasting blood glucose, lipid profile, electrolytes, vitamin B12, and iron.
- Different types of urine samples, representing collection at different times of day and for different durations of time, are used for laboratory analyses.
- 24-hour urine samples need either use of preservative or refrigeration.
- Fecal specimen should be collected in a clean, dry container.
- CSF and other body fluids are collected with use of a local anesthetic, and a resting period following sample collection.
- Semen should be ejaculated in specimen container and should be kept as close to body temperature as possible.
- Sputum should be coughed up from as far down in the lungs as possible.
- Methods used in clinical biochemistry laboratory can be manual, semiautomatic, or full automatic, depends upon flow of patients in laboratory.

- Analyzers can be batch analyzer or random access auto analyzers.
- Test result should be rounded off to the nearest significant figure before reporting.
- Precision is the reproducibility of an analytical method.
- Accuracy defines how close the measured value is to the actual value.
- Sensitivity of an assay is a measure of how little of the analyte the method can detect.
- Specificity of an assay is related to how good the assay is at discriminating between the requested analyte and potentially interfering substances.
- A reference range is prediction interval between which 95% of values of a reference group fall into.
- There are different biological factors affecting the interpretation of results such as age and sex of patient.

PRACTICE QUESTIONS

1. Define clinical biochemistry and biochemical profiling.
2. Differentiate between selective screening and individual screening.
3. Explain with example: Reasons of performing biochemical tests.
4. What is SI? Who and when established it?
5. Why there is need of SI system?
6. Define all seven basic units of SI system.
7. What are derived units? Explain with example.
8. The average volume of blood in an adult male is 4.7 L. What is this volume in milliliters?
9. Perform each conversion.
    a. 101,000 ns to seconds
    b. 32.08 kg to grams
    c. 1.53 grams to cg
    d. 4,300,000 cL to liter
    e. 1.73 hg to dg
    f. 15 nm to km
10. Discuss the different types of glass used to produce laboratory glassware.
11. Name and draw any five laboratory glassware.
12. What do you mean by volumetric glassware? Explain the use of any two volumetric glassware.
13. Discuss the types and use of pipette in clinical laboratory.
14. Write a method to clean: a. New glassware, b. grease on glassware, c. glassware with organic residue.
15. What is phlebotomy? What is the role of phlebotomist in clinical laboratory?
16. What are different methods of blood collection? Distinguish between arterial and venous blood collection.
17. Create a sample of specimen label.
18. Learn and write table given in chapter for order of draw, additives as per cap color of collection bottle.
19. What different sources of sampling errors? Discuss consequences of it.

Chapter 12: Introduction to Clinical Biochemistry

20. For which blood tests, sample is required to be withdrawn in fasting condition? Why?
21. What are the different types of urine samples collected?
22. What is CSF? How it is collected?
23. Why is automation implicated in modern day laboratories?
24. Compare method of working in small laboratories and large laboratories.
25. Discuss the criteria should be kept in mind while reporting/reading laboratory test results.
26. Why reference range should not be considered same as normal values?
27. Discuss biological factors affecting the interpretation of results.

CHAPTER 13

Advanced Analytical Techniques–I

> **Keywords**
> Chromatography, stationary phase, mobile phase eluent, eluate, elution, analyte, column chromatography, isocratic elution technique, gradient elution technique, anion exchange chromatography, ion exchange chromatography cation exchange chromatography, gel chromatography, paper chromatography, Whatman filter paper, gas chromatography (GC), the retention factor (Rf), high-performance liquid chromatography (HPLC), thin layer chromatography (TLC) mass spectroscopy, ionization, acceleration, deflection, detection

■ INTRODUCTION

Analytical technique is a method that is used to determine a chemical or physical property of a chemical substance, chemical element, or mixture. There are a wide variety of techniques used for analysis of clinical samples in clinical biochemistry laboratory. It ranges from simple weighing to advanced techniques using highly specialized instrumentation. Two such advanced techniques, namely, chromatography and mass spectroscopy, are discussed in this chapter.

■ CHROMATOGRAPHY

Chromatography is an important biophysical technique that enables the separation, identification, and purification of the components of a mixture for qualitative and quantitative analysis. Chromatography is based on the principle where molecules in mixture applied onto the surface or into the solid, and fluid stationary phase (stable phase) is separating from each other while moving with the aid of a mobile phase. Important terms and definition related to chromatography are mentioned in **Table 13.1**.

Table 13.1: Important terms and definitions related to chromatography.

Terms	Definitions
Mobile phase or carrier	Solvent moving through the column
Stationary phase or adsorbent	Substance that stays fixed inside the column
Eluent	Fluid entering the column
Eluate	Fluid exiting the column (that is collected in flasks)
Elution	The process of washing out a compound through a column using a suitable solvent
Analyte	Mixture whose individual components have to be separated and analyzed

The factors effective on this separation process include molecular characteristics related to adsorption (liquid–solid), partition (liquid–solid), and affinity or differences among their molecular weights. Because of these differences, some components of the mixture stay longer in the stationary phase, and they move slowly in the chromatography system, while others pass rapidly into the mobile phase, and leave the system faster.

Three components thus form the basis of the chromatography technique.

1. **Stationary phase:** This phase is always composed of a "solid" phase or "a layer of a liquid adsorbed on the surface solid support."
2. **Mobile phase:** This phase is always composed of "liquid" or a "gaseous component."
3. **Separated molecules:** A wide range of chromatographic procedures are available to separate substances on the basis of the presence of characteristics such as size and shape, total charge, hydrophobic groups present on the surface, and binding capacity with the stationary phase. This leads to different types of chromatography techniques, each with their own instrumentation and working principle.

Column Chromatography

Column chromatography is the separation technique where the components in a mixture are separated on the basis of their differential adsorption with the stationary phase, resulting in them moving at different speeds when passed through a column.

It is a solid-liquid chromatography technique in which the stationary phase is a solid and the mobile phase is a liquid or gas.

Principles of Column Chromatography

- This technique is based on the principle of differential adsorption where different molecules in a mixture have different affinities with the absorbent present on the stationary phase.
- The molecules having higher affinity remain adsorbed for a longer time decreasing their speed of movement through the column.
- However, the molecules with lower affinity move with a faster movement, thus allowing the molecules to be separated in different fractions.
- Here, the stationary phase in the column chromatography, also termed the absorbent, is a solid (mostly silica) and the mobile phase is a liquid that allow the molecules to move through the column smoothly.

Steps of Column Chromatography

- The column is prepared by taking a glass tube that is dried and coated with a thin, uniform layer of stationary phase (cellulose and silica).
- Then the sample is prepared by adding the mixture to the mobile phase. The sample is introduced into the column from the top and is allowed to pass the sample under the influence of gravity or by use of pumping system or applied gas pressure **(Fig. 13.1)**.
- The molecules bound to the column are separated by two elution techniques:
    1. *Isocratic elution technique:* Same solvent composition or solvent of same polarity is used throughout the process of separation, e.g., use of chloroform alone.
    2. *Gradient elution technique:* Solvents of gradually increasing polarity or increasing elution strength are used during the process of separation, e.g., initially benzene, then chloroform, then ethyl acetate.
- The separated molecules can further be analyzed for various purposes.

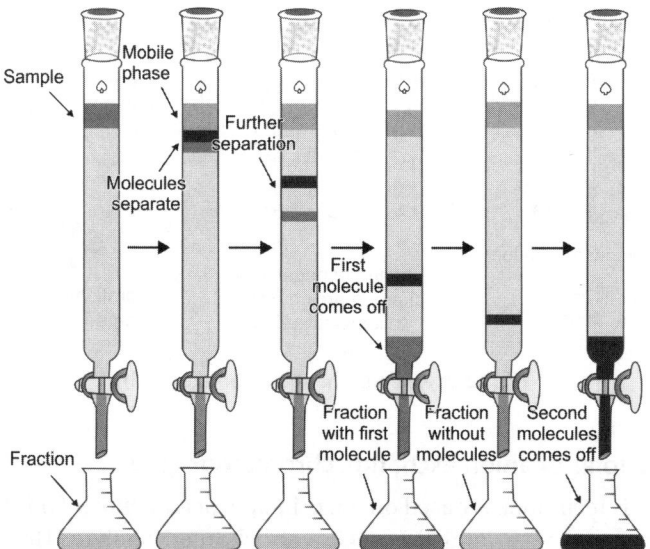

Fig. 13.1: Column chromatography.

Applications

Column chromatography is one of the most useful methods for the separation and purification of both solids and liquids. Its major application in clinical biochemistry is separation of proteins and hemoglobins and isolation of metabolites from biological fluids.

Ion Exchange Chromatography

Ion exchange chromatography (or ion chromatography) is a process that allows the separation of ions and polar molecules based on their affinity to ion exchangers. The principle of separation is thus by reversible exchange of ions between the target ions present in the sample solution to the ions present on ion exchangers.

In this process two types of exchangers, i.e., cationic and anionic exchangers, can be used.

Anion Exchange Chromatography

Anion exchange chromatography is the separation technique for negatively charged molecules by their interaction with the positively charged stationary phase in the form of ion-exchange resin **(Fig. 13.2)**.

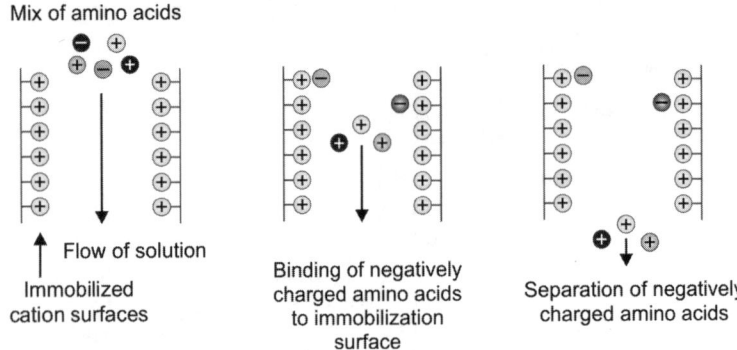

Fig. 13.2: Anion exchange chromatography.

Principles of anion exchange chromatography

- This technique is based on the principle of attraction of positively charged resin and the negatively charged analyte. Here the exchange of positively charged ions takes place to remove the negatively charged molecules.
- The stationary phase is first coated with positive charges where the components of the mixture with negative charges will bind.
- An anion exchange resin with a higher affinity to the negatively charged components then binds the components, displacing the positively charged resin.
- The anion exchange resin-component complex then is removed by using different buffers.

Steps of anion exchange chromatography

- A column packed with positively charged resin is taken as the stationary phase.
- The mixture with the charged particles is then passed down the column where the negatively charged molecules bind to the positively charged resins.
- The anion exchange resin is then passed through the column where the negatively charged molecules now bind to the anion exchange resin displacing the positively charged resin.
- Now an appropriate buffer is applied to the column to separate the complex of anion exchange resins and the charged molecules.

Applications of anion exchange chromatography
- The separation of nucleic acids from a mixture obtained after cell destruction.
- The separation of proteins from the crude mixture obtained from the blood serum.

Cation Exchange Chromatography
Cation exchange chromatography is the separation technique for positively charged molecules by their interaction with negatively charged stationary phase in the form of ion-exchange resin (**Fig. 13.3**).

Principles of cation exchange chromatography
- This technique is based on the principle of attraction of negatively charged resin and the positively charged analyte. Here the exchange of negatively charged ions takes place to remove the positively charged molecules.
- The stationary phase is first coated with negative charges where the components of the mixture with positive charges will bind.
- A cation exchange resin with a higher affinity to the positively charged components then binds the components, displacing the negatively charged resin.
- The cation exchange resin-component complex then is removed by using different buffers.

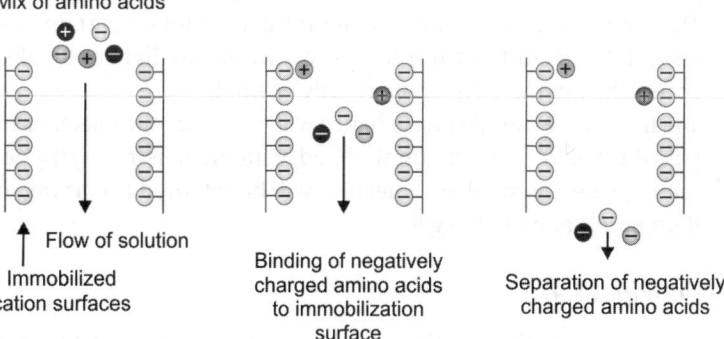

Fig. 13.3: Cation exchange chromatography.

Steps of cation exchange chromatography

- A column packed with negatively charged resin is taken as the stationary phase.
- The mixture with the charged particles is then passed down the column where the positively charged molecules bind to the negatively charged resins.
- The cation exchange resin is then passed through the column where the positively charged molecules now bind to the cation exchange resin displacing the negatively charged resin.
- Now an appropriate buffer is applied to the column to separate the complex of cation exchange resins and the charged molecules.

Applications

- The determination of presence of calcium ions in biological samples.
- To separate organic cations from inorganic salts.

Gel Chromatography

Gel-filtration chromatography is a form of partition chromatography used to separate molecules of different molecular weight or sizes.

Principles

- The stationary phase is a matrix of porous polymer which has pores of specific sizes.
- When the sample is injected with the mobile phase, the mobile phase occupies the pores of the stationary phase (gel).
- The basis of the separation is that molecules above a certain size are totally excluded from the pores, while smaller molecules access the interior of the pores partly or wholly.
- The flow of the mobile phase hence will cause larger molecules to pass through the column unhindered, without penetrating the gel matrix, whereas smaller molecules will be retarded according to their penetration of the gel.

Steps (Fig. 13.4)

- The column is filled with semi-permeable, porous polymer gel beads with a well-defined range of pore sizes.

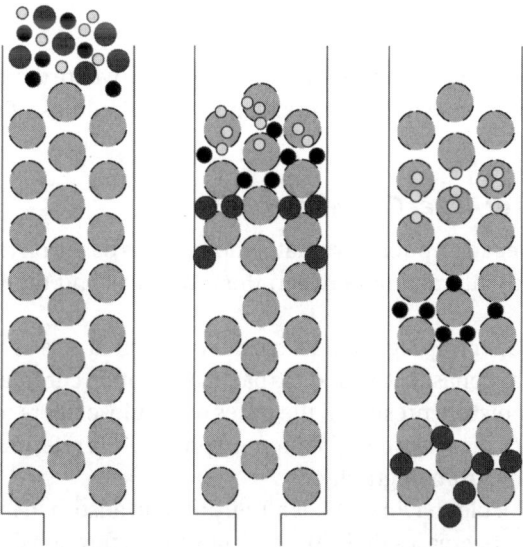

Fig. 13.4: Gel-filtration chromatography.

- The sample, mixed with the mobile phase, is then injected into the column from the top of the column.
- The molecules bound to the column are separated by elution solution where either solution of the same polarity is used (isocratic technique), or different samples with different polarities are used (gradient technique).
- Elution conditions (pH, essential ions, cofactors, protease inhibitors, etc.) can be selected, which will complement the requirements of the molecule of interest.

Applications

- The separation of recombinant human granulocyte colony-stimulating factor (rhG-CSF) from inclusion bodies in high yield by urea-gradient size-exclusion chromatography.
- Gel-filtration chromatography has been used to separate various nucleic acid species such as DNA, RNA, and tRNA as well as their constituent bases, adenine, guanine, thymine, cytosine, and uracil.
- Purification of proteins and peptides from various sources.

Paper Chromatography

Paper chromatography is a separation technique where the separation is performed on Whatman filter paper (with cellulose fibers on a paper).

Principles of Paper Chromatography

- The paper adsorption chromatography that is based on the varying degree of interaction between the molecules and the stationary phase.
  When paper impregnated with silica or alumina acts as adsorbent (stationary phase), it is called as paper adsorption chromatography. When moisture present in the pores of cellulose fibers of the filter paper acts as adsorbent (stationary phase), it is referred as paper partition chromatography.
- The molecules having higher affinity remain adsorbed for a longer time, this decreases their speed of movement through the column. Whereas the molecules with lower affinity will move faster.
- Because of different affinities, molecules are separated in different fractions.
- "Retention factor" is applied during the separation of molecules in the paper chromatography.
- The retention value for a molecule is determined as a ratio of distance traveled by the molecule to the distance traveled by the mobile phase (solvent).
- The retention value of different molecules can be used to differentiate those molecules.

Steps of Paper Chromatography

- The stationary phase is selected as a fine quality cellulosic paper.
- Different combinations of organic and inorganic solvents are taken as the mobile phase.
- About 2-200 µL of the sample solution is injected at the baseline of the paper, and it is allowed to air dry **(Fig. 13.5A)**.
- The sample loaded paper is then carefully dipped into the mobile phase not more than the height of 1 cm **(Fig. 13.5B)**.

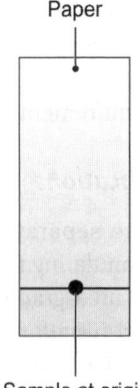

Fig. 13.5A: Whatman paper with sample.

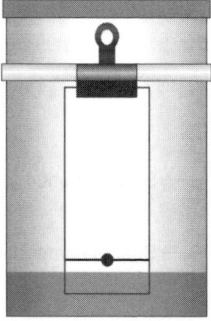 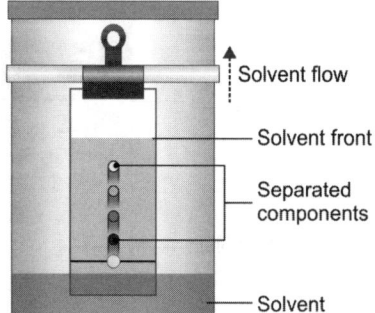

Fig. 13.5B: Paper dipped in a solvent. **Fig. 13.5C:** Components separated.
(For color version, see Plate 4) *(For color version, see Plate 5)*

- After the mobile phase reaches near the other edge of the paper, the paper is taken out **(Fig. 13.5C)**.
- The retention factor (Rf) is calculated, and the separated components are detected by different techniques.

$$R_f = \frac{\text{Distance moved by the component}}{\text{Distance moved by the solvent}}$$

Applications

- Paper chromatography is performed to detect the purity of various pharmaceutical products.
- In clinical biochemistry, it is used to separate amino acids.
- Identification of sugars excreted in urine.

Thin Layer Chromatography

Thin layer chromatography is similar to paper chromatography. Major difference in procedure is in stationary phase. TLC is performed on a TLC plate. It is a sheet of glass, plastic, or aluminum foil, which is coated with a thin layer of adsorbent material, usually silica gel, aluminum oxide (alumina), or cellulose. This layer of adsorbent is known as the stationary phase **(Fig. 13.6)**.

Another thing is, the filter paper should be kept in TLC jar to saturate the air in the jar with the solvent vapors. If the air is not saturated with solvent, the solvent that is rising up the plate will evaporate in an attempt to saturate the air.

Rf value is calculated as discussed in paper chromatography. Retention factor is a unique value for each compound under the same conditions. On the basis of this, compounds are identified.

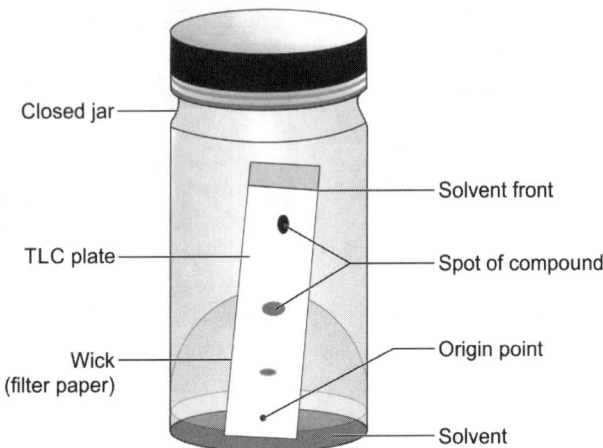

Fig. 13.6: Thin layer chromatography.

Advantages of TLC over paper chromatography: It is less time-consuming, has more sharp separation, and has high sensitivity. It is possible to heat TLC plate and evaluate under UV.

Gas Chromatography

Gas chromatography (GC) is a separation technique in which the molecules are separated on the basis of their retention time depending on the affinity of the molecules to the stationary phase. The sample is either liquid or gas that is vaporized in the injection point **(Fig. 13.7)**.

Principles of Gas Chromatography

- GC is based on the principle that components having a higher affinity to the stationary phase have a higher retention time as they take a longer time to come out of the column.
- However, the components having a higher affinity to the stationary phase have less retention time as they move along with the mobile phase.
- The mobile phase is a gas, mostly helium, that carries the sample through the column.
- The sample once injected in converted into the vapor stage is then passed through a detector to determine the retention time.

Chapter 13: Advanced Analytical Techniques–I

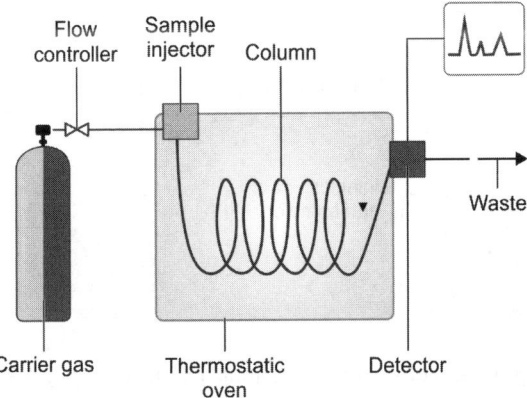

Fig. 13.7: Gas chromatography.

- The components are collected separately as they come out of the stationary phase at different times.

Steps of Gas Chromatography

- The sample is injected into the column where it is vaporized into a gaseous state. The vaporized component than mixes with the mobile phase to be carried through the rest of the column.
- The column is set with the stationary phase where the molecules are separated on the basis of their affinity to the stationary phase.
- The components of the mixture reach the detector at different times due to differences in the time they are retained in the column.

Applications

- This is used in the analysis of air pollutants, oil spills, and other samples.
- GC can also be used in forensic science to identify and quantify various biological samples found in the crime scene.
- The identification of performance-inducing drug in the athlete's urine

Note: Another important form of chromatography is liquid chromatography. The main difference between gas and liquid chromatography is that the mobile phase of GC is a gas, whereas the mobile phase of liquid chromatography is a liquid, which can be either polar or nonpolar.

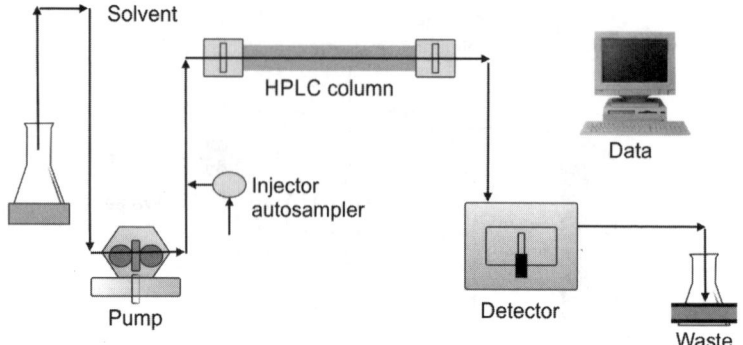

Fig. 13.8: High-performance liquid chromatography (HPLC).

High-performance Liquid Chromatography

High-performance liquid chromatography (HPLC) is a modified form of column chromatography where the components of a mixture are separated on the basis of their affinity with the stationary phase **(Fig. 13.8)**.

Principles of HPLC

- This technique is based on the principle of differential adsorption where different molecules in a mixture have a varying degree of interactions with the absorbent present on the stationary phase.
- The molecules having higher affinity remain adsorbed for a longer time decreasing their speed of movement through the column.
- However, the molecules with lower affinity move with a faster movement, thus allowing the molecules to be separated in different fractions.
- This process is slightly different from the column chromatography as in this case; the solvent is forced under high pressures of up to 400 atmospheres instead of allowing it to drip down under gravity.

Steps of High-performance Liquid Chromatography

- The column is prepared by taking a glass tube that is dried and coated with a thin, uniform layer of stationary phase (cellulose and silica).
- Then the sample is prepared by adding the mixture to the mobile phase. The sample is introduced into the column from the top,

and a high-pressure pump is used to pass the sample at a constant rate.
- The mobile phase then moves down to a detector that detects molecules at a certain absorbance wavelength.
- The separated molecules can further be analyzed for various purposes. A common HPLC detector is a UV absorption detector, as most medium to large molecules absorb UV radiation. Detectors that measure fluorescence and refractive index are also used for special applications.

Uses of High-performance Liquid Chromatography

- The increased speed of this technique makes the process faster and more effective.
- It is used to separate and determine various types of hemoglobin.
- This technique can also be used to separate different biological molecules such as proteins and nucleic acids.
- HPLC has been performed to test the efficiency of different antibodies against diseases such as Ebola.

■ MASS SPECTROSCOPY

Mass spectrometry (MS) is an advanced technique for determining the molecular weight of a compound. The instrument has now a wide range of applications in pharmaceutical (drug discovery, pharmacokinetics, and drug metabolism), clinical (neonatal screening, hemoglobin analysis, and drug testing), environmental (water quality, food contamination, and pollutant determination), and in almost every field.

Principle

The mass spectroscopy is based on the positive-ion generation. The basic principle of MS is to generate ions from either inorganic or organic compounds by any suitable method, to separate these ions by their mass-to-charge ratio (m/z) and to detect them qualitatively and quantitatively by their respective m/z and abundance.

The analyte may be ionized thermally, by electric fields or by impacting energetic electrons, ions, or photons. The ions can be single ionized atoms, clusters, molecules or their fragments or associates.

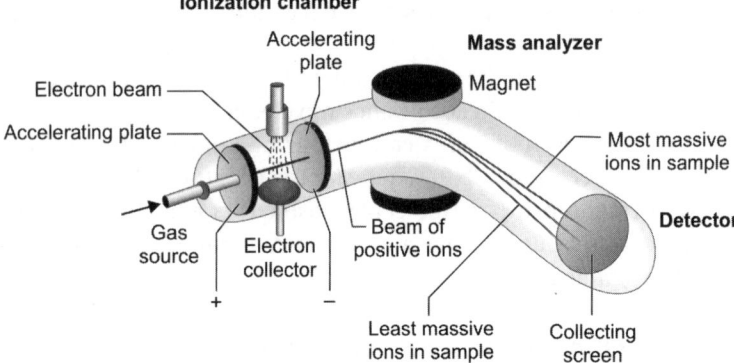

Fig. 13.9: Mass spectroscopy.

Ion separation is effected by static or dynamic electric or magnetic fields.

Instrumentation

The three main parts of a mass spectrometer are the ion source, the mass analyzer, and the detector **(Fig. 13.9)**.

Ionization

The initial sample may be a solid, liquid, or gas. The sample is vaporized into a gas and then ionized by the ion source, usually by losing an electron to become a cation. The sample under investigation is converted into vapor phase and bombarded with electrons having energy sufficient to knock out one electron from it (>10 eV) to produce a positively charged ion called molecular ion or parent ion which is denoted by M^+. Positively charged molecule M^+ is often unstable, and with increase in energy (10–70 eV) according to bond strength, they break into fragments called fragment or daughter ion which is denoted by M_1^{+1} and M_2^{+1}.

$$M + e^- \longrightarrow M^+ + 2e^-$$
$$\downarrow e^-$$
$$M_1^+ \longrightarrow M_2^+$$

Where,
M^+ = molecular ion
M_1^+ and M_2^+ = Fragment ions

The ionization chamber is kept in a vacuum so the ions that are produced can progress through the instrument without running into molecules from air. Ionization is from electrons that are produced by heating up a metal coil until it releases electrons.

Acceleration

The ions placed between a set of charged parallel plates get attracted to one plate and repel from the other plate. This accelerates ionization. The acceleration speed can be controlled by adjusting the charge on the plates. In the mass analyzer, the ions are then accelerated through a potential difference and focused into a beam. The purpose of acceleration is to give all ions or fragments the same kinetic energy.

Deflection

The ion beam passes through a magnetic field which deflects ions based on its charge and mass. If an ion is heavy or has two or more positive charges, then it is least deflected. If an ion is light or has one positive charge, then it is deflected the most.

Detection

The ions with correct charge and mass move to the detector. The ratio of mass to charge is analyzed through the ion that hits the detector. A detector counts the number of ions at different deflections. The data is plotted as a graph or spectrum of different masses. Detectors work by recording the induced charge or current caused by an ion striking a surface or passing by.

Working

In a regular mass spectrometer, the material to be analyzed is ionized to pass through the spectrometer with enough energy. Thus, the sample is bombarded by electrons to ionize it. This ionized beam is now passed through a series of electric or magnetic fields depending on the type of the sample and its properties. The ions are deflected by the field through which they are passed through in such a way that the ions with the same mass to signal ratio will follow the same path to the detector.

These charged and deflected ions are now incident onto a detector which is capable of distinguishing the charged particles falling on it. Based on the mass spectrum produced by the charged ions, we can identify the atoms or molecules constituting the sample by comparing them with known masses or through a characteristic fragmentation pattern.

Applications

- Mass spectroscopy is widely employed in phytochemical analysis due to its capability to identify and measure metabolites having very low molecular weight at very low concentration ranges below nanogram per milliliter (ng/mL). Therefore, it is considered as trace analysis methodology.
- A variety of analyte separation techniques such as capillary electrophoresis (CE), GC, and HPLC are united with mass spectroscopy for simultaneous separation and determination of analytes called CE-MS, GC-MS, and HPLC-MS, respectively.
- Analytes having high molecular weight and temperature sensitive can be efficiently analyzed by HPLC coupled with atmospheric pressure ionization-mass spectrometer (API-MS).
- Mass spectroscopy has an important application in analysis of sequence of amino acids in proteins and peptides, that is, analysis of structure of proteins and peptides.

SUMMARY

- Analytical technique is a method that is used to determine a chemical or physical property of a chemical substance, chemical element, or mixture.
- Stationary phase is composed of a "solid" phase or "a layer of a liquid adsorbed on the surface solid support."
- Mobile phase is composed of "liquid" or a "gaseous component."
- Eluent is fluid entering the column.
- Eluate is fluid exiting the column.
- Elution is the process of washing out.
- Analyte is sample mixture.

- Chromatography is a laboratory technique for the separation of a mixture.
- Chromatography is based on the principle where molecules in mixture applied onto the surface or into the solid, and fluid stationary phase (stable phase) are separating from each other while moving with the aid of a mobile phase.
- Column chromatography is the separation technique where the components in a mixture are separated on the basis of their differential adsorption with the stationary phase, resulting in them moving at different speeds when passed through a column.
- Isocratic elution technique: Same solvent composition or solvent of same polarity is used throughout the process of separation.
- Gradient elution technique: Solvents of gradually increasing polarity or increasing elution strength are used during the process of separation.
- Ion exchange chromatography (or ion chromatography) is a process that allows the separation of ions and polar molecules based on their affinity to ion exchangers. The principle of separation is thus by reversible exchange of ions between the target ions present in the sample solution to the ions present on ion exchangers.
- Anion exchange chromatography is the separation technique for negatively charged molecules by their interaction with the positively charged stationary phase in the form of ion-exchange resin.
- Cation exchange chromatography is the separation technique for positively charged molecules by their interaction with negatively charged stationary phase in the form of ion-exchange resin.
- Gel-filtration chromatography is a form of partition chromatography used to separate molecules of different molecular weight or sizes.
- In paper chromatography, the mixture is spotted onto the paper, dried and the solvent is allowed to flow along the sheet by capillary attraction. As the solvent slowly moves through the paper, the different compounds of the mixture separate into different colored spots.
- TLC is similar to paper chromatography but instead of paper, the stationary phase is a thin layer of an inert substance like silica supported on a flat, unreactive surface like glass plate is used.
- Column chromatography is a technique in which the substances to be separated are introduced onto the top of a column packed with an adsorbent.
- It passes through the column at different rates that depend on the affinity of each substance for the adsorbent and for the solvent or solvent mixture.
- Gas chromatography is a separation technique in which the molecules are separated on the basis of their retention time depending on the affinity of the molecules to the stationary phase. The sample is either liquid or gas that is vaporized in the injection point.

- HPLC is a modified form of column chromatography where the components of a mixture are separated on the basis of their affinity with the stationary phase.
- MS is an advanced technique for determining the molecular weight of a compound.
- The mass spectroscopy is based on the positive-ion generation. The basic principle of MS is to generate ions from either inorganic or organic compounds by any suitable method, to separate these ions by their mass-to-charge ratio (m/z) and to detect them qualitatively and quantitatively by their respective m/z and abundance.
- The four stages in a mass spectrometer are: ionization, acceleration, deflection, and detection.
- A variety of analyte separation techniques are united with mass spectroscopy for simultaneous separation and determination of analytes.

PRACTICE QUESTIONS

1. Define chromatography, stationary phase, mobile phase eluent, eluate, elution, and analyte.
2. Write the principle and procedure of column chromatography.
3. Write the principle and procedure of cation exchange chromatography.
4. Write the principle and procedure of anion exchange chromatography.
5. Write the principle and procedure of gel chromatography.
6. Write the principle and procedure of paper chromatography.
7. Write the principle and procedure of thin layer chromatography (TLC).
8. Write the principle and procedure of gas chromatography.
9. Write the principle and procedure of high-performance liquid chromatography (HPLC).
10. What is Rf? Give the formula for calculation of *Rf* value.
11. Name different types of chromatography and write two applications for each of them.
12. What is the principle of mass spectroscopy?
13. Write the instrumentation and applications of mass spectroscopy.

CHAPTER 14

Advanced Analytical Techniques–II

Keywords
Radioisotopes, enzymes, fluorescent dyes, radioimmunoassay (RIA), ELISA, optical density, indirect ELISA, direct ELISA, sandwich ELISA, competitive ELISA, fluorochromes, autoantibodies, immunofluorescence, agarose gel, DNA ladders, DNA extraction, hybridization, probe detection, polyvinylidene difluoride (PVDF) membrane, horseradish peroxidase (HRP), electrophoresis, buffer, secondary antibody

■ INTRODUCTION

Underlying most human diseases is a change in the amount or function of one or more proteins that in turn triggers changes in cellular, tissue, or organ function. The dysfunction is commonly characterized by a significant change in the biochemical profile of body fluids. The application of quantitative analytical biochemical tests to a large range of biological analytes in body fluids and tissues is a valuable aid to the diagnosis and management of the prevailing disease state. In this chapter, the general biological and analytical principles underlying these tests are be discussed.

■ IMMUNOASSAY

The search for new and better diagnostic aids over the past 10–20 years had led to the application of immunology to diagnostic medicine, creating a new group of tests known as immunoassays. Immunoassays combine the specificity of an antigen–antibody (Ag-Ab) reaction with the sensitivity of an indicator system. For high sensitivities, these immunoassays usually make use of an antigen, hapten, or antibody labeled in some way.

The most common labels are radioisotopes, enzymes, and fluorescent dyes.

The high sensitivity achieved relates to the physical and/or biochemical characteristics of the label, which releases high-energy products or amplifies the signal. Assays employing these labels may be evaluated both quantitatively and qualitatively.

Radioimmunoassay

Radioimmunoassay (RIA) is a laboratory method that measures, with relative accuracy, minute amounts of substances present in the body. It is considered as the blueprint for more advanced methods of laboratory techniques.

Drugs, antigens, and hormones are some of the substances measured by RIA.

Principles

- The target antigen is labeled radioactively.
- It is then made to bind with a known amount of its specific antibodies.
- A sample, e.g., a blood serum, with the same kind of unlabeled antigen (test target) is then added to the above labeled Ag-Ab complex.
- This will initiate a competitive reaction of the labeled antigens from the preparation, and the unlabeled antigens from the serum sample, with the specific antibodies. The competition for the antibodies will release a certain amount of labeled antigen. This amount is proportional to the ratio of labeled to unlabeled antigen.
- The more the concentration of unlabeled antigen, the more it binds to the antibody, displacing the labeled variant.
- The bound antigens are then separated from the unbound ones, and the radioactivity of the free antigens remaining in the supernatant is measured.
- A binding curve can be generated using a known standard, which allows the amount of antigens in the patient's serum to be derived.

Ag-Ab complex + unlabeled antigen gives Ag-Ab complex attached to unlabeled antigen and radiolabeled antigen becomes free **(Fig. 14.1)**.

- Isotopes, such as C^{14} and H^3 have been used as a label to prepare labeled antigen.

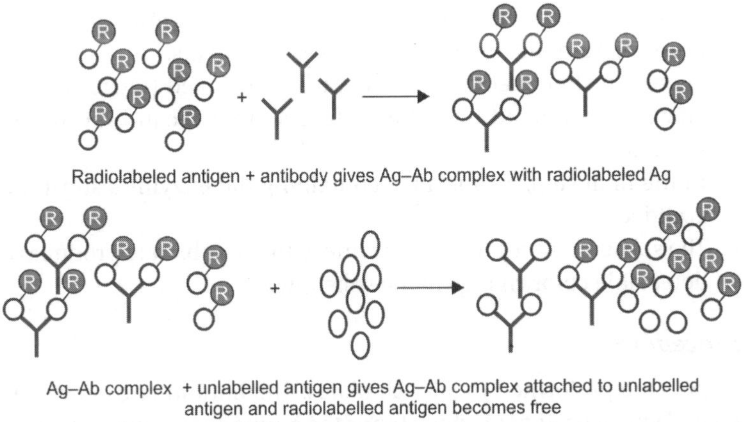

Fig. 14.1: Principle of radioimmunoassay.
(For color version, see Plate 5)

- Double antibody, charcoal, cellulose, chromatography, or solid phase techniques are applied to separate bound and free radiolabeled antigens.
- The bound or free fraction is counted in a gamma counter.
- A calibration or standard curve is generated with samples of known concentrations of the unlabeled standards. The amount of antigen in unknown samples can be calculated from this curve.
- Besides the use of RIA in blood-bank screening for hepatitis, and tracking other viruses, it is also used for other purposes like early detection of leukemia and other cancers, measurement of human growth hormones, and aid in the detection of many kinds of ulcers.

ELISA (Enzyme-linked Immunosorbent Assay)

It is also a type of immunoassay aimed to detect the antigen or antibodies present in an infected individual for proper diagnosis and further treatment.

It can be done rapidity with greater sensitivity and specificity for even small amount of test samples. The reaction is measurable in both qualitative and quantitative terms.

Principles

- The antigens (or antibodies) present in a patient's sample are allowed to stick to a polyvinyl plate.

- Then the plate is washed to separate antigens (or antibodies, if any present) from the remaining sample components.
- Then a further specific antibody, which is inked (tagged) to an enzyme, is applied over the surface so that it can bind to the antigen.
- In the final step, a substance containing the enzyme's substrate is added.
- The subsequent reaction of enzyme with the substrate produces a detectable color change in the substrate.

Procedure

ELISAs are performed in 96-well plates. The bottom of each well is coated with a protein to which binds the antibody (or antigen/ target protein) to be measured. Whole blood is allowed to clot and the cells are centrifuged out to obtain the clear serum with antibodies (or antigen/target protein). These are called as primary antibodies . The serum is incubated in a well, and each well contains a different serum **(Fig. 14.2)**. A positive control serum and a negative control serum would be included among the 96 samples being tested.

After some time, the serum is removed and weakly adherent antibodies are washed off with a series of buffer rinses. To detect the bound antibodies (or antigen/target protein), a secondary antibody (or secondary antigen) is added to each well. The secondary antibody would bind to all human antibodies and is typically produced in a rodent. Attached to the secondary antibody is an enzyme, such as peroxidase or alkaline phosphatase. These enzymes can metabolize colorless substrates (sometimes called chromagens) into colored products. After an incubation period, the secondary antibody solution

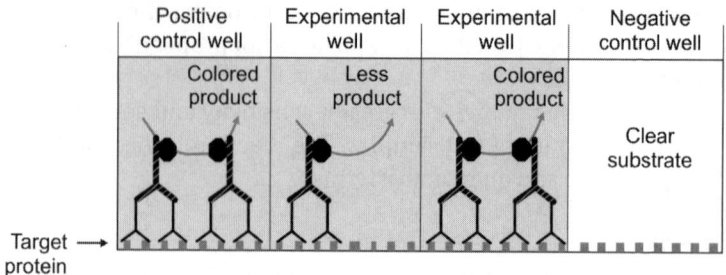

Fig. 14.2: Side view of 4 wells from 96 wells of enzyme-linked immunosorbent assay (ELISA) test.

is removed and loosely adherent ones are washed off as before. The final step is the addition of the enzyme substrate and the production of colored product in wells with secondary antibodies bound.

When the enzyme reaction is complete, the entire plate is placed into a plate reader and the optical density (i.e., the amount of colored product) is determined for each well. The amount of color produced is proportional to the amount of primary antibody bound to the proteins on the bottom of the wells.

Types of ELISA

ELISA is broadly classified as heterogeneous and homogeneous depending upon the state of antigen.
1. **Heterogeneous:** Here the *antigen first added is a solid type*, i.e., it is fixed to the plate and not in liquid form while next antibodies or antigens added are always in liquid phase.
2. **Homogeneous:** Here the *antigens first added are in liquid phase* and the antibodies added on to it are also in liquid phase.

ELISA is further classified into following types:
1. **Direct ELISA:** It is one wherein there is only one set of antigens and one set of antibodies to react. In this method, antigens from the patient sample fixed to the ELISA plates are made to react with an antibodies sample which is tagged to an enzyme, i.e., an enzyme-linked antibody is added directly to the antigen in the test to produce a color reaction with externally added substrate, i.e., ELISA reagent **(Fig. 14.3)**.

    Ag or Ab + Ab or Ag-(e) ⟶ Reaction color.
2. **Indirect ELISA**: *HIV ELISA Test* is done using this principle. This differs from direct ELISA in that *one more additional anti-body*

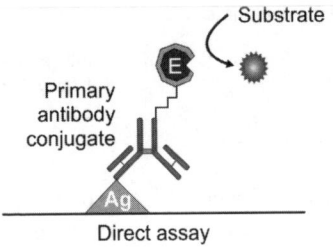

Fig. 14.3: Direct enzyme-linked immunosorbent assay (ELISA).

is added in the reaction. To the antigen (fixed to ELISA plate) an antibody is added. Again secondary antigen is added which is enzyme linked. This requirement is due to the reason that sometimes in patients antigen of disease-causing agent may not be present but a corresponding antibody is available in the patient sample. This can be traced. These are of two types, normal Indirect ELISA and sandwich ELISA.

$$\text{Ag or Ab + Ab or Ag + Ag or Ab-(e)} \longrightarrow \text{Reaction color.}$$

a. *Indirect ELISA procedure:* Here an external antigen of suspected antibody which might be present in patient sample is added to the plate. Then patient sample is added to see if any suspected antibody is present, it reacts with the external antigen fixed in the plate. Then another antibody, which is enzyme-linked, is added to react with antibody from sample and produce color on addition of substrate **(Fig. 14.4)**.

$$\text{Ag + Ab + Ab-(e)} \longrightarrow \text{Reaction color}$$

b. *Sandwich ELISA:* This is also an indirect type of ELISA. The only difference in this ELISA principle is that just like a sandwich, in between two antibodies an antigen is present as seen in the **Fig. 14.5**. The antibody at bottom fixes to the surface of plate, over it antigen is fixed onto which one more antibody (junction) is attached. On this junction antibody, an enzyme-linked

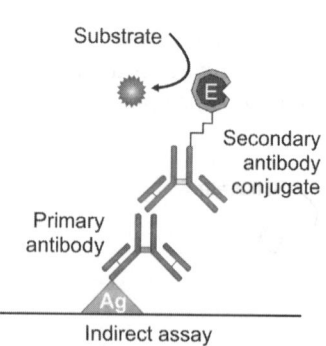

Fig. 14.4: Indirect enzyme-linked immunosorbent assay (ELISA).
(For color version, see Plate 5)

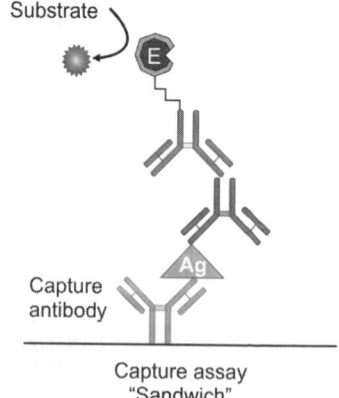

Fig. 14.5: Sandwich enzyme-linked immunosorbent assay (ELISA).
(For color version, see Plate 6)

antibody is present to give the color reaction with substrate added **(Fig. 14.5)**.

Ab + Ag + Ab + Ab-**(e)** ⟶ Reaction color.

3. **Competitive ELISA:** It is not a special type of ELISA but a slight modification to the protocols mentioned in above types of ELISA, such as direct, indirect, sandwich ELISA types. Here one more substance (preferably biotinated substance) is added to compete with Ab and Ag to bind to the already added Ag and Ab during the reaction. The intention of adding this competitor substance is to prevent unnecessary binding of Ab or Ag and see that the binding is only due to greater affinity in between Ag or Ab but not mere addition of them.

An ELISA test may be used to diagnose: HIV (the virus that causes AIDS), lyme disease, pernicious anemia, rocky mountain spotted fever, rotavirus, squamous cell carcinoma, syphilis, toxoplasmosis, varicella zoster virus (which causes chickenpox and shingles), dengue virus, etc.

The scope of ELISA is very wide as it can detect very minute amount of antigen and antibodies qualitatively as well as quantitatively. The patient in window period can be detected by ELISA. It can also help to monitor progress of disease in a patient. ELISA is not cheaper, but is cost effective and very reliable in terms of results.

Immunofluorescence Immunoassay

- Immunofluorescence is an antigen-antibody reaction where the antibodies are tagged (labeled) with a fluorescent dye and the antigen-antibody complex is visualized using ultraviolet (fluorescent) microscope. Fluorochromes are dyes that absorb ultraviolet rays and emit visible light. This process is called fluorescence. Fluorescence is the property of certain molecules or fluorophores to absorb light at one wavelength and emit light at longer wave- length (emission wavelength) when it is illuminated by light of a different wavelength.
- The incident light excites the molecule to a higher level of vibrational energy. As the molecules return to the ground state, the excited fluorophore emits photon (= fluorescence emission).

Commonly used fluorochromes are Acridine Orange, Rhodamine, Lissamine and Calcofluor white. However, these fluorochromes are used for general fluorescence. When fluorescein (FITC) is excited by a blue (wavelength 488 nm) light, it will emit a green (520 nm) color. Phycoerythrin (PE) emits an orange (570 nm) color. The fluorochromes commonly used in immunofluorescence are fluorescein isothiocyanate (green) and tetramethyl rhodamine isothiocyanate (red).

Types of Immunofluorescence
1. Direct immunofluorescence
2. Indirect immunofluorescence

Direct immunofluorescence

This technique is used to detect antigen in clinical specimens using specific fluorochrome labeled antibody. The steps involved are: Fixation of smear on the slide, treating with labeled antibody, incubation, washing to remove unbound excess labeled antibody and visualization under fluorescent microscope. When viewed under fluorescent microscope, the field is dark and areas with bound antibody fluoresce is green **(Fig. 14.6)**.

This technique can be used to detect viral, parasitic, tumor antigens from patient specimens or monolayer of cells. Another application is identification of anatomic distribution of an antigen within a tissue or within compartments of a cell.

Indirect immunofluorescence

Indirect immunofluorescence is employed to detect antibodies in patient serum. The antigen on smear are made to react with specific

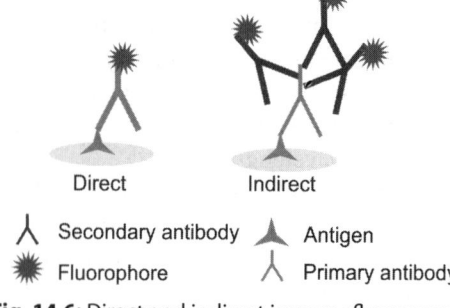

Fig. 14.6: Direct and indirect immunofluorescence.
(For color version, see Plate 6)

unlabeled antibody (raised in mouse) and washed. The unbound antibody gets washed off. The presence of specific mouse antibody bound to the antigen on smear is detected by adding another antibody. The second antibody is labeled anti-gamma globulin (rabbit antibody against mouse antibody) antibodies. This antibody binds to Fc portion of first antibody and persists despite washing. The presence of the second antibody is detected by observing under fluorescent microscope. It is often used to detect autoantibodies. Commonly used in the detection of anti-nuclear antibodies (ANA) found in the serum of patients with SLE **(Fig. 14.6)**.

Advantages of indirect immunofluorescence
- Gives an amplification effect—more tag or label (signal) per molecule of target protein
- Requires only one labeled antibody to identify many proteins. Same labeled secondary antibody can be used to bind to ("light up") many different proteins (preparation of labeled antibody is difficult and expensive).
    a. A different primary antibody is used for each target protein, (not labeled–no tag). Variable part of primary antibody binds to specific part of target protein.
    b. The secondary antibody binds to the constant part of the primary antibody. Therefore, a sample of the same (labeled or tagged) batch of secondary antibody can bind to many different (unlabeled) primary antibodies.

Application

The enzyme-linked immunosorbent assay (ELISA) is a biomolecular technique that utilizes the specificity of an antibody, as well as the sensitivity of enzyme assays, to detect and quantify molecules such as hormones, peptides, antibodies, and proteins.

■ ELECTROPHORESIS

Gel Electrophoresis

Gel electrophoresis is a technique used to separate DNA fragments (or other macromolecules, such as RNA and proteins) based on their size and charge.

As the name suggests, gel electrophoresis involves a gel—a slab of jelly-like material made out of a polysaccharide called agarose, placed in a gel box. One end of the box is hooked to a positive electrode while the other end is hooked to a negative electrode. The main body of the box, where the gel is placed, is filled with a salt-containing buffer solution that can conduct current. The buffer should be filled up in the gel box to a level where it just barely covers the gel **(Fig. 14.7)**.

At one end of the box, it has wells to hold DNA samples to be examined. One well is reserved for a DNA ladder, a standard reference that contains DNA fragments of known lengths. The end of the gel with the wells is positioned toward the negative electrode. The end without wells is positioned toward the positive electrode. Next, the power to the gel box is turned on, and current begins to flow through the gel. The DNA molecules have a negative charge because of the phosphate groups in their sugar-phosphate backbone, so they start moving through the matrix of the gel toward the positive electrode. When the power is turned on and current is passing through the gel, the gel is said to be running.

As the gel runs, shorter pieces of DNA will travel through the pores of the gel matrix faster than longer ones. After the gel has run for a while, the shortest pieces of DNA will be close to the positive end of the gel, while the longest pieces of DNA will remain near the wells.

Visualizing the DNA fragments

Once the fragments have been separated, different sizes of bands are found on it. When a gel is stained with a DNA-binding dye and placed

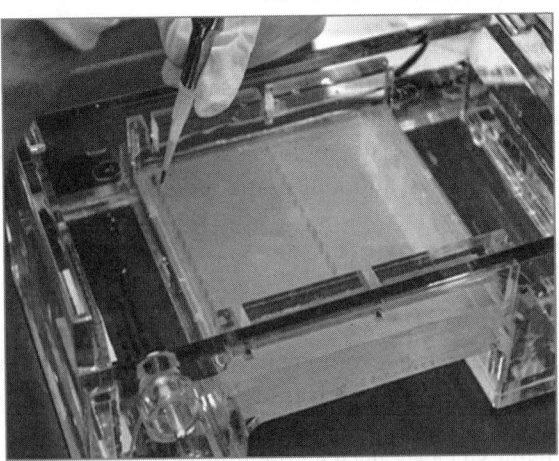

Fig. 14.7: Sample loading in wells.

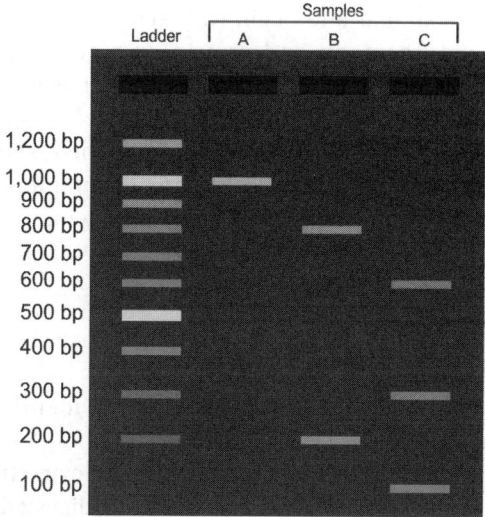

Fig. 14.8: Bands of electrophoresis.

under UV light, the DNA fragments will glow, allowing us to see the DNA present at different locations along the length of the gel.

This well-defined "line" of DNA on a gel is called a band. Each band contains a large number of DNA fragments of the same size that have all traveled as a group to the same position. By comparing the bands in a sample to the DNA ladder, we can determine their approximate sizes. The reference sample is called ladder as it contains various nucleotide sequences that form bands which resemble a "ladder." Commercial DNA ladders come in different size ranges; one with good "coverage" of the size range of our expected fragments is to be chosen **(Fig. 14.8)**.

Application
Electrophoresis is used to separate DNA, RNA, or protein molecules based on their size and electrical charge. An electric current is used to move molecules to be separated through a gel. Pores in the gel work like a sieve, allowing smaller molecules to move faster than larger molecules.

■ BLOTTING TECHNIQUES

Different blotting techniques are used to identify unique proteins and nucleic acid sequences. Southern, Northern, and Western blotting procedures are similar and begin with electrophoretic separation of nucleic acid fragments and protein on a gel, which are then transferred to a membrane, where they are immobilized. This enables radiolabeled or enzymatically labeled antibody or DNA probes to bind the immobilized target, and the molecules of interest may then be visualized with various methods. Blotting techniques are selected based on the target molecule: DNA, RNA, or protein.

Southern Blot

- It is based on the principle of specific base pairing rule of complementary nucleic acid strands.
- Southern blots are used to determine the identity, size, and abundance of specific DNA sequences.
- The Southern blot protocol begins with DNA extraction from the cells or tissues, which is then enzymatically digested to produce DNA fragments.
- The fragments are separated by size on an agarose or polyacrylamide gel via electrophoresis. Smaller fragments will migrate farther on the gel than larger ones.
- Following electrophoresis, the DNA on the gel is transferred to a Nylon membrane.
- The membrane is incubated with a nucleic acid probe that has a sequence homologous to the target sequence and is labeled with radioactivity, fluorescent dye, or an enzyme capable of generating a chemiluminescent signal. Hybridization of complementary sequences occurs during incubation, and the unhybridized probe is removed by washing with buffer.
- The fully hybridized labeled probe molecules will remain bound to the blot. Based on the probe label, different detection methods are in use.

Southern Blot Procedure (Fig. 14.9)

1. DNA isolation
2. **Restriction digestion:** Digest the DNA with a restriction enzyme and, if necessary, concentrate digested DNA.
3. **Gel electrophoresis:** Prepare an agarose gel and either tris-acetate EDTA (TAE) or tris-borate-EDTA (TBE) buffer (buffer selection

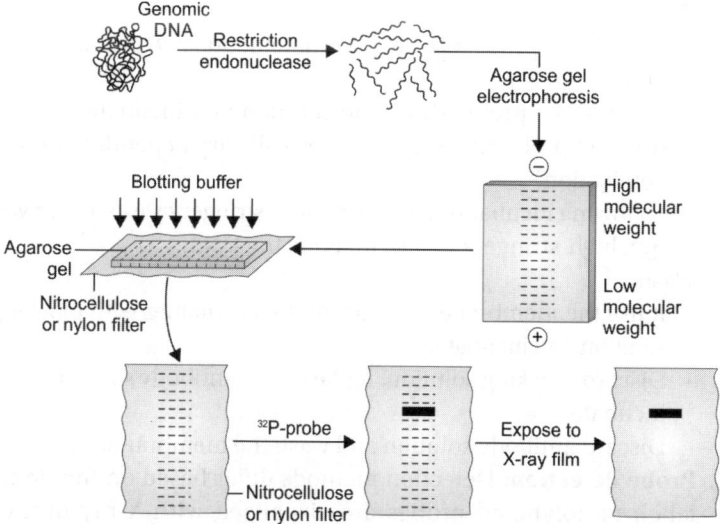

Fig. 14.9: Southern blotting.

will depend on the duration of the run and the size of the DNA fragments). Load samples into wells and include a DNA molecular weight marker. Run the gel.

4. **Transfer (blotting):**
   - Place the gel in a container with denaturing solution and wash twice for 15 minutes on a shaker.
   - Rinse with water and then wash with neutralization solution.
   - During the previous step, begin to prepare Whatman paper and nylon membrane for the transfer.
   - Assemble the transfer apparatus with the membrane, Whatman paper, and gel and transfer insaline-sodium citrate (SSC) or saline sodium phosphate EDTA (SSPE) buffer.
   - When transfer is complete, cross-link DNA in a cross-linker and then rinse the membrane.
5. **Prehybridization (blocking):** Blocking reduces nonspecific binding to the membrane. Prepare the prehybridization solution and add sample DNA. Remove the blot from the cross-linker, add the prehybridization solution, and incubate at 80°C for 2–3 hours or expose to ultraviolet radiation to permanently attach the transferred DNA onto the membrane.

6. **Hybridization:**
   - Prepare the probe mixture (a complementary DNA strand) and buffer.
   - Remove the prehybridization solution and incubate the blot with the probe (incubation times will vary depending on the application).
   - Following incubation, perform a low-stringency wash followed by a high-stringency wash to refine the DNA.
7. **Wash:**
   - Rinse the membrane and transfer to a container with blocking solution and incubate.
   - Discard blocking solution, replace with antibody solution, and incubate.
   - Discard antibody solution and wash the membrane.
8. **Probe detection:** Detection methods differ based on the probe label; radiolabeled probes are visualized with X-ray film or phosphor imaging and enzymatically labeled probes are visualized with chemiluminescent substrate.

Northern Blot

- It is based on the principle of the RNA-DNA hybridization technique.
- Northern blots are used to determine the identity, size, and abundance of specific RNA sequences.
- Northern blot protocols begin with RNA isolation, and separation techniques vary depending on the RNA size. Large RNAs are separated by electrophoresis on a formaldehyde agarose gel or glyoxal agarose gel, which prevents normal base paring and maintains RNA in a denatured state. Small RNAs are separated on a denaturing (urea) polyacrylamide gel.
- The RNA is then transferred from the gel to a Nylon membrane, which is then incubated with a radioactively or nonisotopically labeled RNA, DNA, or oligodeoxynucleotide probe.
- The unhybridized probe is removed by washing with buffer. Radiolabeled probes are visualized with X-ray film, and enzymatically labeled probes are visualized with chemiluminescence.

Northern Blot Procedure

1. RNA isolation
2. **Electrophoresis:**
   - *For a formaldehyde agarose gel:* Prepare the gel and insert the gel tray into the apparatus. Fill with MOPS [3-(N-Morpholino) propane sulfonic acid] buffer, load the samples, and include a molecular weight marker. Run the gel and then trim the gel prior to blotting.
   - *For a glyoxal agarose gel:* Prepare the gel and insert the gel tray into the apparatus. Fill with MOPS buffer, prepare samples, and load into wells along with RNA ladder.
   - *For a denaturing polyacrylamide gel:* Cast the gel and mount it in the electrophoresis unit. Prepare samples, load into the gel, and run with TBE running buffer.
3. **Transfer:**
   - *For a formaldehyde agarose gel or glyoxal agarose gel:* Wash the gel in SSC and then assemble the transfer unit with the gel, filter paper, and nylon membrane. When transfer is complete, place the membrane in a UV cross-linker.
   - *For a denaturing polyacrylamide gel:* Assemble the transfer unit including gel, filter paper, and Nylon membrane ensuring that they are flooded with TBE. When transfer is complete, place the membrane in a UV cross-linker to fix the RNA to the membrane.
4. **Prehybridization (blocking):** Prehybridize the membrane in hybridization solution (same as that of Southern blot).
5. **Hybridization:**
   - Add probe to the hybridization solution and incubate.
   - Wash the membrane in low-stringency washes to remove hybridization solution and unhybridized probe, and in high-stringency washes to remove partially hybridized molecules.
6. **Probe detection:** Detection methods differ based on the probe label (same as that of Southern blot).

Western Blot

- It is based on the principle of Ag-Ab reaction.
- Western blots are used to determine the identity, size, and abundance of specific proteins within a sample.

- The western blot protocol begins with sample lysate preparation from tissue or cell culture and separation on a polyacrylamide gel via electrophoresis.
- The separated proteins are then transferred to a nitrocellulose or polyvinylidene difluoride (PVDF) membrane.
- The membrane is incubated with a blocking agent to prevent nonspecific binding, followed by incubation with a primary antibody to bind the protein of interest. There are two detection methods—direct and indirect.
- Direct detection (**Fig. 14.10**) relies on a labeled primary antibody, whereas indirect detection requires a primary antibody directed against the target protein and a secondary antibody directed against the primary antibody's species (**Fig. 14.11**).
- Visualization methods include colorimetric assays in which a colored precipitate is produced, chemiluminescence, and fluorescence.

Western Blot Procedure

1. Prepare lysate from cell culture or tissue. Cell lysate is the most common sample for western blotting. Protein is extracted from the cell by mechanical or chemical lysis of the cells.
2. **Sample preparation:**
   - Determine the protein concentration of each sample with a protein quantification assay (i.e., Bradford assay).
   - Add an equal volume of 2X Laemmli sample buffer to each sample.

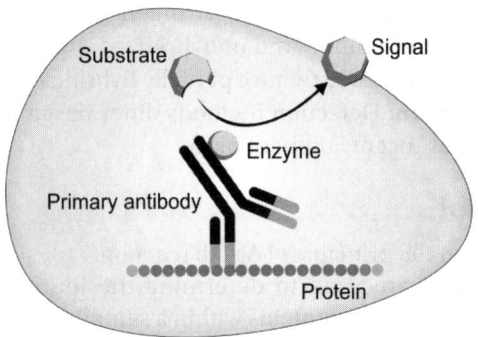

Fig. 14.10: Direct detection relies on a labeled primary antibody.

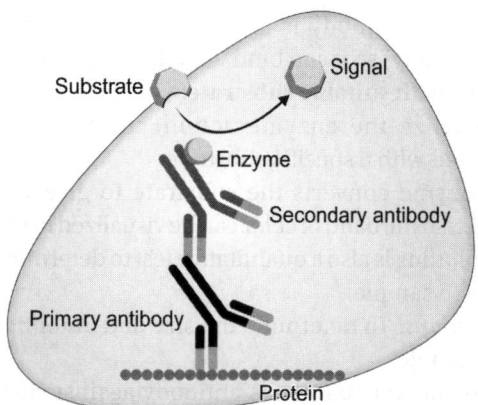

Fig. 14.11: Indirect detection relies on a primary antibody and a labeled secondary antibody.

- Some samples may need to be reduced or denatured; this is achieved by boiling samples in buffer.
3. **Electrophoresis:**
   - Prepare an SDS-PAGE (sodium lauryl sulfate-polyacrylamide gel electrophoresis gel) and load samples along with molecular weight marker.
   - Run the gel in running buffer.
4. **Transfer:**
   - Following electrophoresis, assemble the transfer unit including the gel, PVDF or nitrocellulose membrane, and filter paper.
   - Transfer the proteins to the membrane with transfer buffer.
5. **Antibody Staining (indirect detection):**
   - Blocking is a very important step in western blotting.
     - Antibodies are also protein so they are likely to bind the nitrocellulose paper. So before adding the primary antibody, the membrane is nonspecifically saturated or masked by using casein or Bovine serum albumin (BSA). The primary antibody is specific to the desired protein so it forms the Ag-Ab complex.
6. **Treatment with secondary antibody:**
   - The secondary antibody is enzyme labeled. For example, alkaline phosphatase or horseradish peroxidase (HRP) is labeled with secondary antibody.

- Secondary antibody is antibody against primary antibody (antiantibody) so it can bind with the Ag-Ab complex.
7. **Treatment with suitable substrate:**
   - To visualize the enzyme action, the reaction mixture is incubated with a specific substrate.
   - The enzyme converts the substrate to give visible colored product, so the band of color can be visualized in the membrane.
8. Western blotting is also a quantitative test to determine the amount of protein in sample.
   - *Applications:* To determine the size and amount of protein in given sample.
   - *Disease diagnosis:* Detects antibody against virus or bacteria in serum
   - Western blotting technique is the confirmatory test for HIV. It detects anti-HIV antibody in a patient's serum.
   - Useful to detect defective proteins, e.g., Prion disease.
   - Definitive test for Creutzfeldt-Jakob disease, Lyme disease, Hepatitis B and Herpes (**Table 14.1**).

Table 14.1: Comparisons between southern, northern, and western blot.

Criteria	Southern blot	Northern blot	Western blot
Target molecule	DNA	RNA	Protein
Sample preparation	DNA extraction enzymatic digestion	RNA isolation	Protein extraction
Separation	Electrophoresis	Electrophoresis	Electrophoresis
Membrane material	Nylon	Nylon	Nitrocellulose or PVDF
Probe	Nucleic acid probe with sequence homologous to target	RNA, DNA, or oligodeoxynucleotide	Primary antibody
Probe label	Radiolabel, enzyme	Radiolabel, enzyme	Enzyme
Detection methods	X-ray film, chemiluminescence	X-ray film, chemiluminescence	Film, cooled CCD, camera, LED

Application

The blotting techniques can be used for the detection and determination of hormones, enzymes, viral antigens, allergens, receptors, autoantibodies, DNA binding proteins, apolipoproteins, glycoproteins, oncogens, etc.

SUMMARY

- Immunoassays are used to test for the presence of a specific antibody or a specific antigen in blood or other fluids.
- Radioimmunoassay (RIA) is performed by using Ab-Ag binding and radioactive antigen. The basic principle of RIA is competitive binding reaction, where the antigen from the test sample competes with the radiolabeled antigen for binding to the fixed antibody.
- Enzyme-linked immunosorbent assay (ELISA) is performed by using Ab-Ag binding and enzyme-labeled antigen. ELISA is based on the principle that specific antibodies bind to their target antigen only when the interaction occurs. The substrate will be able to bind to the enzyme and substrate conversion will be seen, thus giving a positive result.
- The four main types of ELISAs are indirect, direct, sandwich, and competitive.
- In a direct ELISA, an antigen or sample is immobilized directly on the plate and a conjugated detection antibody binds to the target protein.
- In an indirect ELISA, first, a primary detection antibody is added and binds to the specific antigen. A secondary antibody directed against the primary antibody is then added. The substrate then produces a signal.
- Two specific antibodies are used to sandwich the antigen, commonly referred to as matched antibody pairs. Capture antibody is coated on a microplate, sample is added, and the protein of interest binds and is immobilized on the plate. A conjugated-detection antibody is then added and binds to an additional epitope on the target protein. A substrate is added which produces a signal.
- In competitive ELISAs, competitor substance is added to prevent unnecessary binding of antibody or antigen.
- In immunofluorescence immunoassay, specific antibodies bind to the antigen of interest.
- Fluorescent dyes are coupled to these Ag-Ab complexes in order to visualize the antigen of interest using microscopy.
- Immunofluorescence immunoassay may be of two types—direct immunofluorescence and indirect immunofluorescence.
- Gel electrophoresis is a technique used to separate deoxyribonucleic acid (DNA) fragments. When a gel is stained with a DNA-binding dye and placed under ultraviolet (UV) light, the DNA fragments will glow.

- Blotting technique procedures are similar and begin with electrophoretic separation of nucleic acid fragments and protein on a gel, which are then transferred to a membrane, where they are immobilized.
- This enables radiolabeled or enzymatically labeled antibody or DNA probes to bind the immobilized target, and the molecules of interest may then be visualized with various methods.
- Southern, northern, and western blotting techniques are selected based on the target molecule: DNA, ribonucleic acid (RNA), or protein, respectively.
- Southern blot is based on the principle of specific base pairing rule of complementary nucleic acid strands.
- Northern blot is based on the principle of the RNA–DNA hybridization technique.
- Western blot is based on the principle of Ag-Ab reaction.
- The blotting techniques can be used for the detection and determination of hormones, enzymes, viral antigens, allergens, receptors, autoantibodies, DNA-binding proteins, apolipoproteins, glycoproteins, oncogene, etc.

PRACTICE QUESTIONS

1. What are immunoassays? Mention its types.
2. Write a note on RIA.
3. Expand ELISA. Mention its principle.
4. Define heterogeneous ELISA and homogeneous ELISA.
5. Differentiate between direct ELISA and indirect ELISA.
6. Draw a diagrammatic representation of sandwich ELISA. Explain why it is called so.
7. Write a note on immunofluorescence immunoassay.
8. Differentiate between direct immunofluorescence and indirect immunofluorescence.
9. Write a note on:
    i. Process of electrophoresis
    ii. DNA ladder
10. Name a technique to identify DNA sequences. Explain the steps involved in it.
11. Discuss the method to isolate RNA.
12. Write a note on Western blot technique.
13. Enlist the applications of different blotting techniques.

CHAPTER 15

Enzyme Assay

Keywords
Coenzyme, cofactor, apoenzyme, holoenzyme, isoenzyme, substrate, oxidoreductases, transferases, hydrolases, lyases, isomerases, ligases, lock and key model, induced-fit model, enzyme inhibition, denaturation of enzymes, amylase, iodometric method, visible kinetic method, caraway unit, lipase, pancreatitis, lactate dehydrogenase (LDH), King's method, alkaline phosphatase, acid phosphatase (ACP), Gutman and Gutman method, creatine phosphokinase (CPK), CKBB, CKMM, CKMB, electrophoresis, ELISA

■ INTRODUCTION

Enzymes are organic molecules synthesized by cells of all living organisms. The term enzyme was first introduced by Kuhne in 1878 (i.e., En = in and Zyme = Yeast) while working on fermentation. All the life processes are biochemical reactions. Enzyme acts like catalyst and accelerates the rate of these biochemical metabolic reactions, without being utilized in the overall process. The substance on which enzyme acts to form a specific end product is known as substrate. Only a small quantity of enzyme is needed to exercise its effect on a reaction. Enzymes play a very important role as they carry out processes such as digestion, respiration, protein synthesis, coagulation defense mechanism, and muscular activities.

■ PROPERTIES OF ENZYME
- All enzymes are protein in nature.
- Enzymes are usually named by the suffix "–ase" with the name of the substrate. For example, enzyme acting on urea is known as urease.
- Enzymes show substrate specificity. This means, a particular enzyme acts only on a particular substrate with specific chemical

grouping. For example, enzyme urease acts only on urea, not on other substrate.
- Some enzymes are also named by adding "ase" as suffix to the activity brought about by them. For example, isomerization is brought by isomerases, decarboxylation is brought by decarboxylases.

UNIT OF ENZYME

The enzyme unit, or international unit for enzyme (symbol U/IU) is a unit of enzyme's catalytic activity. 1 IU (μmol/min) is defined as the amount of the enzyme that catalyzes the conversion of one micromole of substrate per minute under the specified conditions of the pH and temperature of assay method.

COENZYMES AND COFACTORS

Coenzymes and cofactors are molecules that help an enzyme or protein to function appropriately **(Fig. 15.1)**. Coenzymes are organic molecules and quite often bind loosely to the active site of an enzyme and aid in substrate recruitment, whereas cofactors do not bind the enzyme. Cofactors are "helper molecules" and can be inorganic or organic in nature. These include metal ions and are often required to increase the rate of catalysis of a given reaction catalyzed by the specific enzyme. These coenzymes and cofactors play an integral role in a number of cellular metabolism reactions playing both structural and functional roles to aid in the catalysis.

Coenzymes are nonprotein dialyzable organic compounds, which are noncovalently bound to the enzyme protein and are responsible for the catalytic activity of several enzymes. Many enzymes catalyze reactions only in the presence of particular coenzyme. A biochemically active compound formed by the combination of an enzyme with a coenzyme and/or cofactor is called holoenzyme **(Fig. 15.1)**. Coenzymes are particularly involved in the reactions involving group transfer, oxidation-reduction, conversion of isomers, and the reactions resulting in the formation of covalent bond.

Coenzymes are generally derived from the water-soluble B-complex vitamins and carry out transfer of hydrogen or any other group of substrate in an enzymatic reaction. For example,

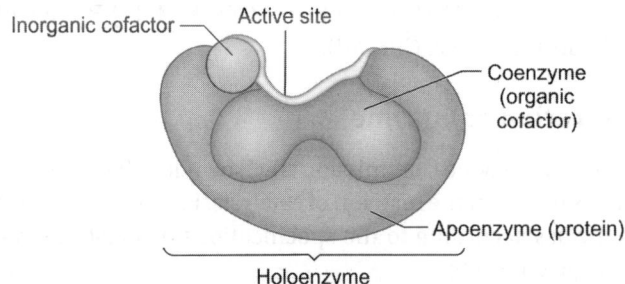

Fig. 15.1: Structure of holoenzyme.

nicotinamide adenine dinucleotide (NAD), nicotinamide adenine dinucleotide phosphate (NADP), flavin mononucleotide (FMN), flavin adenine dinucleotide (FAD), and coenzyme P participate in transfer of hydrogen atoms (electrons).

Thiamine pyrophosphate (TPP) participates in transfer of aldehydes.

Coenzyme A and lipoamide participate in transfer of acyl groups:
For example, Lactate + NAD$^+$ → pyruvate + NADH + H$^+$.

LDH Reaction

$$\text{Lactate} + \text{NAD} \xrightarrow{\text{LDH}} \text{NADH} + \text{H}^+$$

In this reaction, NAD is coenzyme, which transfers hydrogen ion. Enzyme lactate dehydrogenase (LDH) cannot act on substrate lactate in the absence of coenzyme NAD. In reverse reaction, NADH acts as a coenzyme.

CK Reaction

$$\text{Creatine} + \text{ATP} \xrightleftharpoons{\text{CPK}} \text{Phosphocreatine} + \text{ADP}$$

Isoenzyme

Isoenzymes are different forms of same enzyme having same enzymatic activity. They are from different sources. They may differ in physical, biochemical, and immunological properties. They also differ in molecular weights and affinity for substrates and coenzymes.

For example, different sources of Isoenzymes are

Creatine phosphokinase (CPK) has three forms. It is a dimer. Two units of CPK recognized are M (muscle) and B (brain).

Isoenzyme are: (1) Skeletal muscle CPK-MM, (2) Brain CPK-BB, and (3) Cardiac muscle CPK-MB.

Classification of Enzyme

International Enzyme Commission (IEC) has classified enzymes into six classes based on the reaction of catalysis. Each class is subdivided into subclass according to the specifications of substrate, reactive group, coenzyme, etc.

1. **Oxidoreductases:** These enzymes bring about oxidation and reduction reactions and hence are called oxidoreductases. In these reactions, electrons in the form of hydride ions or hydrogen atoms are transferred. Deydrogenases or reductases remove hydrogen atoms from the substrate whereas oxidases donate hydrogen atom to the substrate.

$$\underset{\text{Reduced}}{A} + \underset{\text{Oxidized}}{B} \xrightleftharpoons{\text{Oxidoreductase}} \underset{\text{Oxidized}}{A} + \underset{\text{Reduced}}{B}$$

$$\text{Succinic acid} \xrightleftharpoons{\text{Succinate dehydrogenase}} \text{Fumaric acid}$$

2. **Transferases:** These enzymes are responsible for transferring functional groups from one molecule to another. The groups usually transferred by these enzymes are methyl, ethyl, amino, phosphate, etc. Transaminases catalyze the transfer of amino group, and kinases catalyze the transfer of a phosphate group.

$$A - B + C \xrightleftharpoons{\text{Transferases}} A + C - B$$

$$\text{Alanine + Oxaloacetic acid} \xrightleftharpoons{\text{Transaminase}} \text{Pyruvic acid + Aspartic acid}$$

3. **Hydrolases:** These enzymes catalyze reactions that involve the process of hydrolysis. They break single bonds by adding water. Some hydrolases function as digestive enzymes which bring out hydrolysis of lipids, proteins, and carbohydrates.

$$A - B + H_2O \xrightleftharpoons{\text{Hydrolases}} A - H + B - OH$$

$$\text{Starch} + H_2O \xrightleftharpoons{\text{Amylase}} \text{Glucose}$$

4. **Lyases:** These enzymes catalyze reactions where functional groups are added to break double bonds in molecules or where double bonds are formed by the removal of functional groups.

Example: Pyruvate decarboxylase is a lyase that removes CO_2 from pyruvate.

$$A = B \xrightleftharpoons{\text{Lyases}} A - B$$

$$ATP \xrightleftharpoons{\text{layse}} cAMP + PPi$$

Adenosine Hiphosphate to cyclic adenosine monophosphate + phosphate

5. **Isomerases:** These enzymes catalyze the reactions where a functional group is moved to another position within the same molecule such that the resulting molecule is actually an isomer of the earlier molecule.

$$A - B - C \xrightleftharpoons{\text{Isomerase}} A - C - B$$

$$\text{Dextrose} \xrightleftharpoons{\text{Isomerase}} \text{Fructose}$$

6. **Ligases:** Ligases catalyze the condensation (joining) of two molecules with the expense of energy from adenosine triphosphate (ATP) hydrolysis.

$$A + B + ATP \xrightleftharpoons{\text{Ligase}} A - B + ADP + Pi$$

$$\text{L-glutamate} + NH_4^+ + ATP \xrightleftharpoons{\text{Ligase}} \text{Orthophosphate} + \text{L-glutamine} + ADP$$

Mechanism of Enzyme—Substrate Action

Enzyme-catalyzed reactions occur in at least two steps. In the first step, an enzyme molecule (E) and the substrate molecule or molecules (S) collide and react to form an intermediate compound called the *enzyme-substrate* (E–S) *complex.*

$$S + E \rightarrow E\text{-}S$$

This step is reversible because the complex can break apart into the original substrate or substrates and the free enzyme. Once the E–S complex forms, the enzyme is able to catalyze the formation of product (P), which is then released from the enzyme surface:

$$E\text{-}S \rightarrow P + E$$

This is explained by two models:
i. **Lock and key model (Fig. 15.2):** Hydrogen bonding and other electrostatic interactions hold the enzyme and substrate together in the complex. The structural features or functional groups on

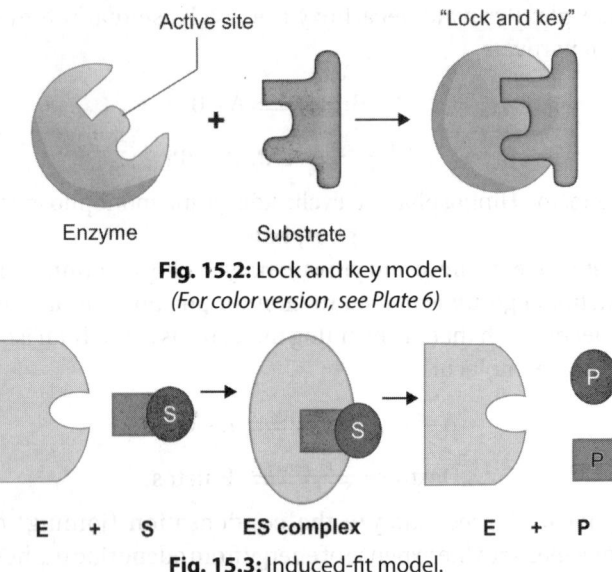

Fig. 15.2: Lock and key model.
(For color version, see Plate 6)

Fig. 15.3: Induced-fit model.
(For color version, see Plate 7)

the enzyme that participate in these interactions are located in a cleft or pocket on the enzyme surface. This pocket, where the enzyme combines with the substrate and transforms the substrate to product, is called the active site of the enzyme. It possesses a unique conformation (including correctly positioned bonding groups) that is complementary to the structure of the substrate, so that the enzyme and substrate molecules fit together in much the same manner as a key fits into a tumbler lock. In fact, an early model describing the formation of the enzyme-substrate complex was called the lock-and-key model. This model portrayed the enzyme as conformationally rigid and able to bond only to substrates that exactly fit the active site.

ii. **Induced-fit model:** The current theory, known as the induced-fit model, says that enzymes can undergo a change in conformation when they bind substrate molecules, and the active site has a shape complementary to that of the substrate only *after* the substrate is bound, as shown in **Figure 15.3**.

Enzyme Inhibition

Enzyme activity is inhibited by certain substances called as enzyme inhibitors and the process is called as enzyme inhibition.

There are two types of enzyme inhibition:
1. Competitive inhibition
2. Noncompetitive inhibition

1. **Competitive inhibition:** Inhibitor substance competes with substrate for the active site of enzyme. This is due to structural similarity of inhibitor with substrate. This yields enzyme inhibitor complex instead of enzyme-substrate complex. Enzyme-inhibitor complex does not yield any product and prevents further enzyme activity.

$$E + S \longrightarrow E - S \longrightarrow E + \text{product}$$
$$E + I \longrightarrow E - I \longrightarrow \text{No product}$$

   It can be reversed by enhancing the concentration of substrate.
   For example, succinate dehydrogenase is an enzyme whose substrate is succinic acid. Malonic acid, oxalic acid, and glutaric acid with structural similarity to succinic acid can inhibit the activity of the enzyme succinate dehydrogenase.

2. **Noncompetitive inhibitor:** It binds to a different site on the enzyme; it does not block substrate binding, but it causes other changes in the enzyme so that it can no longer catalyze the reaction efficiently.
   For example, aspirin inhibits a cyclo-oxygenase so that prostaglandins may not be synthesized, thereby reducing pain, fever, inflammation, blood clotting, etc.

■ FACTORS AFFECTING ENZYME REACTION

Following factors influence the enzyme action:
1. **Contact between enzyme and substrate:** Contact between enzyme and substrate is essential for enzyme action to take place. Enzyme being a protein forms colloidal solution. Hence substrate also must be a water-soluble substance.
2. **Concentration of substrate:** Keeping the concentration of enzyme constant, enzyme action is directly proportional to the concentration of substrate.
3. **Concentration of enzyme:** Enzyme action is directly proportional to the concentration of enzyme. However, after saturation point, increase in concentration of enzyme will not have any effect on the rate of reaction.

4. **Concentration of product:** Product being accumulated lowers enzyme activity. Thus, there exists inverse relation between enzyme and product. Prompt removal of the product prevents this effect.
5. **Effect of pH:** There is optimum pH for maximum activity of any enzyme above and below which enzyme activity declines. Generally, this pH range is from 5 to 9.
6. **Effect of temperature:** There will be optimum temperature for maximum activity of any enzyme above and below which enzyme activity declines or becomes nil. For human enzymes, optimal temperature is body temperature (37°C). Increase in temperature results in breaking of secondary bond that holds the enzyme in its catalytic active state. This is called denaturation of enzymes.
7. **Effect of oxidizing substances:** Activity of enzymes depends on some functional group. For example, sulfhydryl (SH) group present in dehydrogenases and many other enzymes. If such group is oxidized, enzyme activity is lost.
8. **Effect of inhibitors:** Presence of inhibitors reduces the enzyme action, e.g., heavy metals are enzyme inhibitor.

■ IMPORTANCE OF ENZYMES

Medicinal and Pharmaceutical Significance

1. Sulfonamides kill pathogenic organisms by inhibiting folic acid synthetase enzyme.
2. Allopurinol, used in the treatment of gout, acts by inhibiting the enzyme xanthine oxidase.
3. Enzyme asparaginase is used in the treatment of tumors.
4. Enzyme galactosidase is used in the treatment of lactose intolerance in children.
5. Penicillin acylase is used in manufacture of 6-amino penicillanic acid.
6. Aminoacylase is used in preparation of alpha-amino acid.
7. Glucose isomerase is used in manufacture of fructose syrup.
8. Papain is used in the production of protein hydrolysate.
9. Amylase is also used in manufacturing process.

Diagnostic Significance

I. **Determination of enzymes useful in diagnosis of various conditions:**
   Determination of different enzymes is useful in diagnosis of various conditions.

Some of them are as follows:
1. Determination of lipase in plasma is useful in diagnosis of pancreatitis, pancreatic carcinoma, liver disease, diabetes mellitus and vitamin A deficiency. Values are elevated in pancreatitis and pancreatic carcinoma whereas they are decreased in liver disease, vitamin A deficiency and diabetes mellitus.
2. Trypsin is elevated in pancreatic disease.
3. Low plasma levels of cholinesterase are seen in liver disease, malnutrition, and anemia. Infection in cardiac muscle causes lowering of plasma activity of this enzyme.
4. Determination of LDH is significant for diagnosis of myocardial infarction.
5. Serum ACP is elevated in males with prostatic cancer with metastases. Its elevation is moderate in Paget's disease and hyperparathyroidism.
6. Serum alkaline phosphatase is elevated moderately in hepatic conditions.
7. Serum glutamic oxaloacetic transaminase (SGOT) is increased rapidly in myocardial infarction.
8. Serum glutamic pyruvic transaminase (SGPT) is slightly elevated in cardiac necrosis. Its elevation is high in both hepatic and posthepatic conditions.
9. Determination of CPK is significant in diagnosis of myocardial infarction. CPK is elevated in myocardial infarction, muscular dystrophy, polymyositis, motor neuron disorders, and acute cerebrovascular accidents.

II. **Use of enzymes as reagents:**
Enzymatic methods are advantageous owing to their reasonable cost, time saving, avoidance of corrosive, and multiple reagents.
For example,
1. Glucose oxidase and peroxidase enzymes are used in the determination of glucose by glucose oxidase peroxidase (God-Pod) method.
2. Uricase is used in enzymatic method of determination of uric acid.
3. Urease is used in enzymatic method of determination of urea.

4. Lipase, glycerol kinase, glycerol phosphate oxidase, and peroxidase are used in enzymatic method of determination of triglycerides.
5. Cholesterol ester hydrolase, cholesterol oxidase, and peroxidase are used in enzymatic method of determination of cholesterol.

AMYLASE

Amylase is a digestive enzyme predominantly secreted by the pancreas and salivary glands. Main function of amylase is to hydrolyze the glycosidic bonds in starch molecules, converting complex carbohydrates to simple sugars.

$$\text{Starch} + \text{Water} \xrightarrow{\text{Amylase}} \text{Sugar(s)}$$

Several isoforms of amylase have been discovered, but the most abundant that exist are pancreatic amylase (P-amylase) and salivary amylase (S-amylase). P-amylase is specifically found in the pancreas and is synthesized by acinar cells then secreted into the gastrointestinal (GI) tract. S-amylase is primarily produced in salivary glands but can also be produced in ovaries, fallopian tubes, GI tract, lungs, striated muscle, and malignant neoplasms. Serum amylase is tightly regulated in the body. There is a balance between the rate of production and the rate of clearance. Elevated amylase may be due to an increase in pancreatic or extrapancreatic production of a decreased rate of clearance.

The amylases normally occurring in human plasma are small molecules. Because of small size, amylase can be easily filtered through the glomeruli. It is cleared via the kidneys and reticuloendothelial system. Amylase is the only plasma enzyme normally found in the urine.

Amylase has a molecular weight of about 50–55 kDa, an optimum physiological pH of 6.7–7.0, and requires calcium and chloride ions for optimal enzyme activity.

There are two types of methods which are discussed below:
1. Iodometric method
2. Visible kinetic method

Iodometric Method

Specimen
Unhemolyzed serum.

Urine sample—24 hours/6 hours urine sample without preservative is collected. Dilute urine 1:5 with normal saline.

Principle
The iodometric (amyloclastic) method is based on the ability of iodide to form a vivid blue color in combination with starch. The starch is hydrolyzed by amylase in the sample to liberate smaller molecules such as dextran, maltose, and some glucose molecules. The smaller sugar molecules do not form a complex with iodide and do not give a blue color. As more starch is broken down, the intensity of the blue color decreases. Substrate (starch) and sample (amylase) are mixed together and incubated for a fixed time. Iodide color solution is added and the starch/iodide color complex is formed. A spectrophotometric measurement is made to determine color intensity (absorbance). The lower the final absorbance (the greater the difference between the blank and test solutions), the higher the serum amylase activity.

Reagent
1. Buffered substrate
2. Stock color reagent

Procedure
- Dilute stock color reagent to 1:10 with distilled water to get working color reagent.
- Take two test tubes. Label it as test and control.
- Add 2.5 mL of buffered substrate in each tube. Keep at 37°C for 5 minutes.
- Add 0.1 mL serum in test.
- Mix and incubate it for 7 minute.
- Add 2.5 mL of working color reagent in each tube.
- Now add 0.1 mL serum in control.
- At last add 20 mL of distilled water in both the tubes.

- Mix thoroughly and read the absorbance of test and std. against distilled water at 660 nm.

Reagent	T	C
Buffered substrate	2.5 mL	2.5 mL
Keep at 37°C for 5 minutes		
Serum	0.1 mL	—
Mix and incubate it for 7 minutes		
Working color reagent	2.5 mL	2.5 mL
Serum	—	0.1 mL
Distilled water	20 mL	20 mL

Calculation

Caraway unit

The serum amylase is expressed in Caraway units. One Caraway unit is the amount of enzyme that will hydrolyze 10 mg of starch in 30 minutes to a colorless stage.

Serum amylase in Caraway unit =

$$\text{Calculation} - \frac{\text{O.D. Blank} - \text{O.D. test}}{\text{O.D. Blank}} \times 400$$

Normal value: Serum—60–180 Caraway units
Urine—50–300 Caraway unit

Visible Kinetic Method

Principle

Amylase hydrolyzes p-nitrophenyl-alpha-D-maltoheptoside (PNPG7) to p-nitrophenyl maltotriose (PNPG3) and maltotetraose. Glucoamylase hydrolyzes PNPG3 to p-nitrophenyl glycoside (PNPG1) and glucose PNPG1 is hydrolyzed by α-glucosidase to glucose and p-nitrophenol, which produces yellow color. The rate of increase in yellow color is proportional to α-amylase activity in the sample and is measured at 405 nm.

$$PNPG_7 \xrightarrow{\alpha-\text{amylase}} PNPG_3 + \text{Maltoterose}$$

$$PNPG_3 \xrightarrow{\text{Glucoamylase}} PNPG_1 + \text{Glucose}$$

$$PNPG_1 \xrightarrow{\alpha-\text{glucosidase}} \text{P-nitrophenol} + \text{Glucose}$$

Reagent

Amylase reagent—the lyophilized reagent is reconstituted with volume of distill water stated on the vial label. This working reagent is stable for 1 month in refrigerator.

Specimen

Unhemolyzed serum.

Urine sample—24 hours/6 hours urine sample without preservative is collected. Dilute urine 1:5 with normal saline.

Procedure

- Take 1 mL of working amylase reagent in a test tube.
- Add 0.02 mL of serum and mix well.
- Read absorbance every 30 seconds for 2 minutes.
- Determine the absorbance difference (ΔA)/min.
- Multiply (ΔA)/min by 7,123 to get serum amylase result.

Calculations

Serum amylase, IU = $\Delta A \times 7,123$.

Normal Value

- In urine—50–300 IU/hour for 24 hours
- In serum—Below 18 year 0–260 U/L
- 18 and above 18 years 35–115 U/L

These test results are for total amylase values that include pancreatic and salivary amylase. To determine pancreatic amylase, salivary amylase is inhibited by specific antibodies and then it is determined by either of the above mentioned method. Salivary amylase is calculated as the difference between the total and pancreatic amylase.

Clinical Significance

The serum amylase levels are high in acute pancreatitis, obstruction of pancreatic duct by—stone/carcinoma, biliary tract disease, acute cholecystitis complications of pancreatitis, pancreatic trauma, altered GI tract permeability, and acute alcohol ingestion. Serum amylase level is also increased in salivary gland disease (like mumps), malignant tumors especially of pancreas, lung, ovary, esophagus, breast and colon, and advanced renal insufficiency. The other causes include—chronic liver disease, ovarian cyst, diabetic ketoacidosis, and splenic rupture. Increased serum amylase with low urine amylase may be seen in renal insufficiency and macroamylasemia.

Decreased serum amylase levels are clinically significant in marked destruction of pancreas, severe liver damage like in hepatitis, severe burns, etc. Low serum amylase is commonly associated with type 1 diabetes and conditions related with insulin resistance.

■ SERUM LIPASE

Lipases are the enzymes that hydrolyze glycerol esters of long-chain fatty acids. It is fully active in presence of bile salts and a cofactor, called co-lipase. Most of the lipase in the serum is produced in the pancreas, but some is also secreted by the lingual glands, and gastric, pulmonary, and intestinal mucosa. Lipase activity is also seen in leukocytes, adipose tissue cells, and milk. Lipase is filtered at the glomeruli but completely reabsorbed by the tubules. Therefore, it is not normally detected in urine.

Method

Colorimetric.

Principle

Serum pancreatic lipase acts on a natural type of substrate, 1, 2-diglyceride to liberate 2-monoglyceride. The 2-monoglyceride is hydrolyzed by monoglyceride lipase (MGLP) to produce glycerol and fatty acid. Glycerol kinase (GK) then acts on the glycerol to produce glycerol-3-phosphatase which is converted to dihydroxyacetone phosphate and hydrogen peroxide in a reaction catalyzed by glycerol-3-phosphate oxidase (GPO). The hydrogen peroxide then reacts with 4-aminoantipyrine and N-ethyl-N-(2-hydroxy-3-sulfopropyl)-m-toluidine sodium salt (TOOS) in a reaction catalyzed by peroxidase (POD) to yield a quinone dye. The rate of increase in absorbance at 550 nm is directly proportional to the lipase activity of the sample.

1, 2-diglyceride + H_2O —— Pancreatic Lipase ⟶ 2-monoglyceride + Fatty acid

2-monoglyceride + H_2O —— MGLP ⟶ Glycerol + Fatty acid

Glycerol + ATP —— GK ⟶ Glycerol-3-phosphatase + ADP

Glycerol-3-phosphatase + O_2 —— GPO ⟶ Dihydroxyacetone phosphate + H_2O_2

$2H_2O_2$ + 4-aminoantipyrine + TOOS —— POD ⟶ Quinone dye + $4 H_2O_2$

Reagent

1. Lipase substrate
2. Lipase substrate buffer
3. Lipase activator

Reagent Preparation

Reconstitute the lipase substrate vial with the amount of lipase substrate buffer indicated on the vial label. Swirl to dissolve. Reconstitute the lipase standard with 3 mL of distilled water.

Specimen

Fasting, nonhemolyzed serum is the preferred.

Procedure

- Take four test tubes. Label them as "Blank," "Standard," "Control," and "Test."
- Pipette 3 mL of reconstituted lipase substrate reagent to all tubes.
- Pipette 0.05 mL of distilled water to the blank tube and 0.05 mL of the appropriate sample to the tubes labeled "Standard" and "Control."
- Mix each tube well and incubate for 3–5 minutes at 37°C.
- After the preincubation, add 1 mL of lipase activator to the blank tube. Mix well and incubate for 3 minutes at 37°C.

- Then measure the rate of increase in absorbance per minute at 550 nm (540–560 nm). Repeat last two steps for all tubes.

Reagent	T	S	B	C
Lipase substrate	3 mL	3 mL	3 mL	3 mL
Distilled water	—	—	0.05 mL	—
Serum	0.05 mL	—	—	—
Std.	—	0.05 mL	—	—
Control serum	—	—	—	0.05 mL
Mix each tube well and incubate for 3–5 minutes at 37°C				
Lipase activator	1 mL	1 mL	1 mL	1 mL

Calculation

$$\text{Serum lipase} = \frac{\Delta A \text{ sample} - \Delta A \text{ blank}}{\Delta A \text{ standard} - \Delta A \text{ blank}} \times \text{Conc of std.}$$

Normal values: 56–200 IU

Clinical Significance

Serum lipase is recognized as an important indicator for the diagnosis, and therapeutic monitoring, of pancreatic diseases. The lipase test is most often used in evaluating inflammation of the pancreas (pancreatitis), but it is also useful in diagnosing kidney failure, intestinal obstruction, mumps, and peptic ulcers. Doctors often order amylase and lipase tests at the same time to help distinguish pancreatitis from ulcers and other disorders in the abdomen. If the patient has acute (sudden onset) pancreatitis, the lipase level usually rises somewhat later than the amylase level—about 24-48 hours after onset of symptoms—and remains abnormally high for 5-7 days. It is also increased in obstruction of pancreatic duct by stone, intestinal infarction, after organ transplant, chronic liver diseases. Two to three times increase in serum lipase is found in 80% patients with acute and chronic renal failure. Alcoholism, diabetic ketoacidosis, increases in lipase.

No clinically significant role has been known in which serum lipase activity is lower.

SERUM LACTATE DEHYDROGENASE

Lactate dehydrogenase activity is present in all cells of the body. It is found in the cytoplasm of the cell. It is present in high concentration in heart, kidney, erythrocytes, and skeletal muscle. Many of the tissues show different isoenzymes composition. The optimum reaction conditions are at 37°C temperature and 8.8–9.8 pH.

Method

King's method.

Specimen

Strictly unhemolyzed serum since red blood cells are rich in LDH.

Principle

Lactate dehydrogenase catalyzes the following reaction:

$$\text{Lactate} + \text{NAD} \xrightarrow{\text{LDH}} \text{Pyruvate} + \text{NADH} + \text{H}^+$$

The products formed react with 2,4-dinitrophenyl hydrazine (DNPH) to give corresponding hydrazone. Hydrazone gives brown color in alkaline medium, which is a measure of LDH.

Reagent

- Glycine reagent
- Buffered substrate
- NAD solution
- NADH solution
- DNPH reagent
- 0.4 N NaOH

Procedure

Part I: Preparation of Standard Curve

Take seven test tubes. Mark them as Blank, 1, 2, 3, 4, 5, and 6 for enzyme activity—0, 167, 333, 500, 667, 883, and 1,000 respectively. Add the reagent as follows:

Reagent	Blank	1	2	3	4	5	6
S. LDH activity, IU	0	167	333	500	667	883	1000
NADH solution	0 mL	0.05 mL	0.10 mL	0.15 mL	0.20 mL	0.25 mL	0.30 mL
Pyruvate	0 mL	0.05 mL	0.10 mL	0.15 mL	0.20 mL	0.25 mL	0.30 mL
Buffered substrate	1.0 mL	0.9 mL	0.8 mL	0.7 mL	0.6 mL	0.5 mL	0.4 mL
NAD solution	0.2 mL	0.2 mL	0.2 mL	0.2 mL	0.2 mL	0.2 mL	0.2 mL
Distilled water	0.1 mL	0.1 mL	0.1 mL	0.1 mL	0.1 mL	0.1 mL	0.1 mL
DNPH reagent	1.0 mL	1.0 mL	1.0 mL	1.0 mL	1.0 mL	1.0 mL	1.0 mL
Mix each tube well and keep at room temperature for 15 minutes							
0.4 N NaOH	10 mL	10 mL	10 mL	10 mL	10 mL	10 mL	10 mL

Mix well and keep at room temperature for exactly 10 minutes, measure the intensities of all the tubes setting against blank at 445 nm. Draw a graph by plotting OD on Y-axis and IU on X-axis.

Part II: Preparation of Test

For sample, take two test tubes—label it as test and control. Add the reagent as follows:

Reagent	T	C
Buffered substrate incubate for 5 minutes at 37°C	1.0 mL	1.0 mL
NAD solution	0.2 mL	0.2 mL
Serum	0.02 mL	—
Mix well and incubate for 15 minutes at 37°C		
DNPH reagent	1.0 mL	1.0 mL
Serum	—	0.02 mL
Mix well and keep at room temperature for 15 minutes		
0.4 N NaOH	10 mL	10 mL

Calculation

Net OD of test = OD of T − OD of C.

From the standard graph, calculate the serum LDH value. Normal value:

Newborn	—	160–1,500 U/L
Infant	—	150–360 U/L
Child	—	150–300 U/L
Adult	—	100–250 U/L

Clinical Significance

Serum lactate dehydrogenase (SLDH) is very nonspecific test. It can be used as a marker of hemolysis in anemia.

It is increased in congestive heart failure, acute myocarditis, rheumatic fever, and in liver diseases such as cirrhosis, obstructive jaundice, and hepatitis. In lung diseases such as pulmonary embolus and infarction, SLDH is increased in 50% of patients with carcinomas, especially in advanced stages, in muscle disease, in renal diseases such as in nephritic syndrome, in acute pancreatitis, and hypothyroidism. LDH is increased in various infections and parasitic diseases.

The only condition in which LDH is known to be decrease is X-ray irradiation.

■ PHOSPHATES

Phosphates belong to the class of enzymes called hydrolyses. Phosphatase is an enzyme that removes a phosphate group from its substrate by hydrolyzing phosphoric acid monoesters into a phosphate ion and a molecule with a free hydroxyl group.

Phosphates of diagnostic importance are of two kinds—alkaline phosphates and acid phosphates. These are differentiated by their reaction in alkaline and acidic medium. The pH for measuring the alkaline phosphates activity is 10 and for acid phosphates, it is 5.

- **Alkaline phosphatase:** This is described in detail in Chapter Liver Function Test.

- **ACP:** A total ACP includes all phosphatase with optimum activity in the range 4–6. ACP is present in lysosomes of all the cells, except erythrocytes. Extralysosomal ACPs are also present in many cells. ACP activity is mainly observed in bone marrow, liver spleen, milk, platelets, and highest in prostate glands.

  The ACPs are unstable above pH 7.0 and temperature 37°C. More than 50% of ACP activity is lost in 1 hour at room temperature. Acidification of the serum specimen to a pH below 6.5 aids in stabilizing the enzyme.

Method

Gutman and Gutman.

Principle

Acid phosphatase from serum converts phenyl phosphatase to inorganic PO_4 and phenol at pH 4.9. Phenol in alkaline medium reacts with 4-aminoantipyrine in the presence of potassium ferricyanide forms orange red-colored complex. The color intensity is directly proportional to enzyme activity. Since tartarate inhibits prostatic fraction of enzyme, the difference in ACP activity with and without tartarate represents prostratic fraction.

■ REACTIONS

Phenyl phosphate + Acid phosphatase $\longrightarrow$ Phenol + Inorganic PO_4

Phenol + 4-aminoantipyrine $\xrightarrow{\text{K ferricyanide}/OH^-}$ Orange red complex

Reagents

- Buffered substrate at pH 4.9
- 0.5 N NaOH
- 0.5 N $NaHCO_3$
- 4-aminoantipyrine
- Potassium ferricyanide
- 1M tartarate
- Phenol standard.

Procedure

Take 5 test tubes, mark them as blank, standard (std.), control, test and tartarate stable.

Add the reagents as follows:

Reagents	B	S	C	T	Ts
Buffered substrate	—	—	1 mL	1 mL	1 mL
Distilled water	2.2 mL	1.2 mL	1 mL	1 mL	1 mL
Mix well and incubate for 3 minutes at 37°C					
Working Std.	—	1 mL	—	—	—
1 M tartarate	—	—	—	—	0.05 mL
Serum	—	—	—	0.2 mL	0.2 mL
Mix well and incubate for 1 hours at 37°C					
0.5 N NaOH	1 mL	1 mL	1 mL	1 mL	1 mL
Serum	—	—	0.2 mL	—	—
0.5 N NaHCO$_3$	1 mL	1 mL	1 mL	1 mL	1 mL
4-aminoantipyrine	1 mL	1 mL	1 mL	1 mL	1 mL
Potassium ferricyanide	1 mL	1 mL	1 mL	1 mL	1 mL

Mix well after addition of each reagent and measure the OD of blank, std., test, control and tartarate stable against distilled water at 510 nm.

Calculations

$$\text{Serum acid phosphatase} = \frac{\text{OD of test} - \text{OD of control}}{\text{OD of std.} - \text{OD of blank}} \times 5$$

$$\text{Prostatic fraction} = \frac{\text{OD of test} - \text{OD of Ts}}{\text{OD of std.} - \text{OD of B}} \times 5$$

Normal values	Males	Females
Total	2.5 to 11 U/L	0.3 to 9U/L
Prostatic	0.2 to 3.5 U/L	0.0 to 0.8 U/L

Clinical Significance

Determination of serum ACP is important in detecting and monitoring carcinoma of the prostate, in prostatic carcinoma with metastasis, total ACP activity may reach 40 to 50 times the upper limit. Moderate elevations in total ACP activity often occur in Paget's disease, hyperparathyroidism and breast cancer. Increased serum ACP levels are also seen Gaucher's disease and in myelocytic leukemia. As it is present in high concentration in semen, it is utilized in forensic medicine in the investigation of rape offences.

■ CREATINE PHOSPHOKINASE ISOENZYMES TEST

Creatine phosphokinase or creatine kinase (CK)—also known as phosphocreatine kinase—is an enzyme which is present in various tissues and cells. All isoenzymes of CK catalyzes the conversion of creatine and utilizes adenosine triphosphate (ATP) to create phosphocreatine (PCr) and adenosine diphosphate (ADP). This CK enzyme reaction is reversible and thus ATP can be generated from PCr and ADP.

The rapid formation of ATP from phosphocreatine and ADP when ATP is needed by the tissue, especially skeletal muscle, brain, photoreceptor cells of the retina, hair cells, spermatozoa, and smooth muscle phosphocreatine serves as an energy reservoir for the rapid buffering and regeneration of ATP. Thus, CPK is an important enzyme in such tissues.

Types of Creatine Phosphokinase

Creatine phosphocreatine is a dimeric enzyme, i.e., it consists of two subunits. The genes for these subunits are located on different chromosomes. There are two common gene products, one coding for the "M" subunit—so named because of its predominance in muscle, and the other for the B subunit—so named because of its predominance in brain tissue. The three common forms of active CK include two homodimers and one heterodimer.

- The first homodimer (CK-1) consists of two B subunits and is referred to as CKBB.
- The second heterodimer (CK-2) consists of one of each subunit and is referred to as CKMB (CK-2).
- The third homodimer (CK-3) consists of two M subunits and is referred to as CKMM (CK-3).

Isoenzyme patterns differ in tissues. Skeletal muscle expresses CPK-MM (98%) and low levels of CPK-MB (1%). The myocardium (heart muscle), in contrast, expresses CPK-MM at 70% and CPK-MB at 25–30%. CPK-BB is predominantly expressed in brain and smooth muscle, including vascular and uterine tissue.

Clinical Significance of Creatine Phosphokinase Isoenzymes

CPK-BB (CK-1)

Diagnostic importance of CPK-BB: CK-1 is found mostly in the brain and lungs, injury to either of these areas can increase CK-1 levels. Increased CK-1 levels may be due to:
- Brain injury, stroke, or bleeding
- Brain cancer
- Seizure [abnormality of central nervous system (CNS)]
- Pulmonary infarction (death to an area of the lung).

CK-MB (CK-2)

Diagnostic importance of CK-MB: CK-2 levels rise 3–6 hours after a heart attack. If there is no further heart muscle damage, the level peaks at 12–24 hours and returns to normal 12–48 hours after tissue death. Levels that drop and then rise again may indicate a second heart attack and/or ongoing heart damage. Increased CPK-2 levels may also be due to:
- Electrical injuries
- Heart defibrillation (purposeful shocking of the heart by medical personnel)
- Heart injury (due to accident)
- Inflammation of the heart muscle usually due to a virus (myocarditis)
- Open heart surgery

CK-MM (CK-3)

Diagnostic importance of CK-MM (CK-3): As CK-MM is mostly found in muscles, increase in level of CK is, depends upon muscle damage severity. Higher-than-normal CPK-3 levels are usually a sign of muscle injury or muscle stress and may be due to:
- Receiving are damaged from a crush injury (when a body part has been squeezed between two heavy objects)
- Muscle damage due to drugs or being immobile for a long time (rhabdomyolysis)
- Myositis (skeletal muscle inflammation)
- Many intramuscular injections
- Recent nerve and muscle function testing (electromyography)
- Recent seizures
- Recent surgery
- Strenuous exercise
- Muscles are inflamed, muscular dystrophy, and muscle trauma (from contact sports, burns, and surgery).

Along with CKMB, significant levels of CKMM activity are found in cardiac muscle and therefore a large increase in "total CK" was once used as a tool in the diagnosis of AMI (acute myocardial infarction). Once the CK isoenzymes were the marker of choice for AMI, but now in many hospitals, it is eventually surpassed by the cardiac troponins.

METHOD OF DIAGNOSIS FOR CREATINE KINASE ISOENZYMES

Sample Preparation

The CK isoenzymes can be analyzed from blood samples, tissue samples, or cell samples.
- **Blood samples:** It should be serum or heparinized plasma. It should be not hemolyzed and assayed within 4 hours of collection if stored at room temperature and 12 hours if samples are stored at 2–8°C.
- **Tissue samples:** It should be rinsed in phosphate-buffered saline, pH 7.4, to remove blood. Take homogenize tissue (50 mg) in 200 µL of 50 mM potassium phosphate buffer, centrifuge for 15 minutes and use cleared supernatant for assay.

Principle

Creatine kinase reversibly catalyzes the transfer of a phosphate group from creatine phosphate to adenosine diphosphate (ADP) to give creatine and adenosine triphosphate (ATP) as products. The ATP formed is used to produce glucose-6-phosphate and ADP from glucose. This reaction is catalyzed by hexokinase (HK) which requires magnesium ions for maximum activity. The glucose-6-phosphate is oxidized by the action of the enzyme glucose-6-phosphate dehydrogenase (G6P-DH) with simultaneous reduction of the coenzyme NADP to give NADPH and 6-phosphogluconate. NADPH so formed is directly proportional to the activity of CK-MB in the sample. The rate of increase of absorbance due to the formation of NADPH is measured at 340/660 nm.

Creatine phosphate + ADP $\xrightarrow{CK}$ Creatine + ATP

ATP + Glucose $\xrightarrow{HK, Mg^{+2}}$ ADP + Glucose-6-phosphate (G-6-P)

G-6-P + NADP$^+$ $\xrightarrow{G\text{-}6\text{-}P\text{-}DH}$ 6-phosphogluconate + NADPH + H$^+$

■ REAGENT COMPOSITION

1. **CK-MB reagent:** It is composed of creatine phosphate 30 mM; adenosine-5'-phosphate 2 mM; NAD 2 mM; hexokinase ≤3,000 U/L; G6P-DH ≥2,000 U/L.
2. **CK-MB diluent:** It is composed of buffer 100 mM, anti-human CK-M antibody (Goat)-sufficient amount to inhibit up to 1,500 U/L of CK-MM at 37°C.

Reconstitute each vial of CK-MB reagent with the volume CK-MB diluent specified on the vial label. Swirl to dissolve. The reconstituted reagent is stable for at least 7 days in refrigerator (2–8°C) and 24 hours at room temperature (15–30°C).

■ PROCEDURE

- Reconstitute CK-MB reagent.
- 1.0 mL of CK-MB reagent into the appropriate test tubes and pre-warm at 37°C for at least 2 minutes.
- Zero spectrophotometer with water at 340 nm.

- Add 0.050 mL (50 µL) of sample to the reagent, mix, and incubate at 37°C for 5 minutes.
- After 5 minutes, read and record the change in absorbance per minute for 2 minutes.
- Calculate the average absorbance difference per minute (ΔAbs./min.).
- The ΔAbs./min. multiplied by the factor 3,376 (see Calculations) will yield CK-B results in IU/L.

■ CALCULATIONS

$CK\text{-}B$ Activity in IU/L = ΔAbs./min. × TV × 1,000
$$= \text{Abs./min.} \times 1.050 \times 1,000 \text{ d} \times \in \times \text{SV1} \times 6.22 \times 0.050$$
$$= \Delta\text{Abs./min.} \times 3,376$$

where,

ΔAbs./min. = Average absorbance change per minute
TV = Total reaction volume (1.050)
1,000 for conversion of IU/mL to IU/L
d = Light path in cm = 1.0
$\in$ = Millimolar absorptivity of NADH = 6.22
SV = Sample volume in mL = 0.050

For *CK-MB Activity:* CK-MB activity is calculated from CK-B activity as follows:

CK-MB Activity (U/L) = CK-B Activity U/L × 2*

*CK-MB molecule is a dimer consisting of a B subunit and an M subunit. Antibody complexing with the M subunit results in loss of half the catalytic activity of the CK-MB molecule. Therefore, CK-MB activity in the sample is equal to twice the CK-B activity.

Total CK activity: Total CK activity is determined by making sum of isoenzymes values. Or determine total CK activity in serum according to the directions provided in the package insert for CK reagent.

Other important methods include:
- **Electrophoresis:** CK isoenzymes (CK-BB, CK-MB, and CK-MM) were separated on agarose gel (Titan Gel Iso-Dot CKIf) in a 2-amino-2 methyl propanol buffer. The ultraviolet visualization of the separated isoenzymes is facilitated by utilizing a substrate with the same catalytic reactions (Titan Gel CK Isoenzyme Reagent).

The developed electrophoretogram is scanned densitometrically to determine the amount of NADH fluorescence which is directly proportional to the relative activity of each of the isoenzymes present. The activity (U/L) of each isoenzyme is calculated based on its percentage of the total sample CK activity. Observe bands as follows (cathode to anode):
- CK (BB)—migrates closely with albumin.
- CK (MB)—migrates between CK-BB and CK-MM
- CK (MM)—remains near the origin

- **The CK-MB ELISA test:** In this test, CK-MB calibrator, patient specimen, or control is first added to a streptavidin coated well. Biotinylated monoclonal and enzyme-labeled antibodies directed against distinct and different epitopes of CK-MB are added and the reactants are mixed. Reaction between the various CK-MB antibodies and native CK-MB forms a sandwich complex that binds with the streptavidin coated to the well. After the completion of the required incubation period, the enzyme-CK-MB antibody bound conjugate is separated from the unbound enzyme-CK-MB conjugate by aspiration or decantation. The activity of the enzyme present on the surface of the well is quantitated by reaction with a suitable substrate to produce color. The essential reagents required for an immunoenzymometric assay include high affinity and specificity antibodies (enzyme conjugated and immobilized), with different and distinct epitope recognition, in excess and native antigen.

Some factors can interfere with test results. These are:
- Drugs—that lower cholesterol, steroids and anesthetics, and amphotericin B (an antifungal—medication)
- Alcohol and cocaine
- Vigorous exercise
- Intramuscular injections and cardiac catheterization
- Recent surgery

Normal Values

- Total CPK level (at 30°C) is—males 35–175 units/L, females 25–140 units/L, and infants two times that of adults
- CPK-BB: 0% of the total CP

- CPK-MB: 0–6% of the total CPK
- CPK-MM: 96–100% of the total CPK

SUMMARY

- Enzyme acts like catalyst and accelerates the rate of these biochemical metabolic reactions, without being utilized in the overall process.
- The substance on which enzyme acts to form specific end product is known as substrate.
- The enzyme unit, or international unit for enzyme (symbol U/IU), is a unit of enzyme's catalytic activity.
- Coenzymes are nonprotein dialyzable organic compounds, which are noncovalently bound to the enzyme protein and are responsible for the catalytic activity of several enzymes.
- Isoenzymes are different forms of same enzyme having same enzymatic activity.
- A biochemically active compound formed by the combination of an enzyme with a coenzyme and/or cofactor is called holoenzyme.
- IEC has classified enzymes into six classes based on the reaction of catalysis, namely oxidoreductases, transferases, hydrolases, lyases, isomerases, and ligases.
- Two steps of enzyme reaction—S + E → E − S and E−S → P + E
- Two models of enzyme substrate reaction—Lock and key model and induced-fit model.
- Enzyme activity is inhibited by certain substances called as enzyme inhibitors and the process is called as enzyme inhibition.
- Several factors affect the rate at which enzymatic reactions proceed—temperature, pH, enzyme concentration, substrate concentration, contact between enzyme and substrate, concentration of product, effect of inhibitors, and effect of oxidizing substances.
- Enzymes have medical, pharmaceutical as well as diagnostic significance. It can be used as reagents.
- Amylase is a digestive enzyme secreted by the pancreas and salivary glands. Main function of amylase is to hydrolyze the glycosidic bonds in starch molecules, converting complex carbohydrates to simple sugars.
- Amylase is the only plasma enzyme normally found in the urine.
- The iodometric (amyloclastic) method is based on the ability of iodide to form a vivid blue color in combination with starch.
- Salivary amylase is calculated as the difference between the total and pancreatic amylase.
- Visible kinetic method is based on the principle that, amylase hydrolyzes PNPG7 to PNPG3 and maltotetraose. Glucoamylase hydrolyses PNPG3 to

PNPG1 and glucose. PNPG1 is hydrolyzed by α-glucosidase to glucose and p-nitrophenol, which produces yellow color.
- Lipases are the enzymes that hydrolyze glycerol esters of long-chain fatty acids. It is fully active in the presence of bile salts and a cofactor, called co-lipase.
- The lipase test is most often used in evaluating inflammation of the pancreas (pancreatitis), but it is also useful in diagnosing kidney failure, intestinal obstruction, mumps, and peptic ulcers.
- LDH is present in high concentration in heart, kidney, erythrocytes, and skeletal muscle.
- It is determined by King's method using colorimeter.
- LDH activity is present in all cells of the body. It is found in the cytoplasm of the cell.
- Phosphatase is an enzyme that removes a phosphate group from its substrate by hydrolyzing phosphoric acid monoesters into a phosphate ion and a molecule with a free hydroxyl group.
- The pH for measuring the alkaline phosphates activity is 10 and for acid phosphates it is 5.
- ACP from serum converts phenyl phosphatase to inorganic PO_4 and phenol at pH 4.9. Phenol in alkaline medium reacts with 4-aminoantipyrine in the presence of potassium ferricyanide forms orange red-colored complex.
- Creatine phosphocreatine is a dimeric enzyme, i.e., it consists of two subunits—M subunit and B subunit.
- All isoenzymes of CK catalyzes the conversion of creatine and utilizes ATP to create phosphocreatine (PCr) and ADP.
- CK isoenzymes (CK-BB, CK-MB, and CK-MM) are separated by electrophoresis on agarose gel.

PRACTICE QUESTIONS

1. What are enzymes? Discuss its properties.
2. Define—coenzyme, cofactor, apoenzyme, holoenzyme, and isoenzyme.
3. Discuss with a neat labeled diagram, different mechanisms of enzyme–substrate action.
4. What is enzyme inhibition? Discuss with examples.
5. Enlist the factors affecting enzyme reaction.
6. Write a short note on—(i) medical and pharmaceutical significance of enzyme and (ii) diagnostic significance of enzymes.
7. With suitable example, prove that enzymes are used as reagents.
8. What are isoenzymes of amylase? Discuss its clinical significance.
9. Discuss the principle and procedure of serum amylase by iodometric method.

10. Discuss the principle and procedure of serum amylase by visible kinetic method.
11. Define caraway unit.
12. Discuss the principle and procedure of serum LDH by King's method.
13. Write a note on clinical significance of LDH.
14. What are phosphatases? Mention their types.
15. Write the principle and procedure to find out serum acid phosphates by Gutman and Gutman method.
16. With reference to isoenzymes of CPK, answer the following questions:
    a. Types of CPK
    b. Clinical Significance
    c. Method of diagnosis
17. Write a note on principle of diagnosis of CPK isoenzymes.

CHAPTER 16

Water and Mineral Metabolism

Keywords
Metabolism, osmotic forces, organic compounds, inorganic electrolytes, thirst, osmoregulatory mechanism, electrolyte, macrominerals, microminerals, iron, ferritin, calcium, hyperthyroidism, phosphorus, sodium, potassium, aldosterone, magnesium, copper, iodine, thyroid gland, manganese, zinc, molybdenum, selenium, chromium, trace minerals

■ INTRODUCTION

Metabolism consists of a series of reactions that occur within cells of living organisms to sustain life. The process of metabolism involves many interconnected cellular pathways to ultimately provide cells with the energy required to carry out their function. Metabolism can be split into a series of chemical reactions that comprise both the synthesis and degradation of complex macromolecules known as anabolism or catabolism, respectively.

■ DISTRIBUTION OF WATER IN THE BODY

Water is the largest constituent of the body. The average body water content is 60–70% of the body weight. In an adult male of 70 kg, the total body water is about 40 L. The amount of water in females is a little less than in males. The distribution of water in the body is as:
1. Intracellular—the fluid within the cells is 50% of the body weight.
2. Extracellular—all of the fluid outside the cell is 20% of the body weight. It can be further divided as:
   i. Plasma—5.5% of the body weight
   ii. Intestinal and lymph fluids—80%
   iii. Dense connective tissue, cartilage, and bone—6.5%

iv. *Transcellular fluids:* It is found in salivary glands, pancreas, liver, thyroid gland, gonads, skin, mucous membranes of the respiratory and gastrointestinal tracts and the kidneys as well as the fluids in spaces within the eye, cerebrospinal fluid (CSF), etc.—5%.

The distribution of water is continuously changing. Osmotic forces are the principal factors for controlling the amount of fluid in the various compartments of the body. These are maintained by the solutes in the body water.

- **Organic compounds of small molecular size (glucose, urea, and amino acids etc.):** If these are present in large amounts, they can help in retaining water.
- **Organic substances of large molecular size (proteins):** These substances can throw effect in the transfer of fluids from one compartment to the other.
- **Inorganic electrolytes:** These inorganic electrolytes are the most important both in the distribution and in the retention of body water.

■ WATER BALANCE

- **Water intake:** Water is supplied to the body by the following processes:
  - Dietary liquids
  - Solid foods
  - *Oxidation of foodstuffs:* It is obtained from the combustion of fats, proteins, and carbohydrates. The oxidation of fats yields 107 mL/100 g, proteins 41 mL/100 g, and carbohydrates 56 mL/100 g.
- **Water output:** Water is lost from the body by the following routes:
  - Urine
  - Respiration
  - Lactation
  - Feces
  - Evaporation from skin and lungs

Additional water losses in disease:

- Water loss is more in diarrhea and vomiting and these losses can be fatal in infants.
- In kidney disease, renal water loss is more.

- In fever, insensible losses may rise much higher than normal.
- Patients in high environmental temperatures also sustain extremely high external water losses.

Equilibrium persists between the intake and output of water in the body. In addition to other factors, certain hormones, such as antidiuretic hormone (ADH), vasopressin, oxytocin, and aldosterone, influence the regulatory mechanism of body water. The balance sheet of water is given below.

Water intake			Water loss		
Drinks	48%	1,350 mL	Lungs	12%	500 mL
Solid	40%	900 mL	Skin	24%	700 mL
Oxidation of food	12%	450 mL	Urine Feces	56% 08%	1,400 mL 100 mL
	100%	2,700 mL		100%	2,700 mL

There is a continuous excretion of water in the form of digestive juices from the body into the alimentary canal and that water is reabsorbed along with the water of food and drink. The amount of this internal secretion is 7–10 L per day. This entire amount is reabsorbed except about 100 mL which is excreted in feces. The secretion of saliva experiences the fact when we have a sore throat.

■ PHYSIOLOGICAL FUNCTIONS OF WATER

1. **Solvent:** One of the most important properties of water is its capacity to dissolve different kinds of substances. It is therefore the most suitable solvent for cellular components. Water brings together various substances in contact when chemical reactions take place.
2. **Catalytic action:** Water accelerates a large number of chemical reactions in the body due to its ionizing power. All chemical reactions in the body proceed in presence of water only.
3. **Lubricating actions:** Water acts as a lubricant in the body and prevents friction in joints, pleura, conjunctiva, and peritoneum.
4. **Heat regulation:** By virtue of its high specific heat, water prevents any significant rise in the body temperature due to heat liberated from body reactions. The loss of heat from the body is also regulated by the evaporation of water from skin and lungs and its removal in urine.

5. **Dielectric constant:** Oppositely charged particles can coexist in water. Therefore, it is a good ionizing medium. This increases the chemical reactions.

■ REGULATION OF PASSAGE OF WATER

Water has self-regulatory mechanism. This can be explained as follows:
- If the capillary pressure is increased, more water will flow into the tissues.
- A fall in blood pressure (BP) helps the passage of water from the tissues to the blood.
- If the plasma proteins are decreased, water will flow into the tissues.
- Dilution of blood by excessive ingestion of water can lower the osmotic pressure of the plasma proteins and thus may increase capillary pressure.

■ THIRST

Thirst is an osmoregulatory mechanism to increase water input. The thirst mechanism is activated in response to changes in water volume in the blood and to changes in blood osmolality. Blood osmolality is primarily driven by the concentration of sodium cations. The urge to drink results from a complex interplay of hormones and neuronal responses that coordinate to increase water input and contribute toward fluid balance and composition in the body. The "thirst center" is contained within the hypothalamus, a portion of the brain that lies just above the brainstem.

■ MINERALS

Minerals are inorganic substances mined from the earth. They exist naturally on and in the earth and many are critical parts of human tissue. There are total 92 naturally occurring elements, out of these, the 13 minerals are termed "essential" nutrients to human health. These minerals are essential for the normal growth, development, and maintenance of health. Therefore, they must be included in the diet. When the intake in the diet of these minerals is below the required amount, deficiency symptoms appear.

Some important roles of minerals in the body are as follows:
- Cofactors and prosthetic groups of certain enzymes
- Constituent of certain important molecules, such as hemoglobin (Hb)
- Constituent of certain structures, such as bone
- Water, electrolyte, and acid–base balance
- Electrical activity of cells.

Essential minerals are divided into major minerals (macrominerals) and trace minerals (microminerals). These two groups of minerals are equally important, but trace minerals are needed in smaller amounts than major minerals. The amounts needed in the body are not an indication of their importance.

Major Elements (or Macrominerals)

Major elements are the ones the dietary requirement of which is >100 mg or their body content is >5 g. Ca, Mg, P, Na, K, Cl, and S are major elements. These are usually measured in milligrams. These are about 80% of total mineral content.

Minor Elements (or Trace Elements or Microminerals)

Minor elements have daily requirement <100 mg or their body content is <5 g. Fe, I, Cu, Mn, Zn, Co, Mo, Se, and F are trace elements. These are usually measured in micrograms [1 microgram (µg) equals 1/1,000th of a milligram (mg)]. These are about 20% of total mineral content.

All minerals are active in the body in their ionic form. Fe and Cu, being transitional elements, can exist both in the oxidized state as Fe^{3+} and Cu^{2+}, and the reduced state as Fe^{2+} and Cu^+. Ca exists in the body both as ionic form (Ca^{2+}) and also as compounds of phosphate in bones and teeth. P and S exist in the body as phosphates and sulfates, respectively. Phosphates and sulfates exist either as free inorganic ions or bound to organic molecules. S atoms, in addition, exist as heteroatoms in organic biomolecules.

Thirteen Essential Minerals

1. **Iron:** Iron is an essential constituent of Hb and certain enzymes such as cytochrome oxidase, catalase, and peroxidase. It

performs two important functions in the body—to transport oxygen to tissues (through Hb) and to take part in oxidation-reduction reactions (cytochrome system).

Deficiency of iron results in various types of anemias:
- *Sources*: Meat, liver, eggs, spinach, and fruits.
- *Absorption*: Dietary intake of iron is mainly in ferric (Fe^{+++}) form as hydroxides or in organic compounds. The action of gastric HCl and of some organic acids liberates free ferric ions, which in turn are reduced to ferrous ions (Fe^{++}) by reducing substances such as cysteine or ascorbic acid. The ferrous form of iron is more soluble and thus easily absorbed. The absorption of iron occurs in duodenum and stomach.
- *Transport and storage*: Iron is transported in plasma in ferric form, which remains firmly bound to a specific β-globulin, transferrin. The normal concentration of protein bound iron in plasma is 50–180 µg/100 mL.

Iron is stored chiefly in mucosal cells of intestine, liver, spleen, and bone marrow as ferritin.
- *Normal range*: Serum iron 75–175 µg/dL (13–31 µmol/L)
- *Daily requirement*: Infants—6–15 mg, children—10–18 mg, adult (male) 10 mg, and female—18 mg.

2. **Calcium:** Calcium is the most important and essential mineral. It performs following functions—builds and maintains bones and teeth; regulates heart rhythm; eases insomnia; helps regulate the passage of nutrients in and out of the cell walls; assists in normal blood clotting; helps maintain proper nerve and muscle function; lowers BP; important to normal kidney function; and in current medical research reduces the incidence of colon cancer, and reduces blood cholesterol levels.
   - *Sources*: Good sources of calcium include milk and milk products, yogurt, ricotta, cheese, oysters, salmon, collard greens, spinach, ice cream, cottage cheese, kale, broccoli, and oranges.
   - *Absorption*: Calcium is taken in diet as calcium phosphate, carbonate tartarate, and oxalate. Its absorption occurs mainly in intestine.
   - *Deficiency*: May result in arm and leg muscles spasms, softening of bones, back and leg cramps, brittle bones, rickets,

poor growth, osteoporosis (a deterioration of the bones), tooth decay, and depression.
- *Toxicity*: Occurs in hypervitaminosis D and hyperthyroidism or idiopathic hypercalcemia. It is characterized by vomiting, abdominal cramps, and nephrocalcinosis.
- *Normal range*: Serum calcium—9.0–11.0 mg/dL (2.25–2.75 mmol/L).
- *Daily requirement*: 1,000 mg/day, women age 51+ and men age 71+: 1,200 mg/day.

3. **Phosphorus:** Phosphorus is widely distributed in the body. It has following functions: Builds and maintains bones and teeth along with calcium, required for the synthesis of phospholipids, nucleotides, phosphoproteins, organic phosphates, and energy-rich compounds [adenosine triphosphate (ATP)].
   - *Sources*: Food sources of phosphorus include protein-rich foods such as meats and dairy products, although some is present in almost all foods.
   - *Absorption*: The absorption of phosphorus is intimately related to calcium absorption. High calcium diet diminishes phosphorus absorption due to the formation of insoluble calcium phosphate.

   In blood, phosphorus occurs in three forms:
   1. Inorganic phosphate (2–5 mg/100 mL)
   2. Organic phosphorus (14–29 mg/100 mL)
   3. Phospholipids (8–18 mg/100 mL)

   Serum levels are regulated by kidney reabsorption. In rickets, serum inorganic phosphate level comes down to about 1–2 mg/100 mL. People taking aluminum hydroxide as an antacid for extended periods of time may develop a phosphorus deficiency since the aluminum prevents phosphorus absorption.
   - *Normal range*: Serum inorganic phosphate—3.0–4.5 mg/dL (1.0–1.5 mmol/L).
   - *Daily requirement*: 700 mg/day.

4. **Sodium:** It is a principal cation in extracellular fluid. It regulates plasma volume, acid–base balance, nerve and muscle function, and Na^+/K^+ adenosine triphosphatase (ATPase).
   - *Source*: The salt added to prepare food is the main source of sodium.

- *Metabolism*: Metabolism is regulated by aldosterone [progesterone and acetylcholine (ACH)].
- *Deficiency*: Deficiency is related to diarrhea, vomiting, Addison's disease, excessive sweating, overuse of diuretics, salt-losing nephritis, and diabetes mellitus. It is characterized by headache, nausea, cramps, fall in BP, oliguria, and increased pulse rate.
- *Toxicity*: Occurs in cardiac failure, hepatic cirrhosis, acute glomerulonephritis, premenstrual phase of cycle, excess of adrenocorticotropic hormone (ACTH), ACH, and testosterone. In hypersensitive individuals, it causes elevation of BP and edema.
- *Normal plasma range*: 135–145 mEq/L.
- *Daily requirement*: 5–15 g.

5. **Potassium:** It works with sodium to regulate the body's waste balance and normalize heart rhythms; aids in clear thinking by sending oxygen to the brain; preserves proper alkalinity of body fluids; stimulates the kidneys to eliminate poisonous body wastes; assists in reducing high BP; and promotes healthy skin.
    - *Sources*: Potassium is widely available in foods, but mostly in unprocessed fresh foods—especially fruits and vegetables and nuts.
    - *Metabolism*: Metabolism is regulated by aldosterone.
    - *Deficiency*: It may result in poor reflexes, nervous disorders, respiratory failure, cardiac arrest, and muscle damage.
    - *Toxicity*: Excess causes cardiac arrest and small bowel ulcers. It is a feature of diabetic ketoacidosis, severe burn, blood loss, acute renal failure, Addison disease, and chronic renal disease.
    - *Normal plasma range*: 3–5 mEq/L.
    - *Daily requirement*: 4 g/day.

6. **Magnesium:** It plays an important role in regulating the neuromuscular activity of the heart; maintains normal heart rhythm; necessary for proper calcium and vitamin C metabolism; and converts blood sugar into energy.
    - *Source*: Good food sources of magnesium include seeds, unrefined grains, beans, and other vegetables.

- *Deficiency*: Deficiency may result in calcium depletion, heart spasms, nervousness, muscular excitability, confusion, and kidney stones.
- *Toxicity*: Depressed deep tendon reflexes and respiration.
- *Normal range*: 1.3–2.1 mEq/L (0.65–1.05 mmol/L).
- *Daily requirement*: 350 mg/day.

7. **Copper:** It is necessary for the absorption and utilization of iron; helps oxidize vitamin C and works with vitamin C to form elastin, a chief component of the elastin muscle fibers throughout the body; aids in the formation of red blood cells; and helps proper bone formation and maintenance.
   - *Sources*: Copper is commonly found in whole grains, nuts, shellfish, liver and dark green, and leafy vegetables.
   - *Deficiency*: May result in general weakness, impaired respiration, and skin sores.
   - *Toxicity*: It is rare. Secondary to Wilson disease characterized by more urinary excretion of copper and less serum copper.
   - *Normal level*: 85–180 µg/dL.
   - *Daily requirement*: 900 µg/day.

8. **Iodine:** It aids in the development and functioning of the thyroid gland; regulates the body's production of energy; helps burn excess fat by stimulating the rate of metabolism; mentality, speech, the condition of the hair, skin, and teeth are dependent upon a well- functioning thyroid gland.
   - *Source:* Iodized salt and sea food is the most common source of this essential trace mineral.
   - *Deficiency:* May result in an enlarged thyroid gland, slow mental reaction, dry skin and hair, weight gain, and loss of physical and mental vigor.
   - Toxicity causes thyrotoxicosis and goiter.
   - *Normal level*: 40–92 ng/mL.
   - *Daily requirement*: 150 µg/day.

9. **Manganese:** An antioxidant nutrient; important in the blood breakdown of amino acids and the production of energy; necessary for the metabolism of vitamin B1 and vitamin E; activates various enzymes which are important for proper digestion and utilization of foods; is a catalyst in the breakdown of fats and cholesterol; helps nourish the nerves and brain;

necessary for normal skeletal development; and maintains sex hormone production.
- *Source:* Grains and cereal products are the best food sources of manganese.
- *Deficiency:* May result in paralysis, convulsions, dizziness, ataxia, loss of hearing, digestive problems, blindness, and deafness in infants.
- *Toxicity* due to inhalation causes psychotic symptoms and Parkinsonism.
- *Normal range:* 4.7–18.3 ng/mL.
- *Daily requirement:* Men: 2.3 mg/day and women: 1.8 mg/day.

10. **Zinc:** It is an antioxidant nutrient; necessary for protein synthesis; wound healing; vital for the development of the reproductive organs, prostate functions, and male hormone activity; it governs the contractility of muscles; important for blood stability; maintains the body's alkaline balance; helps in normal tissue function; and aids in the digestion and metabolism of phosphorus.
    - *Sources*: Meats, fish, beans, whole grains, pumpkin seeds, mushrooms, and brewer's yeast are good food sources of zinc.
    - *Deficiency:* May result in delayed sexual maturity, prolonged healing wounds, white spots on finger nails, retarded growth, stretch marks, fatigue, decreased alertness, and susceptibility to infections.

    Too much zinc can lower copper retention, lower high-density lipoprotein (HDL) (good) cholesterol, gastrointestinal irritation, and vomiting.
    - *Normal range*: 60–120 µg/dL.
    - *Daily requirement*: Men: 11 mg/day and women: 8 mg/day.

11. **Molybdenum:** Molybdenum is involved in the operation of several key enzymes in the body. Readily available throughout the diet, deficiencies of this essential mineral are unusual, although rare deficiencies occur in people who suffer from malabsorption conditions. Milk, beans, cereals, and bread are common food sources of molybdenum. Elevated levels of molybdenum can cause a loss of copper.
    - *Normal range*: 0.28–1.17 ng/mL.
    - *Daily requirement*: 45 µg/day.

12. **Selenium:** A major antioxidant nutrient, protects cell membranes, and prevents free radical generation thereby decreasing the risk of cancer and disease of the heart and blood vessels. Medical surveys show that increased selenium intake decreases the risk of breast, colon, lung, and prostate cancer. Selenium also preserves tissue elasticity; slows down the aging and hardening of tissues through oxidation; helps in the treatment and prevention of dandruff.
    - *Source:* Seafood and organ meats such as liver and kidney are high in selenium, whereas selenium levels in grains and vegetables vary widely, depending on local soil content.
    - *Deficiency:* May result in premature aging, heart disease, dandruff, and loose skin. No >200 μg of selenium daily is recommended for general use, because of possible toxicity. Excessive intakes of selenium can affect the functioning of enzymes and normal bone and cartilage development, selenium in excess can cause nausea, loss of hair and nails, skin abnormalities, and nerve damage.
    - *Normal range*: 70-150 ng/mL.
    - *Daily requirement*: 55 μg/day.
13. **Chromium:** It works with insulin in the metabolism of sugar and stabilizes blood sugar levels; cleans the arteries by reducing cholesterol and triglyceride levels; helps transport amino acids to where the body needs them; helps control the appetite; medical research has shown that persons with low levels of chromium in their bodies are more susceptible to having cancer and heart problems and becoming diabetic.
    - *Source*: The only common food source is brewer's yeast.
    - *Deficiency*: May result in glucose intolerance in diabetics; arteriosclerosis, heart disease, depressed growth, obesity, and tiredness.

    Chromium should not be taken in excess however—there have been reported cases of toxicity when used in high doses (>800 μg/day).
    - *Normal range*: ≤1.4 μg/L.
    - *Daily requirement*: 25-30 μg/day.

Trace Minerals

Minerals that occur in tiny amounts or traces are called as trace minerals. These are cobalt, fluorine, iodine chromium, selenium, manganese, and molybdenum. They play a major role in health, since even minute portions of them can powerfully affect health. They are essential in the assimilation and utilization of vitamins and other nutrients. They aid in digestion and provide the catalyst for many hormones, enzymes, and essential body functions and reactions. They also aid in replacing electrolytes lost through heavy perspiration or extended diarrhea and protects against toxic reactions such as heavy metal poisoning.

SUMMARY

- Metabolism is all chemical reactions involved in maintaining the living state of the cells and the organism.
- Metabolism is divided into two categories: Catabolism—the breakdown of molecules to obtain energy. Anabolism—the synthesis of all compounds needed by the body.
- The average body water content is 60–70% of the body weight. It is present in plasma, inside and outside the cells, and in various body fluids.
- Osmotic forces are the principal factors for controlling the amount of fluid in the body. These are maintained by organic and inorganic substances in the body water.
- Physiological functions of water—as a solvent, in catalytic action, lubricating actions, heat regulation, and as dielectric constant.
- Thirst is an osmoregulatory mechanism to increase water input.
- The "thirst center" is contained within the hypothalamus.
- Thirteen minerals are essential for the normal growth, development, and maintenance of health.
- Macrominerals are with dietary requirement >100 mg/day and body content is >5 g.
- Microminerals are with dietary requirement >100 mg/day and body content is <5 g.
- Iron is an essential constituent of Hb and certain enzymes. It performs two important functions in the body—to transport oxygen to tissues (through Hb) and to take part in oxidation–reduction reactions (cytochrome system).
- Calcium is needed for building and maintaining bones and teeth, regulates heart rhythm, eases insomnia, and assists in blood clotting.
- Phosphorus is needed for the synthesis of phospholipids, nucleotides, phosphoproteins, organic phosphates, and energy-rich compounds such as ATP.

- Sodium is a principal cation in extracellular fluid. It regulates plasma volume, acid–base balance, nerve and muscle function, and Na^+/K^+ ATPase.
- Potassium works with sodium to regulate the body's waste balance and normalize heart rhythms, and aids in clear thinking. It also preserves alkalinity of body fluids.
- Magnesium is required for neuromuscular activity of the heart; maintains normal heart rhythm; necessary for proper calcium and vitamin C metabolism.
- Copper is necessary for absorption of and utilization of iron. It also aids in the formation of red blood cells and helps in proper bone formation and maintenance.
- Iodine aids in the development and functioning of the thyroid gland; regulates the body's production of energy and helps burn excess fat by stimulating the rate of metabolism.
- Manganese is an antioxidant it activates various enzymes important for proper digestion and utilization of food. It also maintains production of sex hormones.
- Zinc is an antioxidant nutrient; necessary for protein synthesis; wound healing and vital for the development of the reproductive organs.
- Molybdenum is involved in the operation of several key enzymes in the body.
- Selenium also preserves tissue elasticity; slows down the aging and hardening of tissues through oxidation; helps in the treatment and prevention of dandruff.
- Chromium works with insulin in the metabolism of sugar and stabilizes blood sugar levels; cleans the arteries by reducing cholesterol and triglyceride levels.
- Minerals that occur in tiny amounts or traces are called as trace minerals. These are cobalt, fluorine, iodine, chromium, selenium, manganese, and molybdenum. They are essential in the assimilation and utilization of vitamins and other nutrients.

PRACTICE QUESTIONS

1. Define metabolism, catabolism, anabolism, and thirst.
2. How much amount of water is present in the body? Discuss its distribution in the body.
3. Explain balance sheet of water in detail.
4. What are physiological functions of water?
5. Write a note on the mechanism of thirst.
6. Minerals play important role in the body. Justify the statement by giving at least ten different examples.
7. Differentiate between macroelements and trace elements.
8. What are the different forms of phosphorus? How it is related to calcium and aluminum?

Section 3: Clinical Biochemistry

9. Why it is suggested to eat iodized salt?
10. What happens if zinc, sodium, calcium, copper, and magnesium are consumed in large quantity?
11. Trace minerals and essential minerals are same or different? Justify your answer.
12. Complete the table:

Mineral	Sources	Deficiency	Important role	Normal range
Iron				
Calcium				
Phosphorus				
Sodium				
Potassium				
Magnesium				
Copper				
Iodine				
Manganese				
Zinc				
Molybdenum				
Selenium				
Chromium				

Inborn Errors of Metabolism

CHAPTER 17

Keywords

Glycogen storage disease, Von Gierke disease, Pompe disease, 1,4-glucosidase, limit dextrinosis, amylopectinosis, McArdle disease, myophosphorylase, Hers disease, phosphofructokinase, Tarui disease, gout, pentosuria, xylitol dehydrogenase, galactosuria, galactose-1-phosphate, uridyltransferase, hereditary fructose intolerance (HFI), aldolase B, mucopolysaccharidoses, pyruvate dehydrogenase, pyruvate carboxylase, alkaptonuria phenylketonuria, maple syrup urine disease (MSUD), homogentisate oxidase, phenylalanine hydroxylase, glutaric acidemia type 1, homocystinuria, homocysteine, Niemann–Pick disease, sphingomyelinase, Tay-Sachs disease, hexosaminidase A, Gaucher disease, glucocerebrosidase, Fabry disease, Lesch–Nyhan syndrome, hereditary xanthinuria, xanthine dehydrogenase

■ INTRODUCTION

Inborn errors of metabolism (IEM) comprise a large class of rare genetic diseases involving disorders of metabolism. The majority are due to defects of single genes that code for enzymes that facilitate conversion of various substrates into products. In most of the disorders, problems arise due to accumulation of substances which are toxic or interfere with normal function, or to the effects of reduced ability to synthesize essential compounds. Depending on the metabolic error involved, the clinical presentation can be severe or lethal with neurodegenerative process, skeletal abnormalities, and/or physiologic dysfunctions.

The global incidence of each particular IEM is low, but considered all together they represent >1 affected individual each 1,000 births. The occurrence of each disease can be significantly different in particular regions.

Some of the important diseases belonging IEM are discussed here.

CARBOHYDRATE METABOLISM

Inborn errors of carbohydrate metabolism occur in following different forms:

Glycogen Storage Disease (Glycogenosis)

It is a group of congenital disorders which occur due to deposition of large amounts of glycogen in several tissues such as liver, kidney, heart, and muscle. Glycogen accumulation in these tissues occurs due to deficiency or lack of enzymes involved in the breakdown of glycogen. On the basis of the deficiency of various enzymes in different tissues, such disorders have been divided into following types:

Type I (Von Gierke Disease)

Enzyme deficiency: Glucose-6-phosphatase.

Glucose-6-phosphatase is an enzyme that hydrolyzes glucose-6-phosphate resulting in the creation of a phosphate group and free glucose. Deficiency of this enzyme impairs the ability of the liver to produce free glucose from glycogen and from gluconeogenesis. Glycogen deposition predominantly occurs in liver and kidney. Since, glucose cannot be derived from glycogen in this condition, children with this disease develop hypoglycemia. Thus, most of the energy requirements of the body are met by fat breakdown and this leads to ketosis and hyperlipidemia.

Symptoms: Hypoglycemia, hyperlipidemia, hepatomegaly, lactic acidosis, and hyperuricemia.

Progression: Growth failure. Children suffering from this disease are generally known to die young, though a number of them survive to adolescence.

Type II (Pompe Disease)

Enzyme deficiency: α-1,4-glucosidase.

Pompe disease is an autosomal recessive metabolic disorder, which damages muscle and nerve cells throughout the body. It is caused by an accumulation of glycogen in the lysosome due to deficiency of the lysosomal acid α-glucosidase enzyme that transforms glycogen into glucose in lysosomes. It is caused by a mutation in a gene (acid α-glucosidase: also known as acid maltase) on long arm of chromosome.

Symptoms: The build-up of glycogen causes progressive muscle weakness (myopathy) throughout the body and affects various body tissues, particularly in the heart, skeletal muscles, and weakness of facial and oral muscles. Trouble with sucking, chewing, and/or swallowing can lead to insufficient caloric intake, problems maintaining a healthy weight, and a general failure to thrive.

Progression: Death by age ~2 years.

Type III (Limit Dextrinosis)

Enzyme deficiency: Debranching enzyme.

Because of the deficient enzyme, breakdown of glycogen after phosphorylase action is affected. Limit dextrin is the remaining polymer produced after hydrolysis of glycogen. Without glycogen debranching enzymes to further convert these branched glycogen polymers to glucose, limit dextrinosis abnormally accumulates in the cytoplasm.

Symptoms: Infancy with hypoglycemia, hepatomegaly, and muscular disease, including hypotonia and cardiomyopathy.

Progression: The persons with limit dextrinosis are known to survive well into adult life.

Type IV (Amylopectinosis)

Enzyme deficiency: Branching enzyme.

Amylopectinosis is a result of the absence of the glycogen branching enzyme, which is critical in the production of glycogen. This leads to very long unbranched glucose chains being stored in glycogen. This has fewer branching points and longer outer chains, thus resembling amylopectin. The long unbranched molecules have a low solubility which leads to glycogen precipitation in the liver. These deposits subsequently build up in the body tissue, especially the heart and liver.

Symptom: Fasting hypoglycemia in infants. The inability to breakdown glycogen in muscle cells causes muscle weakness. The abnormally branched glycogen accumulates as intracytoplasmic nonmembrane-bound inclusions in hepatocytes, myocytes, and neuromuscular system; where it increases osmotic pressure within cells, causing cellular swelling and death.

Progression: The probable end result is cirrhosis and death within 5 years.

Type V (McArdle Disease)

Enzyme deficiency: Myophosphorylase.

Myophosphorylase is muscle isoform of the enzyme glycogen phosphorylase. This enzyme helps break down glycogen into glucose-1-phosphate, so that it can be utilized within the muscle cell.

Symptoms: The onset of this disease is usually noticed in childhood, but often not diagnosed until the third or fourth decade of life. Symptoms include exercise intolerance with myalgia, early fatigue, painful cramps, weakness of exercising muscles, and myoglobinuria. Myoglobinuria, the condition where myoglobin is present in urine, may result from serious damage to the muscles, or rhabdomyolysis, where skeletal muscle cells breakdown rapidly, sending their contents into the bloodstream.

Progression: Some patients learn the limits of their exercise and work within their restrictions, going on to live fairly normal lives. Progression includes renal failure due to myoglobinuria.

Type VI (Hers Disease)

Enzyme deficiency: Phosphofructokinase.

Clinically, it is mild type I glycogenosis. In this condition, there is deficiency of phosphofructokinase enzyme which causes moderate accumulation of glycogen in skeletal muscle. Glucose-6-phosphate and fructose-6-phosphate are also found to accumulate in this disease. Clinically, the picture resembles with that of type 5 glycogenosis.

Of the above-mentioned types of glycogen storage disease (glycogenosis) the most commonly occurring types are type 1, 2, 3, and 6.

Type VII (Tarui Disease)

Enzyme deficiency: Phosphofructokinase.

Tarui disease is a metabolic disorder with autosomal recessive inheritance phosphofructokinase deficiency. In this condition, a deficiency phosphofructokinase enzyme impairs the ability of cells such as erythrocytes and skeletal muscles to use carbohydrates for energy. The mutation impairs the ability of phosphofructokinase to phosphorylate fructose-6-phosphate prior to its cleavage into glyceraldehyde which enters the Krebs cycle, effectively limiting energy production.

Symptom: The disease presents with exercise-induced muscle cramps and weakness, myoglobinuria, as well as with hemolytic anemia causing dark urine. Hyperuricemia is common. High uric acid concentrations that may cause gout.

Individuals with Tarui disease should avoid intensive muscle activity that has many negative consequences for physical and mental health. Clinically, the picture resembles with that of type 5 glycogenosis.

Of the above-mentioned types of glycogen storage disease (glycogenosis) the most commonly occurring types are type I, II, III, and VI.

Pentosuria

Enzyme deficiency: Xylitol dehydrogenase.

Appearance of pentose sugar in urine is called pentosuria. A congenital defect in the enzyme xylitol dehydrogenase catalyzing the conversion of L-xylulose to L-xylitol in the uronic acid pathway in liver is responsible for this IEM. It is characterized by the excessive urinary excretion of the pentose sugar xylitol. It may lead to confusion with diabetes mellitus, which is not related to pentosuria. Pentosuria has been observed almost exclusively in persons of Jewish descent.

No disabilities are incurred, and no dietary or other measures are necessary.

Galactosuria

Enzyme deficiency: Galactose-1-phosphate uridyltransferase.

Galactosuria is a hereditary disorder due to metabolic defect in the conversion of galactose to glucose. It occurs due to deficiency or complete lack of enzyme galactose-1-phosphate uridyltransferase which converts galactose-1-phosphate to glucose-1-phosphate. This results in accumulation of galactose-1-phosphate in tissues and blood. Infants with this condition suffer from malnutrition, mental retardation, galactosuria, and eventually hepatomegaly and cirrhosis may also develop. Increased level of galactose reduces blood glucose concentration. On removal of milk from the food, however, the clinical symptoms of this disorder can be removed.

Hereditary Fructose Intolerance

Enzyme deficiency: Aldolase B.

Hereditary fructose intolerance (HFI) is a metabolic disease caused by the absence of an enzyme called aldolase B. In people with HFI, ingestion of fructose (fruit sugar) and sucrose (cane or beet sugar, table sugar) causes severe hypoglycemia (low blood sugar) and the buildup of dangerous substances in the liver. HFI may be relatively mild or a very severe disease. The condition is caused by mutations in the *ALDOB* gene. It is inherited in an autosomal recessive pattern.

In this disorder, the body is missing an enzyme that allows it to use fructose and sucrose. As a result, a by-product of fructose accumulates in the body, blocking the formation of glycogen and its conversion to glucose for use as energy. Ingesting more than tiny amounts of fructose or sucrose causes low blood sugar levels (hypoglycemia), with sweating, confusion, and sometimes seizures and coma. Children who continue to eat foods containing fructose develop kidney and liver damage, resulting in jaundice, vomiting, mental deterioration, seizures, and death.

For most types of this disorder, early diagnosis and dietary restrictions started early in infancy can help prevent these more serious problems.

The diagnosis is made when a chemical examination of a sample of liver tissue determines that the enzyme is missing.

Mucopolysaccharidoses

Mucopolysaccharidosis refers to a group of inherited conditions in which the body is unable to properly breakdown mucopolysaccharides (long chains of saccharides molecules that are found throughout the body). As a result, these sugars buildup in cells, blood, and connective tissue which can lead to a variety of health problems. Seven distinct forms and numerous subtypes of mucopolysaccharidosis have been identified. Associated signs and symptoms and the severity of the condition vary significantly by form. In general, most affected people appear healthy at birth and experience a period of normal development, followed by a decline in physical and/or mental function. As the condition progresses, it may affect appearance; physical abilities; organ and system functioning; and, in most cases, cognitive development. The underlying genetic cause varies by form. Most cases are inherited in an autosomal recessive manner, although one specific form (Type II) follows an X-linked pattern of inheritance.

Symptoms: During infancy and childhood, short stature, hairiness, and abnormal development become noticeable. The face may appear coarse. Some types of mucopolysaccharidoses cause intellectual disability to develop over several years. In some types, vision or hearing may become impaired. The arteries or heart valves can be affected. Finger joints are often stiff.

The presence of a mucopolysaccharidosis in other family members also suggests the diagnosis. Urine tests may help but are sometimes inaccurate. X-rays may show characteristic bone abnormalities.

■ PYRUVATE METABOLISM

Pyruvate is a substance that is formed in the processing of carbohydrates and proteins and that serves as an energy source for cells. Problems with pyruvate metabolism can limit a cell's ability to produce energy and allow a buildup of lactic acid, a waste product. Many enzymes are involved in pyruvate metabolism. A hereditary deficiency in any one of these enzymes results in one of a variety of disorders, depending on which enzyme is missing. Symptoms may develop any time between early infancy and late adulthood. Exercise and infections can worsen symptoms, leading to severe lactic acidosis. These disorders are diagnosed by measuring enzyme activity in cells from the liver or skin.

Pyruvate Dehydrogenase Complex Deficiency

This disorder is caused by a lack of a group of enzymes needed to process pyruvate. This deficiency results in a variety of symptoms, ranging from mild to severe. Some newborns with this deficiency have brain malformations. Other children appear normal at birth but develop symptoms, including weak muscles, seizures, poor coordination, and a severe balance problem, later in infancy or childhood. Intellectual disability is common.

This disorder cannot be cured, but some children are helped by a diet that is high in fat and low in carbohydrates.

Absence of Pyruvate Carboxylase

Pyruvate carboxylase is an enzyme. A lack of this enzyme causes a very rare condition that interferes with or blocks the production of glucose from pyruvate in the body. Lactic acid and ketones build up in the blood. Often, this disease is fatal. Children who survive have seizures and severe intellectual disability, although there are recent reports of children with milder symptoms. There is no cure, but some children are helped by eating frequent carbohydrate-rich meals and restricting dietary protein.

■ PROTEIN METABOLISM

Inborn errors of protein metabolism occur in following different forms which are described here.

Alkaptonuria

Enzyme deficiency: Homogentisate oxidase.

Alkaptonuria is a congenital metabolic disorder associated with the abnormal metabolism of tyrosine. It is characterized by the presence of large amounts of homogentisate in urine, which turns black due to oxidation in air. It is also known as black urine disease. Alkaptonuria is caused by the absence of homogentisate oxidase which catalyzes the conversion of homogentisate to maleylacetoacetate which leads to the formation of fumarate and acetoacetate in the body as shown in **Flowchart 17.1.**

Although, large amounts of homogentisate (or alkapton) are excreted in urine daily. Alkaptonuria does not produce any important clinical manifestation. However, in some cases, darkening of cartilage and tendons (ochronosis) has been observed. This may occur due to the deposition of oxidized homogentisate.

Flowchart 17.1: Abnormal metabolism of tyrosine.

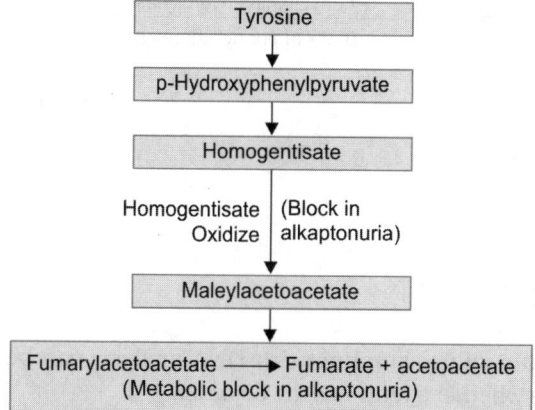

Phenylketonuria

Enzyme deficiency: Phenylalanine hydroxylase.

Phenylketonuria (PKU) is a congenital metabolic disorder, which is characterized by the excretion of phenylpyruvate with good amounts of phenyllactate and phenylacetate, and large amounts of phenylalanine and phenylacetylglutamine in urine.

Phenylketonuria occurs due to the absence of the enzyme phenylalanine hydroxylase which catalyzes the conversion of phenylalanine to tyrosine in human liver. In this condition, phenylalanine is metabolized through an alternate pathway, which results in the formation and excretion of large quantities of its pyruvate and acetate derivative as shown in **Flowchart 17.2**.

Symptom: It can cause problems with brain development, leading to progressive mental retardation, brain damage, and seizures. Other symptoms include seizures, nausea and vomiting, an eczema-like rash, lighter skin and hair than their family members, aggressive or self-injurious behavior, hyperactivity, and sometimes psychiatric symptoms. Untreated children often give off a mousy body and urine odor as a result of a by-product of phenylalanine (phenylacetic acid) in their urine and sweat.

Diagnosis: PKU is usually diagnosed with a routine screening test. PKU occurs in most ethnic groups. If PKU runs in the family and DNA is available from an affected family member, amniocentesis

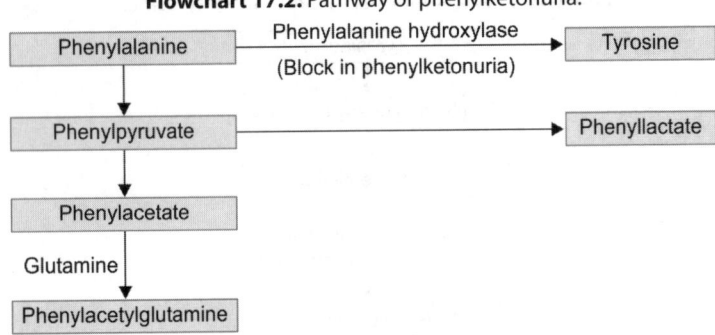

Flowchart 17.2: Pathway of phenylketonuria.

or chorionic villus sampling with DNA analysis can be done to determine whether a fetus has the disorder.

Maple Syrup Urine Disease

Enzyme deficiency: Enzyme complex branched-chain alpha-keto acid dehydrogenase.

Maple syrup urine disease (MSUD) is also called branched-chain ketoaciduria and it is an autosomal recessive metabolic disorder affecting branched-chain amino acids. It is one type of organic acidemia. MSUD is caused by a deficiency of the branched-chain alpha-keto acid dehydrogenase complex (BCKDH), leading to a buildup of the branched-chain amino acids (leucine, isoleucine, and valine) and their toxic by-products in the blood and urine. The disease is characterized in an infant by the presence of sweet-smelling urine, with an odor similar to that of maple syrup.

Symptom: From early infancy, symptoms of the condition include poor feeding, vomiting, dehydration, lethargy, seizures, hypoglycemia, ketoacidosis, pancreatitis, coma, and neurological decline. Infants with this disease seem healthy at birth but if left untreated suffer severe brain damage and eventually die.

Glutaric Acidemia Type 1

Glutaric acidemia type 1 ("Glutaric aciduria"/"GA1") is an inherited disorder in which the body is unable to break down completely the amino acids lysine, hydroxylysine, and tryptophan. This results in accumulation of excessive levels of their intermediate breakdown products such as—glutaric acid, glutaryl-coenzyme A (CoA), 3-hydroxyglutaric acid, and glutaconic acid. GA1 causes secondary carnitine deficiency, as glutaric acid, like other organic acids, is detoxified by carnitine.

Symptom: It can cause damage to the brain (and also other organs), but particularly the basal ganglia, which are regions that help regulate movement. Mental retardation may also occur.

Homocystinuria

Homocystinuria (HCU) is an inherited disorder of the metabolism of the amino acid methionine due to a deficiency of cystathionine beta-synthase or methionine synthase. It is an inherited autosomal recessive trait, which means a child needs to inherit a copy of the defective gene from both parents to be affected.

This disorder can cause a number of symptoms, including decreased vision and skeletal abnormalities. Children with homocystinuria are unable to metabolize the amino acid homocysteine. Homocysteine, a sulfur-containing amino acid, is a metabolite of the essential amino acid methionine.

Homocysteine, along with certain toxic by-products, builds up to cause a variety of symptoms. Symptoms may be mild or severe, depending on the particular enzyme defect.

Infants with this disorder are normal at birth. The first symptoms, including dislocation of the lens of the eye, causing severely decreased vision, usually begin after 3 years of age. Most children have skeletal abnormalities, including osteoporosis. Children are usually tall and thin with a curved spine, chest deformities, elongated limbs, and long, spiderlike fingers. Without early diagnosis and treatment, mental (psychiatric) and behavioral disorders and intellectual disability are common. Homocystinuria makes the blood more likely to clot spontaneously, resulting in strokes, high blood pressure, and many other serious problems.

A test measuring enzyme function in liver or skin cells confirms the diagnosis.

Tyrosinemia

Tyrosinemia is caused by lack of the enzyme needed to metabolize tyrosine. The most common form of this disorder mostly affects the liver and the kidneys.

There are two main types of tyrosinemia: Type I and type II.

Type I Tyrosinemia

Tyrosinemia type I is a rare autosomal recessive genetic metabolic disorder characterized by lack of the enzyme fumarylacetoacetate hydrolase (FAH), which is needed for the final break down of the amino acid tyrosine.

Children with this disorder typically become ill sometime within the first year of life with dysfunction of the liver, kidneys, and nerves, resulting in irritability, rickets, or even liver failure and death. Restriction of tyrosine in the diet is of little help. Often, children with type I tyrosinemia require a liver transplant.

Type II Tyrosinemia

Tyrosinemia type 2 is caused by a deficiency of the enzyme tyrosine aminotransferase, one of the enzymes required for the multi-step process that breaks down tyrosine. This enzyme shortage is caused by mutations in the TAT gene. This condition is inherited in an autosomal recessive manner. It is less common. Affected children sometimes have intellectual disability and frequently develop sores on the skin and eyes.

■ LIPID METABOLISM

Accumulation of abnormal quantities of certain lipids characterizes some diseases (lipidosis) which occur due to metabolic defect in lipid metabolism. Inborn errors of lipid metabolism occur in following different forms:

Niemann–Pick Disease

Enzyme deficiency: Sphingomyelinase.

Niemann–Pick disease is a condition that affects many body systems. It has a wide range of symptoms that vary in severity.

Niemann-Pick disease is divided into four main types: Type A, type B, type C1, and type C2. These types are classified on the basis of genetic cause and the signs and symptoms of the condition.

Niemann-Pick disease types A and B are caused by mutations in the *SMPD1* gene. This gene provides instructions for producing an enzyme called acid sphingomyelinase. This enzyme is found in lysosomes, which are compartments within cells that break down and recycle different types of molecules. Acid sphingomyelinase is responsible for the conversion of a fat (lipid) called sphingomyelin into another type of lipid called ceramide. Mutations in *SMPD1* lead to a shortage of acid sphingomyelinase, which results in reduced break down of sphingomyelin, causing this fat to accumulate in cells. This fat buildup causes cells to malfunction and eventually die. Over time, cell loss impairs function of tissues and organs including the brain, lungs, spleen, and liver in people with Niemann-Pick disease types A and B.

Mutations in either the *NPC1* or *NPC2* gene cause Niemann-Pick disease type C. The proteins produced from these genes are involved in the movement of lipids within cells. Mutations in these genes lead to a shortage of functional protein, which prevents movement of cholesterol and other lipids, leading to their accumulation in cells. Because these lipids are not in their proper location in cells, many normal cell functions that require lipids (such as cell membrane formation) are impaired. The accumulation of lipids as well as the cell dysfunction eventually leads to cell death, causing the tissue and organ damage seen in Niemann-Pick disease types C1 and C2.

Symptoms: The disease primarily affects the—liver, spleen, brain, and bone marrow. This leads to enlargement of the spleen and neurologic problems. Affected organs, symptoms, and treatments vary based on the particular type of Niemann-Pick disease. However, every type is severe and can shorten a person's life expectancy. Clinically, it is manifested as anemia and leukocytosis.

Tay-Sachs Disease

Enzyme deficiency: Hexosaminidase A.

Tay-Sachs disease is a rare, neurodegenerative disorder in which deficiency of an enzyme (hexosaminidase A) results in excessive accumulation of certain lipids known as gangliosides in the brain and nerve cells. This abnormal accumulation of gangliosides leads to progressive dysfunction of the central nervous system. This disorder is categorized as a lysosomal storage disease. When hexosaminidase A, an enzyme within lysosomes that break down fats, is missing or ineffective, they build up in the lysosomal. This is called abnormal "storage." When too much fatty material builds up in the lysosome, it becomes toxic destroying the cell and damaging surrounding tissue.

Symptoms: As the disease progresses, affected infants and children may develop cherry-red spots within the middle layer of the eyes, gradual loss of vision, and hearing loss, increasing muscle stiffness and restricted movements (spasticity), eventual paralysis, uncontrolled electrical disturbances in the brain (seizures), and deterioration of cognitive processes (dementia). The classical form of Tay-Sachs disease occurs during infancy. This is the most common form and is usually fatal during early childhood.

Gaucher Disease

Enzyme deficiency: Glucocerebrosidase.

Gaucher disease is a genetic disease caused by a hereditary deficiency of the enzyme glucocerebrosidase. The enzyme acts on a fatty substance glucocerebroside (also known as glucosylceramide). When the enzyme is defective, glucocerebroside accumulates, particularly in white blood cells (mono and lymphocyte). Glucocerebroside can collect in the spleen, liver, kidneys, lungs, brain, and bone marrow.

Symptoms: Painless hepatomegaly, splenomegaly, mental retardation, and rapid and premature destruction of blood cells, leading to anemia. Accumulations of glucocerebrosidase in the eyes cause yellow spots called pinguecula to appear. Accumulations in the bone marrow can cause pain and destroy bone.

Fabry Disease

In Fabry disease, glycolipid, which is a product of fat metabolism, accumulates in tissues. Because the defective gene for this rare disorder is carried on the X chromosome, the full-blown disease occurs only in males. The accumulation of glycolipid causes noncancerous (benign) skin growths (angiokeratomas) to form on the lower part of the trunk. The corneas become cloudy, resulting in poor vision. A burning pain may develop in the arms and legs, and children may have episodes of fever. Children with Fabry disease eventually develop kidney failure and heart disease, although most often, they live into adulthood. Kidney failure may lead to high blood pressure, which may result in stroke.

Fabry disease can be diagnosed in the fetus by chorionic villus sampling or amniocentesis. The disease cannot be cured or even treated directly, but researchers are investigating a treatment in which the deficient enzyme is replaced by transfusion. Treatment consists of taking analgesics to help relieve pain and fever or anticonvulsants. People with kidney failure may need a kidney transplant.

■ NUCLEIC ACID METABOLISM

Inborn errors of nucleic acid metabolism occur in following different forms:

Lesch–Nyhan Syndrome

Enzyme deficiency: Hypoxanthine-guanine phosphoribosyltransferase enzyme (HGPRT).

Its inherited (X-linked recessive) disorder is caused by a deficiency of the hypoxanthine-guanine phosphoribosyltransferase enzyme (HGPRT), produced by mutations in the *HPRT* gene. The HGPRT deficiency causes a build-up of uric acid in all body fluids. This results in both hyperuricemia (uric acid in blood) and hyperuricosuria (uric acid in urine).

Symptom: Severe gout and kidney problems, neurological signs include poor muscle control and moderate mental retardation. These complications usually appear in the first year of life.

Hereditary Xanthinuria

Enzyme deficiency: Xanthine dehydrogenase.

Hereditary xanthinuria type I is caused by mutations in the XDH gene. This gene provides instructions for making an enzyme called xanthine dehydrogenase. This enzyme is involved in normal breakdown of purines, which are building blocks of DNA and RNA.

Specifically, xanthine dehydrogenase carries out the conversion of xanthine to uric acid (which is excreted in urine and feces). Because xanthine is not converted to uric acid, affected individuals have high levels of xanthine and very low levels of uric acid in their blood and urine.

Symptom: The excess xanthine can accumulate in the kidneys and other tissues. In the kidneys, xanthine forms tiny crystals that occasionally build up to create kidney stones. These stones can impair kidney function and ultimately cause kidney failure. Related symptoms can include abdominal pain, recurrent urinary tract infections, and blood in the urine (hematuria). Less commonly, xanthine crystals build up in the muscles, causing pain and cramping.

DIAGNOSIS OF INBORN ERRORS OF METABOLISM

The identification of specific enzymes and metabolic pathways, metabolic diseases can be diagnosed in many cases with routine biochemical blood tests and metabolic screening of urine, such as ferric chloride test, DNPH test, Rothera's test, cyanide nitroprusside test, etc. High performance liquid chromatography (HPLC) can be used for analysis of amino acids, organic acids, or other metabolites in blood. However, specific diagnosis requires enzyme assays, DNA analysis, etc. Nowadays prenatal diagnostic techniques are also available. Radioimmunoassay (RIA), enzyme-linked immunosorbent assay (ELISA), fluorescence-based assays, and gas chromatography mass spectrometry (GCMS) are widely used for diagnosis of IEM.

The introduction of tandem mass spectrometry was a turning point in the history of newborn screening (NBS) for metabolic diagnosis and treatment. A tandem mass spectrometry (TANDEM MS) is a two-step technique used to analyze a sample either by using two or more mass spectrometers connected to each other or a single mass spectrometer by several analyzers arranged one after another. TANDEM MS (MS/MS) contains two or three quadrupoles and a time-of-flight (TOF) analyzer. Tandem mass spectrometry (TM) employs a single assay for multiple disorders, has increased efficiency with low cost per sample, although the initial cost of the equipment is high.

It has replaced classic screening techniques of one-analysis, one-metabolite, and one-disease with one analysis, many-metabolites, and many-diseases.

Since dried blood spot remains stable for many years, the mode of collection should be capillary blood from the heel, impregnation of drops of blood into filter paper, drying of these blood spots and transport of the specimens to a central screening laboratory. The ideal time of sampling for our set up, to take the sample after first 24 hours of life.

Early diagnosis, treatment, and dietary management can reduce the morbidity and mortality. The combination of protein restriction and medical food is used. These dietary modifications may involve substrate restriction, replacement organic acidurias of deficient products, and removal of toxic metabolites or stimulation of residual enzymes.

SUMMARY

- IEM comprise a large class of rare genetic diseases involving disorders of metabolism.
- Glycogen storage disease (glycogenosis) is a group of congenital disorders which occur due to deposition of large amounts of glycogen in the body.
- Type I (Von Gierke disease) is because of enzyme deficiency glucose-6-phosphatase.
- Type II (Pompe disease) is because of enzyme deficiency—α-1,4-glucosidase. It is an autosomal recessive metabolic disorder, which damages muscle and nerve cells.
- Type III (limit dextrinosis) is because of enzyme deficiency—debranching enzyme. It affects breakdown of glycogen after phosphorylase action.
- Type IV (amylopectinosis) is because of deficiency of branching enzyme. This leads to very long unbranched glucose chains being stored in glycogen.
- Type V (McArdle disease) is because of enzyme deficiency—myophosphorylase. This enzyme helps break down glycogen into glucose-1-phosphate within the muscle cell.
- Type VI (Hers disease) is because of enzyme deficiency: Phosphofructokinase which causes moderate accumulation of glycogen in skeletal muscle.
- Type VII (Tarui disease) is metabolic disorder with autosomal recessive inheritance of enzyme phosphofructokinase deficiency.
- Deficiency of enzyme xylitol dehydrogenase causes appearance of pentose sugar in urine is called pentosuria.

- Galactosuria is because of enzyme deficiency—galactose-1-phosphate uridyltransferase. This is a hereditary disorder caused due to metabolic defect in the conversion of galactose to glucose.
- HFI enzyme deficiency—aldolase B. It causes severe hypoglycemia.
- Mucopolysaccharidosis refers to a group of inherited conditions in which the body is unable to properly breakdown mucopolysaccharides.
- Pyruvate is a substance that is formed in the processing of carbohydrates and proteins and that serves as an energy source for cells.
- Pyruvate dehydrogenase complex deficiency is a disorder caused by a lack of a group of enzymes needed to process pyruvate.
- Absence of pyruvate carboxylase interferes with or blocks the production of glucose from pyruvate in the body.
- Alkaptonuria is because of enzyme deficiency—homogentisate oxidase. It is a congenital metabolic disorder associated with the abnormal metabolism of tyrosine.
- PKU is because of enzyme deficiency—phenylalanine hydroxylase. It is characterized by the excretion of large amount of phenylalanine and phenylacetylglutamine in urine.
- MSUD is because of deficiency of enzyme complex BCKDH leading to a buildup of the branched-chain amino acids.
- Glutaric acidemia type 1 is an inherited disorder in which the body is unable to break down completely the amino acids lysine, hydroxylysine, and tryptophan.
- Homocystinuria or HCU is an inherited disorder of the metabolism of the amino acid methionine due to a deficiency of cystathionine beta-synthase or methionine synthase.
- Tyrosinemia is caused by lack of the enzyme needed to metabolize tyrosine. The most common form of this disorder mostly affects the liver and the kidneys.
- Niemann–Pick disease is because of enzyme deficiency—sphingomyelinase caused by gene mutation.
- Tay–Sachs disease is because of enzyme deficiency—hexosaminidase A. It is a rare, neurodegenerative disorder which results in excessive accumulation of certain lipids known as gangliosides.
- Gaucher disease is because of enzyme deficiency—glucocerebrosidase which results in accumulation of glucocerebroside.
- In Fabry disease, glycolipid, which is a product of fat metabolism, accumulates in tissues.
- Lesch–Nyhan syndrome is because of enzyme deficiency—hypoxanthine-guanine phosphoribosyltransferase enzyme (HGPRT). It is an inherited (X-linked recessive) disorder.
- Hereditary xanthinuria is because of enzyme deficiency xanthine dehydrogenase. It results in high levels of xanthine and very low levels of uric acid in their blood and urine.

Chapter 17: Inborn Errors of Metabolism

- Most tests are done to a urine or blood sample to detect amino acids or other substances that might be present in the body. Sometimes, test is performed on tissues from the liver, brain, muscles, bone marrow, or skin; or they may request specific DNA testing.

PRACTICE QUESTIONS

1. What is inborn error of metabolism?
2. Name deficient enzyme in case of:
   i. Von Gierke disease
   ii. Tarui disease
   iii. Gaucher disease
   iv. Alkaptonuria
   v. Hereditary xanthinuria
   vi. McArdle disease
3. Name the disease for deficiency of following enzymes:
   i. Xylitol dehydrogenase
   ii. Xanthine dehydrogenase
   iii. Phenylalanine hydroxylase
   iv. Myophosphorylase
   v. Galactose-1-phosphate
   vi. Glucocerebrosidase
   vii. uridyltransferase
4. Write the symptoms of following diseases:
   i. Maple syrup urine disease (MSUD)
   ii. Hers disease
   iii. Tay–Sachs disease
   iv. Hereditary fructose intolerance (HFI)
   v. Fabry disease
   vi. Lesch–Nyhan syndrome
5. What is pyruvate? What are the conditions associated with its metabolism?
6. Write different methods of diagnosis of IEM.

CHAPTER 18

Endocrine Glands and Hormones

> **Keywords**
> Metabolism homeostasis lipophilic hormone, hydrophilic hormone, immediate stimuli, feedback mechanism, stimulus, adenohypophysis, neurohypophysis, growth hormone, acromegaly, gigantism, thyroid-stimulating hormone, adrenocorticotropic hormone, prolactin, gonadotropins, vasopressin oxytocin, adrenal gland, corticosteroids, Cushing syndrome, catecholamines, epinephrine, dopamine, islets of Langerhans, glucagon, pineal gland, melatonin, testis, testosterone, androgen estrogen, progesterone, ectopic pregnancy, gastrin atrial natriuretic factor (ANF), juxtaglomerular cells, renin, erythropoietin, leptin, cholecalciferol

■ INTRODUCTION

The endocrine system consists of a number of different endocrine glands that are situated in various parts of the body. Their secretions are called hormones. The glands are ductless glands and their secretion is released directly into the bloodstream. The organ on which the hormone acts is called as target organ. The hormones are carried away from gland (site of production) to the target organ through blood. Hormones act as chemical regulators. They are specific in their action so that one hormone can regulate only a particular metabolic process in a particular organ.

■ FUNCTIONS OF HORMONES

Hormones can affect many aspects of the body and its state of health. The main functions of hormones are as follows:

1. **Metabolism:** Some hormones regulate the rate of basal metabolisms, e.g., thyroxin of thyroid gland.
2. **Homeostasis:** Internal environmental factors including temperature regulation, water and ion balance, blood glucose levels, etc., are maintained by hormones.

3. **Growth and maturation:** Hormones control growth by addition of segments. Hormones also control maturation, e.g., growth hormone (GH).
4. **Secondary sexual characters and reproductive activities:** Hormones secreted by gonads produce secondary sexual characters and reproductive activities. For example, testosterone in male produces male characters and maturation of sperms.
5. **Control of other endocrine glands:** In some cases, hormones secreted by one gland controls the secretary activity of other endocrine glands. For example, trophic hormones of anterior pituitary control the secretion of thyroid, adrenal cortex, gonads, etc.
6. **Adaptations:** Adaptation to external factors such as visual adaptations to light intensities and control of physiological color changes are regulated by hormones.

■ CHEMICAL NATURE OF HORMONES

There are three classes of hormones:
1. Peptide hormones
2. Lipid-derived hormones
3. Monoamine hormones

Peptide Hormones

Peptide hormones consist of short chains of amino acids, such as vasopressin, that are secreted by the pituitary gland and regulate osmotic balance; or long chains, such as insulin, that are secreted by the pancreas, which regulates glucose metabolism.

Some peptide hormones contain carbohydrate side chains and are termed glycoproteins, such as the follicle-stimulating hormone (FSH). All peptide hormones are hydrophilic and are therefore unable to cross the plasma membrane alone.

Lipid-derived Hormones

Lipid- and phospholipid-derived hormones are produced from lipids such as linoleic acid and arachidonic acid. Steroid hormones, which form the majority of lipid hormones, are derived from carbohydrates, for example, testosterone is produced primarily in the testes and plays a key role in development of the male reproductive system.

Eicosanoids are also lipid hormones that are derived from fatty acids in the plasma membrane. Unlike other hormones, eicosanoids are not stored in the cell—they are synthesized as required. Both are lipophilic and can cross the plasma membrane. For example, cortisol.

Monoamine Hormones

Monoamine hormones are derived from single aromatic amino acids such as phenylalanine, tyrosine, and tryptophan. For example, the tryptophan-derived melatonin that is secreted by the pineal gland regulates sleep patterns.

■ MECHANISM OF HORMONE ACTION

The glands of the endocrine system secrete hormones directly into the extracellular environment. The hormones then diffuse to the bloodstream via capillaries and are transported to the target cells through the circulatory system. This allows hormones to affect tissues and organs far from the site of production or to apply systemic effects to the whole body.

Hormone-producing cells are typically specialized and reside within a particular endocrine gland, such as thyrocytes in the thyroid gland. Hormones exit their cell of origin through the process of exocytosis or by other means of membrane transport.

On reaching the target cell, there are two different ways through which it brings about the effect. Depending upon this mechanism of action, hormones are divided into two broad categories:

1. Water-soluble hormones/hydrophilic hormones **(Fig. 18.1)**:
   - Water-soluble hormones dissolve in water.
   - They are formed from amino acids (peptide hormone).
   - They cannot pass through the target cell membranes (which include fatty components).
   - They affect cells by binding to receptors on the surface of the target cell.
   - The hormone molecule attaches (binds) to a receptor molecule protruding from the surface of the target cell.

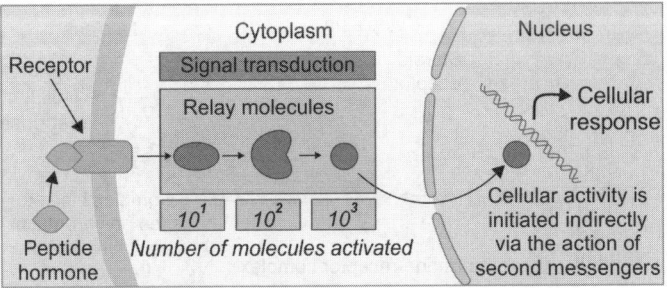

Fig. 18.1: Mechanism of action—hydrophilic hormone.

- Binding of the hormone to the receptor "triggers" a chemical "response" inside the cell without the hormone molecule itself ever entering the cell.
- Receptors come on the surface of the cell, which are typically coupled to internally anchored proteins, known as relay molecules (e.g., G proteins).
- The receptor and hormone molecule form a receptor complex, which activates a series of relay molecules also called as second messengers, which initiate cell activity.
- This process is called signal transduction, because the external signal (hormone) is transduced via internal intermediaries.
- Examples of second messengers include cyclic adenosine monophosphate (cAMP), calcium ions (Ca^{2+}), nitric oxide (NO), and protein kinases.
- The use of second messengers enables the amplification of the initial signal (as more molecules are activated).
- The receptor complex is transported to nucleus, where it binds to receptor sites on chromatin (DNA) activating mRNA transactions.
- Water-soluble hormones include insulin, glucagon, leptin, antidiuretic hormone (ADH), and oxytocin.

2. Fat-soluble hormones/lipophilic hormones **(Fig. 18.2)**:
   - Fat-soluble hormone dissolves in fats. These are usually formed from cholesterol. Also called as steroid hormone.
   - Fat-soluble hormones can pass through cell membranes (see also functions of cell membranes).
   - They affect cells by binding to receptors inside the target cell.

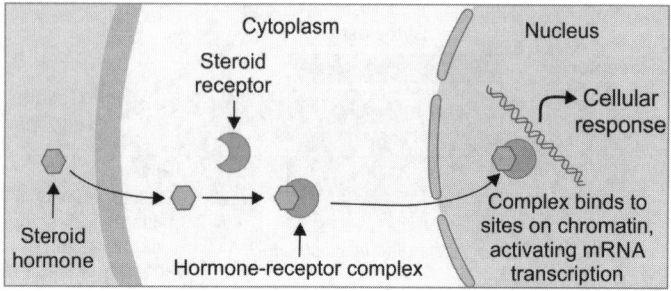

Fig. 18.2: Mechanism of action—hydrophobic hormone.

- The hormone molecule passes through the cell membrane then attaches (binds) to a receptor that can move around inside the cell. When the hormone binds to the receptor, the combination of these two parts is called the "hormone-receptor complex."
- The hormone-receptor complex moves to the nucleus of the cell.
- After it has entered the cell nucleus, the hormone-receptor complex binds to a region of DNA (deoxyribonucleic acid), activating mRNA transactions.

■ CONTROL OF HORMONE SECRETION

There are two ways by which body controls secretion of hormones:
1. By immediate stimuli
2. By feedback mechanism.

Immediate Stimuli

There are three factors stimulating production and release of hormones which are described below.

Specific Molecules in the Blood

The presence or level (concentration) of specific molecules in the blood, e.g., certain minerals or nutrients—referred to in biochemistry such as electrolyte and metabolite.
- **Example:** Low levels of calcium (Ca^{2+}) ions in the blood stimulate the parathyroid glands to release parathyroid hormone.
- Increasing levels of blood glucose contribute to stimulation of the secretion of the hormone insulin from the pancreas.

Stimulation by Other (Specific) Hormones

This is brought about by leading to the rhythmic release of hormones, i.e., hormone levels rising and falling in a predictable pattern. A hormone that stimulates hormone secretion (i.e., that causes endocrine cells to release hormones) is called a tropic hormone.

For example,

- **Growth hormone-releasing hormone (GHRH)** produced in the hypothalamus stimulates the anterior pituitary to release human growth hormone (HGH).
- **Thyroid-stimulating hormone (TSH)** from the anterior pituitary stimulates the thyroid to produce triiodothyronine and thyroxin.

Stimulation by Signals from the Nervous System

This is brought about by leading to hormone release in short bursts or spurts as required—as opposed to in a steady rhythm. For example,

- Sympathetic preganglionic neurons (part of the sympathetic nervous system) stimulate the adrenal glands to release the hormone adrenaline.
- Neurosecretory cells in the hypothalamus have the usual features of nerve cells (e.g., dendrites, axons, and terminals) and act as endocrine cells by secreting hormones into the bloodstream. Release of hormones from the neurosecretory cells of the hypothalamus is regulated by the nerve cells that form synapses with the dendrites of the individual neurosecretory cells. In this way, the nervous system controls the release of hormones from the hypothalamus.
- Secretion of insulin from the β cells of the pancreas is regulated by both the sympathetic and the parasympathetic divisions of the autonomic (i.e., involuntary) nervous system. Parasympathetic input to the pancreatic β cells stimulates insulin secretion. Sympathetic input to the pancreatic β cells inhibits insulin secretion.

Feedback Mechanism

A feedback mechanism is a cycle of events in which the state of a specific aspect of the body's condition like hormone level is continually monitored and adjusted as appropriate to keep the value of that hormone within a safe range so that the body continues to function successfully—as opposed to sustaining damage.

Constant monitoring and making adjustments to keep hormone levels stable is particularly important in the case of hormone levels because:
- Hormones can affect target organs at low concentrations so even a small quantity can sometimes be too much.
- The length of time during which hormones remain active is limited so more hormones must be secreted as necessary to replace those that are inactivated.

Feedback systems are an ideal means of controlling hormone levels. A feedback mechanism *is a loop in which a product feeds back to control its own production. Most hormone feedback mechanisms involve* negative feedback loops. Few of them also have a positive feedback that keeps the concentration of a hormone within a narrow range.

Terms Used to Describe Feedback Systems

- **Controlled condition**: The aspect of the body's condition that the particular feedback mechanism is regulating, e.g., "level of glucocorticoids in body."
- **Stimulus:** Any disturbance (to the internal or external environment) that causes a change in the controlled condition. Some feedback systems involve more than one stimulus.
- **Receptor**: A structure of the body that detects changes in the controlled condition and sends information about it (called "input") to the control center.
- **Control center:** A processing center that receives input from receptors, which may be located in one region or throughout the body), sends ("outputs") instructions to effectors—causing them to take specific actions to change the value of the controlled condition, as appropriate.
- **Effector:** A structure of the body that receives signals output by the control center and responds to them by taking or producing actions ("effectors" produce effects!) that affect the controlled condition.

Example of a General Feedback System: Regulating a Glucocorticoid Hormone

- **Controlled condition:** Level of glucocorticoid in the blood.
- **Stimulus**: Blood level of glucocorticoid decreases.
- **Receptor**: Neurosecretory cells in the hypothalamus send input signals in the form of:
  - increased hypothalmic releasing hormone
  - decreased glucocorticoid
- **Control center**: Anterior pituitary gland sends output signals in the form of: Increased adrenocorticotropic hormone (ACTH).
- **Effector**: Adrenal cortex—secretes glucocorticoids.

As a result of the adrenal cortex (the effector) secreting glucocorticoids, the level of glucocorticoid in the blood (controlled condition) is brought back into balance.

Negative Feedback

Negative feedback occurs when a product feeds back to decrease its own production. This type of feedback brings things back to normal whenever they start to become too extreme.

Example: The thyroid gland is regulated by a negative feedback loop. The loop includes the hypothalamus and pituitary gland in addition to the thyroid (**Fig. 18.3**).

- When level of thyroid gland hormone T_4 and T_3 increases
- The hypothalamus secretes thyrotropin-releasing hormone or TRH
- TRH stimulates the pituitary gland to produce thyroid-stimulating hormone or TSH.
- TSH, in turn, stimulates the thyroid gland to secrete its hormones, T_4 and T_3.
- When the level of thyroid hormones T_4 and T_3 is high enough, the hormones feedback to stop the hypothalamus from secreting TRH and the pituitary from secreting TSH.
- Without the stimulation of TSH, the thyroid gland stops secreting its hormones.

Negative feedback also controls insulin secretion by the pancreas.

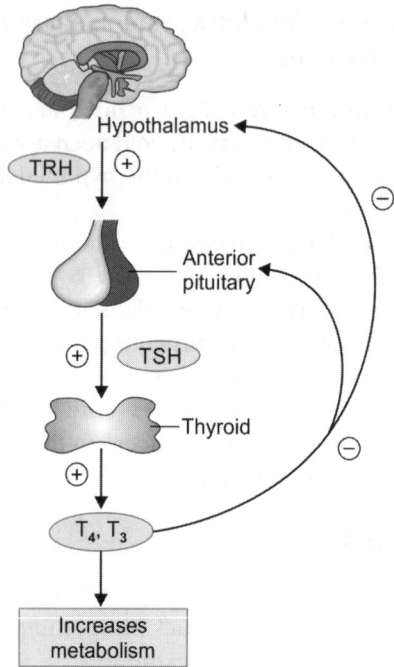

Fig. 18.3: Regulation of thyroid gland by a negative feedback loop.
(TRH: thyrotropin-releasing hormone; TSH: thyroid-stimulating hormone)

Positive Feedback

Positive feedback occurs when a product feeds back to increase its own production. This causes conditions to become increasingly extreme. Positive feedback will continue to amplify the initial change until the stimulus is removed.
- An example of positive feedback is milk production by a lactating mother. As the baby suckles, nerve messages from the nipple cause the pituitary gland to secrete prolactin.
- Prolactin, in turn, stimulates the mammary glands to produce milk, so the baby suckles more.
- This causes more prolactin to be secreted and more milk to be produced.
- This will continue until baby stops feeding.

This example is one of the few positive feedback mechanisms in the human body.

■ ENDOCRINE GLANDS

The endocrine glands and hormone producing diffused tissues/cells are located in different parts of our body which constitute the endocrine system. Hypothalamus and pituitary, pineal, thyroid, adrenal, pancreas, parathyroid, thymus, and gonads (testis in males and ovary in females) are the organized endocrine bodies in our body. In addition to these, some other organs, e.g., gastrointestinal tract, liver, kidney, and heart also produce hormones.

Hypothalamus and Pituitary Gland

The pituitary gland has been called the "master gland" of the human endocrine system because it secretes some hormones that control other endocrine glands by stimulating them to release specific hormones. However, the pituitary gland itself also has a "master," which is the hypothalamus. Hypothalamus is the region of the brain that regulates the interaction of the endocrine system and the nervous system. The pituitary gland and hypothalamus act as a unit, regulating the activity of most of other endocrine glands.

The hypothalamus makes up the lower region of the diencephalon and lies just above the brain stem. The pituitary gland (hypophysis) is attached to the bottom of the hypothalamus by a slender stalk called the infundibulum.

The hypothalamus oversees many internal body conditions. It receives nervous stimuli from receptors throughout the body and monitors chemical and physical characteristics of the blood, including temperature; blood pressure; and nutrient, hormone, and water content. When deviations from homeostasis occur or when certain developmental changes are required, the hypothalamus stimulates cellular activity in various parts of the body by directing the release of hormones from the anterior and posterior pituitary glands.

The hypothalamic hormones are released into blood vessels that connect the hypothalamus and the pituitary gland (i.e., the hypothalamic-hypophyseal portal system). Because they generally promote or inhibit the release of hormones from the pituitary gland, hypothalamic hormones are commonly called releasing or inhibiting

hormones. The major releasing and inhibiting hormones include the following:
- Corticotropin-releasing hormone (CRH):
  - Target organ—anterior pituitary
  - Action—stimulates release of ACTH
- Gonadotropin-releasing hormone (GnRH):
  - Target organ—anterior pituitary
  - Action—stimulates release of luteinizing hormone (LH) and FSH
- TRH:
  - Target organ—anterior pituitary
  - Action—stimulates release of TSH and GH
- GHRH:
  - Target organ—anterior pituitary
  - Action—stimulates release of GH
- Growth hormone-inhibiting hormone (GHIH)/somatostatin:
  - Target organ—anterior pituitary
  - Action—inhibits release of GH
- Prolactin-releasing hormone (PRH):
  - Target organ—anterior pituitary
  - Action—stimulates release of PRL
- Prolactin-inhibiting hormone (PIH)/dopamine:
  - Target organ—anterior pituitary
  - Action—inhibits release of PRL
- ADH:
  - Target organ—posterior pituitary
  - Action—stimulates water reabsorption by kidneys
- Oxytocin:
  - Target organ—anterior pituitary
  - Action—stimulates uterine contractions during childbirth

Pituitary Gland

Location

The pituitary gland is a pea-sized oval structure located close to the ventral aspect of the brain below the hypothalamus. It is attached to the hypothalamus by hypophyseal stalk (also known as pituitary stalk/infundibulum) just behind the optic chiasma. It is well-protected in a depression of the sphenoid bone of skull called sella turcica (Turkish saddle).

Morphology

Anatomically, the pituitary gland is a "two-in-one" structure consisting of the anterior pituitary and the posterior pituitary **(Fig. 18.4)**. These parts have different embryonic origins and function very differently.

Anterior Lobe/Adenohypophysis

The anterior lobe is known as adenohypophysis. It is the largest lobe and forms 75% of the gland. It is derived from an outpouching of the roof of the pharynx, called Rathke's pouch. It is composed of glandular epithelium and secretes a number of hormones. The lobe can be further divided into three parts:
1. Pars anterior—the largest part, responsible for hormone secretion.
2. Pars intermedia—a thin epithelial layer that separates the pars anterior from the posterior lobe of pituitary gland. It is reduced, less developed, and non-functional in human beings.
3. Pars tuberalis—an upward extension of the pars anterior that surrounds the anterolateral aspect like a collar of the infundibulum.

The release of hormones is under the control of the hypothalamus, which communicates with the gland via neurotransmitters secreted

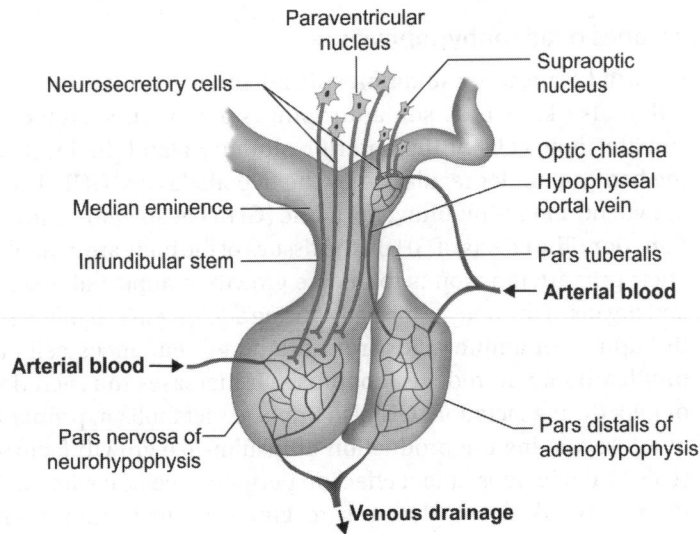

Fig. 18.4: Morphology of pituitary gland.
(For color version, see Plate 7)

into the hypophyseal (infundibulum) portal vessels. These vessels ensure that the hypothalamic hormones remain concentrated, rather than being diluted in the systemic circulation.

Posterior Lobe/Neurohypophysis

The posterior lobe is known as neurohypophysis. It is an extension of the hypothalamus. It arises from the embryonic forebrain, and consists of nervous tissue. Neurohypophysis is smaller and constitutes 25% of pituitary. Two hormones are released by neurohypophysis. It is divided in three parts:
1. **Median eminence:** It is the swollen median part of hypothalamus where infundibulum is attached.
2. **Infundibulum:** It is the hypophyseal stalk and helps in attachment of pituitary gland to the hypothalamus. It contains mainly the axonic fibers of neurosecretory cells present in hypothalamus.
3. **Pars nervosa:** It is the lowermost, larger region of neurohypophysis and contains axons in between pituicytes. Axonic fibers end in knobs called Herrings bodies.

Hormones of Pituitary Gland

Hormones of adenohypophysis
1. **Growth hormone or somatotropic hormone:** Growth hormone (GH), also known as somatotropin, is a protein secreted by somatotropic cells of the anterior pituitary gland. Its levels in the body are under regulation by the hypothalamus, GHRH, and growth hormone-inhibiting hormone (GHIH or somatostatin).
Function: The effects of GH on the tissues of the body are anabolic. Their primary function is to induce growth in almost all tissues and organs of the body, especially during adolescence. It increases the uptake of amino acids from the blood, enhances cellular proliferation, and reduces apoptosis. It increases the secretion of milk during lactation. GH also impacts metabolism, primarily by up-regulating the production of insulin-like growth factor-1 (IGF-1) and its subsequent effect on peripheral cells. It stimulates liver to break down glycogen to glucose. Furthermore, GH stimulates lipolysis, breaking down stored fat. Subsequently,

many tissues switch from glucose to fatty acid as their main energy source, resulting in increased levels of glucose in the bloodstream. It increases intestinal absorption of calcium as well as its excretion. In addition to calcium, sodium, potassium, magnesium, phosphate, and chloride ions are also retained.

Disorders of Growth Hormone: Dysfunction of the endocrine system control and release of GH can result in several disorders. Hypersecretion of GH can cause acromegaly and gigantism, both of which are most commonly caused by a GH secreting adenoma of the pituitary gland.

- *Acromegaly:* Acromegaly typically is caused by a GH secreting pituitary adenoma that occurs after the closure of the epiphyseal growth plate in adults. It results in impaired glucose tolerance and growth of bones in the face, hands, and feet in response to excessive levels of GH in individuals who have stopped growing. An increased IGF-1 level establishes the diagnosis.
- *Gigantism:* Gigantism occurs in children when due to hypersecretion of GH before the fusion of long-bone epiphysis. It is characterized by tall stature and should be suspected when the patient's height is three standard deviations above normal mean height.
- *Growth hormone deficiency:* The effect of GH deficiency depends on the age at which the deficiency occurs. Onset in childhood is associated with decreased growth of all skeletal structures, subsequently leading to dwarfism. Frolic dwarf are mentally abnormal child while Lorain dwarf are mentally normal. Adult-onset deficiency is more difficult to diagnose as it does not have a single identifying pathogenomic factor. It usually presents with increased fat mass in visceral tissues and decreased skeletal muscle, as well as decreased bone density and remodeling, leading to osteoporosis. Hyposecretion of GH in adults causes Simmonds disease.

Diagnosis: The specimen preferred is serum. While collecting specimen, it should be taken care that GH is released in pulses. The size and duration of the pulses varies with time of day, age, and gender.

Immunoassays and receptor assays are used for the determination of serum GH.

The normal range for GH level is:
- For adult males: 0.4–10 ng/mL
- For adult females: 1–14 ng/mL
- For children: 10–50 ng/mL

2. **Thyrotrophic hormone/thyroid-stimulating hormone:** Thyroid-stimulating hormone is a peptide hormone secreted by the basophilic thyrotropes of the anterior pituitary gland. The hypothalamus regulates its release.

Function: Thyroid-stimulating hormone binds and activates the thyroid-stimulating hormone receptor (TSHR) found on the basolateral surface of thyroid follicle cells. TSH triggers the secretion of thyroid hormones thyroxin, or T_4 and triiodothyronine, or T_3 by stimulating receptors found in the follicular cells of the thyroid gland. Subsequently, the thyroid hormones promote bone and central nervous system maturation, increase basal metabolic rate, and heat production. TSH is also necessary to maintain the size of the thyroid follicles and their continued ability to produce thyroid hormones.

Disorders of TSH: A TSH assay is the recommended screening test for thyroid disease.
- Low levels of TSH (hyperthyroidism) are either drug-induced or congenital. Graves' disease is common pathology that presents with low TSH levels and is due to an autoimmune disorder, which stimulates the thyroid gland to make excess thyroid hormones. The increased thyroid hormones cause feedback inhibition of TSH secretion (in attempt to compensate excess of thyroid hormone) by the anterior pituitary gland.
- High TSH levels indicate thyroid gland is not producing enough thyroid hormones, a condition called hypothyroidism. Congenital hypothyroidism (previously known as cretinism) is a severe deficiency of thyroid hormone in newborns. It causes impaired neurological function, stunted growth, and physical deformities. Hashimoto's disease is an autoimmune disorder that can cause hypothyroidism.

Diagnosis:
Normal values: 0.5–5 µU/mL.
Thyroid-stimulating hormone values can vary during the day. It is best to have the test early in the morning. For further details of TSH, *see* Chapter 19.

3. **Adrenocorticotropic hormone or corticotropin**: The ACTH is a polypeptide hormone secreted by the basophilic corticotropic cells of the anterior pituitary gland. The hypothalamus regulating its production is in response to the corticotropin-releasing hormone.
   Function: ACTH primarily functions to regulate cortisol and androgen production. The ACTH released from the anterior pituitary acts on its target organ, the adrenal gland, and stimulates the production of glucocorticoids from the zona fasciculata and androgens from the zona reticularis.
   Disorders of adrenocorticotropic hormone: Pathophysiology of ACTH can stem from either dysfunction of the pituitary, the adrenal glands, or ectopic secretions from a pathogenic source.
   - Common causes of decreased ACTH include pituitary insufficiency due to an adenoma compressing the pituitary gland, pituitary apoplexy, the sudden hemorrhage into the pituitary gland causing loss of ACTH, or Sheehan syndrome, a condition of pituitary infarction after blood loss during childhood. Hyposecretion of ACTH leads to Addison's disease (adrenal failure) which affects carbohydrate metabolism leading to weakness and fatigue.
   - The hypersecretion lead to excessive growth of adrenal cortex causing Cushing disease.

   Diagnosis: Adrenocorticotropic hormone results might be different depending on what time of day the test was taken. ACTH is measured in picograms per milliliter (pg/mL) of blood.
   Adults normally have ACTH levels of 10–50 pg/mL at 8 AM.
   The number drops to below 5–10 pg/mL at midnight.
   The sample preferred is serum. Determination of serum ACTH can be performed in the laboratory by RIA (radioimmunoassay) or ELISA (enzyme-linked immunosorbent assay) methods that use specific antibodies to ACTH.

4. **Prolactin or luteotropic hormone:** Prolactin is a protein hormone secreted by lactotropic cells of the anterior pituitary gland. Chemically, prolactin is composed of amino acids. The secretion of prolactin by the anterior pituitary is inhibited by dopamine from the hypothalamus and stimulated by TRH, estrogen, dopamine antagonist (antipsychotics), and multiple factors including suckling, stress, and sleep.

Function: Prolactin is best known for its multiple actions on the mammary gland with its two main functions, including stimulation of milk production and development of breast tissues. During pregnancy, it contributes to the development and growth of the breast tissue with estrogen and progesterone and stimulates the enlargement of the alveoli in preparation for lactation. Prolactin stimulates milk production by inducing the enzyme that synthesizes the constituents of milk, such as lactose (the carbohydrate of milk), casein (the protein of milk), and lipids. It reduces chances of pregnancy during lactation period.

Several functions are assigned to prolactin, therefore have many names such as:

Development of mammary glands (mammotropin), milk secretion by mammary glands (lactogenic hormone), maintenance of corpus luteum which secretes progesterone during pregnancy (luteotropin).

Prolactin initiates its effect by binding to the prolactin receptor found on various tissues across the body, including but not limited to mammillary glands, ovaries, skeletal muscle, uterus, and thymus.

Disorders of prolactin:
- Prolactin deficiency, most commonly due to pituitary destruction, presents with failure to lactate.
- Increased levels of prolactin can be physiological, pathological, or drug-induced. Physiological causes include pregnancy, exercise, sleep, stress, neonatal period, nipple stimulation and lactation, and sexual intercourse. Physiological hyperprolactinemia is transient and adaptive, and most patients may remain asymptomatic. Pharmacological and pathological hyperprolactinemia are symptomatic conditions (hypogonadism and galactorrhea) that have unwanted long-term consequences. Galactorrhea is the production of breast milk in men or in women who are not breastfeeding. It is mainly due to a tumor in the pituitary gland.

Diagnosis: The normal values for prolactin are:
- Men: <20 ng/mL
- Nonpregnant women: <25 ng/mL
- Pregnant women: 80–400 ng/mL

The sample preferred is serum. Determination of serum ACTH can be performed in the laboratory by using electrochemiluminescence method.

5. **Gonadotropic hormones or gonadotropins:** Gonadotropic hormones (GTHs) are of two types: FSH and LH or interstitial-cell-stimulating hormone (ICSH). The secretions of gonadotropin are regulated by gonadotropin-releasing factor (GHRF) of hypothalamus.

   These are glycoprotein hormones secreted by the gonadotropin cells of the adenohypophysis. They both are glycoproteins made up of an α and β subunit. The α subunits are identical between the two hormones, but the β subunit of each is different and gives each hormone its biological specificity.

   The gonadotropins primarily regulate reproductive function and sexual development in both males and females. In the case of females, the onset and cessation of reproductive capacity are also dependent on these hormones.

   FSH stimulates the production and maturation of sex cells, sperm in males, and ova in females. It also promotes follicular maturation in females during the ovarian cycle; these follicles then release estrogen in the female ovaries. In males FSH stimulates germinal epithelium of seminiferous tubules for spermatogenesis and production of mature sperms.

   Luteinizing hormone triggers ovulation in women and causes the release of progesterone from the corpus luteum after ovulation. Furthermore, it causes the release of estrogen and progesterone from the ovaries. In males, LH stimulates the release of testosterone from the Leydig cells of the testes. It is required for development of secondary sexual characters in males.

   Disorder of Follicle-stimulating hormone and luteinizing Hormone:
   - Hyperfunctioning pituitary adenomas or unresponsive gonads can lead to increased FSH and LH. High level of progesterone in female signals negative feedback to pituitary and stops secretion of LH. In males, high level of testosterone in blood gives negative feedback signal to pituitary so that ICSH secretion is stopped.
   - Decreased levels of FSH and LH can stem from pathology within either the hypothalamus or anterior pituitary. Deficiency of FSH leads to infertility in both the sexes.

Diagnosis: Normal FSH levels will differ, depending on a person's age and sex.

Male:
- Before puberty: 0–5.0 IU/L
- During puberty: 0.3–10.0 IU/L
- Adult: 1.5–12.4 IU/L

Female:
- Before puberty: 0–4.0 IU/L
- During puberty: 0.3–10.0 IU/L
- Women who are still menstruating: 4.7–21.5 IU/L
- After menopause: 25.8–134.8 IU/L

The sample preferred is serum. The method used is chemiluminescence.

Hormones of neurohypophysis

Neurohypophysis does not secrete any hormone but stores the hormones which are secreted by hypothalamic neurons. It stores and releases two hormones—antidiuretic hormone or vasopressin and oxytocin.

Vasopressin, also known as antidiuretic hormone (ADH), is synthesized in the supraoptic nuclei of the hypothalamus while oxytocin synthesis occurs in the paraventricular nuclei of the hypothalamus. Both the posterior pituitary hormones are packaged in secretory granules and move down the axon where they are stored in the Herring bodies. These bodies are neurosecretory granules that represent the terminal ends of the axons coming from the hypothalamus.

1. **Antidiuretic hormone or vasopressin**: Vasopressin acts as a water-saving hormone. It is released into the bloodstream to vasoconstrict and reabsorb water from the kidney's collecting duct; this ensures the equilibrium of intracellular and extracellular contents. Absorption of water from the ultrafiltrate and regulation of water balance of body fluids, thereby decreasing the urine output and helps for water conservation. ADH also controls constriction of arterioles to increase blood pressure in kidney which facilitates ultrafiltration hence also called as vasopressin. Its secretion is regulated by increase or decrease of osmotic pressure of blood in feedback manner. The osmotic pressure is detected by osmoreceptors in the hypothalamus.

Disorder of ADH:
- Deficiency of ADH causes diabetes insipidus, i.e., loss of large quantity of water through urine (polyuria or dieresis). It results in polydipsia (increased thirst).
- Hypersecretion causes antidiuresis (less urine formation) and stimulates water retention in body fluids.

Diagnosis: The specimen preferred is serum. Immunoassays and receptor assays are used for the determination of serum.

Normal values for ADH can range from 1 to 5 pg/mL (0.9–4.6 pmol/L).

2. **Oxytocin:** The polypeptide hormone oxytocin is commonly released in females during the process of childbirth. It allows the uterus to contract, which advances the fetus into the vagina for delivery. During lactation, oxytocin also releases milk from the breast tissue into the baby's oral cavity. Finally, oxytocin is also present in males during ejaculation and stimulates contraction of the vas deferens to push the semen and sperm forward.

Disorder of oxytocin:
- Oxytocin insufficiency is not a common pathology but can occur rarely. Decreased levels of oxytocin slow down uterine contractions and reduce milk ejection during the birthing process. Panhypopituitarism, a pathology in which both anterior and posterior hormone levels are below normal, can be the cause of oxytocin hyposecretion.
- Excess oxytocin is also rarely seen and causes an overactive uterus causing hypertrophy, which further leads to difficulty in maintaining pregnancy due to insufficient space for holding the fetus.

Diagnosis: Although there are several immunoassays for the determination of oxytocin, its clinical application is limited.

The level of oxytocin increases at the time of labor in females.

The preferred sample is plasma. The normal range of oxytocin in men and normal women is was 1.80 +/−0.07 microunits/mL.

Adrenal Gland

Location

Adrenal glands, also known as suprarenal glands, are small, triangular-shaped glands located on the top of both kidneys. The adrenal glands are made up of glandular and neuroendocrine tissue with rich blood supply.

Morphology

The adrenal gland consists of an outer cortex of glandular tissue and an inner medulla of nervous tissue **(Fig. 18.5)**. The cortex itself is divided into three zones—zona glomerulosa (outermost layer), the zona fasciculata (middle layer), and the zona reticularis (innermost layer). Each region secretes its own set of hormones.

The zona glomerulosa produces mineralocorticoids, the zona fasciculata produces glucocorticoids, and the zona reticularis produces androgen precursors.

Hormones of Adrenal Glands

The adrenal cortex secretes many hormones collectively called as corticoids controlling several vital body functions. Chemically, all the cortical hormones are steroid.

Zona glomerulosa, which produces a group of hormones collectively referred to as mineralocorticoids because of their effect on body minerals, especially sodium and potassium. These hormones are essential for fluid (osmotic) and electrolyte balance. Aldosterone is the main mineralocorticoids. It helps in the maintenance of electrolytes, body fluid volume, osmotic pressure, and blood pressure.

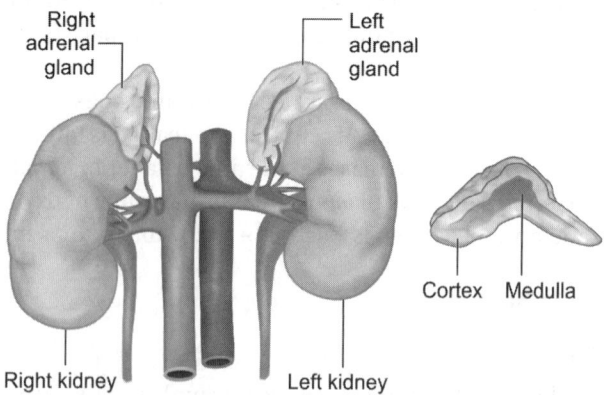

Fig. 18.5: Adrenal gland.
(For color version, see Plate 8)

Glucocorticoids are involved in carbohydrate metabolism. Cortisol is the main glucocorticoid, which stimulates gluconeogenesis, lipolysis, proteolysis, and red blood cell (RBC) production. It is also involved in anti-inflammatory reactions and suppresses the immune response.

The third group of steroids secreted by the adrenal cortex is the gonadocorticoids, or sex hormones. These are secreted by the innermost region. Male hormones, androgens, and female hormones, estrogens, are secreted in minimal amounts in both sexes by the adrenal cortex, but their effect is usually masked by the hormones from the testes and ovaries. In females, the masculinization effect of androgen secretion may become evident after menopause, when estrogen levels from the ovaries decrease.

Small amounts of androgenic steroids play a role in the growth of axial hair, pubic hair, and facial hair during puberty.

Disorders of Adrenal Gland Hormones

Hypersecretion of corticosteroids results in Cushing syndrome—changes in carbohydrate and protein metabolism resulting in high blood glucose levels and the accumulation of lipid deposits on the face and neck—a puffy appearance. In extreme cases, changes such as "buffalo hump" and "moon face" occur. Chronically elevated glucocorticoids compromise immunity, and memory. It can result in rapid weight gain and hair loss.

Hyposecretion of glucocorticoids and mineralocorticoids may results in Addison's disease—hypoglycemia, sodium and potassium imbalance, dehydration, hypotension, rapid weight loss, abdominal pain, nausea, vomiting, sweating, and cravings for salty food. Death occurs with lack of treatment.

Diagnosis

Immunoassay techniques and other methods based on separation techniques are used for the determination of steroids in body fluids. These methods are—liquid chromatography, gas chromatography, high-performance liquid chromatography (HPLC), capillary electrophoresis, etc. Steroids are measured in blood, urine, and saliva specimen.

Sample—serum is needed. Heparinized plasma can be used.

Urine 24 hours is collected with boric acid, and during collection, it is refrigerated.
- Cortisol total
  Serum: Child 1–16 years at 8 AM = 3–21 µg/dL
  Adult at 8 AM = 5–23 µg/dL
  at 4 PM = 3–16 µg/dL
  Urine cortisol (free): Adult = 20–90 µg/day/(<100 µg/day)
  Child = 2–27 µg/day
- Aldosterone in serum
  Children 1–2 years = 7–54 ng/dL
  Children 2–10 years: Supine position = 3–35 ng/dL
  Upright position = 4–48 ng/dL
  Adult: Supine position = 3–16 ng/dL
  Upright position = 7–30 ng/dL
- Estrogen total in serum
  Male: 20–80 pg/mL.
  Female: Luteal phase = 160–400 pg/mL
  Follicular phase = 60–200 pg/mL
  Postmenopausal = <130 pg/mL

Hormones of Adrenal Medulla

Adrenal medulla develops from neural tissue. Catecholamines are class of aromatic amines which includes a number of neurotransmitters. The hormones secreted by adrenal medulla are catecholamines. These are of following three types:
1. **Adrenaline (epinephrine):** It has many effects. These include: Action of heart increased, rate and depth of breathing increased, metabolic rate increased, onset of muscular fatigue delayed, and blood supply to the bladder and intestine reduced, their muscular walls relaxed, and the sphincters contract.
2. **Noradrenaline (norepinephrine):** It has effects similar to adrenaline. It brings about contraction of small blood vessels leading to increased blood pressure and increase in rate and depth of breathing. It increases alertness, papillary dilation, piloerection (hair erection), sweating, etc.
3. **Dopamine:** It is strongly associated with pleasure and reward. Dopamine is involved in neurological and physiological

functioning. It is a contributing factor in motor function, mood, and even our decision-making. It is also associated with some movement and psychiatric disorders.

These hormones are rapidly secreted in response to stimulation by sympathetic nerve, particularly during stressful situations hence are called as emergency hormones or hormones of fight or flight.

A lack of hormones from the adrenal medulla produces no significant effects. Hypersecretion of epinephrine and norepinephrine is the condition of hypertension, hyperglycemia, nervousness, and sweating. Complete exhaustion occurs. Hypersecretion, usually from a tumor, causes prolonged or continual sympathetic responses.

Diagnosis

Serum epinephrine, norepinephrine, and dopamine can be determined by RIA, enzyme immunoassay (EIA), and HPLC methods.

Sample

Plasma in heparin or ethylenediaminetetraacetic acid (EDTA) is needed. Urine may be collected for 24 hours. Add 6 mL hydrochloric acid (HCl) and refrigerate during collection.

Normal value: Epinephrine: <50 pg/mL
Urine epinephrine: 0–20 µg/day
Norepinephrine: 110–410 pg/mL
Urine norepinephrine: 15–80 µg/day
Dopamine: <87 pg/mL
Urine dopamine: 65–400 µg/day

Pineal Gland

The pineal gland is one of the smallest and most important endocrine glands in the body. It is located in the center of the brain close to the pituitary gland. The pineal gland gets its name from its characteristic pine cone shape.

Physiologically, in conjunction with the hypothalamus gland, the pineal gland controls the sex drive, hunger, thirst, and the biological clock which determines the body's normal aging process. It secretes hormone melatonin.

Melatonin

The primary function is that pineal gland secretes melatonin. This hormone is the primary one that controls sleepiness and wakefulness. Natural light tends to turn this gland on. When the pineal gland is activated, brain moves from sleeping to a state of wakefulness. This process is sometimes referred to as the awakening of the "third eye"—a common name for the pineal gland.

Clinical Significance and Normal Level

In normal young adults, the average daytime and peak night time values are 10 and 60 pg/mL.

Deficiency of melatonin results in signs of restlessness, a poor stress response, insomnia, and waking up too early in the morning.

Higher doses of melatonin can reset circadian rhythms, bring on sleepiness, and lower core body temperature.

■ HORMONES SECRETED BY ORGANS

Pancreas

Pancreas is a dual gland exocrine as well as endocrine. The endocrine pancreas is called "Islets of Langerhans" which show three types of cells known as α cells, β cells, and δ cells.

- **Glucagon:** This hormone is secreted by α cells. Glucagon is a hyperglycemic hormone. It is a peptide which acts mainly on the liver cells where it stimulates hepatocytes for glycogenolysis leading to increased level of blood glucose (hyperglycemia). It also stimulates gluconeogenesis which contributes to hyperglycemia. Glucagon also reduces the cellular glucose uptake and utilization. This way glucagon increases blood glucose level.
- **Insulin:** Hormone is secreted by β cells. It is also a peptide hormone, which plays a major role in maintenance of blood glucose level. Insulin stimulates hepatocytes and adipocytes for cellular glucose uptake and utilization. Therefore, glucose from the blood decreases (hypoglycemia) conversion of glucose to glycogen (glycogenesis) occurs in target cells. This way insulin decreases blood glucose level.

The blood glucose level is thus maintained by joint action of insulin and glucagon. Prolonged hyperglycemia leads to diabetes mellitus due to insufficient insulin level. In this condition, cells are unable to utilize glucose. Blood having high level of glucose results in excretion of glucose in urine. Diabetes can be treated with hypoglycemic drugs or insulin therapy.

δ cells of pancreas secrete somatostatin hormone, which inhibits glucagon and insulin secretion.

Diagnosis of these hormones is discussed in chapter Diabetic profile.

Testis

A pair of testis is present in the scrotal sac outside the abdomen in male individuals. Testes are primary reproductive organ as well as an endocrine gland. Testis is composed of numerous seminiferous tubules and interstitial clusters of endocrine cells called Leydig cells.

The hormones produced by Leydig cells are called androgens which are steroids. The most significant androgen is the testosterone.

Testosterone/Androgen

Testosterone is responsible for the development of primary sexual development, which includes testicular descent, spermatogenesis, enlargement of the penis and testes, and increasing libido. Androgen regulates and stimulates the development, maturation, and functions of the male reproductive organs such as seminiferous tubules, epididymis, vas deferens, seminal vesicles, prostate glands, and urethra. They stimulate secondary sex characteristics such as muscular growth, growth of facial and axillary hairs, aggressiveness, low pitch of voice, etc. They stimulate seminiferous tubules for the process of spermatogenesis.

Clinical Significance and Diagnosis

During childhood, excessive production of testosterone induces premature puberty in boys and masculinization in girls. In adult women, excess testosterone production results in varying degrees of virilization, including hirsutism, acne, oligo-amenorrhea, or infertility. Mild-to-moderate testosterone elevations are usually asymptomatic in males but can cause distressing symptoms in females. The exact causes for mild-to-moderate elevations in testosterone often remain obscure. Common causes of pronounced elevations of testosterone include genetic conditions (e.g., congenital adrenal hyperplasia); adrenal, testicular, and ovarian tumors; and abuse of testosterone or gonadotropins by athletes.

Decreased testosterone in females causes subtle symptoms. These may include some decline in libido and nonspecific mood changes. In males, it results in partial or complete degrees of hypogonadism. This is characterized by changes in male secondary sexual characteristics and reproductive function. In adult men, there is a gradual modest, but progressive, decline in testosterone production starting between the fourth and sixth decades of life.

Techniques commonly used for estimation of testosterone are: RIA, ELISA, and chemiluminescence.

Normal range:
For males: 260–1,000 ng/dL.
For females: 14–76 ng/dL.

Ovary

The ovaries are two almond-shaped structures present on either side of the uterus. The ovaries are primary reproductive organs of female which are also endocrine glands. Ovaries secrete two steroid hormones:

i. **Estrogen:** The estrogen is secreted by the developing ovarian follicles. It has multiple roles in stimulation of growth reproductive organs such as ovaries, oviduct, uterus, and vagina. It also controls female secondary sexual characteristics like high pitch of voice, development of mammary glands, broadening of pelvis, pubic hairs, and deposition of subcutaneous fats to produce feminine stature. The estrogen also regulates female sexual behavior.

Genetic defects, a family history of hormone imbalances, or certain diseases can cause low estrogen levels. Low estrogen levels can interfere with sexual development and sexual functions. They can also increase risk of obesity, osteoporosis, and cardiovascular disease.

High levels of estrogen can lead to weight gain, particularly around the hips and waist. Excess estrogen can also cause menstrual problems, such as irregular periods and heavy bleeding.

In males, symptoms of high estrogen can include: Erectile dysfunction, enlarged breasts, or gynecomastia and infertility.

Serum samples are preferred. It is done on 3rd day of women's menstrual cycle.

Normal values are:
- 30–400 pg/mL for premenopausal women
- 0–30 pg/mL for postmenopausal women
- 10–50 pg/mL for men

ii. **Progesterone:** After ovulation, the empty Graafian follicle is converted into a structure called corpus luteum which secretes a hormone known as progesterone. Progesterone is a progestational hormone which maintains the pregnancy. It can also act on the mammary glands and stimulate them for milk-forming apparatus, milk secretion, and ejection.

Progesterone levels vary during a woman's menstrual cycle. The levels start out low, and then increase after the ovaries release an egg. In pregnancy, progesterone levels will continue to rise as body gets ready to support a developing baby.

Higher-than-normal levels may be due to: Pregnancy, ovulation, adrenal cancer, ovarian cancer, and congenital adrenal hyperplasia (rare).

Lower-than-normal levels may be due to: Amenorrhea [no periods as a result of an ovulation (ovulation does not occur)], ectopic pregnancy, irregular periods, fetal death, and miscarriage.

Serum sample is required. Since progesterone levels increase toward the end of menstrual cycle, the test is done during the luteal phase of menstrual cycle (just before it starts.).

Normal value:

Men: <1.0 ng/mL
Women: Prepubertal = 0.1–0.3 ng/mL
Follicular phase = 0.1–0.7 ng/mL
Luteal phase = 2–25 ng/mL

Pregnancy: As it increases in pregnancy, in third trimester, it reaches 65–290 ng/mL.

Gastrointestinal Tract

There are scattered endocrine cells in different parts of alimentary canal. These secrete peptide hormones:
- **Gastrin:** It stimulates gastric glands for secretion of HCl and pepsinogen.
- **Secretin:** It acts on exocrine pancreas and stimulates secretion of water and bicarbonate ions to form pancreatic juice.
- **Cholecystokinin (CCK):** It acts on pancreas and gallbladder and stimulates secretion of pancreatic enzymes and bile juice respectively.
- **Gastric inhibitory peptide (GIP):** It inhibits gastric secretion.
- **Ghrelin:** It stimulates secretion of GH and also supposed to stimulate appetite.
- **Motilin:** It helps to stimulate the movements of gastrointestinal tract contractions and also stimulates secretion of pepsin.

Heart

The atrial wall of the heart secretes a peptide hormone known as atrial natriuretic factor (ANF). This hormone is secreted when blood pressure increases. It causes dilation of the blood vessels due to which blood pressure decreases.

Kidney

The juxtaglomerular cells of the kidney secrete hormones.
- **Renin:** It converts angiotensin I into angiotensin II which brings about vasoconstriction and hence blood pressure.
- **Erythropoietin:** It stimulates bone marrow for production of RBCs (erythropoiesis).

Skin

It secretes cholecalciferol—this hormone increases blood calcium levels by increasing absorption of dietary calcium.

Adipose Tissue

It secretes hormone leptin—this regulates intake and expenditure of energy, including hunger and metabolism.

SUMMARY

- Hormones are secretions of ductless endocrine glands.
- Hormones are made of short chain of amino acids/lipid and phospholipid/derived from single aromatic amino acids.
- Hydrophilic hormones are poorly lipid soluble and cannot pass through membranes—they bind with receptors on the outer cell membrane surface.
- Lipophilic hormones pass easily through the phospholipid layer of the target cell membrane—they bind with receptors inside.
- There are two ways by which body controls secretion of hormones are:
  1. By immediate stimuli
  2. By feedback mechanism
- The pituitary gland and hypothalamus act as a unit, regulating the activity of most of other endocrine glands.
- Hypothalamic hormones are commonly called releasing or inhibiting hormones.
- The anterior lobe of pituitary gland is known as adenohypophysis, whereas the posterior lobe is known as neurohypophysis.
- The primary function of growth hormone (GH) is to induce growth in almost all tissues and organs of the body. Simmonds disease, gigantism, and acromegaly are conditions associated with it.
- TSH is a peptide hormone secreted by pituitary gland. TSH triggers the secretion of T_4 and T_3.
- The ACTH primarily functions to regulate cortisol and androgen production.
- Prolactin stimulates milk production and development of breast tissues.
- GTHs are of two types: FSH and LH or ICSH.
- FSH stimulates the production and maturation of sex cells, sperm in males, and ova in females.
- LH triggers ovulation in women and causes the release of progesterone from the corpus luteum after ovulation.
- Vasopressin reabsorbs water from the kidney's collecting duct.
- Oxytocin is commonly released in females during the process of childbirth.
- Adrenal glands are small, triangular-shaped glands located on top of both kidneys.
- Aldosterone is the main mineralocorticoids. It helps in the maintenance of electrolytes, body fluid volume, osmotic pressure, and blood pressure.
- Cortisol is the main glucocorticoid, which stimulates gluconeogenesis, lipolysis, proteolysis, and RBC production.
- Male hormones, androgens, and female hormones, estrogens, are secreted by the adrenal cortex.
- Catecholamines are class of aromatic amines which includes a number of neurotransmitters.
- The main hormones secreted by the adrenal medulla include epinephrine (adrenaline) and norepinephrine (noradrenaline), which have similar

functions. It increases alertness, papillary dilation, piloerection (hair erection), sweating, etc.
- Dopamine is strongly associated with pleasure and reward.
- Glucagon and insulin are two hormones secreted by Islets of Langerhans of pancreas. The blood glucose level is thus maintained by joint action of insulin and glucagon.
- The pineal gland is situated in brain close to the pituitary gland. It secretes hormone melatonin, which is responsible for sleepiness and wakefulness.
- Testosterone is produced by Leydig cells of testis which is responsible for the development of primary sexual development.
- Estrogen is secreted by the developing ovarian follicles. It has multiple role in stimulation of growth of female reproductive organs.
- Progesterone is a progestational hormone which maintains the pregnancy.
- There are scattered endocrine cells in different parts of alimentary canal. These secrete peptide hormones.
- The atrial wall of the heart secretes a peptide hormone known as atrial natriuretic factor (ANF).
- The juxtaglomerular cells of the kidney secrete hormones renin and erythropoietin.
- Skin secretes cholecalciferol, which increases blood calcium.
- Adipose tissue secretes hormone leptin, which regulates intake and expenditure of energy, including hunger and metabolism.

PRACTICE QUESTIONS

1. Name the glands:
    i. Master of all endocrine glands
    ii. Third eye gland
    iii. Endocrine as well as exocrine gland
    iv. Master of master gland
    v. Triangle shaped gland
2. What are hormones? Enlist their functions.
3. With suitable example, discuss chemical nature of hormones.
4. Differentiate between hydrophilic and lipophilic hormones.
5. With suitable example, explain control of hormone secretion by immediate stimuli.
6. With suitable example, explain control of hormone secretion by feedback mechanism.
7. Differentiate between negative feedback and positive feedback.
8. Explain in detail how hypothalamus and pituitary gland are interconnected.
9. With neat labeled diagram, explain morphology of pituitary gland.
10. Which cells secrete GH? Discuss its functions and disorders.
11. Describe the role of TSH. What are the conditions associated with hyperthyroidism and hypothyroidism?

Chapter 18: Endocrine Glands and Hormones

12. Which cells secrete ACTH? Describe its functions and disorders.
13. Which hormone is secreted by lactotropic cells? Describe its functions and disorders.
14. What are gonadotropic hormones? Discuss its importance.
15. What is the role of neurohypophysis? Discuss the hormones associated with it.
16. With neat labeled diagram, discuss morphology of adrenal gland.
17. Write a note on:
    i. Cushing syndrome
    ii. Mineralocorticoids
    iii. Gonadocorticoids
    iv. Catecholamines
    v. Dopamine
    vi. Islets of Langerhans
    vii. Melatonin
18. Discuss the role of testis in secreting hormones.
19. What are two hormones secreted by ovaries? Discuss its importance.
20. Write the function and origin of following hormones:
    i. Gastrin
    ii. Secretin
    iii. Gastric inhibitory peptide (GIP)
    iv. Ghrelin
    v. Motilin
    vi. Atrial natriuretic factor (ANF)
    vii. Renin
    viii. Erythropoietin
    ix. Cholecalciferol
    x. Leptin

CHAPTER 19

Thyroid Function Tests

Keywords

Thyroid follicles, colloid, isthmus, thyroglobulin, peroxidase enzymes, iodine, triiodothyronine, cretinism, myxedema goiter, Graves' disease, thyrocalcitonin, parathyroid gland, tetraiodothyronine, thymosins, thyroxine-binding globulin (TBG), thyrotropin-releasing hormone (TRH), immunoradiometric assay, tetramethylbenzidine (TMB), horseradish peroxidase (HRP), chemiluminescent microparticle immunoassay (CMIA), relative light units (RLUs), chorionic gonadotropin (hCG)

■ INTRODUCTION

Thyroid gland is the largest endocrine gland in the body weighing 25–30 g and measures about 5 cm in length and 3 cm in width. It is reddish-brown in color.

LOCATION AND MORPHOLOGY OF THYROID GLAND

Thyroid gland is located in the anterior region of the neck just below the larynx, ventrolateral to the trachea. It varies in size as per age, sex, and diet. It is bilobed and highly vascular. The two lobes, right and left, are joined by connective tissue called isthmus which is at 2nd to 4th tracheal cartilage.

The structural and functional units of thyroid gland are the thyroid follicles. Externally, the gland is covered by this connective tissue capsule. From the capsule arises number of septa called trabeculae which divide the interior of gland into the lobules **(Figs. 19.1A and B)**. Each lobule consists of many thyroid follicles. Total numbers of thyroid follicles are about 3 million. The follicles are made up of a central cavity filled with a sticky fluid called colloid. Surrounded by

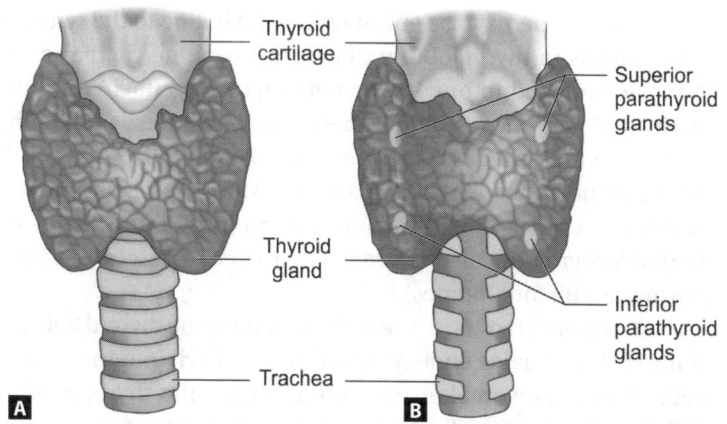

Figs. 19.1A and B: (A) Front view—thyroid gland; (B) Back view—parathyroid gland.
(For color version, see Plate 8)

a wall of epithelial follicle cells, the colloid is the center of thyroid hormone production.

SYNTHESIS AND RELEASE OF THYROID HORMONES

Thyroglobulin is a glycoprotein secreted into colloid by the follicle cells. When atoms of the mineral iodine attach to thyroglobulin, it forms hormones. The following steps outline the synthesis and release of thyroid hormones:

- Thyroid-stimulating hormone (TSH) is released by pituitary gland in the blood. It binds to receptors in the follicle cells of the thyroid gland. This binding causes the cells to actively transport iodide ions (I^-) across their cell membrane, from the bloodstream into the cytosol. As a result, the concentration of iodide ions "trapped" in the follicular cells is many times higher than the concentration in the bloodstream.
- Iodide ions then move to the lumen of the follicle cells that border the colloid. There, the ions undergo oxidation (their negatively charged electrons are removed). The oxidation of two iodide ions ($2\ I^-$) results in iodine (I_2), which passes through the follicle cell membrane into the colloid.

- In the colloid, peroxidase enzymes link the iodine to the tyrosine amino acids in thyroglobulin to produce two intermediaries: A tyrosine attached to one iodine and a tyrosine attached to two iodines. When one of each of these intermediaries is linked by covalent bonds, the resulting compound is triiodothyronine (T_3), a thyroid hormone with three iodines. Much more commonly, when two copies of the second intermediary bond, it forms tetraiodothyronine, also known as thyroxine (T_4). It is a thyroid hormone with four iodines.
- These hormones remain in the colloid center of the thyroid follicles until TSH stimulates endocytosis of colloid back into the follicle cells. There, lysosomal enzymes break apart the thyroglobulin colloid, releasing free T_3 and T_4, which diffuse across the follicle cell membrane and enter the bloodstream.
- In the bloodstream, <1% of the circulating T_3 and T_4 remain unbound. These free T_3 and T_4 can cross the lipid bilayer of cell membranes and be taken up by cells. The remaining 99% of circulating T_3 and T_4 is bound to specialized transport proteins called thyroxine-binding globulins (TBGs), to albumin, or to other plasma proteins. This "packaging" prevents their free diffusion into body cells. When blood levels of T_3 and T_4 begin to decline, bound T_3 and T_4 are released from these plasma proteins and readily cross the membrane of target cells. T_3 is more potent than T_4, and many cells convert T_4 to T_3 through the removal of an iodine atom.
- There are some situations in which TBGs could change their level in the blood, producing changes in the T_4 and T_3 levels. It happens frequently during pregnancy, women who take birth control pills, etc.

■ HORMONES OF THYROID GLAND

T_3 and T_4 Hormone

Function

T_3 and T_4 are the majority of hormone secreted by thyroid gland. These hormones are responsible for increase in the basal metabolic rate (BMR). They have effect on sympathetic nerves; thereby increase heart rate, respiratory rate, digestive secretions, and maturity of brain. Thyroid hormone affects fertility, ovulation, and menstruation. In children, thyroid hormones act synergistically with growth hormone to stimulate bone growth.

Disorders

Dietary iodine deficiency can result in the impaired ability to synthesize T_3 and T_4, leading to a variety of severe disorders. Hypothyroidism can cause symptoms, such as fatigue, weakness, weight gain, depression, slow heartbeat, constipation, and increased sensitivity to cold. Hashimoto's disease, an autoimmune condition, is the most common cause of hypothyroidism. Deficiency of thyroxine in childhood causes cretinism. The symptoms are retardation of physical and mental growth. Deficiency of thyroxine in adults causes myxedema. Symptoms are thickening and puffiness of the skin and subcutaneous tissue particularly of face and extremities. Patients are with low BMR. It also causes mental dullness, loss of memory, and slow action. Simple goiter is caused due to deficiency of iodine in diet or drinking water. It causes enlargement of thyroid gland.

Hyperthyroidism is an overactive thyroid gland that is producing excessive levels of thyroid hormones. It is physically characterized by an enlarged thyroid, rapid heartbeat, high blood pressure (BP), and bulging eyes. Anxiety, irritability, and frequent bowel movements may also occur. Excessive secretion of thyroxine causes exophthalmic goiter (Graves' disease). It is an autoimmune disease. There is slight enlargement of thyroid gland. It increases BMR, heart rate, pulse rate, and BP. Deposition of fats in eye sockets, muscular weakness, and weight loss occur.

Thyrocalcitonin

Thyrocalcitonin (TCT) is secreted by parafollicular cells. It regulates blood calcium level. This hormone stimulates bones to take up (Ca^{++}) from the blood for deposition of calcium phosphates in the bones; thereby decreasing blood (Ca^{++}) level. Increased calcium level of blood stimulates "C" cells to secrete TCT and vice versa.

■ PARATHYROID GLAND

Parathyroid gland is located on the back side of the thyroid gland. There are two pairs of parathyroid glands present one pair in each lobe. Parathyroid glands secrete a peptide hormone known as parathyroid hormone (PTH). The level of Ca^{++} in the blood regulates the secretion of PTH. This hormone increases the Ca^{++} level in the blood. PTH is hypercalcemic hormone. Thus, the calcium balance is maintained by TCT and PTH.

■ THYMUS

Thymus is located on the dorsal side of the heart and aorta **(Fig. 19.2A)**. It is formed of lobules **(Fig. 19.2B)**. The thymus plays a major role in the development of immune system. The peptide hormones known as thymosins are secreted by thymus which plays an important role in the differentiation of T lymphocytes. These cells produce cell-mediated immunity. The thymosins also promote production of antibodies by providing humoral immunity. After puberty, the thymus starts to slowly shrink and become replaced by fat.

■ THYROID FUNCTION TESTS

The key assays that are used to detect thyroid dysfunction are serum TSH and the main circulating thyroid hormones thyroxine (T_4) and triiodothyronine (T_3), either as total or estimated free concentrations **(Table 19.1)**. TBGs are also determined by similar immunoassays.

■ THYROID-STIMULATING HORMONE TEST

Thyroid-stimulating hormone production is controlled by hypothalamic-derived thyrotropin-releasing hormone (TRH).

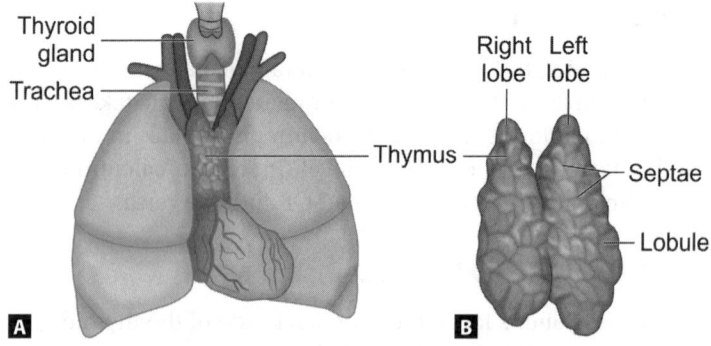

Figs. 19.2A and B: (A) Location of thymus gland; (B) Thymus gland.
(For color version, see Plate 9)

Table 19.1: Reference range and abbreviation for thyroid function test.

Test	Abbreviation	Reference range*
Serum thyroxine	T_4	4.6–12 µg/dL
Free thyroxine	FT_4	0.7–1.9 ng/dL
Serum triiodothyronine	T_3	80–180 ng/dL
Free triiodothyronine	FT_3	230–619 pg/dL
Serum thyrotropin	TSH	0.5–6 uIU/mL
Thyroxine-binding globulin	TBG	12–20 µg/dL T_4 +1.8 µg

*Normal values of hormones differ as per age, sex, and health status (pregnancy). The values given here are indicatory.

Circulating TSH in the blood is the primary determining factor that regulates the secretion of the thyroid hormones thyroxine (T_4) and triiodothyronine (T_3) from the thyroid. The level of thyroid hormones in the blood has an effect on the pituitary release of TSH; when the levels of T_3 and T_4 are low, the production of TSH is increased, and conversely, when levels of T_3 and T_4 are high, TSH production is decreased. This effect creates a regulatory negative feedback loop.

Determination of Thyroid-stimulating Hormone by Immunoradiometric Assay (IRMA)

Principle

The IRMA is a solid-phase immunoradiometric assay, based on monoclonal and polyclonal anti-TSH antibodies, i.e., I^{125}-labeled anti-TSH polyclonal antibody in liquid phase (say antibody 1) and monoclonal anti-TSH antibodies immobilized to the wall of a polystyrene tube (say antibody 2).

Procedure

- TSH (in patient's serum) is captured between antibody 2 and antibody 1.
- Unbound I^{125}-labeled anti-TSH antibody is removed by decanting the test tube.
- The TSH concentration is directly proportional to the radioactivity present in the tube, which is counted by the gamma counter. The

concentration of TSH in the sample is obtained by the standard curve, made with the set of calibrators provided with the kit.

Determination of Thyroid-stimulating Hormone by ELISA

Thyroid-stimulating hormone is a glycoprotein hormone; it is a heterodimer comprised of a common α subunit and a hormone-specific β subunit. The α subunit of TSH is identical to that of human chorionic gonadotropin (hCG), luteinizing hormone (LH), and follicle-stimulating hormone (FSH). The β subunit is TSH-specific, and therefore determines its function.

Principle

The quantitative immunoenzymatic determination of TSH is based on the ELISA (enzyme-linked immunosorbent assay) technique. The assay system utilizes two monoclonal antibodies specific for different antigenic determinants of the TSH β subunit. The first antibody is immobilized on the surface of the microtiter wells. In the second step, antibody is conjugated to horseradish peroxidase. The test sample is allowed to react simultaneously with the two antibodies, resulting in the TSH molecules being sandwiched between the solid phase and the enzyme-linked antibodies. After an incubation step, the wells are washed with washing solution to remove all unbound material. The immune complex is visualized by adding tetramethylbenzidine (TMB) substrate which gives a blue reaction product. The intensity of this product is proportional to the concentration of TSH in the specimen. Sulfuric acid is added to stop the reaction. This produces a yellow endpoint color. Absorbance at 450 nm is read using an ELISA microwell plate reader. The color intensity is directly proportional to the concentration of TSH present in the test sample.

Reagents

- The ready to use break apart snap-off strips are coated with monoclonal antibodies to TSH.
- **Anti-TSH conjugate:** It is a solution with anti-TSH horseradish peroxidase, buffer, stabilizers, preservatives, and an inert red dye.

- Standards vials labeled with Standards A, B, C, D, E, F, and G contain a ready-to-use standard solution. The standards are with following concentrations: Standard A: 0.0 µIU/mL, Standard B: 0.2 µIU/mL, Standard C: 0.5 µIU/mL, Standard D: 2.5 µIU/mL, Standard E: 5.0 µIU/mL, Standard F: 10.0 µIU/mL, and Standard G: 20.0 µIU/mL.
- Washing solution (20× conc.). The bottle contains 50 mL of a concentrated buffer, detergents, and preservatives.
- Working dilute washing solution is prepared as—1:19 with distilled water (e.g., 10 mL washing solution + 190 mL distilled water).
- **TMB substrate solution:** It contains a TMB/hydrogen peroxide system.
- **Stop solution:** It is 0.2 M sulfuric acid solution.
  Sample: Serum or citrate plasma is used for assay.
  Procedure: Please read the test protocol carefully before performing the assay. Every kit may have some differences in procedure. Washing guidelines are to be followed strictly as any error may cause false results.
- Allocate at least 1 well (e.g., A1) for the substrate blank.
- Seven wells (e.g., B1, C1, etc.) for Standards A, B, C, D, E, F, and G. It is recommended to determine standards and patient samples in duplicate and then use mean absorbance of it.
- Perform all assay steps in the order given and without any appreciable delays between the steps.
- Dispense 50 µL of each Standard (A, B, C, D, E, F and G) and samples into their respective wells.
- Leave well A1 for the substrate blank.
- Dispense 100 µL conjugate into all wells except for the blank well (e.g., A1).
- Cover wells with the foil.
- Incubate for 1 hour ± 5 minutes at 37 ± 1°C.
- When incubation has been completed, remove the foil, aspirate the content of the wells, and wash each well five times with 300 µL of washing solution. The soak time between each wash cycle should be >5 seconds. At the end carefully remove remaining fluid by tapping strips on tissue paper prior to the next step.

  Note: Washing is critical! Insufficient washing results in poor precision and falsely elevated absorbance values.
- Dispense 100 µL TMB substrate solution into all wells.

- Incubate for exactly 15 minutes at room temperature (20–25°C) in the dark.
- Dispense 100 µL stop Solution into all wells in the same order and at the same rate as for the TMB substrate solution. After adding this, any blue color developed during the incubation turns into yellow.
- Measure the absorbance of the specimen at 450/620 nm within 30 minutes after addition of the stop solution.

Calculation of results: In order to obtain quantitative results in µIU/mL, plot the (mean) absorbance values of the Standards A–G (Y-axis) on graph paper in a system of coordinates against their corresponding concentrations (X-axis) and draw a standard calibration curve. Read results from this standard curve employing the (mean) absorbance values of each patient specimen. All suitable computer programs available can be used for automated result reading and calculation.

T_3 AND T_4 TESTS

The major form of thyroid hormone in the blood is thyroxine (T_4) and triiodothyronine (T_3). T_4 is present in 50-folds excess in human plasma. It gets converted to T_3 (the metabolically active form) and is thus considered as a prohormone for T_3.

Only 0.02–0.04% of the total T_3 is present is in the unbound form also known as free T_3 (FT_3). Rest is present in the bound form, i.e., bound to TBG, prealbumin, and albumin. Similarly, FT_4 is also a minute fraction of total T_4.

T_4 and T_3 can be measured as free T_4 and free T_3 which are indicators of thyroxine and triiodothyronine activities in the body. It provides the best indication of thyroid dysfunction, since free T_4 is less sensitive to changes in the serum-binding proteins.

They can also be measured as total thyroxine and total triiodothyronine, which also depend on the thyroxine and triiodothyronine that is bound to thyroxine-binding globulin (TBG).

Methods of Estimations of T_3 and T_4

For the estimation of serum thyroid hormones, radioimmunoassay (RIA) and ELISA are commonly used. For this purpose, serum is used and the fasting specimen is not essential.

Determination of T_3 by Radioimmunoassay

Principle

It is a solid-phase RIA, where I^{125}-labeled T_3 competes with T_3 in patient's serum for the specific antibody sites for a fixed time. This reaction takes place in the presence of blocking agents which liberate bound T_3 from the carrier proteins. After incubation, the supernatant is decanted and the antibody bound fraction of the radiolabeled T3 can be measured using gamma counter.

Procedure

RIA diagnostic kits are available which contain: Total T_3 antibody-coated tubes and I^{125}- labeled T_3 and six human serum calibrators for T_3 (A to F) with concentration ranging from 0 to 600 ng/dL. Procedure is followed as per the kit insert and a standard curve is plotted, from which the patient's serum T_3 value is calculated.

Determination of T_4 by Radioimmunoassay

Principle

It is based on the same principle as for T3, determination except for the fact that I^{125}-labeled T4 is used. The antibody bound I^{125}-T4 can be measured by the gamma counter and is inversely related to patient's T4 concentration

T4 by ELISA

In this immunological reaction, enzymes along with the labeled antibodies are used.

In the first step, serum T_3/T_4 and peroxidase (POD) labeled T_3/T_4 compete with the limited quantity of T_3/T_4-specific antibodies coated onto the inside of test vial, respectively. The T_3/T_4-POD conjugate not bound by the antibodies is removed in the separation step.

In the second incubation step, addition of hydrogen peroxide and chromogen (ATBS: diammonium-2, 2-azinobis-3-ethylbenzothiazoline-6-sulfonate) result in the formation of colored complex, which can be measured at 405 nm. The absorbance is proportional to the enzyme activity of antibody-T_3/T_4.

Determination of Free T_4

Historically, the diagnosis of thyroid function has involved performing a total T_4 assay in addition to a thyroxine uptake (TU) assay of the same sample. The mathematical combination of these two assays produces a free thyroxine index (FTI) which provides an indirect proportional estimate for free T_4.

fT_4 by ELISA

The fT_4 is a solid-phase competitive ELISA. The samples, assay buffer, and T_4 enzyme conjugate are added to the wells coated with anti-T_4 monoclonal antibody. fT_4 in the patient's serum competes with a T_4 enzyme [horseradish peroxidase (HRP)] conjugate for binding sites. Unbound fT_4 and T_4 enzyme conjugate is washed off by washing buffer. Upon the addition of the substrate, the intensity of color is inversely proportional to the concentration of fT_4 in the samples. A standard curve is prepared relating color intensity to the concentration of fT_4. It is measured at 450 nm within 15 minutes after adding the stop solution.

Free T_3

Only 0.2–0.4% of the total T_3 is present in solution as unbound or free T_3. This free fraction represents the physiologically active thyroid hormone. Free T_3 is typically elevated to a greater degree than free thyroxine (T_4) in Graves' disease. Occasionally, free T_3 alone is elevated (T_3 thyrotoxicosis) in about 5% of the hyperthyroid population. In contrast, levels of free T_4 are elevated to a greater degree than free T_3 in toxic multinodular goiter and excessive T_4 therapy. Serum free T_3 is useful in distinguishing these forms of hyperthyroidism. Free T_3 may also be important in monitoring patients on antithyroid therapy where treatment is focused on reducing the T_3 production and the T_4 conversion to T_3. Serum free T_3 may also be useful in assessing the severity of the thyrotoxic state.

Determination of Free T_3 by Chemiluminescent Microparticle Immunoassay (CMIA)

Principle

Free T_3 assay is a two-step immunoassay to determine the presence of free (unbound) T_3 in human serum and plasma using

CMIA technology with flexible assay protocols, referred to as chemiflex.

In the first step, sample and anti-T_3-coated paramagnetic microparticles are combined. Free T_3 (unbound) present in the sample binds to the anti-T_3 coated microparticles. After washing, T_3 acridinium-labeled conjugate is added in the second step. Pre-trigger and trigger solutions are then added to the reaction mixture; the resulting chemiluminescent reaction is measured as relative light units (RLUs). An inverse relationship exists between the amount of free T_3 in the sample and the RLUs detected by the optical system.

By Autoanalyzers

Determination of T_3, T_4, and TSH can also be done by using an autoanalyzer.

■ CLINICAL INTERPRETATION (TABLE 19.2)

Combination of these three tests determines whether the abnormality arises centrally from the thyroid gland (primary), peripherally from the pituitary (secondary), or hypothalamus (tertiary—changes in TRH).

■ THYROID FUNCTION TESTS IN PREGNANCY

- In pregnancy, estrogen levels increase and TBG concentrations rise—this leads to an increase in total T_4 and T_3.
- In the first trimester, serum TSH also falls due to the effect of hCG and there may be a small fall in FT_4. In the second and third trimesters, FT_4 and FT_3 decrease, sometimes below the nonpregnant women's reference level.
- Always use trimester-related reference ranges for TSH and total and free thyroid hormones to assess pregnant patients' thyroid status.
- Changes in the immune system during and after pregnancy may alter the course of pre-existing autoimmune thyroid disease and predispose to relapse or to developing novel autoimmune thyroid disease.

Table 19.2: Results of thyroid function tests in various clinical situations.

Physiologic state	Serum TSH	Serum free T_4	Serum T_3
Dysfunction of the hypothalamus and the pituitary gland	High	High	High
Hypopituitarism	Low	Low	Low
Hyperthyroidism			
Untreated	Low*	High	High
T_3 toxicosis	Low	Normal	High
Hypothyroidism			
Primary, Untreated	High	Low	Low/Normal
Secondary/pituitary disease	Low/Normal	Low	Low/Normal
Euthyroidism			
Patient taking iodine	Normal	Normal	Normal
Patient taking exogenous thyroid hormone	Normal	Normal in patient taking T_4, low in patient taking T_3	High in patient taking T_3, normal in patient taking T_4
Patient taking estrogen	Normal	Normal	High
Euthyroid sick syndrome	Normal/Low/High	Normal/Low	Low

(TSH: thyroid-stimulating hormone).

*TSH is low in patients with hyperthyroidism except in the rare instance when the etiology is a TSH-secreting pituitary adenoma or pituitary resistance to the normal inhibition by thyroid hormone.

Hypothyroid Pregnancies

Increased fetal loss and intelligence quotient (IQ) deficits in infants are associated with mothers who had undiagnosed or undertreated hypothyroidism during pregnancy. Thyroxine requirements are also likely to change during pregnancy. The thyroid status of pregnant hypothyroid patients should be checked at regular intervals.

Hyperthyroid Pregnancies

In those receiving antithyroid drugs, TFTs should be checked prior to conception and drugs adjusted to a minimum dose of antithyroid drug only. Thyroid levels are monitored at regular intervals.

SUMMARY

- Thyroid gland is located in the anterior region of the neck just below the larynx. It is bilobed and highly vascular.
- The two lobes right and left are joined by connective tissue called isthmus.
- Lobule in thyroid gland consists of many thyroid follicles which are made up of a central cavity filled with a sticky fluid called colloid.
- Thyroglobulin is a glycoprotein secreted into colloid by the follicle cells. When atoms of the mineral iodine attach to thyroglobulin, it forms hormones.
- T_3 and T_4 are the majority of hormones secreted by thyroid gland. These hormones are responsible for increase in the BMR.
- Deficiency of thyroxine in childhood causes cretinism. Deficiency of thyroxine in adults causes myxedema.
- Excessive secretion of thyroxine causes exophthalmic goiter (Graves' disease).
- TCT is secreted by parafollicular cells. It regulates blood calcium level.
- The peptide hormones known as thymosins are secreted by thymus which plays an important role in the differentiation of T lymphocytes.
- TSH in the blood is the primary determining factor that regulates the secretion of the thyroid hormones thyroxine (T_4) and triiodothyronine (T_3) from the thyroid.
- Most of the T_3 and T_4 hormones are found in bound form. These are bounded to TBG. Very few of them exist in free form.
- T_3, T_4, and TSH are measured by different assay techniques such as RIA, CMIA, and ELISA.
- Combination of these three tests determines whether the abnormality arises centrally from the thyroid gland (primary), peripherally from the pituitary (secondary), or hypothalamus (tertiary—changes in TRH).
- In pregnancy, estrogen levels increase and TBG concentrations rise—this leads to an increase in total T_4 and T_3.

PRACTICE QUESTIONS

1. Where is the thyroid gland located?
2. Draw a neat labeled diagram of thyroid gland and discuss its morphology.
3. Describe the process of synthesis and release of thyroid hormones.
4. Mention the functions and disorders related to T_3 and T_4 hormones.

Section 3: Clinical Biochemistry

5. What is the role of thyrocalcitonin?
6. Write a note on: (1) Parathyroid gland and (2) Thymus.
7. Describe the importance of TSH in thyroid function tests.
8. Write the principle and the procedure to determine TSH by IRMA.
9. Write the principle and the procedure to determine TSH by ELISA.
10. What is the difference between free and bound thyroid hormones?
11. Describe the principle and the procedure of determination of T_3 and T_4.
12. Describe the principle and the procedure of determination of free T_3 and T_4.
13. Compare the levels of different hormones in hypothyroid and hyperthyroid conditions.
14. What is euthyroidism?
15. Why it is necessary to perform thyroid function tests in pregnancy?

Diabetic Profile

CHAPTER 20

Keywords
Diabetes mellitus, gestational diabetes, prediabetes, insulin-dependent diabetes, insulin non-dependent diabetes, Folin–Wu method, O-toluidine, glucose oxidase, glucometer, glucose tolerance test (GTT), insulin, hypoglycemia, hyperglycemia, C-peptide, HbA1c, Benedict's test, islet cell antibody (ICA), urine ketone test, Rothera's test

■ INTRODUCTION

Diabetes mellitus is derived from the Greek word diabetes meaning to pass through and the Latin word mellitus meaning honeyed or sweet. This is because in diabetes excess sugar is found in blood as well as the urine.

Diabetes mellitus is chronic disorder of carbohydrate metabolism, in which body cannot regulate the amount of glucose in the blood.

After a meal, food mainly carbohydrate is broken down into glucose, which is carried by the blood to cells throughout the body. Cells use insulin, a hormone made in the pancreas, to convert blood glucose into energy. People with diabetes mellitus have problems in converting glucose to energy.

People develop diabetes mellitus in two conditions—because the pancreas does not make enough insulin or because the cells in the muscles, liver, and fat do not use insulin properly, or both. As a result, the amount of glucose in the blood increases while the cells are starved of energy. Over the years, high blood glucose, also called hyperglycemia, damages nerves and blood vessels, which can lead to complications such as heart disease and stroke, kidney disease, blindness, nerve problems, gum infections, and amputation.

■ TYPES OF DIABETES

The three main types of diabetes are: type 1, type 2, and gestational diabetes.

1. **Type 1/juvenile diabetes/insulin-dependent diabetes mellitus (IDDM)**
   - Type 1 diabetes, formerly called juvenile diabetes, is usually first diagnosed in children, teenagers, or young adults. In this form of diabetes, the beta cells of the pancreas no longer make insulin because the body's immune system has attacked and destroyed them.
   - Autoimmune pancreatic beta-cell destruction possibly triggered by an environmental exposure in genetically susceptible people. Destruction progresses subclinically over months or years until beta-cell mass decreases to the point that insulin concentrations are no longer adequate to control plasma glucose levels.
   - Type 1 diabetes accounts for < 10% of all cases of diabetes mellitus.
   - It is not known what causes this autoimmune reaction to occur, but it is believed that certain viruses or environmental factors, lifestyle changes such as dietary factors and stress as well as genetic factors are play a part in the development of the condition.

2. **Type 2/adult-onset diabetes/noninsulin-dependent diabetes mellitus (NIDDM)**
   - Type 2 diabetes, formerly called adult-onset diabetes, is the most common form. People can develop it at any age, even during childhood. This form of diabetes usually begins with insulin resistance, a condition in which muscle, liver, and fat cells do not use insulin properly. Because insulin cannot work properly, blood glucose levels keep rising, releasing more insulin. For some people with type 2 diabetes this can eventually exhaust the pancreas such that, it loses the ability to secrete enough insulin in response to meals. Less insulin, causing even higher blood sugar levels.
   - People with type 2 diabetes require insulin injections
   - Type 2 diabetes involves a more complex interplay between genetics and lifestyle. Type 2 diabetes has a stronger hereditary

profile as compared to type 1. The majority of patients with the disease have at least one parent with type 2 diabetes. Obesity and weight gain and lifestyle are important determinants of insulin resistance in type 2 diabetes.
- Age is also an important factor, with the condition most commonly occurring after the age of 40 years. As people age, beta cells become less efficient and the cells in the body become less able to use the insulin made by the pancreas.
- It is the most common form of diabetes affecting approximately 90% of all people with diabetes.

Signs and symptoms: The onset of symptoms in type 1 diabetes is typically quite sudden and symptoms can be severe. However, the symptoms of type 2 diabetes tend to manifest gradually, so much so that they may go unnoticed. When hyperglycemia occurs, the body tries to get rid of the excess glucose by excreting it in the urine. This increases urine output and can lead to dehydration. At the same time the body's cells are starved of the glucose energy they need. The combination of these factors produces the common symptoms of diabetes.

These may include: weight loss, excessive thirst, excessive urination, fatigue, nausea, irritability, yeast infections blurry vision, skin wounds or infections that are slow to heal, numbness and tingling in the feet.

Complications: People with diabetes mellitus may experience many serious, long-term complications. Some of these complications begin within months of the onset of diabetes, although most tend to develop after a few years. Most of the complications gradually worsen.
- Most complications of diabetes are the result of problems with blood vessels. Complex sugar-based substances build up in the walls of small blood vessels, causing them to thicken and leak. Over time, narrowing of blood vessels can harm the heart, brain, legs, eyes, kidneys, nerves, and skin, resulting in angina, heart failure, strokes, leg cramps during walking (claudication), poor vision, chronic kidney disease, damage to nerves (neuropathy), and skin breakdown.
- Poor control of blood glucose levels causes the levels of fatty substances in the blood to rise, resulting in atherosclerosis and

- decreased blood flow in the larger blood vessels. Atherosclerosis leads to heart attacks and strokes.
- Hypoglycemia is abnormally low levels of sugar (glucose) in the blood. Hypoglycemia is most often caused by drugs taken to control diabetes. A fall in blood glucose causes symptoms such as hunger, sweating, shakiness, fatigue, weakness, and inability to think clearly, whereas severe hypoglycemia causes symptoms such as confusion, seizures, and coma.

3. **Gestational diabetes:** Gestational diabetes is a type of diabetes that develops only during pregnancy.
   - During pregnancy, body makes more hormones and goes through other changes, such as weight gain. In this period, the placenta, (which connects baby to mother for blood supply), produces high levels of various other hormones. Almost all of them impair the action of insulin in cells, raising the level of blood sugar. Modest elevation of blood sugar after meals is normal during pregnancy.
   - As baby grows, the placenta produces more and more insulin-blocking hormones. In gestational diabetes, the placental hormones provoke a rise in blood sugar to a level that can affect the growth and welfare of baby. These changes cause body's cells to use insulin less effectively, a condition called insulin resistance. Insulin resistance increases body's need for insulin. If pancreas cannot make enough insulin, it will cause gestational diabetes.
   - However, during pregnancy, some women develop higher than normal levels of glucose in their blood, which insulin cannot bring under control.
   - Gestational diabetes usually develops in the third trimester (after 28 weeks) and usually disappears after the baby is born. However, women who develop gestational diabetes are more likely to develop type 2 diabetes later in life.

Diagnosis: Gestational diabetes often does not cause any symptoms. Screening test is done for the condition by a venous glucose sample, at around weeks 8-12 of pregnancy.

If increased risk of gestational diabetes is found, a glucose tolerance test (GTT) is done during weeks 24-28 of pregnancy or sooner.

High blood glucose (hyperglycemia) can cause some symptoms as that of diabetes.

Chances of getting gestational diabetes increases if a person—is overweight, have had gestational diabetes before, have given birth to a baby weighing more than 9 pounds, have a parent, brother, or sister with type 2 diabetes, have prediabetes and have a hormonal disorder called polycystic ovary syndrome, also known as PCOS.

Complications: Most women who have gestational diabetes deliver healthy babies. However, gestational diabetes that's not carefully managed can lead to uncontrolled blood sugar levels and cause problems for mother and baby, including an increased likelihood of needing a C-section to deliver.

- A mother's high blood sugar may increase her risk of early labor and delivering her baby before its due date. Babies born early may experience respiratory distress syndrome—a condition that makes breathing difficult.
- *Low blood sugar (hypoglycemia):* Sometimes babies of mothers with gestational diabetes develop low blood sugar (hypoglycemia) shortly after birth because their own insulin production is high.

Complications that may affect mother: Gestational diabetes may also increase the mother's risk of:

- *High blood pressure and preeclampsia:* Gestational diabetes raises risk of high blood pressure, as well as, preeclampsia—a serious complication of pregnancy that causes high blood pressure and other symptoms that can threaten the lives of both mother and baby.
- *Future diabetes:* If mother have gestational diabetes, she is more likely to get it again during a future pregnancy, also more likely to develop type 2 diabetes.

4. **Prediabetes:** In prediabetes, blood sugar levels are slightly higher than normal, but still not as high as in diabetes. This is a border line situation of diabetes.

The rise in blood sugar levels that is seen in prediabetes starts when the body begins to develop a problem called "insulin resistance". If usual amounts of insulin cannot trigger the body to move glucose out of the bloodstream into cells, this condition is called insulin resistance.

Once insulin resistance begins, it can worsen over time. In period of prediabetes, body makes extra insulin to keep sugar levels near to normal. Insulin resistance can worsen with age, and weight gain. If insulin resistance progresses, eventually it cannot compensate well enough by making extra insulin. When this occurs, sugar levels will increase, leading to diabetes.

Depending on what a blood sugar test finds, prediabetes can be more specifically called "impaired glucose (sugar) tolerance" or "impaired fasting glucose." Impaired fasting glucose means that blood sugar increase after 8–10 hours of fasting. Impaired glucose tolerance means that blood sugar levels reach a surprisingly high level after eating sugar. To diagnose impaired glucose tolerance, a glucose tolerance test is used.

Prediabetes has increased risk of diabetes, and for heart disease.

Symptoms: Prediabetes is often called a "silent" condition because it usually has no symptoms. Or it may show few symptoms of diabetes. Prediabetes can remain undiagnosed for several years. Certain risk factors increase the chances of prediabetes are:
- Being overweight, being 45 years or older, a family history of diabetes, low levels of high-density lipoprotein (HDL) cholesterol (the "good" cholesterol), high triglycerides, high blood pressure, a history of gestational diabetes

Diagnosis: The same blood sugar tests that are used for diabetes are used to diagnose prediabetes.

Reference range for prediabetes:
- *Fasting glucose test:* Between 100 and 125 mg/dL
- *Oral glucose tolerance test:* Between 140 and 199 mg/dL
- *Hemoglobin A1C test:* Between 5.7% and 6.4%

Note: Diabetes insipidus is not related to diabetes mellitus (type 1 and type 2 diabetes). Diabetes insipidus is caused by problems related to the antidiuretic hormone (ADH) or its receptor and causes frequent urination.

■ DIAGNOSIS OF DIABETES

Group of tests that are used to diagnose diabetes or its complications, it includes:
1. **Blood glucose (types: FBS, PPBS, RBS):**
    - *Fasting blood sugar (FBS):* This is done after minimum 8 hours of fasting.

- *Post meal plasma blood sugar (PPBS):* Patient must complete meal within 15–20 minutes specimen is collected after exactly 2 hours from beginning meal.
- *Random blood sugar (RBS):* It can be collected at any random time.
2. Glucose tolerance test (GTT)
3. HbA1c
4. C-peptide
5. Islet cell antibody (ICA) for type I
6. Insulin (hormone test)
7. Urine test for presence of glucose and ketone bodies.

Positive test results should be confirmed by repeating the fasting plasma glucose test or the oral glucose tolerance test on a different day.

Blood Glucose

Blood glucose can be determined at different times. As stated above, it may be fasting, post meal or random.

Specimen: Sreum, plasma, or whole blood can be used. Serum should be separated from blood clot within half hour of blood collection. For plasma preparation, fluoride with oxalate is used as an anticoagulant.

There are three important methods to determine plasma glucose level.
1. Folin-Wu method
2. O-Toluidine method
3. Glucose oxidase method

Folin-Wu Method

It is economical, simple and convenient method.

Principle

Glucose on boiling with alkaline copper solution reduces copper from the cupric to cuprous state. The cuprous oxide so formed reduces phosphomolybdic acid to blue colored molybdenum blue, which is measured colorimetrically. The intensity of blue color is proportional to glucose concentration.

Reagents

1. 10% sodium tungstate
2. 0.66 N sulfuric acid
3. Alkaline copper sulfate solution
4. Phosphomolybdate solution
5. Stock glucose standard
6. Working standard—dilute 1 mL of glucose stock standard with 9 mL of distill water to give 100 mg % working standard. Prepare this every day.

Procedure

Part I: Preparation of Protein Free Filtrate

In a 10 mL test tube take 3.5 mL distill water and 0.1 mL of plasma/serum, followed by 0.2 mL of 10% sodium tungstate. Mix and add slowly 0.2 mL of 2/3 N sulfuric acid. Mix well stand for 5 minutes. Filter or centrifuge.

Part II: Color Development

Folin blood sugar test tubes are recommended for this test. The tubes are specially designed to prevent contact of atmospheric oxygen with the reaction mixture, which affects the result.

1. Take four Folin-Wu tubes **(Fig. 20.1)** and label it as blank (B), Standard (S), Control (C) and Test (T). Add 1 mL of distilled water, glucose standard, protein free filtrate of control serum and test serum in respective tubes.
2. Add 1 mL of alkaline copper reagent to each tube.
3. Transfer the tubes to boiling water bath for 10 minutes.
4. Cool the tubes for 2–3 minutes under running tap water without shaking.
5. After cooling add 2 mL phosphomolybdate reagent to each tube.
6. Mix well by inversion and dilute the contents of each tube up to 12.5 mL with distilled water.
7. Set the wavelength of photometer to 620 nm and measure the OD.

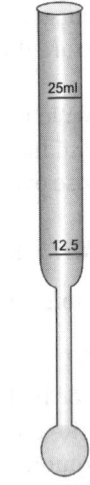

Fig. 20.1: Folin-Wu's blood sugar tube.

Following table shows Folin-Wu procedure:

Reagent	Blank	Standard	Control	Test
Distilled water	1 mL	—	—	—
Glucose standard	—	1 mL	—	—
Filtrate of 'C'	—	—	1 mL	—
Filtrate of 'S'	—	—	—	1 mL
Alkaline Cu reagent	1 mL	1 mL	1 mL	1 mL
Boiling water bath for 10 minutes				
Phosphomolybdate	2 mL	2 mL	2 mL	2 mL

O-toluidine Method

Principle

The aldehyde group of glucose condenses with O-toluidine in glacial acetic acid, which on heating gives an emerald-blue green color which is measured photometrically. The intensity of color is directly proportional to the glucose concentration.

Reagents

1. O-toluidine reagent
   Orthotoluidine: 60 mL
   Thiourea: 1.5 g
   Glacial acetic acid: 1,000 mL
2. Glucose stock standard (200 mg/dL in 0.2% benzoic acid solution)
3. Glucose working solution.

Procedure

1. Take three test tubes and label them as blank, standard and test.
2. Transfer 1 mL distilled water, 1 mL working standard, and 1mL test serum to respective tube.
3. To each tube, add 0.9 mL of distilled water and 7 mL of O-toluidine reagent. Cover the tubes with loose cap or aluminium foil.
4. Place in a boiling water bath for 10 minutes work inside the hood as it gives strong smell, which is injurious.
5. Cool the tubes for 2–3 minutes under running tap water.
6. Read the absorbance within 30 minutes of cooling at 630 nm.

Following table shows O-toluidine procedure:

Reagent	Blank	Standard	Test
Distilled water	1 mL	—	—
Glucose standard	—	1 mL	—
Test serum	—	—	1 mL
Distilled water	0.9 mL	0.9 mL	0.9 mL
O-toluidine reagent	7 mL	7 mL	7 mL

Glucose Oxidase Method

Principle

Glucose oxidase (GOD) oxidizes glucose to gluconic acid. Hydrogen peroxide is produced in this reaction. In presence of peroxide hydrogen peroxidase (POD) reacts with 4-aminoantipyrine and phenol to form red colored quinoneimine dye. The intensity of color is directly proportional to the glucose concentration. This method is highly specific for glucose and does not involve any other sugar.

$$Glucose + H_2O \xrightarrow{GOD} Gluconic\ acid + H_2O_2$$

$$H_2O_2 + phenol + 4\text{-aminoantipyrine} \xrightarrow{POD} Quinoneimine\ dye$$

Reagents

1. Glucose oxidase reagent
2. Phenol solution
3. Glucose stock standard (200 mg/dL in 0.2% benzoic acid solution)
4. Glucose working solution.

Procedure

1. Take three test tubes and label them as blank, standard and test.
2. Add 2 mL of glucose oxidase reagent into the three test tubes.
3. Add 0.5 mL of distilled water; 0.5 mL of ten times diluted serum, 0.5 mL of working standard in blank, test and serum respectively.
4. Add 2 mL of phenol reagent into the three test tubes.
5. Shake well and allow it to stand for 30 minutes at room temperature or 15 minutes at 37°C.
6. Read the absorbance at 515 nm.

Following table shows glucose oxidase procedure:

Reagent	Blank	Standard	Test
Glucose oxidase	2 mL	2 mL	2 mL
Glucose standard	—	0.5 mL	—
Diluted test serum	—	—	0.5 mL
Distilled water	0.5 mL	—	—
Phenol reagent	2 mL	2 mL	2 mL

Calculation

$$\text{Glucose mg}/100 \text{ mL} = \frac{\text{OD of test}}{\text{OD of std.}} \times \text{Conc. of std.}$$

Normal values

- Fasting: 65–110 mg/dL
- Post meal: 120–140 mg/dL
- Random: 70–140 mg/dL

Clinical significance

Blood glucose level is mainly determined to diagnose diabetes mellitus. It provides the valuable information about the course, severity and therapeutic control of diabetes mellitus.

With the FPG test, a fasting blood glucose level between 100 and 125 mg/dL signals prediabetes. A person with a fasting blood glucose level of 126 mg/dL or higher has diabetes. The early symptoms of untreated diabetes mellitus are related to the elevated blood glucose levels. Excess glucose in the blood ultimately results in high levels of glucose being present in the urine (glucosuria). This increases the urine output, which leads to dehydration and increased thirst. Other symptoms include extreme tiredness, weight loss, blurred vision, itchy skin and repeated minor infections such as thrush and boils.

Beside the diabetes, blood sugar level is also increased in:

With increased circulatory epinephrine, pancreatitis, some CNS lesions, or effects of drugs like alcohol, phenytoin, etc.

Decreases in—extrapancreatic tumors, hepatic disease, endocrine disorders, pediatric abnormalities, enzyme diseases and malnutrition.

Glucometer

A glucose meter (or glucometer) is a medical device for determining the approximate amount of glucose in a drop of blood obtained by pricking the skin with a lancet. Glucose meters are portable and designed for use by laypersons, including those with diabetes mellitus or with proneness to hypoglycemia.

There are now dozens of models of glucose meters are available which also differ in their principle. Most of them are based on colorimetric or amperometric principle.

Typical features common to most of the glucose meters are given below:
- The average size is now approximately the size of the palm of the hand. They are battery powered.
- A consumable element containing chemicals, which react with glucose in the drop of blood, is used for each measurement. For most models this element is a plastic test strip with a small spot impregnated with glucose oxidase and other components. Each strip can only be used once and is then discarded.
- The glucose value in mg/dL or mmol/L displayed in a small window.
- Glucose levels in plasma are generally 10–15% higher than glucose measurements in whole blood (and even more after eating). This is important because home blood glucose meters measure the glucose in whole blood while most laboratory tests measure the glucose in plasma.
- Current "count times" range from 5 to 60 seconds for different models.
- The size of the drop of blood needed by different models currently varies from 0.3 to 10 µL.
- All meters now include a clock, which must be set for date and time, and a memory for past test results. The memory is an important aspect of diabetes care, as it enables the person with diabetes to keep a record of management and look for trends and patterns in blood glucose levels over days. Most memory chips can display an average of recent glucose readings.
- Many meters have now had more sophisticated data handling capabilities. Many can be downloaded by a cable or infrared to a computer which has software to display the test results in a variety of formats. Some meters allow entry of additional data throughout

the day, such as insulin dose, amounts of carbohydrates eaten, or exercise.
- A number of meters have been combined with other devices, such as insulin injection devices, PDAs. A radio link to an insulin pump allows automatic transfer of glucose readings to a calculator that assists the wearer in deciding on an appropriate insulin dose. One model also measures beta-hydroxybutyrate in the blood to detect ketoacidosis.
- Special glucose meters for multi-patient hospital use are now used. These provide more elaborate quality control records, and the data handling capabilities are designed to transfer glucoses into electronic medical records and the laboratory computer systems for billing purposes.

Principle

- Most of the glucometers are based on electrochemical technology which use electrochemical test strips to perform the measurement.
- Each glucometer test strip contains an enzyme called glucose oxidase. This enzyme then reacts with the glucose in the blood sample and creates an acid called gluconic acid.
- The gluconic acid thus formed then reacts with another chemical in the testing strip called ferricyanide. The ferricyanide and the gluconic acid then combine with each other and forms ferrocyanide.
- As soon as the ferrocyanide has been formed the device (i.e., glucometer) runs an electronic current through the blood sample on the strip.
- This current thus generated is able to read the ferrocyanide and identify the amount of glucose present in the blood sample on the testing strip.
- That number is then displayed on the screen of the glucometer.

Procedure

1. Clean the finger and proceed as per manufacturer's instructions.
2. A small drop of the blood is to be tested is placed on a disposable test strip of the glucometer for glucose measurement.

Accuracy of glucose meters is a common topic of clinical concern. Nearly all of the meters have similar accuracy (±10–15%) when used optimally. However, a variety of factors can affect the accuracy of a test. Factors affecting accuracy of various meters have included calibration of meter, ambient temperature, pressure use to wipe off strip, size of blood sample, high levels of certain drugs in blood, hematocrit, dirt on meter, humidity, and aging of test strips.

Glucose Tolerance Test

Glucose tolerance test (GTT) means ability of the body to utilize glucose in blood circulation. Glucose tolerance decreases in certain diseases like diabetes mellitus and endocrine disorders.

Blood glucose in case of normal individual remains fairly constant throughout the day. Except, after meals, there is temporary rise, which comes to normal within 2-3 hour of meal. In decreased tolerance level however, the blood sugar level does not return to normal within 2-3 hours of meal. Glucose tolerance test determines the degree and duration of hyperglycemia after an oral intake of known quantity of glucose.

The patient is prepared for the test by being kept on a diet containing 300 g of carbohydrate a day for three days before the test. Patient should come to laboratory in the morning after overnight fasting of 12-16 hours. Patient is not allowed to have tea/coffee/medicine/smoke/tobacco chew.

Procedure

1. First, collect the fasting urine and blood sample. If glucose is present in urine, do not perform GTT, instead take a post meal sample.
2. If glucose is absent, give patient 75 to 100 g glucose (1.50 g/kg body weight) dissolved in water. Note the time.
3. Thereafter, the blood and urine samples are collected for every 30 minutes for two and half hour.
4. Determine blood and urine sugar.
5. Prepare a glucose tolerance curve by plotting time on X-axis and glucose values on Y-axis **(Fig. 20.2)**.

Interpretation

1. **Glucose tolerance curve No. 1:** This is a normal type of curve. It shows fasting glucose within normal limits. Maximum blood

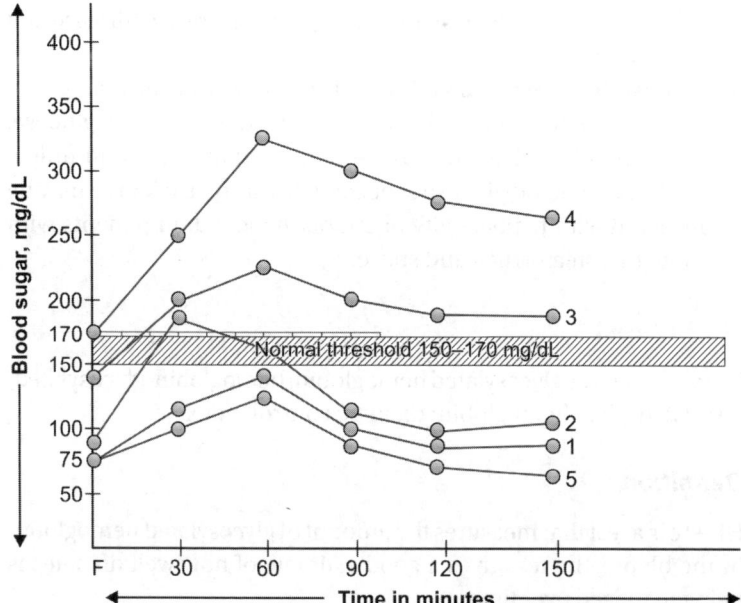

Fig. 20.2: Glucose tolerance test curves: (1) Normal; (2) Lag type; (3) Mild diabetic; (4) Severe diabetic; (5) Low glucose level.

glucose level is reached either half or one hour after taking glucose. Within 2 hours it comes rapidly to normal limits. Glucose should not present in any of urine sample.

2. **Glucose tolerance curve No. 2:** This type of curve is termed as lag curve. Here, the peak of blood glucose level may be higher than normal but the 2 hour value is within normal limits or often low. The increase in blood glucose level is due to delay in insulin mechanism coming into action. If the blood glucose level at peak of the curve is above the renal threshold level, glucose appears in next urine sample. Such a curve is seen in—normal individuals, after gastrectomy and in severe liver disease.

3. **Glucose tolerance curve No. 3 and 4:** This is present when ability of body to utilize glucose decreases. The rise in blood glucose is greater than in normal persons and the return of blood glucose to normal fasting level is delayed. GTC No. 3 indicates mild diabetes and GTC No. 4 indicates severe diabetes. This type of curve may

be seen in hyperactivity of hormones, very severe liver disease and severe infection.
4. **Glucose tolerance curve No. 5:** This curve indicates increased glucose tolerance, i.e. ability of the body to utilize more glucose. The fasting blood sugar may be below usual limits and only a small rise in blood glucose is observed. This type of curve may be observed with hypoactivity of endocrine gland, in patients with idiopathic steatorrhea and sprue.

HbA1c Test

It is also called as glycosylated hemoglobin; hemoglobin-glycosylated; A1c; GHb; glycohemoglobin; diabetic control index.

Definition

HbA1c is a test that measures the amount of glycosylated hemoglobin in the blood. The test gives a good estimate of how well diabetes is being managed over time.

Normally, only a small percentage of the hemoglobin (Hb) molecules in red blood cells become glycosylated (that is, chemically linked to glucose). The percent of glycosylation increases over time, and is higher if there is more glucose in the blood. Therefore, older red blood cells will have a greater percent of glycosylated hemoglobin, and diabetics whose blood glucose has been too high will have a greater percent of glycosylated hemoglobin.

This test measures blood sugar control over an extended period in people with diabetes. In general, the higher the HbA1c value, the higher the risk that a person will develop problems such as eye disease, kidney disease, nerve damage, heart disease, and stroke. This is especially true if the HbA1c remains elevated for more than one occasion.

Normal Values

HbA1c is normal if it is 5% or less. The test can show that the blood glucose levels have not been well-regulated over a period of weeks to months. If the HbA1c value is above 7%, it means diabetes is poorly controlled. High values indicate greater risk of diabetic complications. This test is recommended usually every 3 or 6 months.

C-Peptide Test

C-peptide is the abbreviation for connecting peptide, it is a 31-amino acid peptide, that is released into the blood as a byproduct of the formation of insulin by the pancreas. This test measures the amount of C-peptide in a blood or sometimes a urine sample.

In the beta cells of pancreas, proinsulin, a biologically inactive molecule, is split apart to form one molecule of C-peptide and one molecule of insulin. When insulin is released from the beta cells into the blood in response to increased levels of glucose, equal amounts of C-peptide are also released. Since C-peptide is produced at the same rate as insulin, it is useful as a marker of insulin production.

Specimen: Fasting of 8–10 hours is needed. Serum/EDTA-plasma/urine sample are used for c-peptide determination.

Principle of Test

Like other enzymes and hormones, C-peptide is determined by several immunoassays such as RIA, ELISA or CMIA.

The C-peptide ELISA assay kit is designed, developed and produced for the quantitative measurement of human C-peptide in serum and/or samples. The C-peptide ELISA assay kit utilizes the "sandwich" technique with selected antibodies that bind to various epitopes of C-peptide.

Assay standards, controls and samples are added directly to wells of a microplate that is coated with an anti-human C-peptide specific antibody. Simultaneously, a horseradish peroxidase-conjugated monoclonal C-peptide specific antibody is added to each well. After the first incubation period, the antibody on the wall of the microtiter well captures human C-peptide in the sample. A "sandwich" of "anti-C-peptide antibody—human C-peptide—HRP conjugated tracer antibody" is formed. The unbound tracer antibodies and other matrix protein from the test sample are removed in the subsequent washing step. For the detection of this immunocomplex, the well is then incubated with a substrate solution in a timed reaction and then measured in a spectrophotometric microplate reader. The enzymatic activity of the immunocomplex bound to human C-peptide on the wall of the microtiter well is directly proportional to the amount of C-peptide in the sample. A standard curve is generated by plotting the absorbance versus the respective human C-peptide concentration for each standard on point-to-point or 4 parameter curve fit. The concentration of human C-peptide in test samples is determined directly from this standard curve.

Clinical Interpretation

- C-peptide testing can be used to help evaluate the production of insulin made by the body (endogenous) and to help differentiate it from insulin taken in as diabetic medication (exogenous) which not generates C-peptide. This test may be done in conjunction with an insulin test or a glucose test.
- In vitro determination of insulin and C-peptide level help in differential diagnosis of liver disease, acromegaly, Cushing syndrome, familial glucose intolerance, insulinemia, renal failure, ingestion of accidental oral hypoglycemic drugs or C-peptide induced factitious hypoglycemia.
- It is helpful to differentiate between type 1 diabetes or type 2 diabetes. The pancreas of patients with type 1 diabetes is unable to produce insulin, so a decreased level of C-peptide, while C-peptide levels in type 2 patients is normal or higher than normal.
- C-peptide assays may be analytically more sensitive than insulin assays.
- Insulin and C-peptide are secreted into portal circulation in equimolar concentrations, fasting levels of C-peptide are 5–10 fold higher than those of insulin owing to the longer half-life of C-peptide. The liver does not extract C-peptide however; it is removed from the circulation by degradation in the kidneys with a fraction passing out unchanged in urine. Hence the urine C-peptide levels correlate well with fasting C-peptides levels in serum.
- A C-peptide test can also help find the cause of low blood sugar (hypoglycemia), such as excessive use of medicine to treat diabetes or a noncancerous growth (tumor) in the pancreas (insulinoma). A person with a low blood sugar level from taking too much insulin will have a low C-peptide level but a high level of insulin. An insulinoma causes the pancreas to release too much insulin, which causes blood sugar levels to drop (hypoglycemia). A person with an insulinoma will have a high level of C-peptide in the blood when they have a high level of insulin.

Result

The level of C-peptide in the blood must be read with the results of a blood glucose test. Both these tests should be done at the same time. A test to measure insulin level also may be done.

Normal value: Fasting: 0.51–2.72 nanogram per milliliter (ng/mL) or 0.17–0.90 nanomoles per liter (nmol/L).

High values are found in type 2 diabetes or insulin resistance (such as from Cushing's syndrome), hypoglycemia, insulinoma or that the use of certain medicines such as sulfonylureas (for example, glyburide) is causing the high C-peptide level.

Low values are found in liver disease, a severe infection, Addison's disease, or insulin therapy like in Type 1 diabetes and in complete removal of the pancreas (pancreatectomy).

Islet Cell Antibody for Type I

Islet cells are specialized cells in the pancreas that produce and secrete one of several hormones that affect certain body functions; some examples include alpha cells that produce glucagon and beta cells that produce insulin.

After a diagnosis of diabetes is made, islet cell antibody (ICA) for type 1 test is done to help distinguish autoimmune type 1 diabetes from type 2 diabetes.

Diabetes-related autoantibodies are proteins produced by the immune system that have been shown to be associated with type 1 diabetes. Testing can detect the presence of one or more of these autoantibodies in the blood.

Type 1 diabetes is a condition characterized by a lack of insulin due to autoimmune processes that destroy the insulin-producing beta cells in the pancreas. Diabetes-related autoantibodies reflect the destruction of beta cells, the loss of beta cell function, and inadequate production of insulin that are features of type 1 diabetes, but they are not thought to be the cause of type 1 diabetes. In contrast, type 2 diabetes primarily results from the body's resistance to the effects of insulin (insulin resistance) and does not involve autoimmune processes.

When autoimmune type 1 diabetes is present, one or more of the diabetes autoantibodies will be present in about 95% of those affected at the time of initial diagnosis. With type 2 diabetes, the autoantibodies are typically absent.

Four of the most common diabetes-related autoantibody tests include:
- Islet cell cytoplasmic autoantibodies (ICA)
- Glutamic acid decarboxylase autoantibodies (GADA)
- Insulinoma-Associated-2 Autoantibodies (IA-2A)
- Insulin autoantibodies (IAA).

Test	Abbr	Description	Comments
Islet cell cytoplasmic autoantibodies	ICA	Measures a group of islet cell autoantibodies targeted against a variety of islet cell proteins (*Note:* beta cells are one type of islet cell)	One of the most common islet cell autoantibodies detected at onset of disease; detected in about 70–80% of newly diagnosed type 1 diabetics
Glutamic acid decarboxylase autoantibodies	GADA	Tests for autoantibodies directed against beta cell protein (antigen) but is not specific to beta cells	Also one of the most commonly detected autoantibodies in newly diagnosed type 1 diabetics (about 70–80%)
Insulinoma-associated-2 autoantibodies	IA-2A	Tests for autoantibodies directed against beta cell antigens but is nonspecific	Detected in about 60% of type 1 diabetics
Insulin autoantibodies	IAA	Autoantibody targeted to insulin; insulin is the only antigen thought to be highly specific for beta cells	Detected in about 50% of type 1 diabetic children; not commonly detected in adults. IAA test does not distinguish between autoantibodies that target the endogenous

Contd...

Contd...

Test	Abbr	Description	Comments
			(produced in body) insulin and antibodies produced against exogeneous (externally incorporated) insulin

The autoantibodies seen in children are often different than those seen in adults. IAA is usually the first marker to appear in young children. As the disease evolves, this may disappear and ICA, GADA and IA-2A become more important. IA-2A is less commonly positive at the onset of type 1 diabetes than either GADA or ICA. Whereas about 50% of children with new-onset type 1 diabetes will be IAA positive, IAA positivity is not common in adults.

If ICA, GADA, and/or IA-2A are present in a person with symptoms of diabetes, the diagnosis of type 1 diabetes is confirmed. Likewise, if IAA is present in a child with diabetes who is not insulin-treated, type 1 diabetes is the cause.

Islet autoantibodies may also be seen in people with other autoimmune endocrine disorders such as Hashimoto thyroiditis or autoimmune Addison disease.

If no diabetes-related autoantibodies are present, then it is unlikely that the diabetes is type 1.

Diagnosis

Autoimmunity laboratories use immunoassays as the basic technique for the determination of autoantibodies. The central and main procedure principle for all autoantibody diagnostic assays is the capture of autoantibodies from serum using immobilized autoantigens immunofluorescence, the enzyme-linked immunosorbent assay (ELISA), multiplexed immunoassays.

Multiplexed immunoassays support the identification of multiple autoantibodies from a single determination in the same time.

Because GADA and IA-2A assays are automated, these tests are generally more available than ICA testing, which is labor-intensive and requires considerable expertise in interpretation.

Insulin (Hormone Test)

The traditional test methods for insulin and other indicators in clinical diagnosis, which include enzyme-linked immunosorbent assay (ELISA), radioimmunoassay, and various chemiluminescence-based techniques, are usually based on microplates and large automatic biochemistry analyzers.

Principle of the ELISA Method

The human insulin ELISA kit is a solid phase sandwich ELISA. The assay uses monoclonal antibodies (mAbs) directed against distinct epitopes of insulin. Samples including standards of known insulin content, control specimens, and unknowns are pipetted into the wells. A detector monoclonal antibody labeled with horseradish peroxidase (HRP) is added. After an incubation period, the microtiter plate is washed to remove unbound enzyme-labeled antibody and a substrate solution [tetramethylbenzidine (TMB)-H_2O_2] is added and incubated. The reaction is stopped with HCl and the microtiter plate is read spectrophotometrically. The intensity of color is directly proportional to the concentration of insulin in the original specimen.

Normal range:
- Adult = 6–26 μU/mL (43–186 pmol/L)
- Newborn = 3–20 μU/mL
- Possible critical value = >30 μU/mL

Increased insulin level is seen in:
- Insulinoma
- **Acromegaly:** Overproduction of growth hormone in these patients gives rise to constant stimuli for the production of insulin.
- **Cushing's syndrome:** Raised level of glucose by the overproduction of cortisol.
- Pancreatic islet cell hyperplasia.
- **Obesity:** There is a constant raised level of insulin.
- Fructose or galactose intolerance.

Decreased insulin level is seen in:
- Diabetes mellitus type 1 (maybe total lake or very low)
- Diabetes mellitus type 2, there is a low level of resistance to insulin.
- Hypopituitarism.

Urine Test for Presence of Glucose and Ketone Bodies

Urine Sugar Test

Examination of urine for glucose is rapid, noninvasive, and inexpensive for screening the urine. When blood sugar level exceeds 170 mg/dL, glucose appears in urine. This condition is called glycosuria. Increased concentration of glucose in urine indicates proportionate increase in blood sugar level.

Qualitative test for sugar determination test for glucose (or reducing substances such as fructose, lactose, galactose, pentose)

- *Benedict's test (Qualitative):* Take 5 mL of Benedict's qualitative reagent in test tube and add 0.5 mL of urine. Boil the content of tube. Let it stand on the rack for 5–10 minute. The appearance of yellow or red deposits indicates the presence of reducing substances, i.e., sugar. Cupric sulfate is reduced to cuprous oxide by boiling with reducing agents.

  Report: A slight green color, light turbidity or a bluish white precipitate (ppt) or no change is reported as negative. A greenish color with a little yellow deposit is reported as a trace (+), green yellowish (++), orange (+++) and brick red (++++) **(Fig. 20.3)**.

- Nowadays, paper strips are available commercially which are dipped in urine as directed and the color produced is matched against the color chart supplied. Glucose-specific enzyme glucose oxidase is used in strips. It is as instant screening method for urine sugar.

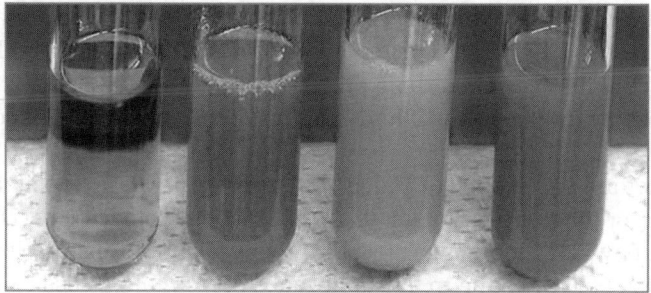

Fig. 20.3: Test tubes showing results of Benedict's test.
(For color version, see Plate 9)

Quantitative test for sugar determination

Reducing sugars (glucose) reacts with Benedict's quantitative reagent. Here, glucose reduces cupric ions to cuprous ions which react with potassium thionate in the reagent to form white ppt. This is very sharp reaction and easy to detect.

Procedure

- Pipette 5 mL of the Benedict's quantitative reagent in a porcelain dish.
- Add 2–3 g anhydrous sodium carbonate and mix well.
- Heat the mixture to the boiling point.
- Add urine drop wise with constant stirring with glass rod till the blue color of the reagent disappears and white ppt is formed.
- Note the titration reading.

Calculations:

$$\text{Urinary glucose (mg/dL)} = \frac{10 \times 10}{\text{Titration reading (mL)}}$$

Normal value: 0–0.3 g/24 hour.

Causes of Glycosuria: Diabetes mellitus, nondiabetic glycosuria includes emotional disturbances, hyperthyroidism, pregnancy, after ingestion of considerable carbohydrates, either anesthesia, in some infections, like pneumococcal pneumonia, etc.

Urine Ketone Test

A ketone test checks for presence of ketones in urine. Ketones are substances that are made when the body breaks down fat for energy. Normally, body gets the energy it needs from carbohydrates diet. But stored fat is broken down and ketones are made if diet does not contain enough carbohydrate to supply the body with sugar (glucose) for energy or if body cannot use blood sugar (glucose) properly.

Ketones are done to judge the severity of the acidosis and monitor the response to the treatment. Diabetic ketoacidosis (DKA) occurs when blood sugar levels are very high and insulin levels are low. In DKA, due to low or absence of insulin, glucose cannot get into the cells, so it builds up, resulting in high blood sugar levels.

Diagnostic methods:
- Urine ketones are usually measured as a "spot test" using a dipstick coated with chemicals that react with ketone bodies. The dipstick is dipped in the urine sample. Color change indicates the presence of ketones.
- **Rothera's test:** It is method of detecting acetone and acetoacetic acid in urine **(Fig. 20.4).**

Principle: Nitroprusside used in this test reacts with both acetone and acetoacetic acid in presence of alkali (NH_4OH) to produce permanganate calomel red ring at the junction.

Procedure:
- Saturate about 10 mL of urine with Rothera's mixture*.
- Add 2 mL of strong liquid ammonia slowly so that it floats over the urine.
- Wait for 5 minutes a purple (potassium permanganate) color indicates positive reaction.

Clinical significance:
In urine normal value: Ketone bodies are not present in normal urine.

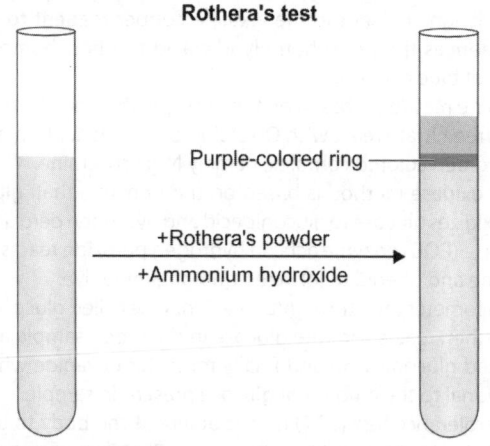

Fig. 20.4: Rothera's test.
(For color version, see Plate 9)

Composition of Rothera's mixture: Ammonium sulfate 99 parts + sodium nitroprusside 1 part. Grind and mix well.

Diabetic ketoacidosis (DKA) can occur when a diabetic's blood sugar is significantly increased, with illness severe infection, pregnancy, and a variety of other conditions. Diabetic ketoacidosis, if it progresses and worsens without treatment, can eventually cause unconsciousness, from a combination of a very high blood sugar level (more than 500 mg/dL), dehydration and shock, and exhaustion.

SUMMARY

- Diabetes mellitus is chronic disorder of carbohydrate metabolism, in which body cannot regulate the amount of glucose in the blood.
- The three main types of diabetes are type 1, type 2, and gestational diabetes.
- Type 1 diabetes is an autoimmune disease. It occurs when the insulin-producing islet cells in the pancreas are completely destroyed, so the body cannot produce any insulin.
- In type 2 diabetes, the islet cells are still working. However, the body is resistant to insulin.
- Gestational diabetes is a type of diabetes that develops only during pregnancy.
- Prediabetes is a border line situation of diabetes.
- Folin–Wu method of glucose is based on the principle that glucose reduces the cupric ions present in the alkaline copper reagent to cuprous ions, which reduces the phosphomolybdic acid to phosphomolybdous acid, which is of blue colored.
- O-toluidine method is based on the principle that the glucose present in a protein free filtrate react with O-toluidine in a hot acidic medium to form a stable green colored complex, namely N-glycosamine.
- Glucose oxidase method is based on the principle that, glucose oxidase (GOD) oxidizes glucose to gluconic acid and hydrogen peroxide is liberated. Peroxidase (POD) enzyme acts on hydrogen peroxide reacts with 4-amino antipyrine and phenol to form red quinoneimine dye.
- Each glucometer test strip contains an enzyme called glucose oxidase. This enzyme then reacts with the glucose in the blood sample and creates an acid called gluconic acid and finally forms ferrocyanide which is directly proportional to the amount of glucose present in sample.
- Glucose tolerance test (GTT) means ability of the body to utilize glucose in blood circulation. It is done after giving 75–100 g of glucose to patient.
- HbA1c is a test that measures the amount of glycosylated hemoglobin in the blood.
- A C-peptide test measures the level of this peptide in the blood. It is generally found in amounts equal to insulin.
- Islet cells are specialized cells in the pancreas that produce and secrete insulin.

- After a diagnosis of diabetes is made, islet cell antibody (ICA) for type 1 test is done to help distinguish autoimmune type 1 diabetes from type 2 diabetes.
- The traditional test methods for insulin and other indicators in clinical diagnosis, which include ELISA, radioimmunoassay, and various chemiluminescence-based techniques.
- When blood sugar level exceeds 170 mg/dL, glucose appears in urine. This condition is called as glycosuria.
- Urine test for sugars is Benedict's test based on the principle that, cupric sulfate is reduced to cuprous oxide by boiling with reducing agents. Different colors correspond to different grades of urine sugar.
- Diabetic ketoacidosis occurs when blood sugar levels are very high and insulin levels are low.
- Urine ketone test is done by Rothera's test based on the principle that nitroprusside used in this test reacts with both acetone and acetoacetic acid in presence of alkali (NH_4OH) to produce permanganate calomel red ring at the junction.

PRACTICE QUESTIONS

1. Which conditions can lead to diabetes?
2. Differentiate between type 1 and type 2 diabetes.
3. What is gestational diabetes? Discuss its complications.
4. What is prediabetes? Discuss symptoms related to it.
5. Write principle and procedure of Folin–Wu method of glucose detection.
6. Write principle and procedure of O-toluidine method of glucose detection.
7. Write principle and procedure of glucose oxidase method of glucose detection.
8. Why glucometer is considered as user friendly method for detection of glucose at home?
9. Write principle and working of glucometer.
10. What is meant by GTT? Mention procedure for the same.
11. How hemoglobin is related to glucose level in the blood? Write importance of HbA1c test.
12. Write importance of C-peptide test.
13. Write principle of C-peptide test.
14. What are diabetes-related autoantibody tests? Write a note on ICA type I test.
15. Write principle of insulin test.
16. What are urine tests related to diabetes?
17. Write principle, procedure and result observation for Benedict's test.
18. What is diabetic ketosis? Write a method to diagnose it.
19. Make a table of reference ranges of all tests included in diabetic profile.

CHAPTER 21

Liver Function Tests

Keywords

Regeneration, hepatocytes, sinusoids, portal vein, bile, Kupffer cells, bilirubin, unconjugated, conjugated, hepatitis, jaundice, biliverdin, biliary duct, Malloy and Evelyn method, diazotized sulfanilic acid, azobilirubin complex, Jendrassik-Grof method, alkaline tartrate, azobilirubin solution, transamination, alpha ketoacid, alanine aminotransferase (ALT), glutamate pyruvate transaminase (GPT), glutamate oxaloacetate transaminase (GOT), aspartate aminotransferase (AST), L-alanine, α-ketoglutarate, pyruvate, L-Aspartate (Asp), oxaloacetate, L-glutamate (glu), 2-4-DNPH, total protein albumin, globulin, biuret method, bromocresol green method, Kind and King method, alkaline phosphatase, disodium phenylphosphate phenol, 4-minoantipyrine potassium, ferricyanide, bile salts, glycocholic acid, taurocholic acid, hemoglobin, Fouchet's test, barium chloride, Gmelin's test, nitric acid, urobilinogen, Ehrlich's test, P-dimethylaminobenzaldehyde

■ INTRODUCTION

Liver is one of the vital organs of our body with wide range of functions. The liver is located just beneath the right rib cage. Liver is a reddish brown pyramid shaped organ. It weighs around 150 g at birth and increases to 1,200–1,500 g in adult.

■ MORPHOLOGY AND FUNCTIONS

It is the largest internal organ. It has two lobes—the bigger right lobe and smaller left lobe **(Fig. 21.1)**. The left and right lobes are divided by the falciform (sickle-shaped) ligament, which connects the liver to the abdominal wall.

Liver regeneration is the process by which the liver is able to replace lost liver tissue from the growth of the remaining tissue. The liver is the only visceral organ that possesses the capacity to regenerate. If

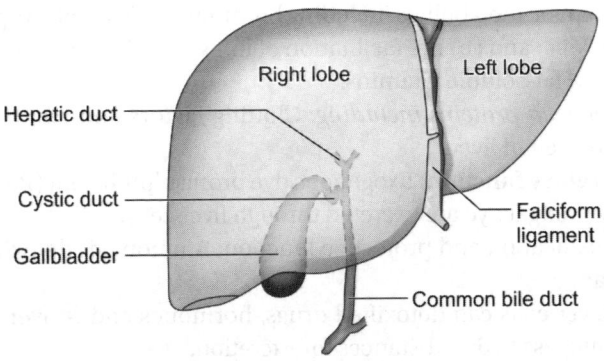

Fig. 21.1: Liver morphology.

75% of liver is removed the remaining 25% could regenerate a full size liver in 8–15 days. The liver can regenerate after either surgical removal or chemical injury.

The liver is made of multiple cells called as hepatocytes. These are functional unit of the liver, arranged in the form of small lobes, termed as lobule. Within the lobule there are spaces between the hepatocytes which are called sinusoids through which the blood flows. 80% of the blood supply to liver comes from portal vein. The portal vein carries blood containing digested nutrients from entire intestine, spleen, and pancreas.

Liver is a central organ of body metabolism and independently involves in many other biochemical functions. Liver perform over 300 diversified functions enumerated as follows:

1. **Metabolic function:** Liver is the key organ and the principal site where the metabolism of carbohydrate, lipids, protein, minerals, and vitamins take place.
    i. Glycogen is either synthesized (glycogenesis) or broken down (glycogenolysis) depending on plasma glucose and insulin
    ii. Fat is stored as triglycerides and hydrolyzed to glycerol and fatty acids,
    iii. Amino acids are transaminated, deaminated and decarboxylated
2. **Secretory function:** Liver secrets proteins, enzymes hormones (IGF-1, angiotensinogen) and other products.
    i. Liver is responsible for the formation and secretion of bile in the intestine. It serves two major purposes—(a) the excretion of

hepatic metabolites including bilirubin, cholesterol, drugs, and toxins; and (b) the facilitation of intestinal absorption of lipids and fat-soluble vitamins.
  ii. *Plasma proteins including:* Clotting factors and albumin are formed in liver.
3. **Excretory function:** Exogenous dye bromsulphthalein (BSP) and Rose Bengal dye are excreted through liver cells.
  Detoxification and protective function: Ammonia is detoxified to urea:
    i. Liver cells can detoxified drugs, hormones and convert them into less toxic substances for excretion.
    ii. Kupffer cells of liver perform phagocytosis to eliminate foreign compounds.
4. **Storage function:** Liver stores carbohydrates as glycogen.
    i. Trace mineral iron and vitamin B12, folic acid D and all fat-soluble vitamins (A, D, E, K) are stored in liver
5. **Acid-base balance:** Liver maintains acid-base balance by producing or consuming large numbers of hydrogen ions.

Liver Function Tests

These includes following tests:
- Serum bilirubin
- Serum glutamic pyruvic transaminase (SGPT)
- Serum glutamic oxaloacetic transaminase (SGOT)
- Serum protein
- Alkaline phosphatase (ALP)
- Urine—bile salts, bile pigments and urobilinogen.

The interpretation of liver function test plays a key role to diagnose jaundice, parenchymal diseases such as hepatitis, cirrhosis, and fatty liver infiltration, chronic hepatitis, altered drug metabolism, endocrine abnormality, nutritional and metabolic abnormality, etc.

■ SERUM BILIRUBIN

Bilirubin is a yellow bile pigment produced through hemolysis (breakdown) of red blood cells. Bilirubin is metabolized prior to excretion through the feces and urine.

Forms of Bilirubin

Bilirubin exists in two forms—(1) unconjugated and (2) conjugated.

Unconjugated bilirubin is insoluble in water. This means it can only travel in the bloodstream if bound to albumin and it cannot be directly excreted from the body.

In contrast, conjugated bilirubin is water soluble. This allows it to travel through the bloodstream without requiring any transport proteins hence; it can also be excreted out of the body.

Metabolism of Bilirubin (Fig. 21.2)

1. **Creation of bilirubin:** Reticuloendothelial cells are responsible for the maintenance of the blood, through the destruction of old or abnormal cells. They take up red blood cells and metabolize the hemoglobin present into its individual components—heme and globin. Globin is further broken down into amino acids which are subsequently recycled. Meanwhile, heme is broken down into iron and biliverdin. This process is catalyzed by enzyme heme oxygenase. The iron gets recycled, while biliverdin is reduced to create unconjugated bilirubin.

   Unconjugated bilirubin is insoluble in water. This means it can only travel in the bloodstream if it is bound to albumin and hence, it cannot be directly excreted from the body.

2. **Bilirubin conjugation:** In the bloodstream, unconjugated bilirubin binds to albumin and it is transported to the liver. In the liver, glucuronic acid is added to unconjugated bilirubin by the enzyme glucuronyl transferase. This forms conjugated bilirubin,

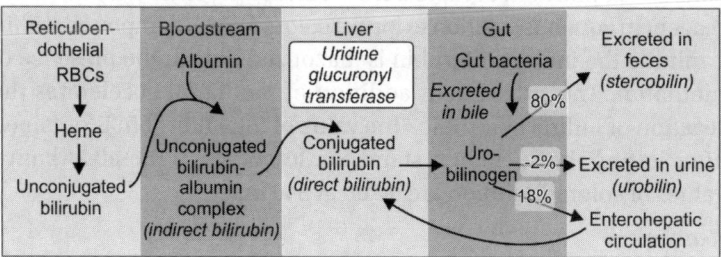

Fig. 21.2: Metabolism of bilirubin.

which is water soluble. This allows conjugated bilirubin to be excreted into the duodenum in bile.
3. **Bilirubin excretion:** From duodenum, bilirubin comes down in the colon. Once in the colon, colonic bacteria deconjugate bilirubin and convert it into urobilinogen. Around 80% of this urobilinogen is further oxidized by intestinal bacteria and converted to stercobilin and then excreted through feces. It is stercobilin which gives feces their color.

Around 20% of the urobilinogen is reabsorbed into the bloodstream as part of the enterohepatic circulation. It is carried to the liver where some is recycled for bile production, while a small percentage reaches the kidneys. Here, it is oxidized further into urobilin and then excreted into the urine.

Estimation of Bilirubin

Specimen: Serum is preferred for determination of bilirubin. It should not be hemolyzed. Protect it from light. Plasma can be used with anticoagulant such as heparin. Generally, fasting samples are preferred.

Note: Conjugated bilirubin also is called direct bilirubin because it reacts directly with the reagent, and unconjugated bilirubin is called indirect because it has to be solubilized first.

Method

Malloy and Evelyn Method

Principle:
Bilirubin couples with diazotized sulfanilic acid to form a purple colored azobilirubin complex. Direct bilirubin reacts with the diazo reagent in aqueous solution to form a colored diazo compound within 1 minute the indirect bilirubin is diazotized only in the presence of methanol. The subsequent addition of methanol accelerates the reaction of indirect bilirubin. The value of total bilirubin is obtained after letting the specimen stand for 30 minutes. The absorbance values of colored solution are taken at 540 nm.

Reagents:
- Diazo reagent A and B
- Methanol

- Conc. HCl
- Working bilirubin standard (std.) (10 mg%)
- Diazo blank reagent (1.5 mL conc. HCl diluted to make 100 mL with distilled water).

Procedure:
- Prepare diazo mixture by adding 5 mL diazo A and 0.15 mL of diazo B.
- Take four test tubes. Label them as, TT (total test), TB (total blank), DT (direct test), and DB (direct blank).
- Add the reagents as—
  - 0.1 mL serum and 0.9 mL distilled water in each tube
  - 0.25 mL Diazo blank in TB and DB
  - 0.25 mL Diazo reagent in TT and TB
  - 1.25 mL distilled water to DT and DB
  - 1.25 mL methanol to TT and TB.
- Mix well and read the OD of DT and DB after 1 minute against distilled water at 540 nm.
- Mix well and keep the tubes TT and TB in dark at room temperature for 30 minutes and read the OD against distilled water at 540 nm.
- Read OD of bilirubin std. (reagent 4) against distilled water.

Table showing Malloy and Evelyn method:

Reagent	TT	TB	DT	DB
Serum	0.1 mL	0.1 mL	0.1 mL	0.1 mL
Distilled water	0.9 mL	0.9 mL	0.9 mL	0.9 mL
Diazo blank	—	0.25 mL	—	0.25 mL
Diazo reagent	0.25 mL	—	0.25 mL	—
Distilled water	—	—	1.25 mL	1.25 mL
Methanol	1.25 mL	1.25 mL	—	—

Calculation:

$$\text{Total bilirubin (A)} = \frac{\text{OD of TT} - \text{OD of TB}}{\text{OD of Std}} \times 10$$

$$\text{Direct bilirubin (B)} = \frac{\text{OD of DT} - \text{OD of DB}}{\text{OD of Std}} \times 10$$

Indirect bilirubin = A – B

Jendrassik-Grof Method

Principle:
Bilirubin reacts with diazotized sulfonilic acid in presence of a strong alkaline tartrate solution gives blue azobilirubin solution. This is a reaction of direct bilirubin. Indirect bilirubin reacts with diazo reagent in presence of the accelerator caffeine benzoate. This reaction represents total bilirubin.

Reagents:
- 0.05 N HCl
- Caffeine benzoate reagent
- Diazo reagent
- Ascorbic acid solution
- Alkaline tartrate
- Normal saline.

Procedure:
Part I: Direct Bilirubin
1. Dilute the specimen by mixing 1 mL of specimen with 4 mL of saline.
2. Take two test tubes. Label them as, DT (direct test), and DB (direct blank).
3. To the tube DT, add 0.5 mL of diazo reagent and exactly after 1 minute add 1.5 mL alkaline tartrate.
4. Add 1 mL of diluted serum and 2 mL of 0.05 N HCl in both the tubes. Mix and after 10 minutes read the absorbance.
5. To DB, add 0.5 mL diazo A, 0.5 mL ascorbic acid and 1.5 mL alkaline tartrate. Mix and take the reading without waiting.

Reagent	DT	DB
Diazo reagent	0.5 mL	0.5 mL
Ascorbic acid	—	0.5 mL
Alkaline tartrate	1.5 mL	1.5 mL
Diluted serum	1 mL	—
0.05 N HCl	2 mL	—

Part II: Total Bilirubin
- Take two test tubes. Label them as, TT (total test), and TB (total blank)
- Place 1 mL of diluted serum and 2.1 mL caffeine benzoate reagent in both the tubes.

- Add 0.5 mL of diazo reagent in test.
- After 10 minutes add 1.5 mL of alkaline tartrate and take the absorbance after 10 minutes.
- In the tube TB, add 0.5 mL diazo A and then 1.5 mL alkaline tartrate.

Reagent	TT	TB
Dilute serum	1 mL	1 mL
Caffeine benzoate	2.1 mL	2.1 mL
Diazo reagent	0.5 mL	—
Alkaline tartrate	1.5 mL	—
Diazo reagent	—	0.5 mL
Alkaline tartrate	—	1.5 mL

Calculation:

$$\text{Total bilirubin (A)} = \frac{\text{OD of TT}}{\text{OD of Std}} \times \% \text{ of Std}$$

$$\text{Direct bilirubin (B)} = \frac{\text{OD of DT}}{\text{OD of Std}} \times \% \text{ of Std}$$

Indirect bilirubin = A − B

Normal values:

Total bilirubin:

Age	Value
Newborn:	up to 5.8 mg/dL
1–2 days:	up to 8.2 mg/dL
3–5 days:	up to 11.7 mg/dL

More than 1 month to adults:
Total bilirubin: Up to 1.0 mg/dL
Direct bilirubin: 0.0–0.2 mg/dL
Indirect bilirubin: 0.4–0.8 mg/dL

Clinical significance: Determination of serum bilirubin is important in diagnosis of diseases of hepatobiliary system and pancreas and other causes of jaundice. Jaundice becomes apparent clinically when serum bilirubin level goes more than 2.5 mg/dL.

Increased direct bilirubin is seen in hepatic cellular damage, liver diseases related to viral, toxic, alcohol or drugs, biliary duct obstruction, infiltrations, space occupying lesions, live metastatic tumor, etc.

Increased indirect bilirubin is seen in hemolytic diseases, ineffective erythropoiesis, blood transfusions, hematomas, hereditary disorders (e.g., Gilbert's disease).

■ TRANSAMINASES

Transamination is a process in which an amino group is transferred from an amino acid to an alpha keto acid. It is an important step in amino acid metabolism. The enzymes responsible for transamination are called transaminases. Two diagnostically useful transaminases are:
i. Glutamate pyruvate transaminase or GPT (also called alanine aminotransferase or ALT), and
ii. Glutamate oxaloacetate transaminase or GOT (also called aspartate aminotransferase or AST).

SGPT/ALT

Alanine aminotransferase (ALT), or the old name was glutamate-pyruvate transaminase (SGPT) which catalyzes the reversible transfer of the amino group between an amino acid and α-ketoacid where vitamin B6 (pyridoxal phosphate) is the cofactor.

Alanine aminotransferase is an enzyme found predominantly in the cytoplasm of liver cells. Any damage to the liver cells, SGPT enzyme, is released into circulation, specifically for liver cell necrosis.

Estimation of SGPT (ALT)

Method: 2-4-DNPH method.

Specimen: Serum is required for the test. Hemolysis should be avoided.

Principle: L-alanine + Oxoglutarate $\xrightarrow{\text{SGPT / ALT}}$ Pyruvate + Glutamate

Pyruvate so formed is coupled with 2, 4-dinitrophenyl hydrazine (2,4-DNPH) to corresponding hydrazone, which gives brown color in alkaline medium. This can be measured colorimetrically.

Reagents
- Buffered alanine α-KG substrate at pH 7.4
- DNPH color reagent
- 4N NaOH
- Working pyruvate std. 2 mm.

Procedure: Dilute 1 mL of 4N NaOH to 10 mL purified water. This makes the working solution.

Part I: Preparation of standard curve: Standardization is done against the standard Karmen unit assay and this is extrapolated to different amounts of pyruvate. The standard graph of enzyme activity (in units/mL) on X-axis versus OD on Y-axis shows that OD increases with increase in enzyme activity at a decreasing rate.

Take five test tubes, mark them as—1, 2, 3, 4, and 5 for corresponding enzyme activity—0, 28, 57, 97 and 150. Add the reagents as follows (table showing SGPT procedure):

Tube no.	1	2	3	4	5
Enzyme activity units/mL	0	28	57	97	150
Buffered alanine at pH 7.4	0.5 mL	0.45 mL	0.4 mL	0.35 mL	0.3 mL
Working pyruvate std. 2 mm	—	0.05 mL	0.1 mL	0.15 mL	0.2 mL
Purified water	0.1 mL	0.1 mL	0.1 mL	0.1 mL	0.1 mL
DNPH color reagent	0.5 mL	0.5 mL	0.5 mL	0.5 mL	0.5 mL

Mix well and allow it to stand at room temperature for 20 minutes. Add 5 mL of diluted NaOH to each tube. Mix well by inversion. Allow it to stand at room temperature for 10 minutes; measure the OD of all the five tubes against purified water on a colorimeter at 505 nm.

Part II: Preparation of test:
- Take 0.25 mL of buffered alanine at pH 7.4 in a test tube. Incubate at 37°C for 5 minutes.

- Add 0.05 mL serum to the test tube and again incubate at 37°C for 30 minutes.
- Now add 0.25 mL DNPH color reagent. Mix well by inversion. Allow to stand at RT for 20 minutes.
- At last add 2.5 mL diluted NaOH. Mix well and allow it to stand at RT for 10 minutes.
- Now measure the OD against purified water on a colorimeter at 505 nm.

Calculations: Mark the OD of test on Y-axis of standard curve and extrapolate it to the corresponding enzyme activity on X-axis.

Normal values:
- 5–45 IU/L
- It is slightly higher in infants and elderly.

Clinical significance:
Determination of SGPT level is important in differential diagnosis of diseases of hepatobiliary system and pancreas. Increased SGPT levels are found in severe preeclampsia, rapidly progressing acute lymphoblastic leukemia, obesity, etc.

Viral hepatitis and liver diseases (may reach 100 times), in cirrhosis (may reach 4–5 times), infectious mononucleosis, biliary duct obstruction (10–20 times).

Above 9,000 U/L are seen in alcohol-acetaminophen syndrome. This level can distinguish from alcoholic or viral hepatitis.

Decreased SGPT levels are found in genitourinary infection malignancy, malnutrition, pregnancy, alcoholic liver disease, etc.

SGOT/AST

This enzyme catalyzes the reversible transfer of amino groups between an amino acid, and α-ketoacids are called aminotransferase or transaminases.

This enzyme is distributed in all tissues (primarily all the tissues), but the highest concentration is found in the liver, heart, and skeletal muscles. The injury to cells leads to the release of the SGOT into the blood circulation and causes an elevation in the SGOT level.

Estimation of SGOT (AST)

Method: 2-4-DNPH method.

Chapter 21: Liver Function Tests

Specimen:
Serum is required for the test. Hemolysis should be avoided.

Principle:
GOT catalyzes following reaction—

L-aspartate + Oxoglutarate $\xrightarrow{\text{GOT / AST}}$ Oxaloacetate + Glutamate

Oxalate so formed is coupled with 2,4-dinitrophenyl hydrazine (2,4-DNPH) to corresponding hydrazone, which gives brown color in alkaline medium. This can be measured colorimetrically.

Reagents:
- Buffered aspirate α-KG substrate at pH 7.4
- DNPH color reagent
- 4N NaOH
- Working oxalate std. 2 mm.

Procedure: Dilute 1 mL of 4N NaOH to 10 mL purified water. This makes the working solution.

Part I: Preparation of standard curve:
Standardization is done against the standard Karmen unit assay and this is extrapolated to different amounts of oxalate. The standard graph of enzyme activity (in units/mL) on X-axis versus OD on Y-axis shows that OD increases with increase in enzyme activity at a decreasing rate.

Take five test tubes, mark them as—1, 2, 3, 4, and 5 for corresponding enzyme activity—0, 24, 61, 114 and 190. Add the reagents as follows (table showing SGOT procedure):

Tube no.	1	2	3	4	5
Enzyme activity units /mL	0	24	61	114	190
Buffered aspartate at pH 7.4	0.5 mL	0.45 mL	0.4 mL	0.35 mL	0.3 mL
Working oxalate std. 2 mm	—	0.05 mL	0.1 mL	0.15 mL	0.2 mL
Purified water	0.1 mL	0.1 mL	0.1 mL	0.1 mL	0.1 mL
DNPH color reagent	0.5 mL	0.5 mL	0.5 mL	0.5 mL	0.5 mL

Mix well and allow it to stand at room temperature for 20 minutes.

Add 5 mL of diluted NaOH to each tube. Mix well by inversion. Allow it to stand at room temperature for 10 minutes measure the OD of all the five tubes against purified water on a colorimeter at 505 nm.

Part II: Preparation of test:
- Take 0.25 mL of buffered aspartate at pH 7.4 in a test tube. Incubate at 37°C for 5 minutes.
- Add 0.05 mL serum to the test tube and again incubate at 37°C for 60 minutes.
- Now add 0.25 mL DNPH color reagent. Mix well by inversion. Allow to stand at RT for 25 minutes.
- At last add 2.5 mL diluted NaOH. Mix well and allow it to stand at RT for 10 minutes.
- Now measure the OD against purified water on a colorimeter at 505 nm.

Calculations: Mark the OD of test on Y-axis of std. curve and extrapolate it to the corresponding enzyme activity on X-axis.

Normal values:
- 5–40 IU/L
- New born and Infants have slightly raised values.

Clinical significance: Determination of SGOT level is important in differential diagnosis of diseases of hepatobiliary system and pancreas.

Increased SGOT levels are found in liver diseases such as cirrhosis, hepatic ischemia biliary obstruction, granulomas, etc. SGOT is also increased in—cerebral infarction, burns, intestinal injury, acute pancreatitis, etc. Marked increase, i.e., above 3,000 U/L is found in acute hypotension, toxic liver injury, liver trauma, viral hepatitis, etc.

Decreased SGOT levels are found in azotemia, chronic renal dialysis, malnutrition, pregnancy, alcoholic liver disease, etc.

SGOT:SGPT

The normal ratio of SGOT/ SGPT is 0.7 to 1.4. It is found increased in—drug hepatotoxicity (>2.0), alcoholic hepatitis (≤6.0), cirrhosis (1.4–2.0) intrahepatic cholestasis (>1.5) and chronic hepatitis.

AST (SGOT) is always is raised in acute myocardial infarction, where ALT (SGPT) will be normal unless there is damage to the liver.

ALT (SGPT) is more raised in acute hepatobiliary obstruction than AST (SGOT).

ALT (SGPT) is more specific than AST (SGOT) for liver cell injury. AST (SGOT) is more sensitive to alcoholic liver cell injury.

■ SERUM PROTEINS

Serum protein test in LFT measures total protein, albumin and A:G ratio.

Two main categories of proteins are found in the blood, albumin, and globulin.

1. Albumin is made by the liver and makes up about 60% of the total protein. Albumin keeps fluid from leaking out of blood vessels, nourishes tissues, and transports hormones, vitamins, drugs, and substances such as calcium throughout the body.
2. Globulins make up the remaining 40% of proteins in the blood. The globulins are a varied group of proteins, some produced by the liver and some by the immune system. They help fight infection and transport nutrients.

The test also compares the amount of albumin with globulin and calculates what is called the A/G ratio. A change in this ratio can provide a clue as to the cause of the change in protein levels.

Estimation of Serum Total Proteins

Method: Biuret method.

Specimen: Serum. Hemolysis is strictly avoided.

Principle: Proteins react with cupric ions in alkaline medium to form a violet colored complex. The intensity of color produced is directly proportional to proteins present in the specimen and can be measured at 530 nm.

Reagents:
- Biuret reagent.
- Protein std. (6 g/dL)

Procedure:
- Take three test tubes. Mark them as T, S and B and add 5 mL of Biuret reagent in each tube.
- Add 0.05 mL of serum, 0.05 mL of protein std. and 0.05 mL of distilled water in test, std. and blank, respectively. Mix thoroughly and keep at room temperature for exactly 10 minutes.
- Measure the intensities of test and std. against blank at 530 nm.

Reagent	T	S	B
Biuret reagent	5 mL	5 mL	5 mL
Serum	0.05	—	—
Protein std.	—	0.05	—
Distilled water	—	—	0.05

Calculations:

OD of T Serum proteins = $\dfrac{\text{OD of T}}{\text{OD of S}} \times 6$

Normal values:
- Adult = 6–8.0 g/dL
- Newborn = 4.6–7.4 g/dL
- Infants = 5.9–7.0 g/dL
- Child = 5.9–7.8 g/dL

Clinical significance: Determination of serum total proteins is useful in screening for nutritional deficiencies and gammopathies.

It is increased in multiple myeloma, dehydration, monoclonal gammopathy, hypergammaglobulinemias, and hypovolemic states. It is often found lower than limits in nutritional deficiency such as Kwashiorkor and Marasmus. Decreased protein synthesis like in case of severe liver disease, increased protein loss like in severe skin disease, GI disease, renal disease, and blood loss. Increased catabolism as in case of fever or inflammation, malignancy, etc.

Estimation of Serum Albumin

Method: Bromocresol green method.

Principle: Albumin binds specifically with bromocresol green at pH 4.1 to form green colored complex. The intensity of color is directly proportional to the amount of albumin present in the sample. The color is measured at 640 nm.

Specimen: Serum.

Reagents:
- Albumin reagent
- All standard (4.0 g/dL)

Procedure:
- Take three test tubes, mark them as test, std. and blank. Add 5 mL albumin reagent, in each tube
- Add 0.05 mL serum, 0.05 mL albumin std. and 0.05 mL distilled water to test, std. and blank, respectively.

Reagent	T	S	B
Albumin reagent	5 mL	5 mL	5 mL
Serum	0.05	—	—
Albumin std.	—	0.05	—
Distilled water	—	—	0.05

- Mix thoroughly and keep at room temperature for exactly 10 minutes.
- Measure the intensity of the test and std. against blank at 640 nm

Calculation:

$$\text{Serum albumin} = \frac{\text{OD of T}}{\text{OD of S}} \times 4$$

Normal values:
- Adult = 3.5–5 g/dL
- Newborn = 3.5–5.4 g/dL
- Infants = 4.4–5.4 g/dL
- Child = 4–5.9 g/dL

Clinical significance: Determination of serum albumin is important in disorders of protein metabolism.

Albumin levels are high in dehydration and intravenous albumin infusions.

Albumin is found to be decreased in—malnutrition, decreased absorption, liver diseases, chronic infection, hyperthyroidism, pregnancy, burns, hemorrhage, etc.

Decreased albumin synthesis seen in liver diseases and decreased amino acid intake. Increased albumin loss is seen in kidney diseases such as nephrotic syndrome, blood loss, and burns. Increased catabolism of albumin seen in malignancy and inflammation resulting in low levels of albumin.

Estimation of Serum Globulin

Serum globulin can be obtained when the values of total protein and serum albumin are known.

Total protein = Serum albumin + Serum globulin

∴ Serum globulin = Total protein − Serum albumin

Normal values:

Age	Values
<1 year:	0.4–3.7
1–3 years:	1.6–3.5
4–9 years:	1.9–3.4
10–49 years:	1.9–3.5

A/G Ratio

$$\text{A/G Ratio} = \frac{\text{Serum albumin}}{\text{Serum globulin}}$$

Normal value = 1.2:1 to 2:1.

Clinical significance: Calculation of A/G ratio is also helpful in diagnostic interpretation for liver disease. An alteration in the A/G ratio and reversal may occur due to the reduction in albumin and or elevation of globulin. The ratio is reduced and often reversed in cirrhosis with jaundice. However, the ratio may be increased in some cases of xanthomatosis or biliary cirrhosis.

■ ALKALINE PHOSPHATASE

Alkaline phosphatase is called alkaline because its function is seen between a pH of 9 to 10 and best at a pH of 9.0.

Alkaline phosphatase is present in most tissues but is present in high concentration in liver, bones, intestines, spleen, placenta and kidney. ALP in the intestine is associated with lipid transport. ALP is also associated with the calcification process of the bone.

In liver, it is involved in transport of phosphate across cell membrane. The ALP's main function is to remove the phosphate group from the proteins and other molecules.

Liver ALP isoenzyme is ALP1. This is derived from the epithelial cells of the biliary tract. The normal route of elimination is its excretion into the intestine as bile.

Method

Kind and King's method.

Specimen

Serum is preferred, but heparinized plasma can also be used. Other anticoagulants inhibit the enzyme activity. Overnight fasting serum is preferred; store the serum in refrigerator if immediate analysis is not possible.

This is because at room temperature, activity of ALP increases by 1% for every 6 hours.

Principle

Alkaline phosphatase from serum converts phenyl phosphate to inorganic phosphate and phenol at pH 10. Phenol so formed reacts in alkaline medium with 4-aminoantipyrine in presence of the oxidizing agent potassium ferrocyanide and forms an orange-red colored complex which can be measured colorimetrically. The color intensity is proportional to enzyme activity.

Reaction

$$\text{Phenyl phosphate} \xrightarrow{\text{Alkaline phosphatase}} \text{Phenol} + \text{Phosphate}$$

$$\text{Phenol} + \text{4-amino antipyrine} \xrightarrow[\text{OH}^-]{\text{Pot. ferricyanide}} \text{Orange red}$$

Reagents

- Substrate: Disodium phenyl phosphate
- Bufffer: $NaHCO_3 + Na_2CO_3$ (pH 10)
- Phenol std: 0.01 mg/mL
- NaOH
- 4-aminoantipyrine
- Potassium ferricyanide (oxidizing agent).

Procedure

Take four test tubes. Mark them as—test, control, std. and blank. Add the reagents according to following table.

Reagents	T	C	S	B
Buffer substrate	1 mL	1 mL	—	—
Buffer	1 mL	1 mL	1.1 mL	1.1 mL
Phenol std.	—	—	1 mL	—
Distilled water	—	—	—	1 mL
Serum	1 mL	—	—	—
Incubate at 37°C for 15 minute				
NaOH	0.8 mL	0.8 mL	0.8 mL	0.8 mL
Serum	—	0.1 mL	—	—
4- amino antipyrine	1 mL	0.8 mL	1 mL	1 mL
Potassium ferricyanide	1 mL	0.8 mL	1 mL	1 mL

Mix after addition of each reagent and measure the OD of T, C, S and B against distilled water at 540 nm after 10 minutes.

Calculations

$$\text{Serum ALP} = \frac{\text{OD of test} - \text{OD control}}{\text{OD std.} - \text{OD blank}} \times 0.10$$

Age up to 29 days = 70 to 380 IU/L
Age 29 days–16 years = 60 to 425 IU/L
Age more than 16 years = 30 to 130 IU/L

Clinical Significance

Determination of ALP is important in diagnosis of causes and monitoring of course of cholestasis (e.g., neoplasm, drugs). It is also helpful in diagnosis of various bone disorders (e.g., Paget's disease).

Alkaline phosphatase is increased in—bone disorders such as osteomalacia, Hodgkin's disease, increased deposition of calcium, etc. Liver diseases such as liver infiltrates, nodules in liver, hepatic congestion due to heart disease 44% of diabetic patients have 40% increase of ALP. 15-20 times increase in ALP is found in primary cirrhosis and liver cancer. 1-2 times raised level may be seen in various liver parenchymal diseases like hepatitis and cirrhosis.

In extrahepatic obstruction, ALP increases three times the normal. In the case of complete obstruction, ALP may be raised 10–12 times. In the case of infectious diseases, ALP rises two times normal value.

ALP is decreased in—excess vitamin D ingestion, celiac disease, malnutrition, scurvy, zinc deficiency, magnesium deficiency, and hypothyroidism. In one-third patients of pernicious anemia, ALP level is decreased.

URINE ANALYSIS: BILE SALT, BILE PIGMENT, AND UROBILINOGEN

Random urine sample is required to test bile salts, bile pigment, and urobilinogen. The principle components of bile are cholesterol, bile salts, and the pigment bilirubin.

Metabolism of Bile Salts

Bile acids are synthesized in the hepatocytes from cholesterol. These are excreted into the bile and then pass into the duodenum. The primary bile acids are—cholic acid and chenodeoxycholic acid. These primary bile acids pass into the duodenum, by the bacterial action are converted to secondary bile acids. Secondary bile acids are—deoxycholic acid and lithocholic acid. The bile acid can conjugate with glycine and taurine and form bile salts. Bile salts help in stimulating the bile flow and are a potent antibacterial.

Detection of Bile Salts (Hay's Test)

Principle: Bile salts consist of glycocholic acid and taurocholic acid. They lower the surface tension of the fluid and thus cause sulfur particles to sink **(Fig. 21.3)**.

Procedure:
- Take about 3–5 inch column of urine in a small beaker or in a test tube.
- Sprinkle finely powered dry sulfur over the surface from a height of about half-inch.
- If bile salts are present, the sulfur powder will sink at bottom.

The presence of bile salts indicates obstructive jaundice.

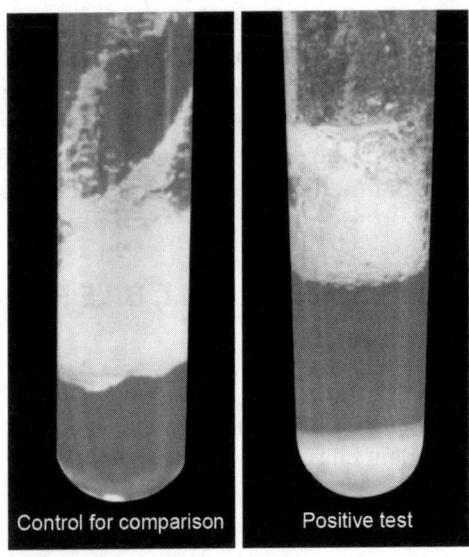

Figs. 21.3A and B: (A) Control for Hay's test: (B) Positive Hay's test.
(For color version, see Plate 10)

Metabolism of Bile Pigments

The primary bile pigments are due to catabolism of the hemoglobin (as discussed earlier) are:
- Bilirubin is orange or yellow in color.
- Biliverdin is green in color.
- Urobilinogen is converted to the yellow pigmented urobilin apparent in urine.

The leading site of the formation of bile pigments is liver. Ultimately these leave the body in feces and a small amount in the urine.

Detection of Bile Pigments

For bile pigments, following two tests are most common:
1. **Fouchet's test:**
   Principle: Bile pigments present in urine solution reacts with barium chloride ($BaCl_2$) to form white precipitate. When this is dried and reacted with Fouchet's reagent green or bluish green color precipitate is obtained due to formation of complex derivative. This is the most sensitive test.

Procedure:
- If the urine is alkaline or neutral, acidify it with few drops of 2% acetic acid.
- To about 10 mL of acidic urine, add about 5 mL of 10% barium chloride solution. Mix well and filter.
- To the residue (white ppt.) on the filter paper add a drop of Fouchet's reagent.
- A green or blue color indicates presence of bile pigments, i.e., biliverdin and bilirubin, respectively.

2. **Gmelin's test:**
Principle: Nitric acid oxidizes bilirubin to biliverdin giving different colors from green to violet.
Procedure:
- Take about 5 mL of concentrated HNO_3 in a test tube.
- Add an equal volume of urine carefully so that the two liquids do not mix.
- At the junction of two liquids various colored rings will be formed.
- *Color formed are yellow*-bilirubin/green-biliverdin/red-bilifushchin/violet-bilicyanin

Detection of Urobilinogen

Urobilinogen is colorless. The intestinal bacteria oxidize urobilinogen to urobilin, which is a brown pigment. Metabolism of urobilinogen is discussed earlier.

Ehrlich's Test

Principle: The test for urobilinogen is based on the Ehrlich aldehyde reaction.

P-dimethylaminobenzaldehyde in an acid medium with a color enhancer reacts with urobilinogen to form a pink-red color.

Note: To avoid interference, if the urine sample contains bile pigment, it should be removed by addition of 1 part of 10% aqueous solution of calcium chloride to four parts of urine and filtering it.

Procedure:
- To 10 mL of fresh urine, add 1 mL of Ehrlich aldehyde reagent.
- Allow it to stand for 3 minutes.

- If red/cherry color is obtained, it indicates presence of urobilinogen in urine.
- Intensity of color developed depends on the amount of urobilinogen present.
- For feces, the same method can be used except:
    - Stool aqueous extract is treated with the alkaline ferrous hydroxide to reduce urobilin to urobilinogen. Then Ehrlich's reagent is added.

Normal value:
Random sample = < 1 mg/dL
24 hours sample = 0.5–4 mg/dL

Clinical Significance

- **Bile salts:** Positive bile salt test is seen in:
    - Obstructive jaundice
    - Liver diseases with the appearance of jaundice
- **Bile pigments:** Positive bile pigment test is seen in:
    - Hepatitis and liver diseases are caused by infection or exposure to toxic agents (cirrhosis)
    - Obstructive biliary tract disease/liver or biliary tract tumor
    - Septicemia, hyperthyroidism
    - Presence of gallstones
    - Metastatic tumor in the liver
    - Urine bilirubin is negative in hemolytic disease.
- **Urobilinogen:** Increased urobilinogen is seen in:
    - Cirrhosis (due to alcoholic cirrhosis, viral diseases, chemicals)
    - Biliary obstruction/biliary tract infection, cholangitis
    - Hepatotoxic drugs, e.g., aminosalicylic acid, phenothiazine, and penicillin
    - Due to increased RBCs destruction (hemolytic anemia/pernicious anemia/malaria/drugs)
    - Acute hepatitis, pulmonary infarction
    - Hematoma, excessive ecchymosis
- Decreased urobilinogen is seen in:
    - Presence of gallstones
    - Biliary obstruction/severe biliary tract infection
    - Pancreatic cancer

Table 21.1: Presence of urine bilirubin and urobilinogen in various conditions.

Test	Normal person	Hemolytic anemia	Liver disease	Biliary obstruction
Urine bilirubin	Negative	Negative	Positive/negative	Positive (+++)
Urine urobilinogen	Negative	Positive (+++)	Positive (+++)	Absent (Low)

- Drugs such as aspirin, chloramphenicol, insulin, etc.
- Its absence indicates obstructive jaundice.

Table 21.1 shows the presence of urine bilirubin and urobilinogen in various conditions.

SUMMARY

- Liver is the largest internal organ of the human body. It has two lobes—the bigger right lobe and smaller left lobe.
- Liver regeneration is the process by which the liver is able to replace lost liver tissue from the growth of the remaining tissue.
- Liver perform over 300 diversified functions including metabolic of organic molecules, secretion of enzymes and hormones, excretion of some dyes and drugs, storage of minerals and vitamins and maintaining acid base balance.
- Bilirubin exists in two forms—unconjugated and conjugated. Unconjugated bilirubin is insoluble in water while conjugated is soluble.
- Bilirubin is metabolized prior to excretion through the feces and urine. Bilirubin metabolism can be summarized as a series of steps, including: (1) production, (2) uptake by the hepatocyte, (3) conjugation, (4) excretion into bile ducts, and (5) delivery to the intestine.
- Bilirubin concentration is detected by Malloy and Evelyn method— bilirubin couples with diazotized sulfanilic acid to form a purple colored azobilirubin complex.
- Bilirubin concentration is detected by Jendrassik-Grof method—bilirubin reacts with diazotized sulfonilic acid in presence of a strong alkaline tartrate solution gives blue azobilirubin solution.
- Transamination is a process in which an amino group is transferred from an amino acid to an alpha ketoacid.
- Alanine aminotransferase (ALT), or (SGPT) catalyzes—
    - L-alanine + α-ketoglutarate ⇌ pyruvate + L-glutamate
    whereas, AST or SGOT catalyzes—
    - L-Aspartate (Asp) + α-ketoglutarate ⇌ oxaloacetate + L-glutamate (Glu)
    Both are determined by 2-4-DNPH method. ALT (SGPT) is more specific than AST (SGOT) for liver cell injury.

- Serum total protein includes albumin (60%) and globulin (40%).
- *Total protein by Biuret method*: Proteins react with cupric ions in alkaline medium to form a violet.
- Albumin concentration is measured by Bromocresol green method. Albumin binds specifically with Bromocresol green at pH 4.1 to form green colored complex.
- Alkaline phosphatase is involved in transport of phosphate across cell membrane. It has hydrolytic and phosphate transferase activity.
- Kind and King method for ALP: At an alkaline pH it hydrolyzes disodium phenylphosphate to form phenol. The phenol formed reacts with 4-aminoantipyrine in the presence of potassium ferricyanide, as an oxidizing agent, to form a red colored complex.
- *Bile salts in urine:* Bile salts consist of glycocholic acid and taurocholic acid. They lower the surface tension of the fluid and thus cause sulfur particles to sink.
- Bilirubin and biliverdin are two important bile pigments formed in the decomposition of hemoglobin.
- Bilirubin presence in urine is detected by Fouchet's test with 10% barium chloride and Gmelin's test with nitric acid.
- Urobilinogen is detected by Ehrlich's test. P-dimethylaminobenzaldehyde in an acid medium with a color enhancer reacts with urobilinogen to form a pink-red color.

PRACTICE QUESTIONS

1. Write location and morphology of liver.
2. What is meant by regeneration? Explain it with reference to liver.
3. Enlist various functions of liver.
4. Write a note on how bilirubin is metabolized in the body.
5. Differentiate between:
   i. Conjugated and unconjugated bilirubin
   ii. Albumin and globulin
   iii. AST and ALT
6. Write principle and procedure for Malloy and Evelyn method of bilirubin estimation.
7. Write principle and procedure for Jendrassik-Grof method of bilirubin estimation.
8. What is transamination? Explain role of enzymes involved in this.
9. Write principle and procedure for estimation of AST.
10. Write principle and procedure for estimation of ALT.
11. What are serum protein tests? Give its clinical importance.
12. Write principle and procedure for estimation of serum total proteins.
13. Write principle and procedure for estimation of albumin

14. What is role of alkaline phosphatase? Give its clinical significance.
15. Write principle and procedure for estimation of alkaline phosphatase.
16. Explain metabolism of bile salts and tests to determine presence of bile salts in urine.
17. What are bile pigments? How they are metabolized in the body?
18. Explain tests to determine presence of bile pigments in body.
19. What is urobilinogen? Write principle and procedure to detect its presence in urine.
20. Make a table of all liver function tests with its reference values.

CHAPTER 22

Renal Function Tests

> **Keywords**
> Fibrous capsule, cortex, medulla, nephron, glomerulus, Bowman's capsule, renal pyramids hilum proximal convoluted tubule, loop of Henle, distal convoluted tubule, calcitriol, urea, erythropoietin, blood urea nitrogen, urease, ammonia, α-ketoglutarate glutamate dehydrogenase (GLDH), Berthelot reaction, hypochlorite, indophenol, diacetyl monoxime, urea clearance test, hemodialysis, creatinine, creatine phosphate, alkaline-picrate method, creatinine clearance test, uric acid, Henry–Caraway method, glomerular filtration rate (GFR), urinary calculi, nephrolithiasis, ureterolithiasis, cystolithiasis, calcium, magnesium ammonium phosphate, cystine, Fourier transform infrared (FTIR) spectroscopy

■ INTRODUCTION

A renal function tests are a group of tests that may be performed together to evaluate kidney (renal) function. These mainly include urine and blood tests for urea, uric acid and creatinine.

The kidneys lie on the posterior abdominal wall, one on each side of the vertebral column. They extend from T12 to L3 vertebrae and in this way they get protection from lower ribs. The right kidney is slightly lower than the left one because of the space occupied by the liver. These are bean-shaped organ of about 11 cm long, 6 cm wide and 3 cm thick. It weighs around 150 g.

■ STRUCTURE AND FUNCTIONS OF KIDNEY

The kidney is divided in three sections **(Fig. 22.1A)**:
1. Outer fibrous capsule that surrounds the kidney.
2. The cortex is the reddish-brown tissue which is middle layer present just below the capsule and outside the renal pyramids.
3. The medulla is the innermost layer, which consists of pale conical shaped structure known as renal pyramids.

Chapter 22: Renal Function Tests

The hilum is a small opening located on the inner edge of the kidney, where it curves inward. It is an opening where the blood vessels, lymph vessels, ureters and nerves enter.

The kidney contains 1-2 millions of nephrons which are the functional units of kidneys.

Nephrons

The nephron is like tubule which is closed at one end and joins to the collecting duct at the other end (**Fig. 22.1B**). The closed end of

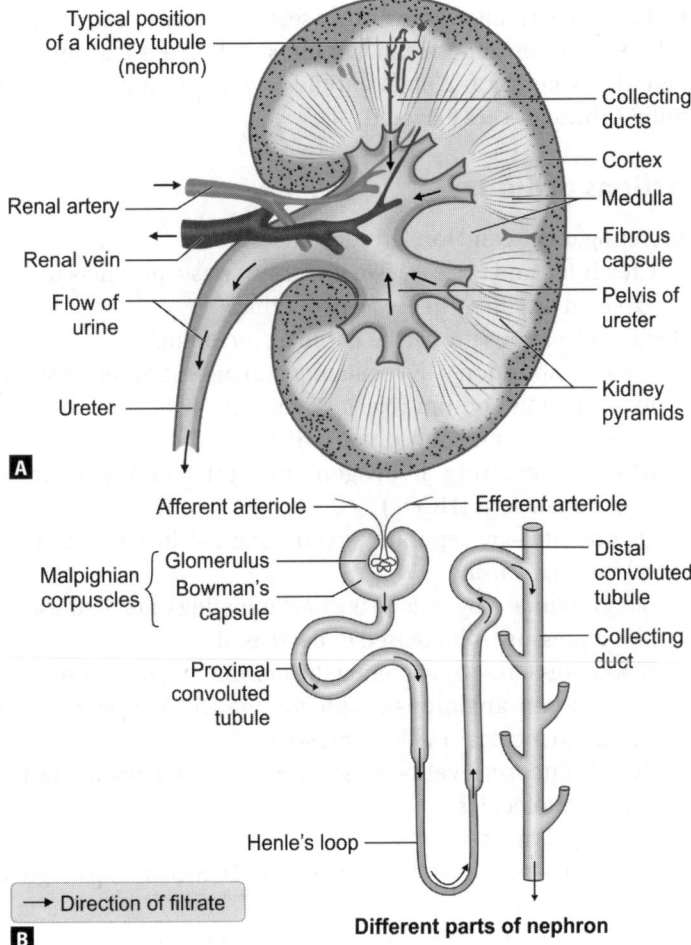

Figs. 22.1 A and B: Structure of the kidney and nephron.

nephron is a cup-shaped structure known as glomerular capsule or Bowman's capsule. This is a place where blood is initially filtered. It completely surrounds the network of tiny capillaries known as glomerulus. Continuing the glomerular capsule is the remaining nephron which is about 3 cm long and is divided in three parts:

1. **Proximal convoluted tubule (PCT):** Folded structure connected to the Bowman's capsule where selective reabsorption occurs.
2. **Loop of Henle:** A selectively permeable loop that descends into the medulla and establishes a salt gradient.
3. **Distal convoluted capsule (DCT):** A folded structure connected to the loop of Henle where further selective reabsorption occurs.

All essential substances and 178 liters of fluid are reabsorbed in the tubules, whereas 1–2 liters of fluids, waste products, and other harmful substances are excreted.

Functions of Kidney

- Excreting wastes and foreign substances:
    - Creatinine and urea are two important waste products that are excreted by kidney in the form of urine.
- Regulating various properties of blood, including:
    - Ionic composition—by regulating the concentrations of several ions, such as sodium (Na^+), potassium (K^+), calcium (Ca^{2+}), chloride (Cl^-) and phosphate (HPO_4^{2-})
    - pH—by excreting hydrogen ions (H^+) and conserving bicarbonate ions (HCO_3^-)
    - Osmolarity—by separately regulating the loss of water and solutes in the urine
    - Blood volume—by conserving or eliminating water in the urine, blood pressure is increased or decreased
    - Blood pressure—by secreting the enzyme renin, a component of the renin-angiotensin-aldosterone (RAA) system; renin causes an increase in blood pressure
    - Blood glucose levels—by synthesizing and releasing new glucose molecules
- Producing hormones
    - Calcitriol—the active form of vitamin D, which helps regulate calcium levels
    - Erythropoietin (EPO)—which stimulates the production of red blood cells.

RENAL FUNCTION TESTS

Proteins cannot be stored in the body when these are in excess then surplus amino acids are catabolized for energy. Breakdown of the proteins and nucleic acid gives rise to a non-protein nitrogenous compound in the blood and these are urea, amino acids, urates, ammonia, and creatinine. All these products are harmful and must be removed from the body.

The important blood and urine parameters that are measure of kidney functions are—urea, uric acid and creatinine.

Urea: Blood and Urine Test

Urea Metabolism

Urea is the major end product of nitrogen metabolism in humans. Ammonia, the product of oxidative deamination reactions, is toxic in even small amounts and must be removed from the body. The urea cycle or the ornithine cycle describes the conversion reactions of ammonia into urea. Since these reactions occur in the liver, the urea is then transported to the kidneys where it is excreted. The overall urea formation reaction is:

2 Ammonia + Carbon dioxide + 3 ATP → Urea + Water + 3 ADP

Estimation of blood urea nitrogen

Urea constitutes the major non-protein nitrogen (NPN) of the blood. It represents 45–50% NPN of the blood. It is also the major NPN substance excreted in the urine. In some countries, blood urea is represented as blood urea nitrogen (BUN). BUN reflects only the nitrogen (molecular weight 28) content of urea (molecular weight 60). Therefore, urea measurement reflects the whole of the molecule urea is approximately twice (60/28 = 2.14) that of BUN.

mg % Urea = BUN × 2.14

Thus BUN 10 mg/dL is equivalent to urea 21.4 mg/dL.

If BUN has to be calculated from urea %, it is multiplied by 0.467 (28/60 = 0.467).

BUN = Urea (mg%) × 0.467

Urea is estimated by following methods:
- Rate of reaction method—UV kinetic
- Berthelot reaction method (end-point reaction)
- Diacetylmonoxime method (DAM method)

Note: When urea standard is used, the value comes out is blood urea (or serum urea) and if urea nitrogen standard is used the value is in terms of BUN.

Rate of reaction method—UV kinetic

Principle: Urea is hydrolyzed to ammonia and carbon dioxide by urease. In presence of ammonia α-ketoglutarate and glutamate dehydrogenase (GLDH), NADH is reduced to NAD⁺.

The rate of decrease in OD is measured at the interval of 30 seconds up to 3 minutes at 340 nm. This is directly proportional to the urea concentration in the specimen.

$$\text{Urea} + H_2O \xrightarrow{\text{Urease}} 2NH_3 + CO_2$$

$$NH_3 + \alpha\text{-Ketoglutarate} + NADH + H^+ \xrightarrow{\text{GLDH}} \text{Glutamate} + NAD^+$$

Specimen: Serum.

Reagent:
1. Enzyme vials
2. Diluent (at pH8)
3. Urea nitrogen std. (20 mg/dL)

Procedure:
- Prepare working reagent by mixing contents of one enzyme vial with 20 mL of the diluent. It is stable at 2–4°C for 20 days.
- Take 1 mL of working reagent in a cuvette, add 0.01 mL serum, mix well, and note the change in OD/min (Δ AT) after every 30 second up to 3 min.
- Then take 1 mL of working reagent in a cuvette and add 0.01 mL of urea nitrogen standard (std.) (20 mg/dL). Mix well and note the change in OD/min (Δ AS) after 30 seconds up to 3 min.

$$\text{BUN} = \frac{\Delta AT}{\Delta AS} \times 20$$

Berthelot reaction method (end-point reaction)

Principle: The principle is based on the Berthelot reaction. Urease splits urea into ammonia and carbon dioxide. The ammonia reacts with phenol in the presence of hypochlorite to form indophenol, which with alkali gives a blue colored compound. The intensity of colored compound can be measured at 546 nm.

Specimen: Serum or heparinized plasma.

Reagents:
1. Urease/Buffer reagent
2. Phenol reagent
3. Hypochlorite reagent
4. Std. urea nitrogen (20 mg/dL)

Procedure:
- Take three test tubes. Label them as T, S, and B. Add 0.5 mL of urease reagent in each tube.
- Add 0.02 mL of serum in test and 0.02 mL of standard in std. Mix well and keep at 37°C for 10 minutes. Add 1 mL of phenol reagent and 1 mL of hypochlorite reagent in each tube. Mix well and keep at 37°C for 10 minutes.
- Now add 5 mL of distilled water in each tube. Mix thoroughly and read optical densities of test and standard against blank at 546 nm.

Reagent	Test	Std.	Blank
Urease/buffer reagent	0.5 mL	0.5 mL	0.5 mL
Serum/plasma	0.02 mL	—	—
Std. urea nitrogen (20 mg/dL)	—	0.02 mL	—
Mix well and keep at 37°C for 10 minutes			
Phenol reagent	1 mL	1 mL	1 mL
Hypochlorite reagent	1 mL	1 mL	1 mL
Mix well and keep at 37°C for 10 minutes			
Distilled water	5 mL	5 mL	5 mL

Calculations:

$$\text{Serum urea nitrogen} = \frac{\text{OD of T}}{\text{OD of S}} \times 20$$

Diacetylmonoxime method:

Principle: Urea reacts with diacetylmonoxime in hot medium (100°C) and in the presence of thiosemicarbazide and ferric ions to form a pink colored compound. The color intensity is directly proportional to amount of urea in specimen. It is measured at 520 nm.

Specimen: Serum is preferred; however, heparinized plasma or fluoride plasma can be used.

Reagents:
1. DAM-TSC reagent (diacetylmonoxime thiosemicarbazide)
2. Uric acid reagent
3. Stock urea std. 1 g%
4. Urea working std. (50 mg%)

Procedure: Take 3 test tubes, mark them as T, S and B, for test, std. and blank, respectively.
Add the reagents as per following table:

Reagent	Blank	Std.	Test
Distilled water	3.6 mL	3.5 mL	3.5 mL
Blood	—	—	0.1 mL
Urea working std. (50 mg %)	—	0.1 mL	—
10% sodium tungstate	0.2 mL	0.2 mL	0.2 mL
2/3 N sulfuric acid	0.2 mL	0.2 mL	0.2 mL

Mix well and allow to stand for 5 min. Centrifuge and pipette out into three test tubes as follows:

Reagent	Blank	Std.	Test
Supernatant	2 mL	2 mL	2 mL
DAM-TSC reagent	3 mL	3 mL	3 mL
Urea acid reagent	3 mL	3 mL	3 mL

Mix it. Plug with cotton and place it in a boiling water bath for exactly 15 min. Cool and take the reading at 520 nm.

Calculation:

$$\text{Serum urea} = \frac{\text{OD of test} - \text{OD of blank}}{\text{OD of std} - \text{OD of blank}} \times 50$$

Reference Range:
- Urea = 20 to 40 mg/dL
- Blood urea nitrogen = 10–20 mg/dL
    - Children (BUN) = 5–18 mg/dL
    - Infants = 5–18 mg/dL
    - Newborn = 3–12 mg/dL
    - Cord blood = 21–40 mg/dL
- Elderly people may have a higher level than the adult.

Clinical significance: Determination of BUN is used in diagnosis of renal insufficiency. A BUN of 50-150 mg/dL implies serious impairment of renal function. Markedly increased BUN (150-250 mg/dL) indicates severely impaired glomerular function. BUN is also increased in hemorrhage to GI tract, stress, shock, congestive heart failure, acute myocardial infraction, vomiting, diarrhea, etc. Postrenal causes of increase in BUN are—ureteral obstruction from stones, tumors, or congenital abnormality. Bladder outlet obstruction from prostatic hypertrophy and cancer are also responsible for high BUN.

BUN is found to be lowered in overhydration, severe liver damage, increased utilization of proteins for synthesis, malnutrition low protein diet, poisoning, hepatitis, etc.

Urine urea

This test is mainly used to assess the protein balance and the amount of dietary protein needed by severely ill patients. Urine urea serves this purpose, as it is a measure of protein breakdown in the body.

Urea is excreted by the kidneys, so excretion of urea can reflect kidney function. The urine urea excretion is also measured to obtain a ratio between the plasma (blood) urea and the urine urea. This ratio (U/P urea) is an indicator of how well the kidneys are able to filter and excrete urea from the bloodstream.

Specimen and method:
Urine urea test can be done with random urine sample or 24 hours urine sample.

For 24 hours urine sample: Discard the first urine sample and note the time. Start collecting urine in container for next 24 hours. 10 g of boric acid can be used as preservative/24 hours. Alternatively, it can be stored in a refrigerator.

Diacetylmonoxime method (as described for serum urea) can be applied for urine sample.

For the determination of urine urea nitrogen 24 hours of urine sample diluted to 1:20 is used.

$$\text{Urine urea nitrogen} = \frac{\text{OD of test} - \text{OD of blank}}{\text{OD of std} - \text{OD of blank}} \times 200 \times \text{dilution of urine}$$

Normal value:
Urine urea nitrogen = 12-20 g/day (428.4-714 mmol/day).

Clinical Significance:
Low levels usually indicate: Malnutrition (inadequate protein in diet), kidney dysfunction and increased reabsorption or low protein diet.
High levels usually indicate: Excessive protein intake and increased protein breakdown in the body.

Urea clearance

Urea clearance is the hypothetical amount of blood from which kidney clears urea in 1 minute. This is measured by measuring the concentration of urea in blood, concentration of urea in urine and amount of urine excreted over a 1 hour interval. Urea clearance is less than its glomerular filtration as some of the urea that is filtered at the glomerulus is reabsorbed at the tubules.

Urea clearance is defined the volume of the blood cleared of urea per minute by either renal clearance or hemodialysis.

- To measure urea clearance first the patient should void urine and then made to drink two glasses of water.
- The urine is collected after an hour and a blood specimen is also collected at the same time.
- Then second urine sample is collected after another hour.
- The urea level in the two urine samples and the blood sample is measured.
- The urine volume is calculated as urine output per minute.

When there is a good flow of urine that is, more than 2 mL/min, the proportion of urea, which is reabsorbed, is fairly constant and the clearance is calculated by the usual formula. The value obtained is then called the maximum urea clearance (C_m).

$$C_m = \frac{UV}{P}$$

where,
V = Urine volume in mL per min.
U = Urine urea conc. in mg/100 mL
P = Plasma urea conc. in mg/100 mL

With maximum clearance, normal range is 64–99 mL/min.

If urine flow is less than 2 mL per min., the high concentration of urea in the renal tubules causes increased reabsorption. To compensate for the lower clearances observe with the reduced urine flow with a different formula is applied.

$$C_s = \frac{U\sqrt{V}}{P}$$

With standard clearance, normal is 40–68 mL/min.

Clinical significance:

The urea clearance values fall progressively with increasing renal failure. If the clearance falls below 20% it is considered to be severe renal failure. Below 5% uremic comas may be present.

Creatinine: Blood and Urine Test

Creatinine is a non-protein nitrogenous compound that is produced by the breakdown of creatine. It is present in muscle, brain and blood in free form as well as in the form of creatine phosphate. Creatinine is largely formed in muscle by irreversible and non-enzymatic removal of water from creatine phosphate.

It is filtered out of the blood by the kidneys and then excreted by body in urine. It is filtered at the glomeruli and secreted by the tubules. Creatinine is produced at a steady rate and is affected very little by diet or normal physical activities. If the kidneys are damaged and cannot function normally, the amount of creatinine in the urine decreases while the amount of creatinine in the blood increases. Thus estimation of creatinine directly reflects the kidney function.

Estimation of Serum Creatinine

Method: *Alkaline-picrate method (Jaffe reaction)*

Principle: Creatinine reacts with picric acid in alkaline medium to form a reddish yellow complex. Intensity of which is directly proportional to the concentration of creatinine in the specimen. It is measured at 520 nm.

Specimen: Serum or plasma.

Reagents:

1. 0.04 M picric acid reagent
2. 10 g/dL sodium hydroxide
3. Working creatinine std. 1 mg/dL—this is prepared in 0.01 N HCl by using stock creatinine std. 100 mg/dL.

4. 2/3 N sulfuric acid
5. Alkaline picrate*

Procedure: Part I. Preparation of protein free filtrate
Take two test tubes. Mark them as test and std. Add the reagents as follows:

Reagent	Test	Std.
Distilled water	3 mL	4 mL
Serum	1 mL	—
Standard (1 mg/dL)	—	1 mL
2/3 N sulfuric acid	0.5 mL	—
10 g/dL Sodium tungstate	0.5 mL	—

Centrifuge the content in the test and get clear filtrate.

Part II. Formation of color
Take three test tubes and label it as T, B, and S. Add the reagents as per following table.

Reagent	Test	Std.	Blank
Distilled water	3 mL	3 mL	3 mL
Filtrate	2 mL	—	—
Diluted Std.(part I)	—	2 mL	—
Alkaline picrate reagent	1 mL	1 ml	1 mL

Mix well and keep at room temperature for 20 min. Read the intensities of test and std. at 520 nm against blank.

Calculations:

$$\text{Serum creatinine mg/dL} = \frac{\text{OD of test}}{\text{OD of std}} \times 100$$

Reference range:

Adult:
- Male = 0.6–1.0 mg/dL
- Female = 0.5–1.1 mg/dL
- Elderly = Decrease in muscle masses cause the decreased value
- Child = 0.3–0.7 mg/dL

---

*Prepare alkaline picrate reagent by mixing 4 parts of reagent 1 and 1 part of reagent 2. This working reagent is to be freshly prepared whenever needed.

- Infants = 0.2–0.4 mg/dL
- Newborn = 0.3–1.2 mg/dL

Clinical significance:
Serum creatinine determination is useful in the diagnosis of renal insufficiency. Serum creatinine is more specific and sensitive indication of renal disease than BUN.

Serum creatinine levels is high in ingestion of creatinine (roast meat), muscle disease such as gigantism and acromegaly, prerenal azotemia and postrenal azotemia. Injury to the muscles, postrenal obstruction of urine, congestive heart failure, shock and myasthenia gravis.

50% loss of renal function is needed to increase serum creatinine from 1.0–2.0 mg/dL. Therefore it is not sensitive to mild to moderate renal injury.

The decreased creatinine level are seen in old-age due to decreased muscle mass, pregnancy especially in the first and second trimester, advanced and severe liver disease, and in case of inadequate dietary intake.

BUN/creatinine ratio: It is important to evaluate the renal function.

The normal BUN/creatinine ratio is around 10:1. Having a ratio above this range could mean not getting enough blood flow to kidneys, and could have conditions such as congestive heart failure, dehydration, or gastrointestinal bleeding.

BUN/creatinine ratio decreased is very rare and this may be seen in protein deficiency in the diet and in severe liver disease.

Urine Creatinine

The daily production of creatinine is dependent upon the muscle mass. Women excrete less creatinine than men because of less muscle mass. Creatinine excretion is not affected by protein metabolism or other external factors. Creatinine is raised only when the 50% function of the kidney is lost. There is a minimal amount of creatinine in the urine from tubular secretion. Creatinine amount in the urine increases as the creatinine concentration rises in the blood.

For the determination of urine creatinine, 24 hours of urine sample diluted to 1:10 is used.

Alkaline picrate method (serum creatinine) can be applied. If proteins are present, deproteinization of urine is must.

Calculations:

$$\text{Urine creatinine mg/dL} = \frac{\text{OD of test}}{\text{OD of std}} \times 100$$

For the determination of 24 hours creatinine excretion, measure the urine volume, and calculate the result as follows:

$$\text{Creatinine excretion, mg/24 hours} = \frac{\text{Urine creatinine mg/dL} \times \text{vol. of 24 hours urine}}{100}$$

Normal value:
- Male: 14–26 mg/kg of body weight/24 hour
- Female: 11–20 mg/kg of body weight/24 hour
- Creatinine excretion in the urine decreases with age.

Clinical significance: The amount of creatinine excreted varies with the muscle mass and is nearly constant for individual. Increased excretion of creatinine occurs in tissue metabolism, i.e., in fever. The excretion rate decreases in all kinds of renal diseases and also in postrenal conditions. Decreased excretion of creatinine also occurs in starvation, muscle atrophy and muscular weakness.

Creatinine Clearance Test

Creatinine is filtered at the glomerulus and its reabsorption at the tubular level is insignificant. Because of this creatinine clearance can be used to measure glomerular filtration rate (GFR). It is measured over a period of 24 hours.

Creatinine clearance is defined as the amount of plasma in mL, which would have to be completely cleared of the creatinine, each minute by both the kidneys in order to account for its rate of excretion.

A creatinine clearance test measures how well creatinine is removed from blood by the kidneys. Compared to a blood creatinine level, a creatinine clearance test provides a more precise measure of how well the kidneys are working. A creatinine clearance test is performed both on a blood sample and on a sample of urine collected over 24 hours (24-hour urine sample).

The specimen is 24-hour urine sample. The actual period of urine collection must be accurately timed. The starting and finishing of the test of the patient should be done with an empty bladder. The urine volume is measured and minute volume V is calculated.

$$V = \frac{\text{Total volume of urine in mL}}{\text{Time of collection in minute}}$$

The creatinine concentration of urine (U) and plasma (P) are determined by above methods. In case of any delay in performing the test, specimen should be stored in refrigerator.

$$\text{Creatinine clearance} = \frac{U \times V}{P}$$

Normal value: Clearances vary with body weight. It is generally expressed as 1.73 m² of the body surface area.
- **Male:** 95–140 mL/min
- **Female:** 85–125 mL/min

Clinical significance: Clearance values are decreased in impaired renal function and so provide a rough impression of glomerular damage. It decreases in renal failure with values below 10 mL per minute in severe cases. In less severe failure cases the creatinine clearance will have fallen to about half before a raise in blood creatinine is detectable. Clearance tests are therefore of most value in the diagnosis of early renal disease. They are also useful in monitoring progress, although once the serum creatinine is raised, this estimation alone will be sufficient.

Uric Acid: Blood and Urine Test

Uric Acid Metabolism

Uric acid is the end product of purine metabolism. The first step in the catabolism of purines (adenine and guanine) is their hydrolytic deamination to form xanthine and hypoxanthine. These are then oxidized to uric acid. Uric acid is filtered in the glomeruli and partially reabsorbed by the tubules and then it is excreted in urine. Most of the body purines excreted as uric acid into the urine.

Mainly uric acid is formed in the liver. From liver it is transported to the kidney through the blood.

The blood level of the uric acid depends upon the rate of synthesis in the liver and the rate of excretion by the kidneys.

Estimation of serum uric acid

Henry-Caraway method

Principle: Uric acid in protein free filtrate reacts with phosphotungstic acid reagent in alkaline medium to form a blue colored complex. The intensity of color is measured at 660 nm.

Reagents:
- Deprotenizing reagent
- Sodium carbonate (10 g/d W/V)
- Stock phosphotungstic acid reagent
- Stock uric acid std. (100 mg/dL)

Procedure:
- Dilute stock phosphotungstic acid to 1:10 and stock uric acid std. to 1:200
- In a centrifuge tube, take 5.4 mL of deprotenizing reagent. Add 0.6 mL of serum. Mix well and centrifuge at 3,000 RPM for 10 minutes.
- Now take 3 test tubes, label them as test, std. and blank. Take 3 mL of filtrate, 3 mL of diluted std. and 3 mL of D/W in T, S, and B tubes, respectively.
- Add 1 mL of sodium carbonate and 1 mL of diluted phosphotungstic acid in each tube.
- Mix well and keep in dark for exactly 10 minute.
- Read O.D. of test and std. at 660 nm against blank.

Reagent	T	S	B
Filtrate 3 mL	—	—	
Dilute std.	—	3 mL	—
D/W	—	—	3 mL
Sodium carbonate	1 mL	1 mL	1 mL
Dilute phosphotungstic acid	1 mL	1 mL	1 mL

Calculation:

$$\text{Serum uric acid} = \frac{\text{OD of T}}{\text{OD of S}} \times 5$$

Enzymatic method

Principle: Enzyme uricase converts uric acid to allantoin and hydrogen peroxide. In the presence of peroxidase, hydrogen peroxide reacts with phenolic chromogens to form red colored compound. The intensity of red color is proportional to the amount of uric acid in the sample.

Reaction:

$$\text{Uric acid} + H_2O \xrightarrow{\text{Uricase}} \text{Allantoin} + H_2O_2$$

$$H_2O_2 + \text{Phenolic chromogens} \xrightarrow{\text{peroxidase}} \text{Red color compound}$$

Reagents:
- Uric acid reagent
  Components of uric acid reagent are uricase (100 IU/L), peroxidase (140 IU/L), chromogen (2.5 µMol/L) and buffer (pH 7.5)
- Uric acid std.

Specimen: Serum.

Procedure:
- Take 3 test tubes, mark them as T, S and B. Take 0.025 mL of serum, 0.025 mL of std. and 0.025 mL of distill water in tubes T, S and B, respectively.
- To each tube and 1 mL of uric acid reagent.

Reagent	T	S	B
Serum	0.025 mL	—	—
Std.	—	0.025 mL	—
Distill water	—	—	0.025 mL
Uric acid reagent	1 mL	1 mL	1 mL

- Allow the tubes to stand for 10 minutes at room temperature.
- Measure the OD at 590 nm against blank.

Calculation:

$$\text{Uric acid} = \frac{\text{OD of T}}{\text{OD of S}} \times 5$$

Normal value:

Adult:
- Male = 4.0–8.5 mg/dL
- Female = 2.7–7.3 mg/dL
    - Elderly people = Values may be slightly increased
    - Child = 2.5–5.5 mg/dL
    - Newborn = 2.0–6.2 mg/dL

Clinical significance:

Uric acid levels are very liable and show day-to-day and seasonal variation in some person. It is also increased by emotional stress, total fasting, increased body weight, renal diseases and renal failure. It is found to be increased in gout, leukemia, polycythemia, anemia, psoriasis, hypo- and hyperparathyroidism. It is increased with high protein, weight reduction diet, alcohol consumption, arteriosclerosis and hypertension. Serum uric acid is increased in 80% patients with elevated serum triglycerides.

Serum uric acid levels are decreased in Wilson's disease, Fanconi syndrome, carcinomas, Hodgkin's disease, 5% patients of postoperative state (GI surgery, coronary artery bypass) diabetes mellitus. It is also low in healthy adults with isolated defect in tubular transport of uric acid.

Urine uric acid

The urine uric acid is made up of an exogenous part that is formed from purine rich diet and an endogenous part that is formed from the breakdown of nucleoproteins. Urine uric acid is done to find if kidney stones are due to high uric acid levels in the body and to evaluate uric acid metabolism in gout.

For the determination of urine uric acid, 24 hours of urine sample is collected.

Do not refrigerate the urine; add NaOH (10 mL) to keep the urine alkaline.

Henry–Caraway method (serum uric acid) can be applied. Use dilution 1:200.

If proteins are present, deproteinization of urine is must.

Calculations:

Urine uric acid mg/dL = $\dfrac{\text{OD of test}}{\text{OD of std}} \times 100$

For the determination of 24 hours uric acid excretion, measure the urine volume, and calculate the result as follows:

$$\text{Uric acid excretion, mg/24 hours} = \frac{\text{Urine uric acid (mg/dL)} \times \text{Vol. of 24 hours urine}}{100}$$

Normal value: ≤ 750 mg/24 h.

Clinical significance: A consistently high uric acid excretion is found in gout and leukemia. Viral hepatitis, high purine diet, Wilson's disease, and sickle cell anemia are the condition in which urine uric acid levels are raised. Decreased urine uric acid level seen in long-term alcohol abuse, chronic glomerulonephritis (chronic kidney disease), folic acid deficiency and acidosis.

The uric acid determination is important to find out the possibility of urinary calculi (of uric acid type). The uric acid creatinine ratio is more than 1.0 in most patients with acute renal failure due to hyperuricemia but lower in other causes of acute renal failure.

Glomerular filtration

Glomerular filtration filters out most of the solutes due to high blood pressure and specialized membranes in the afferent arteriole. The blood pressure in the glomerulus is maintained independent of factors that affect systemic blood pressure. The "leaky" connections between the endothelial cells of the glomerular capillary network allow solutes to pass through easily. All solutes in the glomerular capillaries, except for macromolecules such as proteins, pass through by passive diffusion. There is no energy requirement at this stage of the filtration process.

The glomerular filtration rate (GFR) is defined as the volume of glomerular filtrate formed in all the renal corpuscles of both kidneys each minute. GFR is regulated by multiple mechanisms and is an important indicator of kidney function.

In adults, the average is 125 mL/min for men and 105 mL/min for women. Homeostasis of body fluids dictates that a relatively constant GFR is required.

$$\text{Formula for GFR} = \text{eGFR} = K \times \frac{(140 - \text{age in year}) \times \text{weight (kg)}}{\text{Serum creatinin} (\mu mol/L)}$$

K = (1.23 for male and 1.04 for female)

If the GFR is too high, needed substances may pass through the renal tubules and be lost in the urine. If the GFR is too low, all of the filtrate may be reabsorbed and too few waste products excreted.

Urinary calculi

Urinary calculi are solid particles in the urinary system. The urinary system consists of a pair of kidney, pair of the urinary tract, two ureters, the bladder, and the urethra. The kidneys filter waste out of the blood and produce urine, which is transported from the kidneys to the bladder through tube-like ureters. Urine is eliminated from the bladder through the urethra. This is a continual process of waste filtration, urine production, and elimination.

A renal calculus (kidney stone) forms in the kidney from substances that would normally pass out of the body in the urine. When there are large amounts of these substances, they separate from the urine and form kidney stones.

Location: Their location may be—(i) in the kidney (nephrolithiasis), (ii) ureter (ureterolithiasis), or (iii) bladder (cystolithiasis).

Size: A kidney stone can be as small as a grain of sand or as large as a golf ball.

Composition: Chemical composition of stones varies as follows:
- **Calcium (Ca):** About 80% of stones are made up of calcium. Common causes for this type of stone are hypercalciuria, (a hereditary condition present in 50% of men and 75% of women with Ca calculi), hyperparathyroidism, hypocitruria, (urinary citrate <350 mg/day, because citrate normally binds urinary Ca and inhibits the crystallization of Ca salts), and renal tubular acidosis.
    - *Calcium oxalate:* About 70% of calculi are composed of calcium oxalate.
    - *Calcium phosphate:* About 15% of calculi are composed of calcium phosphate.
    - *Uric acid:* About 10% of calculi are composed of uric acid. Most commonly, it develop as a result of increased urine acidity (urine pH <5.5), or rarely with severe hyperuricosuria (urinary uric acid.
    - >1,500 mg/day), which crystallizes undissociated uric acid. Uric acid crystals may comprise the entire calculus or, more

commonly, provide a nidus on which Ca or mixed Ca and uric acid calculi can form.
- **Struvite (magnesium ammonium phosphate):** About 3% of calculi are composed of magnesium ammonium phosphate. Struvite, (infection calculi) indicate the presence of a UTI (urinary tract infection) caused by urea-splitting bacteria (e.g., *Proteus spp., Klebsiella spp.*). The calculi must be treated as infected foreign bodies and removed in their entirety. Unlike other types of calculi, magnesium ammonium phosphate calculi occur three times more frequently in women.
- **Cystine:** About 2% of calculi are composed of cystine. It occurs only in the presence of cystinuria. Cystinuria is an inherited defect of the renal tubules in which resorption of the amino acid cystine is impaired, urinary excretion is increased, and cystine stones form in the urinary tract.

Pathophysiology:
Urinary calculi may remain within the renal parenchyma or renal pelvis or be passed into the ureter and bladder. During passage, calculi may irritate the ureter and may become lodged, obstructing urine flow and causing hydroureter (the swelling of the ureter with urine due to blockage) and sometimes hydronephrosis. Common areas of lodgment include the ureteropelvic junction, the distal ureter, and the ureterovesical junction. Larger calculi are more likely to become lodged. Typically, a calculus must have a diameter more than 5 mm to become lodged. Calculi less than 5 mm are likely to pass spontaneously.

Even partial obstruction causes decreased glomerular filtration, which may persist briefly after the calculus has passed. With hydronephrosis and elevated glomerular pressure, renal blood flow declines, further worsening renal function. Permanent renal dysfunction occurs after about 28 days of complete obstruction. Secondary infection can occur with long-standing obstruction.

Symptoms and signs:
Even large calculi remaining in the renal parenchyma or renal pelvis are usually asymptomatic unless they cause obstruction and/or infection. Severe pain, fever, often accompanied by nausea and vomiting, usually occurs when calculi pass into the ureter, cause obstruction, or both. Sometimes gross hematuria also occurs.

Patients may have symptoms of a urinary tract infection (UTI) such as fever, dysuria, or cloudy or foul-smelling urine.

Pain (renal colic) is of variable intensity but is typically excruciating and intermittent, often occurs cyclically, and lasts 20-60 minutes. Pain in the flank or kidney area that radiates across the abdomen suggests upper ureteral or renal pelvic obstruction. Pain that radiates along the course of the ureter into the genital region suggests lower ureteral obstruction. Suprapubic pain along with urinary urgency and frequency suggests a distal ureteral, ureterovesical, or bladder calculus.

Need of stone analysis:
A kidney stone analysis is done to:
- Find the chemical composition of a kidney stone.
- Guide treatment for a kidney stone.
- Give information on how to prevent the formation of more kidney stones.

Imaging studies:
- Calcium-containing stones are relatively radiodense, and they can often be detected by a traditional radiograph of the abdomen that includes the kidneys, ureters, and bladder.
- CT Scan or ultrasound imaging studies are the diagnostic modality of choice for diagnosis of suspected nephrolithiasis.

Laboratory examination:
- Microscopic examination of the urine, which may show red blood cells, bacteria, leukocytes, urinary casts and crystals. Urinary pH is also important.
- Complete blood count (CBC), looking for increase neutrophil count suggestive of bacterial infection, as seen in the setting of struvite stones or any stone with kidney infection.
- Renal function blood tests (creatinine, urea) to look for loss in renal function.
- Blood test for abnormally high blood calcium blood levels (hypercalcemia).
- 24-hour urine collection to measure total daily urinary volume, magnesium, sodium, uric acid, calcium, citrate, oxalate and phosphate.

Stone analysis

Sample collection

Random urine sample is collected in a clean container with a straining device that has a fine mesh. Microscopic observation is performed looking for crystals.

For a kidney stone that is too large to pass, a health practitioner may perform a surgical procedure to remove it and then send the stone for analysis.

A laboratory will first document the physical characteristics of a stone—its size, shape, weight, color and texture.

Chemical composition of stone can be identified by using one or different combinations of following methods.

Methods to diagnose chemical composition:

Some of the basic principles for chemical analysis are as follows:
- **Carbonate:** Little powdered stone (in mortar with the help of pestle) is acidified with 15N hydrochloric acid. Liberation of carbon indicates the presence of carbonate.
- **Oxalate:** Addition of 20% sodium acetate. A white precipitate indicates the presence of oxalate.
- *Phosphate:* Addition of ammonium molybdate and 1-amino-2-naphthol-4-sulfonic acid solution. A blue color shows the presence of phosphate.
- **Calcium:** Neutralization with, 5N sodium hydroxide alone. If a white precipitate occurs subsequent addition of 4-nitrobenzene-azo-resorcinol produces blue color in the presence of magnesium and a pink color in the presence of calcium.
- **Uric acid:** Neutralization with 5N sodium hydroxide, addition of 15% sodium cyanide and then addition of Folin's uric acid reagent. A blue color indicates the presence of uric acid.
- **Cystine:** Alkalinization with 5N sodium hydroxide, addition of 15% sodium cyanide and then freshly prepared sodium nitroprusside. A deep purplish color is obtained in the presence of cystine.
- **Ammonia:** Neutralization with 5N sodium hydroxide and addition of Nessler's reagent. A yellow brown color is formed in the presence of ammonia.

Limitations of chemical method:
- These methods cannot usually identify a compound as such. These only indicate which ions and radicals are present.
- Chemical methods are destructive and need several milligrams of the sample, so small stones cannot be analyzed with chemical methods.

Fourier Transform Infrared Spectroscopy Analysis
- This method gives fast results and the quantity of sample needed for Fourier transform infrared spectroscopy can be less than 1 μm.
- In FTIR spectral analysis, spectral data is related to the vibrational motions of atoms in bonds.
- Classically, the powdered sample is admixed with powdered potassium bromide, compressed into a nearly transparent wafer, and the IR beam is passed through the wafer.
- The reflected IR beam containing spectral data specific to the sample is then recorded.
- The IR pattern contains absorption bands representing specific energies (presented as wavelengths in units of cm^{-1}, or more commonly known as wavenumbers) corresponding to molecular motions in molecules.

Other methods such as polarizing microscopy, X-ray diffraction, scanning electron microscopy (SEM) and thermal analysis are also helpful to find out chemical composition of a calculus.

SUMMARY

- The kidney is divided in three sections—outer fibrous capsule, middle cortex and inner medulla.
- The nephron is the minute or microscopic structural and functional unit of the kidney.
- Each nephron includes a filter, called the glomerulus within Bowman's capsule, and a tubule which is divided in three parts—proximal convoluted tubule, loop of Henle, and distal convoluted tubule.
- Kidney performs mainly excretory functions. It also produces hormones and regulates various properties of blood.
- Urea is the major end product of nitrogen metabolism in humans.
- Blood urea nitrogen is 2.14 times that of blood urea.
- Urea by rate of reaction method—UV Kinetic—is based on the principle that urea is hydrolyzed to ammonia and carbon dioxide by urease. In

presence of ammonia α-ketoglutarate and glutamate dehydrogenase (GLDH). NADH is reduced to NAD^+.
- End point reaction is based on the Berthelot reaction. Urease splits urea into ammonia and carbon dioxide. The ammonia reacts with phenol in the presence of hypochlorite to form indophenol, with which alkali gives a blue colored compound.
- Diacetylmonoxime (DAM) method is based on principle that urea reacts with diacetylmonoxime in hot medium (1000°C) and in the presence of thiosemicarbazide and ferric ions to form a pink colored compound.
- Urine urea test is mainly used to assess the protein balance and the amount of dietary protein needed by severely ill patients.
- Urea clearance is defined the volume of the blood cleared of urea per minute by either renal clearance or hemodialysis.
- Creatinine is largely formed in muscle by irreversible and non-enzymatic removal of water from creatine phosphate.
- Alkaline-picrate method for creatinine estimation is based on the principle that creatinine reacts with picric acid in alkaline medium to form a reddish yellow complex.
- The normal BUN/creatinine ratio is around 10:1.
- Creatinine in urine is raised only when the 50% function of the kidney is lost.
- Creatinine clearance is defined as the amount of plasma in mL, which would have to be completely cleared of the creatinine, each minute by both the kidneys in order to account for its rate of excretion.
- Uric acid is the end product of purine metabolism.
- Uric acid is estimated by Henry–Caraway method based on the principle that uric acid in protein free filtrate reacts with phosphotungstic acid reagent in alkaline medium to form a blue colored complex.
- Uric acid is estimated by Enzymatic Method based on the principle that enzyme uricase converts uric acid to allantoin and hydrogen peroxide. In the presence of peroxidase, hydrogen peroxide reacts with phenolic chromogens to form red colored compound.
- The glomerular filtration rate (GFR) is defined as the volume of glomerular filtrate formed in all the renal corpuscles of both kidneys each minute.
- Kidney stones are of variable sizes and composition. It may be of calcium, magnesium ammonium phosphate or cystine.
- Urine is examined microscopically for different crystals to identify presence of urinary calculi.
- Chemical composition of stone can be identified by using one or different combinations of methods.
- Fourier transform infrared (FTIR) spectroscopy analysis is the latest method to identify chemical composition of urine.

PRACTICE QUESTIONS

1. With a neat labeled diagram, draw structure of kidney and explain it.
2. With a neat labeled diagram, draw structure of nephron and explain it.
3. Write a note on metabolism of urea.
4. What is the difference in blood urea nitrogen and blood urea content? How they are interrelated?
5. Write principle and procedure of urea estimation by Berthelot reaction method.
6. Write principle and procedure of urea estimation by diacetylmonoxime method.
7. What is urea clearance test? How it is measured?
8. Write importance of BUN/creatinine ratio.
9. Write a note on metabolism of creatinine.
10. Write principle and procedure of creatinine estimation by Jaffe reaction method.
11. What is clearance test? How it is measured?
12. What is glomerular filtration test? How it is measured?
13. Write principle and procedure of uric acid estimation by Henry–Caraway method.
14. What are urinary calculi? Give its location and composition.
15. Why there is a need to analyze kidney stone? Discuss methods to find out its chemical composition.
16. Write a note on:
    i. Renal colic
    ii. Fourier transform infrared (FTIR) spectroscopy analysis for kidney stone.

Cardiac Function Tests

CHAPTER 23

Keywords
Triglycerides, auricles, ventricles, systemic circulation, pulmonary circulation, coronary circulation, cholesterol, low-density lipoprotein (LDL), high-density lipoprotein (HDL), unesterified, esterified, Watson method, acetic anhydride, enzymatic method, chylomicrons, Friedewald equation, total lipids, sulfo-phospho-vanillin method, atherosclerosis, creatine kinase lactate dehydrogenase

■ INTRODUCTION

Lipids are class of organic compounds that are fatty acids or their derivatives and are insoluble in water but soluble in organic solvents. They include many natural oils, waxes, and steroids. Cholesterol and triglycerides are important lipids present in our body. The cardiac function tests helps to evaluate cardiovascular health by analyzing different types of cholesterol and triglycerides in the blood. Too much cholesterol can build up in the blood vessels and arteries, damaging them and heightening the risk of problems, such as heart disease, stroke, and heart attack. Therefore these tests are also called as lipid profile test. A lipid profile test is ordered for screening, monitoring, measuring response to treatment and diagnosis of heart related problems.

■ STRUCTURE AND FUNCTION OF HEART

The human heart is located between the lungs in the thoracic cavity, slightly toward the left of the sternum. Heart is the muscular pumping organ which pushes the blood around the body. Blood delivers oxygen, hormones, nutrients and other components to various parts of the body, including the heart. The heart also ensures that adequate blood pressure is maintained in the body.

Internally, the heart is divided vertically into a left and right portion by a septum. Each half is further divided horizontally into two chambers—upper chamber called auricles and lower chamber called ventricles. The auricles have thin walls, they receive blood from different body parts and pump into the ventricles that are just below them. Ventricles are thick walled and pump blood into lungs and blood vessels that distribute the blood to all parts of body. To maintain flow of blood in one direction, the openings within heart are guarded by valves **(Fig. 23.1)**.

There are two main types of circulation:
1. **Systemic circulation:** The oxygenated blood flows from the left ventricle, provides oxygen to various parts of the body. It takes up carbon dioxide from different parts of body and deoxygenated blood comes to the right atrium.
2. **Coronary circulation:** It is a part of the systemic circulatory system that supplies blood to and provides drainage from the tissues of the heart. Coronary arteries arise from the aorta. Right and left coronary arteries supply blood to the myocardium. The

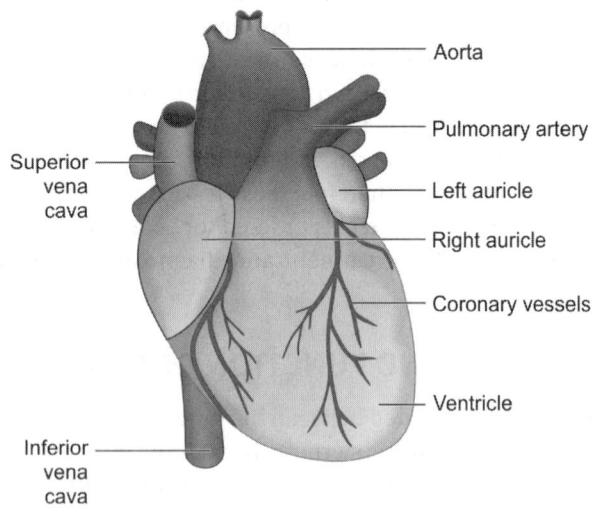

Fig. 23.1: External view of human heart.

left coronary artery gives rise to gives rise to its major branches, the anterior interventricular artery and circumflex artery. Right coronary artery gives rise to the posterior interventricular artery and marginal artery. The great cardiac vein and the middle cardiac vein return blood from myocardial capillaries to the coronary sinus which then returns directly into the right atrium. Most of the heart related problems are associated with coronary circulation.

3. **Pulmonary circulation:** The deoxygenated blood flows from the right ventricle, to the lungs. From lungs, it gets oxygen and gives off carbondioxide. The oxygenated blood now comes to the left atrium.

CARDIAC FUNCTION TESTS

The cardiac function test estimates all the lipid contents of the body. The important lipid profile tests include: total lipids, serum total cholesterol, serum HDL cholesterol, serum triglycerides and low-density lipoprotein (LDL) and very low-density lipoprotein (VLDL).

Cholesterol

Cholesterol is a waxy substance that is present in blood plasma and in almost all the tissues.

Metabolism

Chemically, cholesterol is an organic compound belonging to the steroid family; its molecular formula is $C_{27}H_{46}O$. In its pure state it is a white, crystalline substance that is odorless and tasteless. Cholesterol is essential to life; it is a primary component of the membrane that surrounds each cell, and it is the precursor for (starting material) or an intermediate compound from which the body synthesizes bile acids, steroid hormones, and vitamin D. Cholesterol circulates in the bloodstream and is synthesized 25% by the liver and balance by adrenal glands and reproductive organs. Cholesterol is present in the diet; mostly from the animal source and vegetable oils from a normal diet. Cholesterol is kept in balance by homeostatic mechanisms, higher dietary intake leads to reduced synthesis in the body. It is excreted in the form of the bile acids from the liver. Cholesterol in the colon is metabolized by colonic bacteria which convert it to a non-absorbable sterol that is excreted in the feces.

High levels of cholesterol in the bloodstream are an extremely important cause of atherosclerosis. In this disorder, deposits of cholesterol and other fatty substances circulating in the blood accumulate in the interior walls of the blood vessels. These fatty deposits build up, thicken, and become calcified, eventually converting the vessel walls to scar tissue. The deposits narrow the channels of the blood vessels and thus can constrict the blood flow, causing heart attacks and strokes. High levels of cholesterol in the blood (more than 240 mg of cholesterol per 100 cc of blood plasma) accelerate the buildup of cholesterol deposits in the vessel walls; making it more susceptible to coronary heart disease.

Cholesterol is insoluble in the blood; it must be attached to certain protein complexes called lipoproteins in order to be transported through the bloodstream. Low-density lipoproteins (LDLs) transport cholesterol from its site of synthesis in the liver to the various tissues and body cells, where it is separated from the lipoprotein and is used by the cell. High-density lipoproteins (HDLs) may possibly transport excess or unused cholesterol from the tissues back to the liver, where it is broken down to bile acids and is then excreted, therefore it is also known as good cholesterol. Cholesterol attached to LDLs is primarily that which builds up in atherosclerotic deposits in the blood vessels, therefore it is called as bad cholesterol. HDLs, on the other hand, may actually serve to retard or reduce atherosclerotic buildup.

Total cholesterol = HDL cholesterol + VLDL cholesterol + LDL cholesterol

In the normal biologic process, cholesterol undergoes changes such as synthesis, recycling, and degradation.

Cholesterol exists in two forms: Free cholesterol and esterified cholesterol.
1. Cholesterol is present as unesterified (free cholesterol) is biologically active and has cytotoxic effects.
2. Esterified cholesterol is protective form for storage in the cells and transporting in plasma. 75-85% of the total cholesterol is in the form of esterified cholesterol.

Estimation of Total Cholesterol

Serum total cholesterol includes esterified cholesterol as well as non-esterified cholesterol. There are two methods of serum total cholesterol.
1. Watson method
2. Enzymatic method

Watson Method

Specimen: The best sample is after 12 hours of fast, and that is the morning sample. It should be separated within 2 hours of the collection. Plasma (EDTA) can also be used. However, results with EDTA plasma is 3% lower than serum.

Principle:
Cholesterol reacts with acetic anhydride in the presence of glacial acetic acid and conc. sulfuric acid to form green colored complex. Intensity of the color is proportional to the cholesterol concentration. It is measured at 520–580 nm.

Reagent:
1. Cholesterol reagent—it is prepared by mixing 5.6 g of 2,5-dimethyl benzenesulfonic acid in 200 mL of glacial acetic acid and 300 mL of acetic anhydride. This should be stored in amber colored bottle at room temperature. Cholesterol reagent is highly corrosive so, it should not be pipetted by mouth.
2. Conc. sulfuric acid.
3. Cholesterol standard (200 mg/dL in glacial acetic acid).

Procedure:
- Take three test tubes and mark them as T, S, and B. Add 2.5 mL cholesterol reagent in each tube.
- Add 0.1 mL of serum, 0.1 mL of cholesterol standard and 0.1 mL of distilled water in test, standard and blank respectively.
- This is an exothermic reaction. So, cool the tubes to room temperature by placing in water bath.
- Now carefully add 0.5 mL of sulfuric acid to each tube mix thoroughly and keep in water bath at room temperature for 10 minute.
- Read the absorbance of test and standard against blank at 575 nm.

Reagent	T	S	B
Cholesterol reagent	2.5 mL	2.5 mL	2.5 mL
Serum	0.1 mL	—	—
Cholesterol standard	—	0.1 mL	—
Distilled water	—	—	0.1 mL
Cool to room temperature			
Conc. sulfuric acid	0.5 mL	0.5 mL	0.5 mL

Calculation:

$$\text{Serum cholesterol (mg/dL)} = \frac{\text{OD of T}}{\text{OD of S}} \times 200$$

Enzymatic Method

Specimen: Fasting serum or heparinized plasma.

Principle: Cholesterol esterase hydrolyses cholesterol ester into free cholesterol and fatty acids. In the second reaction, cholesterol oxidase converts free cholesterol to cholest-4-en-3-one and hydrogen peroxide. In presence of peroxidase, hydrogen peroxide reacts with 4-aminoantipyrine and phenol to produce red color. The intensity of red color is directly proportional to the amount of cholesterol present in sample.

Cholesterol ester $\xrightarrow{\text{Cholesterol esterase}}$ Free cholesterol + Fatty acids

Free cholesterol $\xrightarrow{\text{Cholesterol oxidase}}$ Cholest-4-en-3-one + H_2O_2

H_2O_2 + 4-aminoantipyrine + Phenol $\xrightarrow{\text{Peroxidase}}$ Red color

Reagent:
1. Buffer/Enzymes/Chromogen
2. Phenol (30 mg/dL)
3. Cholesterol standard (200 mg/dL)

Procedure:
- Prepare working reagent freshly by mixing 10 mL of reagent 1 and 5 mL of reagent 2, i.e, phenol.
- Take three test tubes and mark them as T, S, and B. Add 1 mL of freshly prepared working reagent in each tube.
- Add 0.1 mL of serum, 0.1 mL of cholesterol standard and 0.1 mL of distilled water in test, standard and blank respectively.
- Mix well and keep at 37°C for 20 minutes.
- Read the absorbance of test and standard against blank at 530 nm.

Reagent	T	S	B
Working reagent	1 mL	1 mL	1 mL
Serum	0.1 mL	—	—
Cholesterol standard	—	0.1 mL	—
Distilled water	—	—	0.1 mL

Calculation:

$$\text{Serum cholesterol (mg/dL)} = \frac{\text{OD of T}}{\text{OD of S}} \times 200$$

Normal value:

Adult
- The desired level to prevent coronary disease is < 200 mg/dL
- Moderate risk is 200–239 mg/dL
- High risk is > 240 mg/dL

Children
- Desirable level is <170 mg/dL
- Moderate risk is 170–199 mg/dL
- High risk is > 200 mg/dL

Clinical significance: Total cholesterol estimation is useful in monitoring for increased risk factor for coronary artery disease, screening and monitoring for hyperlipidemias.

Increased cholesterol (Hypercholesterolemia): It is high in hyperlipoproteinemias, hypothyroidism, gout, nephrosis, pancreatic disease such as diabetes mellitus, chronic pancreatitis, biliary obstruction such as stone, carcinoma, biliary cirrhosis, it is also increased in cholesterol ester storage disease and Von Gierke's disease. Usage of some drugs like birth control pills, amiodarone, or vitamins can also show increased cholesterol value. Stress and alcoholism are associated with high cholesterol.

Decreased cholesterol (Hypocholesterolemia): The serum total cholesterol levels are decreased in severe liver cell damage, hyperthyroidism, chronic anemia, cortisone and ACTH therapy. The levels of total cholesterol are also low in Tangier disease, extensive burns, rheumatoid arthritis, and in some infections.

High-density Lipoproteins

High-density lipoproteins (HDL) are alpha lipoprotein found in the blood. These are mainly protein with the small amount of cholesterol. It is called "good" cholesterol because it removes excess cholesterol from the blood and takes it to the liver. A high HDL level is related to lower risk of heart and blood vessel disease.

Method: Watson method.

Specimen: Fasting serum is preferred:

Principle: In the presence of phosphotungstic acid and magnesium chloride, LDL, VLDL and chylomicrons are precipitated. Centrifugation leaves only HDL in supernatant. Cholesterol in HDL fraction can be tested by usual method.

Reagent:
1. Cholesterol reagent
2. Conc. sulfuric acid
3. Phosphotungstic acid (PTA) reagent
4. Magnesium chloride reagent
5. Cholesterol standard (100 mg/dL)

Procedure:
i. **Precipitation of LDL and VLDL**
   - Take 0.5 mL of serum. Add 0.05 mL of PTA reagent and 0.02 mL of magnesium chloride reagent.
   - Mix well and centrifuge at 3,000 RPM for 20 minutes to obtain a clear supernatant.
   - LDL and VLDL will form precipitate. Only HDL will remain in the supernatant.

ii. **Estimation of HDL**
   - Separate the supernatant by using Pasteur pipette.
   - Take three test tubes and mark them as T, S, and B.
   - Add 2.5 mL cholesterol reagent in each tube.
   - Add 0.1 mL of supernatant, 0.1 mL of cholesterol standard and 0.1 mL of distilled water in test, standard and blank respectively.
   - This is an exothermic reaction. So, cool the tubes to room temperature by placing in water bath.

- Now carefully add 0.5 mL of sulfuric acid to each tube. Mix thoroughly and keep in water bath at room temperature for 10 minutes.
- Read the absorbance of test and standard against blank at 520 nm.

Reagent	T	S	B
Cholesterol reagent	2.5 mL	2.5 mL	2.5 mL
Supernatant	0.1 mL	—	—
Cholesterol standard	—	0.1 mL	—
Distilled water	—	—	0.1 mL
Cool to room temperature			
Conc. sulfuric acid	0.5 mL	0.5 mL	0.5 mL

Calculation: Serum HDL cholesterol (mg/dL) = $\dfrac{\text{OD of T}}{\text{OD of S}} \times 114$

Clinical significance: Estimation of HDL is useful in diagnosis of various lipoproteinemias and to assessment the risk for coronary heart disease (CAD). HDL is inversely proportional to CAD.

It is increased in—increased clearance of triglyceride (VLDL), insulin treatment, vigorous exercise, moderate consumption of alcohol, oral estrogen use, familial lipid disorders with the protection against arteriosclerosis, in hyperalphalipoproteinemias and hypobetalipoproteinemias. HDL also increases in 1 in 20 adults with mild increase in total cholesterol.

There are various secondary causes for decrease in HDL level, e.g., obesity, smoking, diabetes mellitus, stress and recent illness, lack of exercise, hypo- and hyperthyroidism, starvation (nonfasting sample is 10–15% lower). As stated earlier, HDL is inversely proportional to CAD. For every 1 mg/dL decrease in HDL, risk for CAD increases by 2–3%.

HDL normal range:
- Male >50 mg/dL
- Female >55 mg/dL

Total Cholesterol/HDL Ratio

The total cholesterol/HDL-cholesterol ratio is very important to know the risk of coronary heart disease. A high ratio is associated with increased risk.

The risk associated with total cholesterol/HDL ratio is expressed as follows:
- Low-risk: 3.3–4.4
- Average risk: 4.4–7.1
- Moderate risk: 7.1–11.0
- High-risk >11

Very Low-density Lipoprotein

These are prebeta-lipoprotein. These are major carrier of triglyceride (60–70% triglyceride, 10–15% cholesterol). Circulating fatty acids are vitalized by the liver to form triglycerides that are packaged with apoprotein and cholesterol, and exported into blood as very low-density lipoproteins.

Normal value = 7–32 mg/dL.

VLDL can be estimated by Friedewald equation:

$$\text{VLDL} = \frac{\text{Triglycerides}}{5}$$

Note: This formula is applicable only when the triglycerides level is below 400 g/dL.

High VLDL is seen in—nephrotic syndrome, hypothyroidism, chronic liver disease, liver cell carcinoma, and Cushing syndrome.

Decreased VLDL is seen in—hypoproteinemia and hyperthyroidism.

Low-density Lipoproteins

Degradation of VLDL leads to major source of low-density lipoprotein (LDL). LDLs are cholesterol rich remnants of the VLDL. LDL is a lipoprotein found in the blood. It is called "bad" cholesterol because most of the cholesterol carried by the LDL is deposited in the lining of the blood vessels. A high LDL level is related to a higher risk of heart and blood vessel disease. LDL is more prevalent in blood. It is finally catabolized in the liver and possibly in nonhepatic cells as well.

Low-density lipoprotein is measured by ultracentrifugation and by analysis after antibody separation from HDL and VLDL.

LDL can also be estimated by Friedewald equation.

LDL = Total cholesterol – (HDL cholesterol) – (VLDL)

Normal value:
- Adult <130 mg/dL
- Children <110 mg/dL

Clinical significance: Determination of LDL helps in assessment of risk and decides treatment for CAD.

Increase in LDL is directly related to risk of CAD. The LDL is estimated high in—chronic renal failure, hypothyroidism, diabetes mellitus, nephritic syndrome, Wolman's disease, etc.

LDL is low in severe illness, abetalipoproteinemia, chronic pulmonary disease, Reye's syndrome, acute stress like a burn and oral estrogen use.

■ TOTAL LIPIDS

Lipids are usually defined as those components that are soluble in organic solvents (such as ether, hexane or chloroform), but are insoluble in water. This group of substances includes triacylglycerides, cholesterol, LDL and VLDL, HDL lipoproteins, free fatty acids, phospholipids, sterols, and carotenoids.

Method: Sulfo-phospho-vanillin reaction.

Specimen: Fasting serum.

Principle: Lipids react with vanillin in the presence of sulfuric acid and phosphoric acid to form a pink colored complex. This is measured at 546 nm.

Reagent:
1. Total lipid standard (1,000 mg/dL)
2. Phosho-vanillin (color reagent)
3. Conc. sulfuric acid

Reagent 1 and 2 should be kept in refrigerator in amber color bottle.

Procedure:
Take two test tubes. Add the reagents as follows:

Reagent	T	S
Total lipid standard	—	0.05 mL
Serum	0.05 mL	—
Conc. sulfuric acid	2.0 mL	2.0 mL

Mix thoroughly and plug it with cotton. Keep in a boiling water bath for 10 minute. Then cool the tubes and pipette into dry test tubes as follows:

Reagent	T	S	B
From above solution	0.10 mL	0.10 mL	—
Conc. sulfuric acid	—	—	0.10 mL
Color reagent	2.5 mL	2.5 mL	2.5 mL

Mix thoroughly and keep at room temperature for 15 min. Read the absorbance of test and standard against blank at 546 nm.

Calculation:

$$\text{Serum total lipids (mg/dL)} = \frac{\text{OD of T}}{\text{OD of S}} \times 1000$$

Normal value: 400–1,000 mg/dL

Raised levels of lipids are seen in—hypothyroidism, both free and ester-cholesterol is raised. In nephrotic syndrome, β-lipoprotein is greatly raised. It is also seen in lipoid nephrosis, and in the untreated diabetes mellitus.

Serum Triglycerides

Triglycerides are triesters consist of three fatty acids and one molecule of glycerol by ester bond, so-called as triglycerides. Triglycerides are a type of fat present in the blood and transported by the VLDL and LDL. The blood level of this type of fat is most affected by the foods one eat (such as sugar, fat or alcohol) but can also be high due to being overweight, having thyroid or liver disease and genetic conditions. High levels of triglycerides are related to a higher risk of heart and blood vessel disease.

Chapter 23: Cardiac Function Tests

Method: GPO POD/enzymatic method.

Specimen: Fasting serum/plasma (heparin or EDTA).

Principle: Triglycerides are hydrolyzed by lipase to glycerol and fatty acids. Glycerol is phosphorylated by ATP in the presence of glycerol kinase (GK) to glycerol-3-phosphate (G-3-P) which is oxidized by enzyme glycerol-3-phosphate oxidase (G-P-O) producing hydrogen peroxide. Hydrogen peroxide so formed reacts with 4-aminoantipyrine and P-chlorophenol in presence of enzyme peroxidase (POD) to produce a red quinoneimine dye. The intensity of red color is directly proportional to the amount of cholesterol present in sample.

$$\text{Triglycerides} + H_2O \xrightarrow{\text{lipase}} \text{Glycerol} + \text{Fatty acids}$$

$$\text{Glycerol} + \text{ATP} \xrightarrow{\text{GK}} \text{G-3-P} + \text{ADP}$$

$$\text{G-3-P} + O_2 \longrightarrow H_2O_2 + \text{Dihydroxyacetone phosphate}$$

$$H_2O_2 + \text{4-aminoantipyrine} + \text{P-chlorophenol} \xrightarrow{\text{peroxidase}} \text{Red color} + H_2O$$

Reagent:

1. Buffer/Enzymes/Chromogen
2. P-chlorophenol
3. Triglyceride standard (100 mg/dL)

Procedure:

- Prepare working reagent freshly by mixing 10 mL of reagent reagent 1 and 5 mL of reagent 2, i.e. P-chlorophenol.
- Take three test tubes and mark them as T, S, and B. Add 1 mL of freshly prepared working reagent in each tube.
- Add 0.1 mL of serum, 0.1 mL of triglyceride standard and 0.1 mL of distilled water in test, standard and blank, respectively.
- Mix well and keep at 37°C for 20 minute.
- Read the absorbance of test and standard against blank at 530 nm.

Reagent	T	S	B
Working reagent	1 mL	1 mL	1 mL
Serum	0.1 mL	—	—
Triglyceride std	—	0.1 mL	—
Distilled water	—	—	0.1 mL

Calculation:

$$\text{Serum triglyceride (mg/dL)} = \frac{\text{OD of T}}{\text{OD of S}} \times 100$$

Normal value: 80–150 mg/dL.

Clinical Significance:
Triglyceride is the source of energy. When triglyceride is high, it starts depositing in fatty tissue.

Increased triglycerides values are seen in: Hyperlipidemia, nephrotic syndrome, liver diseases, alcoholism (alcoholic cirrhosis), uncontrolled diabetes mellitus, hypothyroidism, gout, and myocardial infarction.

Decreased triglycerides level is seen in: Malnutrition, hyperthyroidism, congenital α-β-lipoproteinemia and malabsorption.

Besides these, enzymes such as creatine kinase and lactate dehydrogenase, or LDH, are also included in cardiac profile tests. These are discussed in chapter on *Enzymes*.

SUMMARY

- Cholesterol and triglycerides are important lipids that are insoluble in water and soluble in organic solvents.
- Heart is four chambered—upper two auricles and lower two ventricles.
- *Systemic circulation*: The oxygenated blood flows from the left ventricle to all parts of the body. This carries oxygen and nutrients to the cells and picks up carbon dioxide and waste products.
- *Pulmonary circulation*: The deoxygenated blood flows from the right ventricle, to the lungs.
- *Coronary circulation*: Supplies blood to the heart and provides drainage from the tissues of the heart.
- Cholesterol is a steroid produced in liver and other organs. It is precursor for bile acids, steroid hormones, and vitamin D. It is excreted through bile and feces.
- The two main types of cholesterol—low-density lipoprotein (LDL), or "bad" cholesterol, and high-density lipoprotein (HDL), or "good" cholesterol.
- Unesterified cholesterol is active whereas esterified cholesterol is storage form.
- Always use 12 hours fasting sample for cholesterol.
- Serum total cholesterol by Watson method is based on the principle that cholesterol reacts with acetic anhydride in the presence of glacial acetic acid and concentrated sulfuric acid to form green colored complex.

- Enzymatic method for cholesterol estimation is based on the principle that, cholesterol oxidase converts free cholesterol to cholest-4-en-3-one and hydrogen peroxide, which then reacts with 4-amino antipyrine and phenol to produce red color.
- For determination of HDL cholesterol, LDL, VLDL and chylomicrons are precipitated in the presence of phosphotungstic acid and magnesium chloride. Centrifugation leaves only HDL in supernatant, which is tested by usual method.
- High total cholesterol/HDL ratio, high is the risk.
- VLDL is major carrier of triglycerides. These are calculated by Friedewald equation.
- LDL is measured by ultracentrifugation and by analysis after antibody separation from HDL and VLDL. It is also estimated by Friedewald equation.
- Total lipids include the components that are soluble in organic solvents.
- Total lipids are estimated by sulfo-phospho-vanillin method, based on principle that lipids react with vanillin in the presence of sulfuric acid and phosphoric acid to form a pink colored complex.
- Triglyceride consists of three fatty acids and one molecule of glycerol by ester bond.
- Triglycerides are hydrolyzed by lipase to glycerol and then estimated by GPO POD method.
- In atherosclerosis, cholesterol and other fatty substances deposits in the interior walls of the blood vessels making it narrow.

PRACTICE QUESTIONS

1. With a neat labeled diagram describe the structure of heart.
2. Enlist the functions of heart.
3. Explain the different types of circulation in body.
4. Write a note on cholesterol metabolism.
5. How many types of cholesterols are there?
6. Why there is good cholesterol and bad cholesterol?
7. Write principle and procedure for estimation of cholesterol by Watson method.
8. Write principle and procedure for estimation of cholesterol by enzymatic method.
9. What action is taken on the sample to prepare it for estimation of HDL?
10. Write a formula to determine concentration of LDL, VLDL and triglycerides.
11. What are total lipids? Write principle and procedure to estimate it.
12. What is meant by triglyceride? Write principle and method of diagnosis.
13. Enlist different cardiac function tests and corresponding normal values.
14. Justify that lipid profile tests are important tool to determine cardiac health.

CHAPTER 24

Electrolytes

> **Keywords**
> Sodium, potassium calcium, magnesium, chloride, bicarbonate, phosphate, flame photometer, Maruna and Trinder's method, turbidimetric method, Cushing's syndrome, Schoenfeld and Lewellen's method, mercuric thiocyanate, Gomori's method, Fanconi's syndrome, O-cresolphthalein complexone (OCPC) method, hypercalcemia, hypokalemia

■ INTRODUCTION AND CLASSIFICATION

Electrolytes are positively and negatively charged molecules, called ions. These are found within cells, between cells, in the bloodstream, and in other fluids throughout the body in the form of dissolved salts. Electrolytes help to move nutrients into and wastes out of the body's cells, maintain a healthy water balance and help stabilize the body's pH level.

Electrolyte panel consists of electrolytes with a positive charge—sodium (Na^+), potassium (K^+), calcium (Ca^{++}), and magnesium (Mg^{++}); the negative ions are chloride (Cl^-), bicarbonate (HCO_3^-; sometimes reported as total CO_2) and phosphate (PO_4^{3-}).

Classifications of Electrolytes

Electrolyte tests are typically conducted on blood plasma or serum, urine, and diarrheal fluids. Electrolytes can be classified in four different ways:
1. Some electrolytes are intracellular, i.e. tend to exist mostly inside cells, while others are extracellular, i.e. tend to be outside cells. Potassium, phosphate, and magnesium are intracellular, while sodium and chloride are extracellular.
2. A second classification distinguishes those electrolytes that participate directly in the transmission of nerve impulses and

those that do not. Sodium, potassium, and calcium are the important electrolytes involved in nerve impulses, and disorders affecting them are most closely associated with neurological disorders.
3. A third classification focuses on electrolytes that are able to form a tight union, or complex, with one another. Calcium and phosphate have the greatest tendency to form complexes with each other. Disorders that cause an increase in either plasma calcium or phosphate can result in the deposit of calcium-phosphate crystals in the soft tissues of the body.
4. A fourth classification concerns those electrolytes that influence the acidity or alkalinity of the bloodstream, also known as the pH. The pH of the bloodstream is normally in the range of 7.35–7.45. A decrease below this range is called acidosis, while a pH above this range is called alkalosis. The electrolytes most closely associated with the pH of the bloodstream are bicarbonate, chloride, and phosphate.

Diagnostic Importance

Electrolyte levels are affected by how much is taken in through the diet, the amount of water in a person's body, and the amount of electrolytes excreted by their kidneys. Balance of the electrolytes in our bodies is essential for normal function of our cells and our organs.

These ions are measured to evaluate symptoms of heart disease and monitor the effectiveness of treatments for high blood pressure, liver disease to assess renal (kidney), endocrine (glandular), and acid-base function, and are components of both renal function and comprehensive metabolic biochemistry profiles.

Knowing which electrolytes are out of balance can help a doctor to determine the cause and treatment to restore proper balance. If left untreated, electrolyte imbalance can lead to dizziness, cramps, irregular heartbeat, and possibly death.

■ SERUM SODIUM AND POTASSIUM

Serum Sodium

Sodium is a major extracellular cation (Na^+) of the body. Sodium salts are necessary to preserve a balance between Ca^{++} and K^+ to maintain normal heart action and equilibrium of the body. Sodium salts regulate the osmotic pressure in the cells and fluids and guard against the excessive loss of water from the tissues. Almost all blood sodium is found in the plasma. There is very little in the red cells.

Method

Modified Maruna and Trinder's method.

Specimen

Serum.

Principle

Sodium from the specimen is quantitatively precipitated as the triple salt uranyl magnesium sodium acetate and the excess of uranyl salt reacts with potassium ferrocyanide to produce brown color. The intensity of brown color produced is inversely proportional to the sodium conc. of the specimen.

Reagent

- Standard sodium chloride solution (equivalent to 300 mg of Na)
- Uranyl magnesium acetate solution
- Acetic acid 1% aqueous solution
- Potassium ferrocyanide 20% solution.

Procedure

Part I: Precipitation step

Take three test tubes and mark them as T, S and B. Add 5 mL of uranyl magnesium acetate solution in each tube. Add 0.1 mL of serum, 0.1 mL of sodium standard and 0.1 mL of distilled water in test, standard and blank, respectively. Mix well and allow it to stand for 5 minutes. Centrifuge for one minute at 3,000 rpm to get clear supernatant.

Reagent	T	S	B
Uranyl magnesium acetate solution	5 mL	5 mL	5 mL
Serum	0.1 mL	—	—
Sodium standard	—	0.1 mL	—
Distilled water	—	—	0.1 mL

Part II: Color formation

Take three test tubes and mark them as T, S, and B. Add 0.2 mL of supernatant from Part 1 in respective tubes. Add 8 mL of acetic acid in each tube. Now add 0.2 mL of potassium ferrocyanide in each tube. Now make up the volume to 10 mL by acetic acid. Read the absorbance of test and standard against blank at 480 nm. Be sure that the readings are taken within 10 minutes of last step.

Reagent	T	S	B
Supernatant from Part I (T)	0.2 mL	—	—
Supernatant from Part I (S)	—	0.2 mL	—
Supernatant from Part I (B)	—	—	0.2 mL
Acetic acid	8 mL	8 mL	8 mL
Potassium ferrocyanide	0.2 mL	0.2 mL	0.2 mL
Acetic acid	1.6 mL	1.6 mL	1.6 mL

Calculation

$$\text{Serum sodium (mg/dL)} = \frac{\text{OD of T}}{\text{OD of S}} \times 300$$

Serum Potassium

Unlike sodium, potassium is the major intracellular cation of the body. Within the cells, it plays an important role in maintenance of acid-base balance, osmotic pressure and water retention. Intracellular potassium is essential for several important metabolic reactions catalyzed by enzymes. It is also very important constituent of the extracellular fluid because it influences muscle activity notably the cardiac muscle.

Method

Turbidometric method.

Specimen

Serum.

Principle

Potassium ions from specimen react with sodium tetraphenyl boron resulting in a turbid suspension. The extent of turbidity is measured photometrically at 620 nm is proportional to the potassium concentration.

Reagent

- Potassium reagent
- Potassium standard (5 mol/L).

Procedure

Take two test tubes and mark them as T and S. Add 3 mL of potassium reagent in each tube. Add 0.1 mL of serum and 0.1 mL of potassium standard in test and standard, respectively. Mix well and allow it to stand for 5 minutes at room temperature. Read the absorbance of T and S against reagent at 620 nm.

Reagent	T	S
Potassium reagent	3 mL	3 mL
Serum	0.1 mL	—
Sodium standard	—	0.1 mL

Another popular method for determination of sodium and potassium is flame photometry.

Reagent

- Stock standard for sodium (1000 mEq/L)
- Stock standard for potassium (100 mEq/L).

Mixed working standards are prepared as follows:
- **Sodium/potassium (120/2.0 mEq/L):** It contains 120 mEq/L of sodium and 2.0 mEq of potassium in 1 liter distilled water. It is prepared by mixing 12 mL stock standard for sodium and 2 mL stock standard for potassium in 86 mL of distilled water.
- **Sodium/potassium (140/4.0 mEq/L):** It contains 140 mEq/L of sodium and 4.0 mEq of potassium in 1 liter distilled water. It is prepared by mixing 14 mL stock standard for sodium and 4 mL stock standard for potassium in 82 mL of distilled water.
- **Sodium/potassium (160/6.0 mEq/L):** It contains 160 mEq/L of sodium and 6.0 mEq of potassium in 1 liter distilled water. It is prepared by mixing 16 mL stock standard for sodium and 6 mL stock standard for potassium in 78 mL of distilled water.

Note: mEq/day = milliequivalents per day.

Specimen

Serum or heparinized plasma.
This test is performed on flame photometer (Refer Chapter 4).

Principle

The solution under test is passed carefully, under controlled conditions as a very fine spray in the air supply to nonluminous flame. In the flame, the solution evaporates and the salt dissociates to give natural ions, which emit light of the characteristic wavelength. The flame is simultaneously monitored by both the channel consists of a detector which views the flame through a narrow band optical filter. The photodetector outputs are connected to two independent digital displays, which are calibrated for direct concentration readouts. Initial calibration is done by using at least three standards of different concentrations.

Procedure

Take four test tubes. Mark them as test, standard 1, standard 2 and standard 3. To each tube add 10 mL of distilled water. Add 0.1 mL of serum to test. Add 0.1 mL of standard (120/2.0 mEq/L), 0.1 mL of standard (140/4.0 mEq/L), 0.1 mL of standard (160/6.0 mEq/L) to standard 1, standard 2 and standard 3, respectively.

Put on the main switch and switch on air compressor and adjust the required air pressure, by adjusting the knob meant for air. Introduce the distilled water through atomizer. Put on gas and control the flame by adjusting the knob meant for gas till the flame is divided into five sharp cones. Adjust the proper filters for the simultaneous determination of sodium and potassium. Make zero adjustment by using distilled water. Introduce the standard 120 /2.0 mEq/L and by using the knob meant for sodium the digits 120.0 and by using the knob meant for potassium the digits 2.0. are adjusted. Introduce the standard 140/4.0 mEq/L. If the standards are accurately prepared the digital display will indicate exact concentration for both sodium and potassium. Introduce the standard 160/6.0 mEq/L and confirm the accuracy of the standard. Now introduce the test and record the readings for sodium and potassium.

Reagent	Test	Standard 1	Standard 2	Standard 3
Distilled water	10 mL	10 mL	10 mL	10 mL
Serum	0.1 mL	—	—	—
Standard (120/2.0 mEq/L)	—	0.1 mL	—	—
Standard (140/4.0 mEq/L)	—	—	0.1 mL	—
Standard (160/6.0 mEq/L)	—	—	—	0.1 mL

Normal Value

Sodium (Na): 135–145 mEq/L
Potassium (K): 1–15 years : 3.7–5.0 mEq/L
16–59 years : 3.6–4.8 mEq/L
≥ 60 years : 3.9–5.3 mEq/L

Clinical Significance

Estimation of serum sodium is useful in diagnosis and treatment of dehydration and overhydration. Changes in sodium more often reflect changes in water balance. Increased sodium values (hypernatremia) are observed in conditions, such as:
- Severe dehydration
- Diabetes insipidus

- Salt poisoning
- Cushing's syndrome
- In certain postrenal conditions like enlarged prostate leading to obstruction of urine flow

Decreased sodium values (hyponatremia) are observed in conditions such as:
- Severe prolonged diarrhea and vomiting
- Salt losing nephritis
- Addison's disease

Estimation of serum potassium is very useful in paralysis, severe fluid and electrolyte loss, diabetic coma, renal failure, etc. Increased potassium values (hyperkalemia) are observed in conditions, such as:
- Addison's disease
- Renal glomerular disease
- In anuria and oliguria
- Familial hyperkalemic paralysis
- Acute acidosis
- Decreased insulin
- Intravascular hemolysis

Decreased potassium values (hypokalemia) are observed in conditions, such as:
- Cushing's syndrome
- Renal tubular damage
- Metabolic alkalosis
- Malnutrition

■ URINE SODIUM AND POTASSIUM

Urine Sodium

To determine urine sodium value, the method used is flame photometry. The procedure is exactly same as that of serum sodium. Use undiluted urine instead of serum.

Calculation

$$24 \text{ hours excretion of urine sodium} = \frac{24 \text{ hours urine volume (mL)}}{100}$$

Normal Value

Urine sodium: 40–220 mEq/24 hour.

Increased in diuretics, high sodium diet, acute tubular necrosis (ATN), salt-losing nephritis, Addison's disease, hypothyroidism, syndrome inappropriate ADH secretion (SIADH), CHF and liver failure.

Decreased in fasting, some fevers and chronic nephritis.

Urine Potassium

To determine urine potassium value, the method used is flame photometry. The procedure is exactly same as that of serum potassium. Use diluted urine (1: 10) instead of serum.

Calculation

Urine potassium, mEq/L = reading × 10

24 hours urine excretion =

$$\frac{\text{Urine potassium (mEq/L)} \times \text{24 hours urine volume (mL)}}{1000}$$

Normal Value

Urine potassium: 25–100 mEq/24 hour.

Increased in primary or secondary aldosteronism, glucocorticoids, alkalosis, renal tubular acidosis, excess potassium intake.

Decreased in acute renal failure, potassium sparing diuretics, diarrhea, and hypokalemia.

■ SERUM AND URINE CHLORIDE

Serum Chloride

Chloride is the major extracellular anion of the body. Its primary role in the body is to maintain proper water distribution, osmotic pressure and normal anion-cation balance in the plasma. In gastric juice, chloride also plays important role in the production of HCl. The chloride ions are ingested through the food (regular salt) and filtered or reabsorbed by the kidney as per the body need.

Method
Modified Schoenfeld and Lewellen's method.

Specimen
Serum or heparinized plasma.

Principle
Chloride ions react with mercuric thiocyanate to form mercuric chloride, an undissociated salt to liberate thiocyanate ions. These thiocyanate ions react with the ferric ions to form ferric thiocyanate, which is colored compound. The color formed is proportional to the chloride content of the specimen. The absorbance can be read at 520 nm. The final color is stable for half an hour:

$$Hg(SCN)_2 + 2Cl^- \longrightarrow HgCl_2 + 2SCN^-$$
$$3\,SCN + Fe^{3+} \longrightarrow Fe(SCN)_3 \text{ (colored compound)}$$

Reagent
- Chloride reagent
- Chloride standard (100 mEq/L)

Procedure
Take three test tubes and mark them as T, S and B. Add 2 mL of chloride reagent in each tube. Add 0.1 mL of serum, 0.1 mL of chloride standard and 0.1 mL of distilled water in test, standard and blank, respectively. Mix well and keep at room temperature for 2 minutes. Read the absorbance of test and standard against blank at 505 nm.

Reagent	T	S	B
Chloride reagent	1 mL	1 mL	1 mL
Serum	0.1 mL	—	—
Chloride standard	—	0.1 mL	—
Distilled water	—	—	0.1 mL

Calculations

Serum chloride (mEq/dL) = $\dfrac{\text{OD of T}}{\text{OD of S}} \times 100$

Normal value: 96–109 mEq/dL

Clinical Significance

Serum chloride is very useful to assess electrolyte, acid-base and water balance. Serum chloride is increased in metabolic acidosis associated with prolonged diarrhea, renal tubular diseases, respiratory alkalosis, some cases of hyperparathyroidism, diabetes insipidus, dehydration, and in conditions causing decreased renal blood flow, i.e. congestive heart failure.

Serum chloride levels are decreased in prolonged vomiting (loss of HCl), salt losing renal diseases, chronic respiratory acidosis, burns, and effect of certain drugs like corticosteroids, bicarbonates, etc.

Urine Chloride

To determine urine chloride value, the method used is modified Schoenfeld and Lewellen's method. The procedure is exactly same as that of serum chloride. Use undiluted urine instead of serum.

Calculation

Chloride excretion, mg/24 hours =

$$\dfrac{\text{Urine chl mEq/L} \times 24\text{ h urine volume (mL)}}{1000}$$

(chl: chloride, h: hours)

Normal Values

The normal range is 20–250 mEq/day. This range is highly dependent on salt intake and the state of the individual's hydration.

Clinical Significance

Increased urine chloride excretion may be caused by—increased salt intake, postmenstrual diuresis, pharmacologic diuresis, salt-losing nephritis, adrenocortical insufficiency.

Decreased urine chloride excretion may occur with—decreased salt intake, adrenocortical hyperfunction, extrarenal fluid loss (such as diarrhea, vomiting, sweating, and gastric suction), salt retention.

■ SERUM AND URINE PHOSPHORUS

Serum Phosphorus

Most of the phosphorus in the blood exists as inorganic phosphate. About 80% of the total phosphorus is combined with calcium in bones and teeth. It is found in every cell of the body. About 10% is combined with proteins, lipids and carbohydrate and other compounds in blood and muscle. The remaining 10% is widely distributed in various chemical compounds.

Method

Gomori's method.

Principle

Protein in serum is first removed by treating with TCA. Protein free filtrate is then treated with an acid molybdate, which reacts with inorganic phosphate to form phosphomolybdic acid. The color reagent, metol reduces phosphomolybdic acid to give a blue colored compound. The intensity of the color is measured at 660 nm.

Reagents

- Trichloroacetic acid (10 g/dL)
- Molybdate reagent
- Color reagent, metol
- Phosphorus standard (5 mg/dL)

Procedure

Take two centrifuge tubes. Mark them as test and diluted standard. Add 4.5 mL TCA reagent in each tube. Add 0.5 mL of serum in test and 0.5 mL of standard in diluted standard tubes. Mix and centrifuge to get clear filtrate. Pipette in the tubes as follows:

Test	Standard	Blank	
Filtrate	2.5 mL	—	—
Diluted standard	—	2.5 mL	—
Distilled water	—	—	2.5 mL
Molybdate reagent	0.5 mL	0.5 mL	0.5 mL
Color reagent	0.5 mL	0.5 mL	0.5 mL

Mix thoroughly and keep in the dark for 10 minutes. Read the intensities at 660 nm.

Calculation

Serum inorganic phosphorus

$$(mg/dL) = \frac{OD\ of\ T}{OD\ of\ S} \times 5$$

Normal Value

Neonates   : 045–100 mg%
1–19 years : 120–240 mg%
20–29 years : 144–275 mg%
30–39 years : 165–295 mg%
40–49 years : 177–350 mg%
50–59 years : 160–330 mg%
> 69 years : 170–300 mg%

Clinical Significance

Decreased serum phosphorus values are observed in preliminary hyperparathyroidism, rickets (vitamin D deficiency) and in Fanconi's syndrome (defect in reabsorption of phosphorus). Increased serum phosphorus levels are found in hypervitaminosis-D, hypoparathyroidism and in renal failure.

Urine Inorganic Phosphorus

The daily excretion of inorganic phosphorus on an average diet is about 1 g. There is increased excretion of phosphorus in urine in hyperparathyroidism, and it is reduced in hypoparathyroidism.

Phosphate excretion is also reduced in rickets, due to impaired absorption of phosphorus.

Method

Gomori's method. Reagents and principle are same as that of serum inorganic phosphate.

Specimen

A 24-hour urine sample with thymol crystals added as a preservative.

Procedure

Dilute the urine sample to 1: 100 in TCA reagent. Also dilute the standard 5 mg/dL in TCA reagent. If proteins are present, a preparation of protein free filtrate is must; if proteins are absent, then directly proceed for the part II step of the serum inorganic phosphate procedure.

Calculation

Urine inorganic phosphorus

$$(mg/dL) = \frac{OD \text{ of } T}{OD \text{ of } S} \times 5$$

Inorganic phosphorus excretion, mg/24 hrs =

$$\frac{\text{Urine calcium (mg/dL)} \times \text{Vol. of 24 hours urine}}{100}$$

Clinical Significance

High urinary phosphorus (i.e. increased renal losses) occurs in primary hyperparathyroidism, vitamin D deficiency, renal tubular acidosis, diuretic use. Phosphates are among the substances, which may be lost in the Fanconi syndrome. Renal loss of phosphate may itself lead to rickets or osteomalacia.

Low in hypoparathyroidism, pseudohypoparathyroidism, vitamin D intoxication.

■ SERUM AND URINE CALCIUM

Serum Calcium

Calcium is the major constituent of bone. Calcium in serum is present in ionized form or as a complex with protein or other inorganic substances like citrate, phosphate and others. Calcium plays many important roles in physiology of the body like it activates many enzymes and plays a key role in blood coagulation.

Method

O-cresolphthalein complexone (OCPC) method.

Specimen

Serum or heparinized plasma. It should be separated as soon as possible.

Principle

Calcium in an alkaline medium reacts with O-cresolphthalein complexone to form an intense chromophore, which is of purple color. Read the absorbance at 575 nm.

Reagents

1. O-cresolphthalein complexone reagent
2. Buffer solution
3. Calcium standard (10 mg/dL)

Procedure

First of all prepare working solution by mixing equal amounts of reagent 1 and reagent 2. This is to be freshly prepared as it is stable only for one day. Take three test tubes and mark them as T, S and B. Add 6 mL of freshly prepared working reagent in each tube. Add 0.05 mL of serum, 0.05 mL of calcium standard and 0.05 mL of distilled water in test, standard and blank, respectively. Mix well and keep at room temperature for exactly 10 minutes. Read the absorbance of test and standard against blank at 575 nm.

Reagent	T	S	B
Working reagent	6 mL	6 mL	6 mL
Serum	0.05 mL	—	—
Calcium standard	—	0.05 mL	—
Distilled water	—	—	0.05 mL

Calculation

$$\text{Serum calcium (mg/dL)} = \frac{\text{OD of T}}{\text{OD of S}} \times 10$$

Normal Value

1–3 years : 8.7–9.8 mg/dL
4–11 years : 8.8–10.1 mg/dL
12–13 years : 8.8–10.6 mg/dL
14–15 years : 9.2–10.7 mg/dL
> 16 years : 8.9–10.7 mg/dL

Clinical Significance

Determination of serum calcium level is useful in diagnosis of parathyroid dysfunction, hypercalcemia of malignancy, 90% of cases of hypercalcemia are due to hyperparathyroidism, neoplasms or granulomatous diseases. Hypercalcemia of sarcoidosis adrenal insufficiency and hyperthyroidism tend to be found in clinically evident disease. Blood calcium should be monitored in renal disease, effects of various drugs, acute pancreatitis, postoperative thyroidectomy and parathyroidectomy.

Calcium levels are found to be low in hypoparathyroidism, malabsorption of calcium and vitamin D, chronic renal disease with uremia, bone disease, late pregnancy, asphyxia, infants of diabetic mothers, cerebral injuries, malignant disease, etc.

Urine Calcium

The same method can be used to determine urine calcium.

Specimen

A 24 hour of urine sample preserved with thymol crystals.

Calculations

Urine calcium (mg/dL) = $\dfrac{\text{OD of T}}{\text{OD of S}} \times 10$

For the determination of 24-hour calcium excretions, measure the urine volume and calculate the result as follows:

Calcium excretion, mg/24 hours =

$$\dfrac{\text{Urine calcium (mg/dL)} \times \text{Vol. of 24 hour urine}}{100}$$

Normal value: 100–300 mg/dL in 24 hour of urine sample.

Clinical Significance

Determination of urine calcium level is useful in diagnosis of hypercalciuria causing renal calculi. High calcium levels in urine are seen in—hyperparathyroidism, excess milk intake, high calcium diet, rapidly progressive osteoporosis, multiple myeloma, Paget's disease, etc. Hypercalciuria without hypercalcemia are due to medullary sponge kidney, renal tubular acidosis, hyperthyroidism, etc.

Low calcium level in urine is due to renal failure, hypoparathyroidism, rickets, osteomalacia, metastatic carcinoma of prostate, etc.

SUMMARY

- Electrolytes are charged molecules that help to move nutrients into and wastes out of the body's cells, maintain a healthy water balance and help stabilize the body's pH level.
- Electrolytes are classified on the basis of location, ability to participate in transmission, ability to form complex and pH.
- Balance of the electrolytes in our bodies is essential for normal function of our cells and organs.
- Sodium and potassium are estimated by flame photometer.
- Sodium estimation is based on the modified Maruna and Trinder method, in which sodium is precipitated as the triple salt, sodium magnesium uranyl

- acetate, with the excess uranium then being reacted with ferrocyanide, producing a chromophore of brown color.
- Potassium estimation is based on turbidimetric method that potassium ions from specimen react with sodium tetraphenyl boron resulting in a turbid suspension.
- Urine sodium and potassium levels are also determined by flame photometer. The levels are decreased in renal failure.
- *Chloride*: Primary role of chloride is to maintain proper water distribution, osmotic pressure and normal anion-cation balance in the plasma.
- Chloride estimation is based on modified Schoenfeld and Lewellen's method that chloride ions react with mercuric thiocyanate to liberate thiocyanate ions, which reacts with the ferric ions to form ferric thiocyanate.
- Most of the phosphorus in the blood exists as inorganic phosphate, combined with calcium in bones and teeth.
- Serum phosphorus is determined by Gomori's method, based on the principle that protein free filtrate is treated with an acid molybdate, reacts with inorganic phosphate to form phosphomolybdic acid. The color reagent, Metol reduces phosphomolybdic acid to give a blue colored compound.
- Calcium in serum is present in ionized form or as a complex with protein or other inorganic substances.
- Calcium estimation is based on the principle that calcium in an alkaline medium reacts with o-cresolphthalein complexone to form an intense chromophore.
- Estimation of electrolytes is critically significant because, sodium, potassium, chloride, and bicarbonate help regulate nerve and muscle function and maintain acid-base balance and water balance.

PRACTICE QUESTIONS

1. What are electrolytes? How they are classified?
2. Discuss clinical significance of each electrolyte.
3. Write principle and procedure to determine sodium ions.
4. Write principle and procedure to determine potassium ions.
5. Write principle and procedure to determine sodium and potassium ions using flame photometry.
6. Write principle and procedure to determine chloride ions.
7. Write principle and procedure to determine phosphorus ions.
8. Write principle and procedure to determine calcium ions.
9. Make a list of all electrolytes and their normal values.

CHAPTER 25

Body Fluids

> **Keywords**
>
> Oligospermia, necrozoospermia, azoospermia, amniocentesis, serous fluid, transudates, exudates, pericarditis, chylous effusion, empyema, chyliform effusion, thoracentesis, markers of pleural tuberculosis (TB), systemic lupus erythematosus (SLE), ascites, paracentesis, arthrocentesis, seminal fluid citric acid, fructose, zinc, acrosome, prostate gland, the seminal vesicles, epididymis, amniotic fluid amniocentesis, bilirubin, creatinine, erythroblastosis fetalis, hepatitis, cerebrospinal fluid (CSF), serous fluid, pericardial fluid, tuberculosis, pleural fluid, amylase, tumor markers, adenosine deaminase (ADA), interferon gamma release assays (IGRAs), peritoneal fluid, serum-ascites albumin gradient (SAAG), synovial fluid, arthritis

■ INTRODUCTION

Body fluids are liquids originating from inside the bodies of living humans and play a vital role within our bodies. They are made up of proteins and are excreted or secreted from the body. There are different types of body fluids that are present in the human body. In healthy adult men, the total body water is about 60% of the total body weight.

The role of different body fluids test is to help detect, isolate, identify any physiological abnormality or other pathogenic microorganisms present in the body. It can also be done on other types of body fluids because they give a better idea of the kind of disease or disorders present in certain parts of the body. Pathologically important body fluids are discussed in this chapter.

■ SEMINAL FLUID

Semen is the bodily fluid in the urethra of the penis which is released during ejaculation. This cloudy, white substance is created by secretions from the male reproductive organs. During ejaculation sperm will move through the ejaculatory ducts to mix with fluid from the prostate, seminal vesicles and bulbourethral glands, forming semen.

The average semen volume in an ejaculation is 2–5 mL. Semen from one ejaculation contain around 40–600 million sperms depending on the length of time the ejaculation lasts and the volume of the ejaculation.

Most of the fluids in semen are made from secretions of male reproductive organs. The contributions and components of semen are given below:

Gland	Approximate (%)	Descriptions
Testes	2–5	Around 200–500 million spermatozoa (sperm) are produced in the testes and released during ejaculation
Seminal vesicle	65–75	Citrate, amino acids, flavins, enzymes, fructose (2–5 mg/mL of semen). This is the main energy source for sperm
Prostate	25–30	Citric acid, acid phosphatase, prostate specific antigen, zinc and proteolytic enzymes. Zinc helps to stabilize chromatin that contains DNA in sperm. Zinc deficiencies can lower fertility because sperm will become more fragile
Bulbourethral glands	Less than 1	Mucus which increases sperm mobility in the cervix and vagina by making the channel more viscous so that the sperm can swim

Sample Collection

- Masturbation
- Sex with a condom
- Sex with withdrawal before ejaculation
- Ejaculation stimulated by electricity

Precautions While Collecting Sample

- Ask patient to avoid ejaculation for 24–72 hours before the test.
- Also to avoid alcohol, caffeine and drugs such as cocaine and marijuana two to five days before the test.

- The semen must be kept at body temperature.
- The semen must be delivered to the testing facility within 30–60 minutes of leaving the body.

Analysis

- The appearance should be whitish to gray and opalescent. Semen that has a red-brown tint could indicate the presence of blood while a yellow tint could indicate jaundice or be a medication side effect.
- The typical volume of semen collected is between 1.5 and 5.5 milliliters (mL) of fluid per ejaculation. Decreased volume of semen would indicate fewer sperm, which diminishes opportunities for successful fertilization and subsequent pregnancy. Excessive seminal fluid may dilute the concentration of sperm.
- The semen should initially be thick and then liquefy within 15–30 minutes. If this does not occur, then it may impede sperm movement.
- Sperm concentration (also called sperm count or sperm density) is measured in millions of sperm per milliliter of semen. Normal is at least 20 million or more sperm per mL, with a total ejaculate volume of 80 million or more. Fewer sperm and/or a lower sperm concentration may impair fertility. Following a vasectomy, the goal is to have no sperm detected in the semen sample.

  Sperm can be counted either manually or by automated methods. Although, automated counting has some advantages for assessment of motility parameters, manual counting is still performed by most clinical laboratories. Hemocytometer (which is used to calculate blood cells) is used to count sperm manually. Calculate the total number of sperm in 5 large squares in both chambers of the hemocytometer. Divide the total number of sperm in the 10 large squares (5 large squares per 2 chambers) by 100 to estimate the number of millions of sperm.
- Motility is the percentage of moving sperm in a sample and graded based on speed and direction travelled. At least 50% should be motile one hour after ejaculation, moving forward in a straight line with good speed. The progression of the sperm, best measured using an automated system, is rated on a basis from zero (no motion) to 4, with 3–4 representing good motility.

Motility can be observed manually by hanging drop technique. Place a drop of semen on a coverslip over cavity slide. Examine with low and high power objective.

Description	Sperm concentration in ejaculate
Mild oligospermia	10 million–20 million sperm/mL
Severe oligospermia	0–5 million sperm/mL
Necrozoospermia	Sperm present but immobile
Azoospermia	0 sperm

Normal sperm morphology: A normal sperm has following parts:
- *Head:* The head is almost conical in shape and is formed of acrosome and nucleus.
    * *Acrosome*: This is found at the anterior tip of the sperm. The acrosome forms a cap like structure called the head cap. The acrosome itself is bounded by a unit membrane. It consists of a number of hydrolytic enzymes such as acid phosphatase, hyaluronidase and others. These enzymes help in tissue lysis (dissolving) and this facilitates the penetration of the sperm into the egg membrane. The enzymes are proteolytic and help in dissolving the egg membrane.
    * *Sperm nucleus*: The nucleus occupies most of the available space of the sperm head.
- *Neck:* The head is followed by a short neck to separate the middle piece of the sperm. The neck consists of just two granules (centrioles).
- *Middle piece:* The middle piece of the sperm consists of the upper portion of the axial filament which contains alpha, beta and gamma fibers. These are the sites of various enzymes.
- *Tail:* The tail usually is the longest part in the sperm.

There are various types of morphological defects found with different parts of sperm like double head, small or no acrosome, neck defects, coiled or short tail, etc. These are analyzed by nigrosin–eosin stain in microscopic analysis.

Biochemical Tests

There are various biochemical markers of accessory gland function, e.g., citric acid, zinc and acid phosphatase for the prostate gland;

Table 25.1: Biochemical variables of semen analysis.

Biochemical tests	Reference value
Total fructose (seminal vesicle marker)	≥13 µmol/ejaculate
Total zinc (prostate marker)	≥2.4 µmol/ejaculate
Total acid phosphatase (prostate marker)	≥200 U/ejaculate
Total citric acid (prostate marker)	≥52 µmol/ejaculate
α-glucosidase (epididymis marker)	≥20 mU/ejaculate
Carnitine (epididymis marker)	0.8–2.9 µmol/ejaculate

fructose and prostaglandins for the seminal vesicles, free L-carnitine, glycerophosphocholine, and alpha-glucosidase for the epididymis. A low secretory function is reflected in a low total output of the specific marker.

Preparation of semen sample for biochemical tests:
Centrifuge seminal fluid at 3,000 rpm for 10–15 min. Stability of the sample is 7 days at 2–8°C. The supernatant is called seminal plasma. Dilute supernatant (1+99) with sodium chloride solution (0.9%) and multiply the result by 100.

- Resorcinol method is used for detection of fructose. In this test, 5 mL of resorcinol reagent (50 mg resorcinol dissolved in 33 mL concentrated hydrochloric acid; dilute up to 100 mL with distilled water) is added to 0.5 mL of seminal fluid. The mixture is heated and brought for boiling. If fructose is present, a red-colored precipitate is formed within 30 seconds. Absence of fructose indicates obstruction proximal to seminal vesicles (obstructed or absent vas deferens) or a lack of seminal vesicles. In a case of azoospermia, if fructose is absent, it is due to the obstruction of ejaculatory ducts or absence of vas deferens, and if present, azoospermia is due to failure of testes to produce sperm.
- Zinc test is based on the principle that zinc reacts with 2-(5-bromo-2-pyridylazo)-5-(N-propyl-N-sulfopropylamino)-phenol (5-Br-PAPS) to form a red chelate complex at pH 9.8. The increase of absorbance measure at 560 nm is proportional to the concentration of total zinc in the sample. Low zinc value indicates prostate dysfunction or ejaculatory duct obstruction.

- Acid phosphatase is enzyme from phosphatase group. It is used as a marker for the presence of prostatic fluid.
- Citric acid is an indicator of prostatic gland function. Decreased citric acid levels may indicate either prostate dysfunction or prostatic duct obstruction. It can be measured using the Boehringer enzymatic, NADH-linked method.
- Seminal plasma contains both neutral α-glucosidase isoenzyme that originated from the epididymis and an acid isoenzyme contributed by the prostate. The latter can be selectively inhibited to allow measurement of neutral α-glucosidase. P-nitrophenol α-glucopyranoside in the presence of α-glucosidase is converted to p-nitrophenol, and the absorbance can be read at 405 nm. Low neutral α-glucosidase isoenzyme indicates dysfunction-obstruction of epididymis.
- L-carnitine is amino acid secreted by epididymis. It is a measure of fertility, determined by various chromatographic methods.
- Besides these markers, pH is also important part of semen analysis. Normal pH of seminal plasma should be 7.2–8.0. Changes in pH influence the health of sperm.

Clinical Significance

A semen analysis is often recommended when couples are having problems getting pregnant. The test will help a doctor determine if a man is infertile. The analysis will also help determine if low sperm count or sperm dysfunction is the reason behind infertility. Men who have had a vasectomy undergo semen analysis to make sure no sperm are in their semen.

Abnormal sperm will have trouble reaching and penetrating eggs, making conception difficult. Abnormal results could indicate—infertility, infection, hormonal imbalance, disease such as diabetes, gene defects or exposure to radiation.

■ AMNIOTIC FLUID

Amniotic fluid is present in the amnion, a membranous sac that surrounds the fetus. It surrounds, protects, and gives nourishment to the fetus during gestation period. Amniotic fluid keeps are increasing throughout the pregnancy. At 10 weeks of gestation, it is about 30 mL whereas, in full term, volume may exceed 1500 mL.

Sample Collection

Amniotic fluid is collected by amniocentesis. Amniocentesis is done during the 14, 16, and 18 weeks of gestation. Amniotic fluid needs to be refrigerated. It is collected in amber colored tube to avoid amniotic fluid from light for the estimation of bilirubin.

The purpose of the test is—to diagnose chromosomal abnormalities, diagnose inherited metabolic disorders like cystic fibrosis. Thus, amniocentesis help for elective abortion in the defective fetus. It also measures bilirubin in Rh sensitization for erythroblastosis fetalis, Analysis of the amniotic fluid for bilirubin level is also useful in the Rh-negative mothers in later weeks of the gestation gives the severity of anemia due to Rh-incompatibility. Genetic abnormalities like sickle cell anemia, thalassemia, and Down's syndrome are diagnosed.

Amniotic fluid is aspirated by the needle into the amniotic sac is called amniocentesis. This is transabdominal amniocentesis. Another route is transvaginal amniocentesis. This method carries a great risk of infection.

30 mL of amniotic fluid is collected in the sterile syringes. The first 2 to 3 mL collected is discarded because this may be contaminated by the maternal blood, tissue fluid, and cells.

Complications of the procedure are there may be a miscarriage, there are chances for injury to the fetus or there may be a leak of amniotic fluid.

Normal Amniotic Fluid Findings

General test	Result
Appearance	Clear, pale to straw yellow
AFP (alpha fetoprotein)	14 to 16 weeks = <5.2 mg/dL, 22 weeks = <3.0 mg/dL
Bilirubin	<0.2 mg/dL
Creatinine	>2.0 mg/dL after 37 weeks
Chromosomal abnormality	Absent
Phosphatidylglycerol	Positive (negative in immature)
Lecithin/Sphingomyelin ratio	Mature >2.0, Immature <2.0, Diabetic mother >3.5
Microscopic examination	There are amniotic epithelial cells from the lining of the sac. Fetal squamous cells originating from fetal skin, oral mucosa, and vagina.

Abnormal Amniotic Fluid Findings

Lab findings	Findings	Clinical significance
Appearance	Yellow	Erythroblastosis (due to the presence of bilirubin)
	Red-brown (dark red-brown)	Indicate fetal death
	Amber color	Indicates bilirubin
	Green color	Due to meconium, fetal hypoxia
	Pink-red (blood-streaked)	Blood contamination, traumatic tap, intra-amniotic hemorrhage
Volume	Increased	Hydramnios due to fetal abnormality
	Decrease	Oligohydramnios is associated with rupture membranes and fetal abnormality, urinary tract deformities
Presence of cells	Long bipolar cells, multiple filamentous pseudopodia, large vacuolated cells with inclusions	Neural tube defect
Bilirubin	At 28 weeks = >0.075 mg/dL	Erythroblastosis fetalis, hepatitis
	At 40 weeks = <0.025 mg/dL	Maternal infection, sickle cell crises
Saturated phosphatidylcholine	>500 µg/L	Respiratory distress syndrome
AFP	Increased, >2.5 MoM	Open spinal defects (neural tube defect)
Creatinine	>2.0 mg/dL	Indicates fetal maturity and the maternal level is normal

■ CEREBROSPINAL FLUID

Cerebrospinal fluid (CSF) is a clear fluid, circulates in the brain and spinal cord. Normal adult has 90–150 mL and newborn 10–60 mL of CSF.

Cerebrospinal fluid acts as buffer, regulates intracranial pressure, carries nutrients to the nervous system and serves as excretory channel for metabolic wastes in the CNS.

Collecting a specimen: Invasive test with potential harm to patient. It is done only for serious reasons like to diagnose meningitis, brain hemorrhage and diagnosis of neurological disease or malignancy. Only a physician collects CSF as it involves risk to patient. Careful handling of specimen is necessary. Three separate tubes of about 5 mL are collected and numbered in sequence.

It acts as blood-brain-barrier. CSF is not an ultrafiltrate of plasma. Many drugs do not enter the CSF from the blood. Some electrolytes are more concentrated, others are less concentrated.

Protein is found only in very small amount. Chemistry tests and microbial examination is done from the first tubes and the last one is for cell counts.

The CSF samples should never be refrigerated. Certain viral studies may require immediate freezing at very low temperatures. Never discard CSF until all tests are done.

Gross appearance: Normal CSF is crystal clear and the consistency of water.

Turbidity: May indicate white cells, bacteria, excess protein or fat. Radiographic dye will give the CSF an oily look. Clotting may be from a traumatic tap.

Color: Bloody fluid—can be from a traumatic tap or may indicate subarachnoid hemorrhage, xanthochromia—may indicate bleeding, lysed RBCs or high protein levels.

CSF cell counts: Normally very few cells are found in CSF—no RBCs, 0–8 WBCs.

PMNs are seen in bacterial infection and lymphocytes are seen in viral infection.

The cells are usually counted manually, with undiluted specimen.

When a cell count is over 30 white cells/microliter a differential count is done smear is made from centrifuged sediment and stained. Cytospin yields better cell count with small amount centrifuged sediment may be used.

Biochemical Tests

- CSF contains same chemicals that are found as in plasma. Normal values are different because of selective filtration.
- **Proteins:** Protein tests and electrophoresis are common tests of many disease states. Normal range is 12-60 mg/dL (less than 1% of plasma concentration).
- Increased protein levels are seen in infections, decreased levels, and leakage of fluid from CNS.
- **Glucose:** Usually about 60-80% of blood glucose should be measured at the same time difference is significant. Bacteria utilize glucose therefore glucose level reduced in bacterial meningitis, but not in viral. Glucose is elevated in diabetic coma.
- **Glutamine:** Indirect measure of waste products. It is seen in some liver disorders, bilirubin and chloride and lactate dehydrogenase.
- **Microbiological examination:** Gram stains and cultures are useful to diagnose acute bacterial meningitis. Organisms can be seen in the Gram stain, acid fast stains for TB, India ink that stains *Cryptococcus*.

Serous Fluid

It includes pleural, pericardial and peritoneal fluids contained within closed cavities of the body. This fluid fills space between layers of cells to lubricate the surfaces as they move against each other. The fluids are formed and reabsorbed as volume is very small. Increased volume is referred as an effusion.

Transudates: Increase in fluid volume (effusion) occurs in many conditions. Transudate is usually the result of a systemic disease. Transudates result from abnormal movement of fluid across a membrane.

Exudates: The effusions result from an inflammatory response serous effusions are classified as transudate or exudate by protein content. Transudates usually have less than 3 g/dL exudates usually over 8 g/dL.

Collection: Strictly antiseptic conditions are needed. It is collected by aspiration. It may be collected for diagnostic purposes or to relieve excess accumulation. EDTA tube for cell counts, morphology and differential, anticoagulated sample for chemical analysis, sterile tube for Gram stain and culture are needed. Keep extra tubes for cytology tumor studies.

■ PERICARDIAL FLUID

Pericardium is a tough double walled sac surrounding the heart. It protects heart from mechanical injuries and external shocks.

Pericardium consists of two membranes, the outer layer is fibrous parietal pericardium and the inner layer is serous visceral pericardium. A fluid is present in between these two layers. It is called as pericardial fluid and the space where it is present is called as pericardial cavity.

Normal values of pericardial fluid:

Pericardial fluid	*Normal value*
Appearance	Clear
Volume	15–50 mL
Color	Pale yellow
Glucose	Parallel serum values
Red blood cell count	None seen
White blood cell count	Less than 300/mm^3
Culture	No growth
Gram stain	No organisms seen
Cytology	No abnormal cells seen

There are two main types of pericardial fluid:
1. **Transudate:** The fluid that accumulates when there is an imbalance between the pressure within blood vessels (which drives fluid out of blood vessels) and the amount of protein in blood (which keeps fluid in blood vessels) in such case, the fluid is called as transudate.

2. **Exudate:** The fluid that accumulates when there is an injury or inflammation of the pericardium, in such case the fluid is called as exudate.

Transudate	Exudate
90% of pericardial fluids are transudates	10% of pericardial fluids are exudates
Fluid appears clear	Fluid may appear cloudy
Albumin level—low	Albumin level—higher than in transudates
Cell count—few cells are present	Cell count—increased
Transudates are most often caused by congestive heart failure or cirrhosis	Exudates may be the result of conditions such as infection (bacterial, viral or fungal), malignancies (metastatic cancer, lymphoma, mesothelioma), or autoimmune disease

Differentiation between the types of fluid is important because it helps diagnose the specific disease or condition. Initial set of tests (cell count, protein or albumin level and appearance of the fluid) is used to distinguish between transudates and exudates.

Pericardiocentesis: It is process of removal of pericardial fluid from the pericardial sac with a needle and syringe. An intravenous (IV) line may be started and the person may be given medications prior to the sample collection. The patient is positioned lying down. A local anesthetic is applied, then the doctor inserts a needle into the space between the ribs (fifth to sixth intercostals space) on the left side of the chest and into the pericardial sac and removes a fluid sample. An ultrasound may be used to help guide the needle.

It can be used to relieve pressure from pericardial effusions or for diagnostic purposes, revealing the cause of abnormalities, such as cancer, cardiac perforation, cardiac trauma and congestive heart failure.

Pericardial Fluid Tests

Following tables interprets different aspects of pericardial fluid analysis.

Gross Appearance

Clear to pale yellow	Normal
Milk-colored (Chylous)	Lymphatic system involvement
Cloudy/turbid	Primary bacterial infection Presence of white blood cells
Bloody tap	Benign or malignant tumor Hemorrhagic pericarditis, perforated ulcer Internal bleeding

In the analysis of pericardial fluid, the first step should be to separate effusions into transudates and exudates.

These are separated on the basis of Light's criteria as described in **Table 25.2**. In practice, biochemistry of pericardial fluid is of less valves as compared to pleural fluid. Lactate dehydrogenase (LDH) and protein content are significant tests.

Pericardiocentesis Biochemistry

- Pericardial adenosine deaminase activity (ADA) >667 nkat/L (40 U/L) suggests tuberculous pericarditis. As cultures are less

Table 25.2: Light's criteria for transudate and exudate.

Characteristics	Transudate	Exudate
Appearance	Clear	Cloudy or turbid
Specific gravity	Less than 1.015	Greater than 1.015
Total protein	Less than 2.5 g/dL	Greater than 3.0 g/dL
Fluid-to-serum protein ratio	Less than 0.5	Greater than 0.5
LDH	Parallels serum value	Less than 200 units/L
Fluid-to-serum LDH ratio	Less than 0.6	Greater than 0.6
Fluid cholesterol	Less than 55 mg/dL	Greater than 55 mg/dL
White blood cell count	Less than 100/mm^3	Greater than 1,000/mm^3

sensitive, this indirect test has become the standard test in the diagnosis of pericardial tuberculosis.
- Pericardial interferon-gamma (IFN-gamma) >200 picograms/L suggests tuberculous pericarditis.

	Levels	Interpretation
Triglyceride	Elevated	Malignant tumor, lymphoma, TB Parasitic infection, hepatic cirrhosis
Glucose	Parallel to serum level	Lowered in case of infection

■ PLEURAL FLUID

Lungs have protective covering of visceral and parietal pleural membranes within the thoracic cavity.

Pleural Effusion

It is excess fluid that accumulates in the pleural cavity, the fluid-filled space that surrounds the lungs. This excess can impair breathing by limiting the expansion of the lungs.

Some pleural effusions are asymptomatic and are discovered incidentally during physical examination or on chest X-ray.

Many cause dyspnea, chest pain, usually a sharp pain that is worse with cough or deep breaths, cough, fever, hiccups, rapid breathing, shortness of breath and fatigue.

Thoracentesis

Once a pleural effusion is diagnosed, the cause must be determined. Pleural fluid is drawn out of the pleural space in a process called thoracentesis, and it should be done in almost all patients who have pleural fluid that is ≥10 mm in thickness on CT, ultrasonography, or lateral decubitus X-ray and that is new or of uncertain etiology. In thoracentesis, a needle is inserted through the back of the chest wall in the sixth, seventh, or eighth intercostal space on the midaxillary line, into the pleural space. The needle used is fine bore (21G) with 50 mL syringe.

Normal Findings

Appearance	Clear
Color	Pale yellow
Amylase	Parallels serum values
Cholesterol	Parallels serum values
CEA	Parallels serum values
Glucose	Parallels serum values
LDH	Less than 200 units/L
Fluid LDH-to-serum LDH ratio	0.6 or less
Protein	3 g/dL
Fluid protein-to-serum protein ratio	0.5 or less
Triglycerides	Parallel serum values
pH	7.37–7.43
RBC count	NIL
WBC count	Less than 1,000/mm^3
Culture	No growth
Gram stain	No organisms seen
Cytology	No abnormal cells seen

(CEA: carcinoembryonic antigen; LDH: lactate dehydrogenase; RBC: red blood cell; WBC: white blood cell)

Pleural Fluid Analysis

Following abnormal findings are associated with different clinical conditions:

Color:
- Milky appearance may point to lymphatic system involvement.
- Reddish pleural fluid may indicate the presence of blood.
- Cloudy, thick pleural fluid may indicate the presence of microorganisms and/or white blood cells.

Biochemical Tests

- **Amylase:** Amylase levels may increase (as compared to upper normal limit for serum) with pancreatitis, esophageal rupture or malignancy.

- **Cholesterol:** Normal cholesterol value runs parallel with serum values. It is above 200 mg/dL in case of pseudochylothorax and usually low in case of chylothorax.
- **Tumor markers:** Normal value of tumor marker runs parallel with serum values.
- For a definite diagnosis a panel of pleural fluid tumor markers including CEA, CA-125, CA 15-3 and CYFRA has been shown to reach a combined sensitivity of only 54%. Thus negative results do not help in investigation or monitoring. Mesothelin is a glycoprotein tumor marker that is present at higher mean concentrations in the blood and pleural fluid of patients with malignant mesothelioma than in patients with other causes of pleural effusion. Positive results have also been recognized in bronchogenic adenocarcinoma, metastatic pancreatic carcinoma, lymphoma and ovarian carcinoma. A positive serum or pleural fluid mesothelin level is highly suggestive of pleural malignancy but a negative result cannot be considered reassuring.
- **Glucose:** In the absence of pleural pathology, glucose diffuses freely across the pleural membrane and the pleural fluid glucose concentration is equivalent to blood. A low pleural fluid glucose level (<3.4 mmol/L) may be found in complicated parapneumonic effusions, empyema, rheumatoid pleuritis and pleural effusions associated with TB, malignancy and esophageal rupture. The most common causes of a very low pleural fluid glucose level (<1.6 mmol/L) are rheumatoid arthritis and empyema.
- **LDH:** Lactate levels can increase with infectious pleuritis, either bacterial or tuberculosis.
- **Triglyceride:** Triglyceride levels may be increased with lymphatic system involvement and in case of chylothorax.
- **pH:** Pleural fluid acidosis (pH <7.30) occurs in malignant effusions, complicated pleural infection, connective tissue diseases (particularly rheumatoid arthritis), TB and esophageal rupture. In isolation, it does not distinguish between these causes. Pleural fluid acidosis reflects an increase in lactic acid and carbon dioxide production. Increased consumption of glucose without replacement in the same conditions means that pleural fluid often has both a low pH and low glucose concentration.
- **Microscopic examination:** Normal pleural fluid has small numbers of white blood cells (WBCs) but no red blood cells (RBCs) or microorganisms.

Diagnostic Markers of Pleural TB

It is desirable to consider diagnosis of tuberculosis in patients with lymphocytic effusions. In patients who are unsuitable for invasive investigations, pleural fluid or blood biomarkers of infection can be useful.
- **Adenosine deaminase (ADA)** is an enzyme present in lymphocytes, and its level in pleural fluid is significantly raised in most tuberculous pleural effusions. Raised ADA levels can also be seen in empyema, rheumatoid disease and occasionally in malignancy. Measurement of isoenzyme ADA-2 can reduce the false positives significantly. ADA is very cheap and quick to perform and remains stable when stored at 48°C for up to 28 days. It is useful in patients with HIV or those immunosuppressed (e.g. renal transplant). Being a highly sensitive test ADA is a useful 'rule out' test in countries with low prevalence of TB.
- **Interferon gamma release assays (IGRAs)** have been studied with sensitivities as high as 90%, but specificity is limited by an inability of the tests to distinguish latent from active TB. The commercial tests are not yet validated for fluids other than blood. Comparatively ADA is easier to perform and cost effective.

■ PERITONEAL FLUID

Peritoneum is a tough semi-permeable membrane lining abdominal and visceral cavities. The organs of abdomen are enclosed in the peritoneum.

The peritoneum is important in osmoregulation.
- It controls passive diffusion of water and solute (up to a certain size).
- It maintains osmotic and chemical equilibrium with blood and lymph.

A fluid is present in between the layers of peritoneum; this is called as peritoneal fluid.

It is produced by mesothelial cells in the abdominal membranes. Peritoneal fluid acts to moisten the outside of the organs and to reduce the friction of organ movement during digestion.

Normal values of peritoneal fluid

Appearance: Light yellow, clear
Volume: Less than 50 mL
RBCs: Negative
WBCs: Less than 300/L
Protein: Less than 4.1 g/dL
Glucose: 70–100 mg/dL
Amylase: 138–404 units/L
Ammonia: Less than 50 mcg/dL
Alkaline phosphatase:
Female less than 45 years old: 76–196 units/L
Female more than 45 years old: 87–250 units/L
Male: 90–240 units/L
Lactate dehydrogenase (LDH): Should equal LDH blood levels
Cytology: Negative for the presence of abnormal cells
Bacteria: Negative
Fungi: Negative
Carcinoembryonic antigen (CEA): Negative for the presence of CEA.

Peritoneal fluid analysis is needed in two conditions:
1. In case of inflammation of the peritoneum called as peritonitis and/or
2. Excessive accumulation of peritoneal fluid called as peritoneal effusion or ascites.

Ascites develops either from:
- **Increased accumulation of fluid:** This happens when there is:
  - Increased capillary permeability
  - Increased venous pressure
  - Decreased protein (oncotic pressure)
- **Decreased clearance of fluid:** This happens when there is:
  - Increased lymphatic obstruction.

There are two main types of peritoneal fluid:
1. **Transudate:** The fluid that accumulates when there is an imbalance between the pressure within blood vessels (which drives fluid out of blood vessels) and the amount of protein in

blood (which keeps fluid in blood vessels) in such case, the fluid is called as transudate.
2. **Exudate:** The fluid that accumulates when there is an injury or inflammation of the peritoneum, in such case the fluid is called as exudate.

Transudate	Exudate
90% of ascitic fluids are transudates	10% of ascitic fluids are exudates
Fluid appears clear	Fluid may appear cloudy
Albumin level—low	Albumin level—higher than in transudates
SAAG values above 1.1 g/dL	SAAG values less than 1.1 g/dL
Cell count—few cells are present	Cell count—increased
Transudates are most often caused by congestive heart failure or cirrhosis	Exudates may be the result of conditions, such as infection (bacterial, viral or fungal), malignancies (metastatic cancer, lymphoma, mesothelioma), or autoimmune disease

Differentiation between the types of fluid is important because it helps to diagnose the likely cause of fluid accumulation. Initial set of tests (cell count, albumin level, and appearance of the fluid) is used to distinguish between transudates and exudates. Once the fluid is determined to be one or the other, additional tests may be performed to further pinpoint the disease or condition causing ascites.

Sample Collection

A sample collection procedure of peritoneal fluid is called as paracentesis.

Paracentesis is the removal of peritoneal fluid from the abdominal cavity with a needle, tubing, and a container that may have a vacuum. The patient is positioned lying down with the head of the bed raised. A local anesthetic is applied and then the doctor inserts the needle into the abdominal cavity and the sample is removed.

Peritoneal Fluid Tests

Following tables interprets different aspects of peritoneal fluid analysis.

Gross Appearance

Clear to pale yellow	Normal
Milk-colored (Chylous)	• Malignant tumor, lymphoma, TB • Parasitic infection, hepatic cirrhosis
Cloudy/turbid	• Peritonitis, primary bacterial infection • Perforated bowel, appendicitis, pancreatitis • Strangulated or infarcted bowel
Bloody tap	• Benign or malignant tumor • Hemorrhagic pancreatitis, perforated ulcer • Internal bleeding

Paracentesis Biochemistry

	Levels	Interpretation
Triglyceride	Elevated	• Malignant tumor, lymphoma, TB • Parasitic infection, hepatic cirrhosis
Protein	• 0.3–4.0 g/dL • >4 g/dL	• Normal • TB, SBP (small bowel perforation)
Glucose	• 7–10 • <6	• Normal • TB and malignancy
Amylase	• 50% of serum level • Increased (up to 5 × serum level)	• Normal • Pancreatitis, pancreatic pseudocyst, pancreatic trauma or Intestinal strangulation
Alkaline phosphatase	Increased	Small bowel perforation and strangulation

Exudate Serum: Ascites Ratios

- **Evidence for these ascites:** Serum ratio is controversial
  - Ascitic fluid protein/serum protein >0.5
  - Ascitic fluid LDH/serum LDH >0.6
  - Ascitic fluid LDH >400.
- Presence of any 2 of these three findings is usually associated with TB, malignancy or pancreatitis.
- Absence of all three usually indicates hepatic cause.

Serum-Ascites Albumin Gradient

- The serum-ascites albumin gradient (SAAG) is the most useful index for evaluating peritoneal fluid and can help distinguish ascites caused by portal hypertension (cirrhosis, portal vein thrombosis, Budd-Chiari syndrome, etc.) from other causes of ascites. In portal hypertension, the SAAG is >1.1 g/dL while ascites from other causes shows SAAG of less than 1.1 g/dL.
- Simple calculation:
  - Serum albumin—ascites albumin = SAAG.

SAAG > 1.1 mg/dL	SAAG < 1.1 mg/dL
- Cirrhosis - Alcoholic hepatitis - Cardiac ascites - "Mixed ascites" - Massive liver metastasis - Fulminant hepatic failure - Budd-Chiari syndrome - Portal vein thrombosis - Veno-occlusive disease - Myxedema - Fatty liver of pregnancy	- Peritoneal carcinomatosis - Tuberculous peritonitis - Pancreatic ascites - Bowel obstruction - Biliary ascites - Nephrotic syndrome - Postoperative lymphatic leak - Serositis in connective tissue disease

Microscopy and Analysis

Red cell count	Interpretation
- None - >100/mL - >100,000/mL	- Normal - Malignancy, TB - Intra-abdominal trauma (DPL-diagnostic peritoneal lavage)

White cell count	Interpretation
- <300/mL - >300/mL - >25% neutrophils - >25% lymphocytes - Mesothelial cells - Gram positive cocci - Gram negative	- Normal - Abnormal - SBP (90%), cirrhosis (50%) - TB or chylous ascites - TB peritonitis - Primary peritonitis - Secondary peritonitis

■ SYNOVIAL FLUID

Synovial fluid is formed as an ultrafiltrate of plasma across the synovial membrane. This is often referred to as joint fluid which is the viscous fluid found in the cavities of the moveable joints. This filtration is nonselective except for the exclusion of high molecular weight proteins. The contents of the synovial fluid are similar to the plasma values. This synovial fluid normally does not clot. But in inflammation due to increased fibrinogen may clot. The synovial cells lining the synovium secrete a mucopolysaccharide containing the hyaluronic acid and a small amount of the protein. This hyaluronic acid causes noticeable viscosity of the synovial fluid. The smooth articular cartilage and synovial fluid reduce friction between the bone during joint movements.

Sample Collection

Synovial fluid analysis is done to diagnose the cause of synovial fluid formation. Swelling and pain are the complaints from patients. It helps to differentiate inflammatory to non-inflammatory causes and arthritis due to crystals like gout and pseudogout. It is also done to monitor chronic arthritic diseases and to study malignant tumor involving the joint.

Synovial fluid is the aspirated fluid from the synovial spaces is called Arthrocentesis.

Collect specimen in three tubes:
1. Tube 1 sterile tube for culture.
2. Tube 2 for microscopy, add heparin and not use EDTA.
3. Tube 3 for chemistry, plain tube.

For glucose, the patient should have 6 hours fast.

Synovial fluid can be aspirated from joint of: Knee, Shoulder, Elbow, Wrist, Ankle, and Hip.

Procedure to collect sample:
- Sterile the area with an antiseptic solution, local anesthesia can be given to decrease the pain.
- Lay the patient on his or her back with the joint fully exposed.
- During aspiration, the joint may be wrapped with an elastic bandage to compress free fluid within a certain area to get maximum fluid.
- Insert a sterile needle into the joint space and get the synovial fluid for analysis.

Synovial fluid is present normally in a very small amount. The amount in the large knee joint is less than 3.5 mL. This fluid collection can increase in the inflammation and maybe around 25 mL. Synovial fluid contains mucopolysaccharides called hyaluronic acid which is responsible for the viscosity of the synovial fluid and lubricates the joints. An increase in a synovial fluid enough to aspirates is due to some disease.

Normal Constituents of the Synovial Fluid

Features	
Physical Features	
Volume	<1.5 mL
Color	Pale yellow
Clarity	Clear
Viscosity	Can form a string 4 to 6 cm long due to high concentration of hyaluronic acid Good mucin clot
Microscopic	
RBC count	<2000/cmm (0 to 2000/cmm)
White cell count	<200 /cmm (0 to 200/cmm)
Polys	<20% of the differential
Lymphocytes	<15% of the differential
Monocytes	65% of the differential
Macrophages	Variable in number
Crystals	Negative
Chemicals	
Glucose	<10 mg/dL lower than the blood level
Total protein	<3 g/dL (1 to 3 g/dL)
Lactate	<250 mg/dL
Uric acid	This is equal to the blood level (male = 2 to 8 mg/dL and female = 2 to 6 mg/dL)
Culture	Negative

Biochemical Tests

- Biochemistry analytes, such as total protein, glucose, albumin, LDH and uric acid are considered clinically important.
- **Glucose:** Typically, under fasting condition, blood and synovial fluid glucose levels are determined. The concentration of glucose

in the synovial fluid should not be more than 0.55 mmol/L and lower than blood value level. Low value of synovial fluid suggests infection or joint inflammation due to glycolytic activities of bacteria of white blood cells. In septic arthritis, this maybe 50% less than the blood glucose level.
- **Protein:** As protein is a large molecule, these molecules are not filtered through the synovial membrane. Normal synovial fluid protein is approximately one-third of blood plasma value. Synovial membrane permeability is altered by inflammation. Thus, the elevation synovial protein value indicates that patients might suffer from hemorrhagic or inflammatory of joint.
- **Lactate dehydrogenase:** LDH is usually raised in condition like rheumatoid arthritis.
- Increased protein and lactate level indicates a bacterial infection.
- **Uric acid:** Synovial fluid uric acid test is performed to verify the diagnosis of gout apart from the result obtained from the serum uric acid test.

Damage to the articular membrane produces pain and stiffness in the joints, this is referred to as arthritis.

There are following types of arthritis:

Etiological classification	Clinical significance
Non-inflammatory	Degenerative joint disease (Osteoarthritis) seen in old age
Inflammatory	An immunologic disorder like Rheumatoid arthritis, and SLE
Septic	Due to microbial infection like TB/viral/fungal
Hemorrhagic	Coagulation factor deficiency, and traumatic injury
Due to crystals	Increased fluid uric acid in gout, increased monocytes

Other Laboratory Tests

- Fluid analysis including:
    - *WBC count:* The differential of the cells.
    - Generally WBCs <200/cmm and RBCs <2000/µL.
    - Rheumatoid arthritis shows more lymphocytes (lymphocytosis).
- Gram stain is done for the diagnosis of gonorrhea.

- AFB stain is done to rule out tubercle bacilli.
- Culture and sensitivity is advised for bacteria and the fungus.
- The calcium pyrophosphate dihydrate crystals are birefringent in pseudogout (blue on red background).
- Complement level is done which is low in—systemic lupus erythematosus and rheumatoid arthritis.

Characteristics of synovial fluid in different type of arthritis.

Test	Non-inflammatory	Inflammatory	Septic	Hemorrhagic
Color	Yellow, clear	Yellow to white	Yellow to green	Red to brown
Viscosity	High (good)	Low	Low	Low
TLC (cmm)	<5000	10,000 to 100,000	10,000 to 200,000	50 to 10,000
Etiology (causative agent)	Degenerative joint disorder	Immunologic, rheumatoid, lupus	Staph. aureus, H. influenzae, Streptococcus pneumococci, Neisseria	Trauma, anticoagulant therapy
Polys (%)	<25	>50	>75	>25
Protein (g/dL)	<3.0	>3.0	>3.0	>3.0
Lactate (mg/dL)	Normal	Normal to high	>250 positive	Normal
Glucose serum/fluid (mg/dL)	<10	>25	>25	<10
Glucose	Normal	Decreased	Decreased	Normal

SUMMARY

- Body fluids are liquids originating from inside the bodies of living humans and play a vital role within our bodies. They are made up of proteins and are excreted or secreted from the body.
- Seminal fluid is produced during ejaculation by accessory glands of male reproductive system.
- Semen contains citric acid, free amino acids, fructose, enzymes, phosphorylcholine, prostaglandin, potassium, and zinc.
- 20 million or more sperms are present in 1 mL. A sperm has head with acrosome at its anterior side, neck, middle piece and tail for movement.

- Semen analysis is done to see morphological defects in sperm, total sperm count, and biochemical markers of accessory gland function.
- Biochemical markers are—citric acid, zinc and acid phosphatase for the prostate gland; fructose and prostaglandins for the seminal vesicles, free L-carnitine, glycerophosphocholine, and alpha-glucosidase for the epididymis.
- Amniotic fluid is present in the amnion, a membranous sac that surrounds the fetus. It is collected by amniocentesis.
- The purpose of the test is to diagnose chromosomal abnormalities, diagnose inherited metabolic disorders like cystic fibrosis.
- Bilirubin, creatinine, and AFP are important biochemical tests of amniotic fluid. These help to diagnose erythroblastosis fetalis, hepatitis, maternal infection and sickle cell crises in fetus.
- Cerebrospinal fluid (CSF) is a clear fluid, circulates in the brain and spinal cord. It is a clear, colorless ultrafiltrate of plasma with low protein content and few cells.
- Chemical tests for CSF include—proteins, glucose, and glutamine.
- Serous fluid is a clear to pale yellow watery fluid that is found in the body in the spaces between organs and the membranes.
- "Transudate" is fluid buildup caused by systemic conditions that alter the pressure in blood vessels, causing fluid to leave the vascular system. "Exudate" is fluid buildup caused by tissue leakage due to inflammation or local cellular damage.
- Pericardial fluid is present in the membranes surrounding heart. It is important to test pericardial fluid to check malignant tumor, lymphoma, TB, parasitic infection, or hepatic cirrhosis.
- Biochemical tests performed on pericardial fluid are triglyceride, glucose, LDH, cholesterol and total protein.
- Pleural fluid is present in the membranes around lungs.
- *Pleural effusion*: It is excess fluid that accumulates in the pleural cavity, the fluid-filled space that surrounds the lungs.
- Biochemical tests performed on pleural fluid are amylase, cholesterol, tumor markers, glucose, LDH, triglyceride, and pH.
- Adenosine deaminase (ADA) and interferon gamma release assays (IGRAs) are considered as diagnostic markers of pleural TB.
- Peritoneal fluid is the liquid in the space surrounding the organs in the abdomen. Paracentesis is the removal of peritoneal fluid from the abdominal cavity.
- The serum-ascites albumin gradient (SAAG) is the most useful index for evaluating peritoneal fluid and can help distinguish ascites caused by portal hypertension (cirrhosis, portal vein thrombosis, Budd-Chiari syndrome, etc.) from other causes of ascites.
- Biochemical tests performed on peritoneal fluid are amylase, glucose, protein, triglyceride and alkaline phosphatase.

Section 3: Clinical Biochemistry

- Synovial fluid is formed as an ultrafiltrate of plasma across the synovial membrane. It is a joint fluid, which is viscous fluid found in the cavities of the moveable joints.
- Biochemistry test of synovial fluid includes total protein, glucose, albumin, LDH and uric acid are considered clinically important.
- Damage to the articular membrane produces pain and stiffness in the joints, this is referred to as arthritis.

PRACTICE QUESTIONS

1. Name the body fluids present in body. Name the procedure to remove each fluid.
2. What are normal contents of seminal fluid?
3. Name different parts of sperm. And describe the terms associated with number of sperms.
4. What is amniotic fluid? What is purpose of its testing?
5. What are normal contents of amniotic fluid?
6. Enlist abnormal findings and their clinical significance for amniotic fluid.
7. What is CSF? Mention its function.
8. What are normal contents of CSF?
9. What is serous fluid?
10. Mention general difference between transudate and exudates.
11. What is pericardial fluid? Mention its function.
12. What are normal contents of pericardial fluid?
13. Which tests are used as markers of pericardial tuberculosis?
14. What are normal contents of pleural fluid?
15. Enlist abnormal findings and their clinical significance for pleural fluid.
16. What are diagnostic markers of pleural TB?
17. Where is peritoneal fluid found in the body? What are normal contents of it?
18. What is meant by SAAG? Give its importance.
19. Where is synovial fluid found in the body? What are normal contents of it?
20. Which condition is responsible for arthritis? Discuss different types of it.
21. Discuss biochemical analytes for synovial fluid.

CHAPTER 26

Blood pH and Buffer System

Keywords
Acidity, alkalinity, indicator strip, pH indicator fluid, pH meter, Nernst equation, potential difference, reference electrode, buffer, chemical buffer system, proteins, hemoglobin, phosphate, bicarbonate, carbonic acid, the respiratory system, carbonic acid, CO_2, the renal system, hydrogen ions (H^+) bicarbonate

■ INTRODUCTION

The pH is a measurement of the acidity of the blood, indicating the number of hydrogen ions [H^+] present. The word pH is acquired from "p," the scientific figure for negative logarithm, and "H," the chemical symbol for Hydrogen. pH is a unit of measure that expresses the level of acidity or alkalinity of a suspension. It is graded on a range of 0 to 14. pH = -log[H^+]. If the H^+ density is higher than OH^-, the substance is acidic, i.e., the pH amount is less than 7. If the OH^- intensity is higher than H^+, the substance is basic, with a pH value higher than 7. If identical quantities of H^+ and OH^- ions are present, the substance is neutral, with a pH of 7.

■ IMPORTANCE OF MAINTAINING BLOOD pH

In order for the body to function normally, the maintenance of the acidity and alkalinity of the body is vital. Human body carefully regulates blood pH, maintaining it within a narrow range of 7.35–7.45 with an average of 7.4. This slightly alkaline blood pH must be maintained to avoid detrimental effects on body. This is because, most biochemical reactions essential to life take place in an aqueous environment. The human body maintains a very delicate pH balance in its fluids, tissues and systems (within a narrow pH range of 7.35–7.45) so that body's immune system is operating in optimal conditions and is able to fight off illness and disease.

■ MEASUREMENT OF pH

- Using an indicator strip which when placed in a solution, changes its color accordingly. The strip is then taken out and its color is matched with a color on the color chart to decide the corresponding pH value. The narrow range pH paper offer high sensitivity and sharp color change for a solution within specified pH range only. There are very narrow pH unit graduations can be used for blood and other body fluids.
- Using a pH indicator fluid where the unknown solution is added to the fluid and the changed color of the fluid is matched with an already available color on the color wheel to decide the pH value. Indicator dyes, such as methyl orange or phenolphthalein, are organic compounds with absorbance in the visible range. They shift their conformation with the activity of hydrogen ions, which causes a change in the absorbance maximum of the compound and hence a change in color, e.g., bromothymol blue is blue at pH 7.6 or above and yellow at pH below 6.0. Thus, it is useful in the pH range of 6.0. to 7.6
- Using a pH sensor such as pH meter, where a probe can be simply inserted inside the solution and pH reading can be done.

■ pH METER

A pH meter is a precise instrument that weighs the hydrogen-ion movement in water-based suspensions, showing its acidity or alkalinity expressed as pH.

It is also called a "potentiometric pH meter" because it measures the variation in electrical potential between a pH electrode and a reference electrode.

The variation in electrical potential directly links to the acidity or pH of the suspension.

pH Meter Working Principle

- A pH meter is made of a few vital components, such as measuring electrode, reference electrode, temperature sensor **(Fig. 26.1)**.

Chapter 26: Blood pH and Buffer System

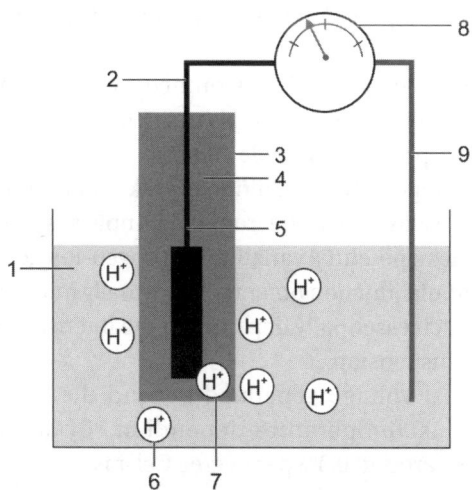

Fig. 26.1: Parts of pH meter.

- The pH meter estimates the voltage of an electrochemical cell and based upon the temperature sensor defines the pH of a suspension.
- Most of the pH meters contain combination electrodes, in which the electrodes and the temperature sensor are fabricated within a single frame.
- The reference electrode contains a neutral solution such as potassium chloride solution with a fixed concentration. It gives a stable voltage.
- On the opposite, the potential of the measuring electrode or glass electrode depends totally upon the pH of the suspension.
- The algebraic total of the potentials of the measuring electrode, reference electrode, and the liquid junction is known as the overall potential or the voltage.
- The potential variation (voltage) between a glass membrane of measuring electrode and a reference electrode which is immersed in the sample liquid to be examined is estimated.
- When the two electrodes are immersed into the sample suspension, the ion-exchange process transpires wherein some of the hydrogen ions flow toward the outside surface of the measuring electrode and displace some of the metal ions within it. Likewise, some of

the metal ions migrate from the glass electrode toward the sample suspension.
- The responsiveness of the reference electrode potential to variation in pH is negligible or it is unaffected by variations in pH and therefore produces a stable voltage.
- An ion-exchange process additionally takes place on the interior surface of the glass electrode from the sample suspension.
- This generates a potential variation (hydrogen-ion activity) among them. The liquid junction potential is normally minute and almost constant which essentially depends on the intensity of the ions in the sample suspension.
- The potential voltage generated beyond the glass electrode membrane is temperature-dependent, by a temperature coefficient of around 0.3% per degree Celsius.
- The pH meters hold provisions to improve the pH measures as the temperature changes and it is termed as automatic temperature compensation (ATC).
- The output of the impedance voltmeter is voltage studies and it possesses to be calibrated to prepare precise pH measurement.
- Calibration is performed by immersing the measuring electrode into buffer liquid of known pH which assists in understanding millivolt reading as pH measurement of the sample suspension at the delivered temperature.

1. The solution being examined.
2. The glass electrode, consisting of a slim layer of silica glass including metal salts, inside which there is a potassium chloride solution; and an internal electrode constructed from silver/silver chloride.
3. Hydrogen ions produced in the experiment solution communicate with the outer surface of the glass.
4. Hydrogen ions produced in the potassium chloride solution communicate with the inside surface of the glass.
5. The meter regulates the variation in voltage between the two surfaces of the glass and turns this "potential difference" into a pH reading.
6. Reference electrode serves as a baseline or reference for the analysis. It is there for simply completing the circuit.

PROCEDURE AND PRECAUTION OF MEASUREMENT OF BLOOD pH

Specimen: Only heparinized plasma should be used for measurement of blood pH.

Note: pH of blood at body temperature (37°C) is different than at room temperature. Therefore, the measurement should be made at 37°C and sample should not be exposed to atmosphere.

Following steps should be followed for pH measurement of blood:
- Turn on the pH meter at least 15 min prior to use. Calibrate the electrode using a standard buffer at 37°C making sure to select the proper pH of buffer at 37°C and to set temperature of pH meter at 37°C. The recommended buffers for plasma pH calibration are 7.384 and 8.841.
- Blood samples must be kept anaerobically to prevent loss of absorption of CO_2. The pH measurement should be made within 15 min after sample collection or sample should be kept on ice and measurement should be made within 2 hours. The samples should be equilibrated to 37°C before measurement.
- To prevent the coating of electrode with the blood sample, the electrode should be flushed with saline solution after each measurement. A residual blood film can be removed by dipping for a few min in 0.1 M NaOH followed by 0.1 M HCl and water or saline.

  Advantages of using pH meter over other methods are as follows:
  - It gives more accurate and precise measurements (up to 1/100th of pH unit)
  - It can be easily used.
  - The pH reading is easier comparatively.
  - These are reusable.

NEED OF BUFFER SYSTEM

Proper physiological functioning of body depends on a very tight balance between the concentrations of acids and bases in the blood. This acid-base balance is measured using the pH scale. The body fluid of living organisms usually has specific pH range. If the pH of the human blood changes by as little as 0.03 pH units or less the functioning of the body will be greatly impaired.

A variety of buffering systems permits blood and other bodily fluids to maintain a narrow pH range, even in the face of perturbations. A buffer is a chemical system that prevents a radical change in fluid pH by dampening the change in hydrogen ion concentrations in the case of excess acid or base. Most commonly, the substance that absorbs the ions is either a weak acid, which takes up hydroxyl ions, or a weak base, which takes up hydrogen ions.

■ BUFFER SYSTEMS IN THE BODY

Human body has several self-regulating control mechanisms—also called homeostatic systems—that protects from wide fluctuations in blood's pH levels. The organs involved in the maintenance of blood pH are the lungs and the kidneys. The buffer systems in the human body are extremely efficient, and different systems work at different rates. Broadly, buffer systems are divided into three categories:
1. Chemical buffer system
2. Respiratory buffer system
3. Renal buffer system

Chemical Buffer System

It takes only seconds for the chemical buffers in the blood to make adjustments to pH. Several buffering agents that reversibly bind hydrogen ions and impede any change in pH exist. Extracellular buffers include bicarbonate and ammonia, whereas proteins and phosphates act as intracellular buffers.

Protein Buffers in Blood Plasma and Cells

Nearly all proteins can function as buffers. Proteins are made up of amino acids, which contain positively charged amino groups and negatively charged carboxyl groups. The charged regions of these molecules can bind hydrogen and hydroxyl ions, and thus function as buffers. Buffering by proteins accounts for two-thirds of the buffering power of the blood and most of the buffering within cells.

Hemoglobin as a Buffer

Hemoglobin is the principal protein inside of red blood cells and accounts for one-third of the mass of the cell. During the conversion of CO_2 into bicarbonate, hydrogen ions liberated in the reaction are buffered by hemoglobin, which is reduced by the dissociation of oxygen. This buffering helps maintain normal pH. The process is reversed in the pulmonary capillaries to reform CO_2, which then can diffuse into the air sacs to be exhaled into the atmosphere.

Phosphate Buffer

Phosphates are found in the blood in two forms—sodium dihydrogen phosphate ($Na_2H_2PO_4^-$), which is a weak acid, and sodium monohydrogen phosphate ($Na_2HPO_4^{2-}$), which is a weak base. When $Na_2HPO_4^{2-}$ comes into contact with a strong acid, such as HCl, the base picks up a second hydrogen ion to form the weak acid $Na_2H_2PO_4^-$ and sodium chloride, NaCl. When $Na_2HPO_4^{2-}$ (the weak acid) comes into contact with a strong base, such as sodium hydroxide (NaOH), the weak acid reverts back to the weak base and produces water. Acids and bases are still present, but they hold onto the ions.

$$HCl + Na_2HPO_4 \rightarrow NaH_2PO_4 + NaCl$$
(strong acid) + (weak base) → (weak acid) + (salt)
$$NaOH + NaH_2PO_4 \rightarrow Na_2HPO_4 + H_2O$$
(strong base) + (weak acid) → (weak base) + (water)

Bicarbonate-Carbonic Acid Buffer

The bicarbonate-carbonic acid buffer works in a fashion similar to phosphate buffers. The bicarbonate is regulated in the blood by sodium, as are the phosphate ions. When sodium bicarbonate ($NaHCO_3$), comes into contact with a strong acid, such as HCl, carbonic acid (H_2CO_3), which is a weak acid, and NaCl are formed. When carbonic acid comes into contact with a strong base, such as NaOH, bicarbonate and water are formed.

$$NaHCO_3 + HCl \rightarrow H_2CO_3 + NaCl$$
(sodium bicarbonate) + (strong acid) → (weak acid) + (salt)
$$H_2CO_3 + NaOH \rightarrow HCO_3^- + H_2O$$
(weak acid) + (strong base) → (bicarbonate) + (water)

As with the phosphate buffer, a weak acid or weak base captures the free ions, and a significant change in pH is prevented. Bicarbonate ions and carbonic acid are present in the blood in a 20:1 ratio if the blood pH is within the normal range. With 20 times more bicarbonate than carbonic acid, this capture system is most efficient at buffering changes that would make the blood more acidic. This is useful because most of the body's metabolic wastes, such as lactic acid and ketones, are acids. Carbonic acid levels in the blood are controlled by the expiration of CO_2 through the lungs. In red blood cells, carbonic anhydrase forces the dissociation of the acid, rendering the blood less acidic. Because of this acid dissociation, CO_2 is exhaled (see equations earlier). The level of bicarbonate in the blood is controlled through the renal system, where bicarbonate ions in the renal filtrate are conserved and passed back into the blood. However, the bicarbonate buffer is the primary buffering system of the surrounding the cells in tissues throughout the body.

$$CO_2 + H_2O \leftrightarrow H_2CO_3 \leftrightarrow H^+ + HCO_3^-$$

Respiratory Regulation of Acid-base Balance (Flowchart 26.1)

The respiratory system contributes to the balance of acids and bases in the body by regulating the blood levels of carbonic acid. CO_2 in the blood readily reacts with water to form carbonic acid. The levels of CO_2 and carbonic acid in the blood are in equilibrium. When the CO_2 level in the blood rises (as it does when you hold your breath), the excess CO_2 reacts with water to form additional carbonic acid, lowering blood pH. Increasing the rate and/or depth of respiration (which you might feel the "urge" to do after holding your breath) results in exhalation of more CO_2. The loss of CO_2 from the body reduces blood levels of carbonic acid and thereby adjusts the pH upward, toward normal levels.

This process also works in the opposite direction. Excessive deep and rapid breathing (as in hyperventilation) removes CO_2 from blood and reduces the level of carbonic acid, making the blood too alkaline. This brief alkalosis can be remedied by rebreathing air that has been exhaled into a paper bag. Rebreathing exhaled air will rapidly bring blood pH down toward normal.

The chemical reactions that regulate the levels of CO_2 and carbonic acid occur in the lungs when blood travels through the lung's pulmonary capillaries. Minor adjustments in breathing are usually sufficient to adjust the pH of the blood by changing how much CO_2 is exhaled. In fact, doubling the respiratory rate for less than 1 minute, removing "extra" CO_2, would increase the blood pH by 0.2. This

Flowchart 26.1: Respiratory regulation of blood pH.

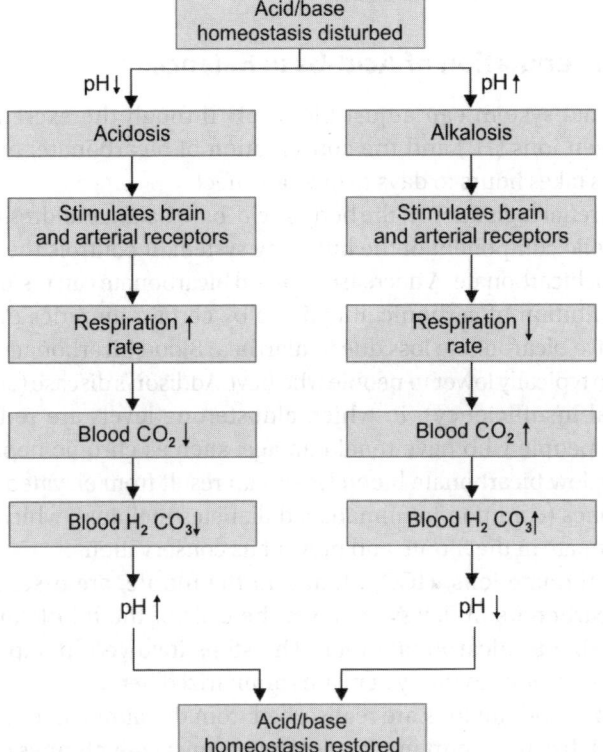

situation is common if strenuous exercise is done for over a period of time. To keep up the necessary energy production, excess CO_2 is produced (and lactic acid if heavy exercising). In order to balance the increased acid production, the respiration rate goes up to remove the CO_2. This helps to prevent acidosis.

The body regulates the respiratory rate by the use of chemoreceptors, which primarily use CO_2 as a signal. Peripheral blood sensors are found in the walls of the aorta and carotid arteries. These sensors signal the brain to provide immediate adjustments to the respiratory rate if CO_2 levels rise or fall. Yet other sensors are found in the brain itself. Changes in the pH of CSF affect the respiratory center in the medulla oblongata, which can directly modulate breathing rate to bring the pH back into the normal range.

The respiratory tract can adjust the blood pH upward in minutes by exhaling CO_2 from the body.

Renal Regulation of Acid-base Balance

The renal system can adjust blood pH through the excretion of hydrogen ions (H^+) and the conservation of bicarbonate, but this process takes hours to days to have an effect.

The renal regulation of the body's acid-base balance addresses the metabolic component of the buffering system. It controls the blood levels of bicarbonate. A decrease of blood bicarbonate can result from the inhibition of carbonic anhydrase by certain diuretics or from excessive bicarbonate loss due to diarrhea. Blood bicarbonate levels are also typically lower in people who have Addison's disease (chronic adrenal insufficiency), in which aldosterone levels are reduced, and in people who have renal damage, such as chronic nephritis. Finally, low bicarbonate blood levels can result from elevated levels of ketones (common in unmanaged diabetes mellitus), which bind bicarbonate in the filtrate and prevent its conservation.

Bicarbonate ions, HCO_3^-, found in the filtrate, are essential to the bicarbonate buffer system, yet the cells of the tubule are not permeable to bicarbonate ions. The steps involved in supplying bicarbonate ions to the system are summarized here:

- **Step 1:** Sodium ions are reabsorbed from the filtrate in exchange for H^+ by an antiport mechanism in the apical membranes of cells lining the renal tubule.
- **Step 2:** The cells produce bicarbonate ions that can be shunted to peritubular capillaries.
- **Step 3:** When CO_2 is available, the reaction is driven to the formation of carbonic acid, which dissociates to form a bicarbonate ion and a hydrogen ion.
- **Step 4:** The bicarbonate ion passes into the peritubular capillaries and returns to the blood. The hydrogen ion is secreted into the filtrate, where it can become part of new water molecules and be reabsorbed as such, or removed in the urine.

It is also possible that salts in the filtrate, such as sulfates, phosphates, or ammonia, will capture hydrogen ions. If this occurs, the hydrogen ions will not be available to combine with bicarbonate ions and produce CO_2. In such cases, bicarbonate ions are not

Chapter 26: Blood pH and Buffer System

conserved from the filtrate to the blood, which will also contribute to a pH imbalance and acidosis.

The hydrogen ions also compete with potassium to exchange with sodium in the renal tubules. If more potassium is present than normal, potassium, rather than the hydrogen ions, will be exchanged, and increased potassium enters the filtrate. When this occurs, fewer hydrogen ions in the filtrate participate in the conversion of bicarbonate into CO_2 and less bicarbonate is conserved. If there is less potassium, more hydrogen ions enter the filtrate to be exchanged with sodium and more bicarbonate is conserved.

Chloride ions are important in neutralizing positive ion charges in the body. If chloride is lost, the body uses bicarbonate ions in place of the lost chloride ions. Thus, lost chloride results in an increased reabsorption of bicarbonate by the renal system.

Disturbances in buffer system of body may results in different pathologic conditions. These are discussed in next chapter.

SUMMARY

- pH is a unit of measure that expresses the level of acidity or alkalinity of a suspension.
- Human body carefully regulates blood pH, maintaining it within a narrow range of 7.35–7.45 with an average of 7.4.
- pH can be measured by using an indicator strip which when placed in a solution, changes its color accordingly.
- Another method is, using a pH indicator fluid where the unknown solution is added to the fluid and the changes color.
- Most suggestible method is—pH meter is a precise instrument that weighs the hydrogen-ion movement in water-based suspensions.
- Using the Nernst equation, the potential difference is used to measure the hydrogen ion concentration indicating the pH of given solution.
- Due to the potential difference between two electrodes, the electron flows and generates current. This generated current is measured by voltmeter. The relationship between the potential difference, generated current and pH has been derived.
- A buffer is a chemical system that prevents a radical change in fluid pH by dampening the change in hydrogen ion concentrations in the case of excess acid or base.
- **Chemical buffer system:** It takes only seconds for the chemical buffers in the blood to make adjustments to pH. Several buffering agents that reversibly bind hydrogen ions and impede any change in pH exist.

Section 3: Clinical Biochemistry

- Chemical buffer system of body includes proteins, hemoglobin, phosphate, bicarbonate-carbonic acid buffer.
- The respiratory system contributes to the balance of acids and bases in the body by regulating the blood levels of carbonic acid, indirectly it is CO_2.
- The renal system can adjust blood pH through the excretion of hydrogen ions (H^+) and the conservation of bicarbonate, but this process takes hours to days to have an effect.

PRACTICE QUESTIONS

1. Define pH.
2. Mention importance of maintaining blood pH.
3. What are three ways to measure pH?
4. Discuss method to measure pH using indicator fluid.
5. Describe working principle of pH meter.
6. With a neat labeled diagram, explain parts of pH meter.
7. What are precautions to be taken during measurement of pH using pH meter.
8. What is meant by buffer? Why there is need of buffer system in the body?
9. Explain, in detail, chemical buffer system of the body.
10. How does respiration regulates acid-base balance?
11. Discuss the role of renal regulation in maintaining body's acid-base balance.

Arterial Blood Gases

CHAPTER 27

Keywords
Allen test, oximeters, spectrophotometry, infrared light, hemoreflector, oxyhemoglobin, oxygen capacity, oxygen content, partial pressure of oxygen, partial pressure of carbon dioxide (pCO_2), Henderson-Hasselbalch equation, Severinghaus electrode, bicarbonates, base excess, blood gas analyzer, respiratory acidosis, metabolic acidosis, metabolic alkalosis, respiratory alkalosis

■ INTRODUCTION

Respiration is exchange of gases. Blood gases are oxygen and carbon dioxide. As blood passes through our lungs, oxygen moves into the blood and transported to cells while carbon dioxide moves out of the blood into the lungs and expelled out.

Determination of blood gases is needed for:
1. Assessment of adequacy of oxygenation
2. Assessment of adequacy of ventilation
3. Assessment of acid-base status

For determination of blood gases, arterial blood is needed rather than venous blood. Reasons for use of arterial blood rather than venous blood are as follows:
1. Arterial blood is a good mixture of blood from all parts of body. Hence it is good to sample arterial blood rather than venous blood which represents that extremity of local area from where it has been collected.
2. Arterial blood gives information of how well oxygenation has taken place in the lungs.

■ COLLECTION OF ARTERIAL BLOOD SPECIMEN

A sample of blood from an artery is taken from the inside of the wrist. The blood supply to hand comes from two arteries (**Fig. 27.1**):

1. The radial artery, which is found on the inner (thumb side) of the wrist and
2. The ulnar artery, which is found on the outer (little finger side) of wrist.

Before drawing blood for an arterial blood gas test, make sure that both arteries are open and working correctly. A procedure called the Allen test may be used to find out if the blood flow to hand is normal.

- For the Allen test, apply pressure to the arteries in wrist for several seconds. This will stop the blood flow to hand, and patient's hand will become cool and pale. When blood is allowed to flow through the artery, patient's hand quickly becomes warm and returns to its normal color. This means that arteries are open and working correctly. If patient's hand remains pale and cold, the Allen test will then be performed on other hand.
- If patient's other hand also remains pale, the blood often will be collected from another artery, usually in the groin (femoral artery) or elbow crease (brachial artery).

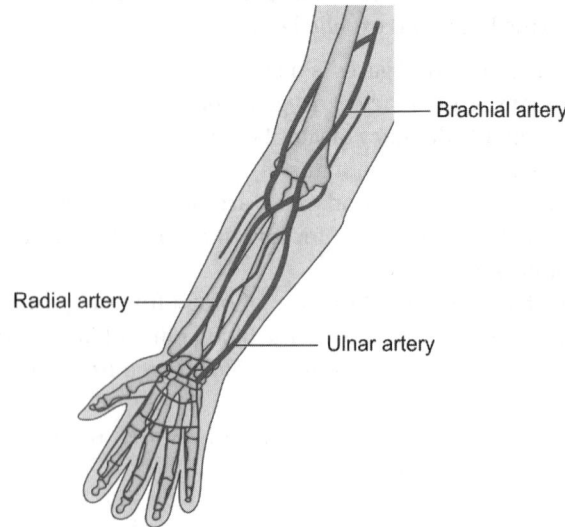

Fig. 27.1: Different arteries for the collection of blood.
(For color version, see Plate 10)

Precautions should be taken that there should not be any air bubble in the sample and patient should breathe normally during procedure of blood collection.
1. Instruct the patient to take supine or sitting or position.
2. Raise the wrist with a pillow and instruct the patient to extend the fingers downward.
3. Palpate the artery.
4. Rotate the patient's hand back and forth until a good pulse is felt.
5. Clean the site of collection with antiseptic agent like betadine.
6. Anesthetize the site of collection with small quantity of 1% xylocaine.
7. Puncture the artery with 20 or 21 gauge sterile needle.
8. Attach pre-heparinized syringe of 12 mL capacity.
9. Draw blood by pulling back the plunger taking care not to pull the needle out of artery.
10. Collect 3-6 mL of sample.
11. Withdraw needle.
12. Keep sufficient absorbent bandage over the site of puncture and apply pressure for about 2 minutes.
13. Cap the syringe and rotate gently to cause proper mixing of blood with heparin.

■ ARTERIAL BLOOD GAS ANALYSIS

Arterial blood gas (ABG) analysis include following tests:
- Blood oxygen analysis
- Blood carbon dioxide analysis
- Base excess (BE)
- pH

Blood Oxygen Analysis

Although oxygen dissolves in blood, only a small amount of oxygen is transported this way. Only 1.5% of oxygen in the blood is dissolved directly into the blood itself. Most oxygen—98.5%—is bound to a protein called hemoglobin and carried to the tissues.

Blood oxygen gas analyses conducted are:
- Determination of oxygen saturation
- Determination of oxygen capacity

- Determination of oxygen content
- Partial pressure of O_2 (PaO_2)

Oxygen Saturation (SaO_2)

Binding sites for oxygen are the heme groups, the Fe^{++}-porphyrin portions of the hemoglobin molecule. There are four heme sites, and hence four oxygen binding sites, per hemoglobin molecule. Heme sites occupied by oxygen molecules are said to be "saturated" with oxygen. The percentage of all the available heme binding sites saturated with oxygen is the hemoglobin oxygen saturation (in arterial blood, the SaO_2). When hemoglobin 92 to 100% carries O_2, then perfusion or oxygen supply to the tissue is normal.

SaO_2 always depends, to a large degree, on the concentration of dissolved oxygen molecules. (i.e., on the PaO_2). With the decrease of the PaO_2 level, the saturation of hemoglobin also decreases. When the O_2 saturation is 70% or low, the tissues cannot get adequate oxygen.

Normally, oxygen saturation on room air is in excess of 95%. With deep or rapid breathing, this can be increased to 98-99%. While breathing oxygen-enriched air (40-100%), the oxygen saturation can be pushed to 100%.

Normal range: O_2 saturation
- Adult/child = 95-100%
- Old people = 95%
- Newborn = 40-90%

Decreased oxygen saturation:
- Inspired oxygen levels are diminished, at increased altitudes.
- Upper or middle airway obstruction exists (such as during an acute asthmatic attack).
- Significant alveolar lung disease exists, interfering with the free flow of oxygen across the alveolar membrane.

Increased oxygen saturation:
- Deep or rapid breathing occurs
- Inspired oxygen levels are increased, such as breathing from a 100% oxygen source

Determination of oxygen saturation:

Two most widely used methods for determination of oxygen saturation are pulse oximetry and spectrophotometrically using a Kipp Hemoreflector.

Pulse oximetry:

Pulse oximetry is a rapid, noninvasive method of estimating oxygenation. It is continuous process, allowing detection of sudden changes in a patient's clinical status.

Principle and working:

Modern pulse oximeters measure the amount of red and infrared light in an area of pulsatile blood flow **(Fig. 27.2)**. Because red light is primarily absorbed by deoxygenated blood and infrared light is primarily absorbed by oxygenated blood, the ratio of absorption can be measured. Because the amount of light absorbed varies with each pulse wave, the difference of measurement between two points in the pulse wave occurs in the arterial blood flow, with more than several hundred measurements per second. This is compared against baseline values, giving both the pulse oximetry oxygen saturation (SpO_2) and the pulse rate.

Pulse oximeters extract and display SpO_2 and heart rate from the photoplethysmographic (PPG) waveform every 3-6 seconds, and some display the PPG waveform. One side of the pulse oximeter probe contains two light-emitting diodes that transmit two wavelengths of light, and the other side contains a photodetector. Red light at 660 nm and near-infrared (NIR) light at 940 nm is transmitted through tissue (skin, arteries, capillaries, veins, bone, and fat), and the light that is not absorbed is detected by the photodetector on the opposite side.

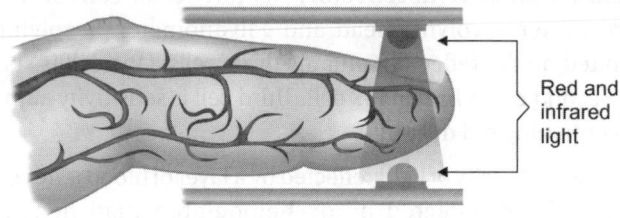

Fig. 27.2: Working of pulse oximeter.
(For color version, see Plate 11)

Construction of instrument: The equipment used for pulse oximetry includes the following:
- Monitoring unit
- Probe sensor

Currently, the two basic types of pulse oximeter probes are transmission probes and reflectance probes.

1. **Transmission probes:** With transmission probes, the light emitter and sensor are placed opposite each other on pulsatile tissue such as a digit or ear. The lights used to measure tissue oxygenation are typically placed across from a detector surrounding approximately 5–10 mm of tissue that contains pulsatile blood flow, such as a fingertip or ear lobe.
2. **Reflectance probes:** With reflectance probes, the light emitter and sensor are placed side by side on a flat body surface. The detector lies adjacent to the light source on a flat surface such as the forehead. This information can be used noninvasively to help evaluate the hemodynamic status of a patient and to detect hypoxemia in various clinical settings.

The probe houses a light source, a light detector, and a microprocessor, which compares and calculates the differences in the oxygen-rich versus oxygen-poor hemoglobin. The microprocessor calculates the differences and converts the information to a digital readout.

Interfering factors include nail polish and artificial fingernails.

Kipp hemoreflector:

The first reflection oximeter for measuring SaO_2, in blood samples was Kipp Hemoreflector, which is still widely being used.

Construction of hemoreflector: Hemoreflector consists of a light source, filter, revolving head and galvanometer. Revolving head mounted on the reflector contains three cells. One cell is specimen cell. Second cell is Indian ink cell. Third cell is sensitivity adjustment cell containing red dye stuff.

Principle: Intensity of light reflected by a layer of blood is determined. Light is more reflected by oxyhemoglobin than hemoglobin. Logarithm of reflected quantity of light is linear function of oxygen saturation.

Chapter 27: Arterial Blood Gases

Requirements:
1. Hemoreflector
2. Dithionate
3. Heparin—used as anticoagulant
4. 2% sodium chloride, is used to dilute the blood specimen
5. 0.3% sodium salicylate, is used to prevent agglutination and sedimentation
6. 0.05% sodium cyanide (NaCN), used to convert any methemoglobin to cyanmethemoglobin
7. Wavelength: 600–680 nm.

Procedure:
1. Adjust the galvanometer reading to zero by placing the compensating cell in the light path.
2. Adjust the galvanometer reading to value given in the calibration certificate by placing dyestuff cell in the light path. The instrument is calibrated using completely saturated and desaturated blood sample.
3. A 0.5 mL heparinized blood sample is transferred anaerobically to a 2 mL syringe previously filled with 0.5 mL of a solution containing 20 g/L NaCl, 3 g/L sodium salicylate and 0.5g/NaCN.
4. The mixture is then injected into an open cylindrical cuvette and the light reflection from the flat cuvette bottom determined immediately. The addition of the reagent solution considerably increases the light reflection of the blood while rouleaux formation is prevented.
5. Place the specimen cell in the light path. The instrument measures the light reflection of undiluted blood. Rouleaux formation being prevented by continuous stirring.
6. Read the value of oxygen saturation from calibration curve supplied.

Oxygen saturation is also calculated by following formula:

$$SaO_2(a) = O_2Hb/(O_2Hb + HHb) \times 100$$

where,
O_2Hb = Concentration of oxygenated hemoglobin in arterial blood
HHb = Concentration of deoxygenated hemoglobin in arterial blood.

Oxygen Capacity

Oxygen capacity is the maximum quantity of oxygen that will combine chemically with the hemoglobin in a unit volume of blood. Normally it amounts to 1.34 mL of O_2 per gram of Hb or 20 mL of O_2 per 100 mL of blood.

Oxygen Content (CaO$_2$)

The oxygen content of blood is the volume of oxygen carried in each 100 mL blood. CaO_2, unlike either PaO_2 or SaO_2, directly reflects the total number of oxygen molecules in arterial blood, both bound and unbound to hemoglobin. In contrast to the other two variables, CaO_2 depends on the hemoglobin content and is directly related to it.

Oxygen content can be measured directly or calculated by the oxygen content equation:

Arterial oxygen content $(CaO_2) = (Hgb \times 1.36 \times SaO_2) + (0.0031 \times PaO_2)$
where,

SaO_2 = % of hemoglobin saturated with oxygen (normal range: 93–100%)

Hgb = hemoglobin [normal range (adults): male: 13–18 g/dL, female: 12–16 g/dL]

PaO_2 = Arterial oxygen partial pressure (normal range: 80–100)

Constant = 1.36, is the amount of oxygen (mL at 1 atmosphere) bound per gram of hemoglobin.

Constant = 0.0031 represents the amount of oxygen dissolved in plasma.

Normal range O_2 content:
- Arterial blood = 15–22 vol%
- Venous blood = 11–16 vol%

Given normal pulmonary gas exchange (i.e., a normal respiratory system), other factors that lower oxygen content are—anemia, carbon monoxide poisoning, methemoglobinemia, or due to conversion of some of hemoglobin into nonfunctional form. It is raised with high hemoglobin content.

Partial Pressure of Oxygen (pO$_2$)

Partial pressure refers to the pressure exerted by a specific gas in a mixture of other gases. This partial pressure of the oxygen gas determines the force it exerts in attempting to diffuse through the pulmonary membrane.

This reflects amount of oxygen passing from pulmonary alveoli into blood. These are those Oxygen molecules which are dissolved in plasma (i.e., not bound to hemoglobin) and are free to impinge on the measuring oxygen electrode. This impingement of free O_2 molecules is reflected as the partial pressure of oxygen. It is influenced by amount of oxygen inhaled. This test measures the pressure exerted by O_2 dissolved in plasma. It gives the effectiveness of lungs in pulling oxygen into the blood stream from the atmosphere. Partial pressure of oxygen can indicate the severity of impairment of lungs to diffuse oxygen across alveolar membrane into circulating blood.

Measurement of pO_2:

$$pO_2 = \frac{(\text{Barometric pressure} - \text{Water vapor pressure})}{100} \times \% \, O_2$$

Normal range of pO_2:
- Adult/child = 80–100 mm Hg
- Newborn = 60–70 mm Hg
- Venous blood = 40–50 mm Hg

Increased pO_2 levels are associated with:
- Increased oxygen levels in the inhaled air
- Polycythemia

Decreased pO_2 levels are associated with: This condition is termed as hypoxemia.
- Decreased oxygen levels in the inhaled air
- Anemia
- Heart decompensation (diseased heart to compensate for its defect)
- Chronic obstructive pulmonary disease
- Restrictive pulmonary disease, pneumonia, shock lung

The partial pressure of oxygen in arterial blood (PaO_2). pO_2 is the indirect measure of O_2 contents of arterial blood represented as PaO_2. The partial pressure of oxygen in the plasma phase of arterial blood (PaO_2), is measured by an electrode that senses randomly-moving, dissolved oxygen molecules. It is known as polarographic (clark) oxygen electrode.

A platinum cathode and a silver/silver chloride anode are placed in a sodium chloride electrolyte solution, and a voltage of 700 mv is applied. The following reactions occur:
- At the cathode: $O_2 + 2H_2O + 4e^- = 4OH^-$
- In the electrolyte: $NaCl + OH^- = NaOH + Cl^-$
- At the anode: $Ag + Cl^- = AgCl + e^-$

Electrons are taken up at the cathode and the current generated is proportional to oxygen tension. A membrane separates the electrode from blood, preventing deposition of protein but allowing the oxygen tension in the blood to equilibrate with the electrolyte solution. The electrode is kept at a constant temperature of 37°C and regular checks of the membrane are required to ensure it is not perforated or coated in proteins. Sampling two gas mixtures of known oxygen tension allows calibration.

Blood Carbon Dioxide Analysis

Carbon dioxide molecules are transported in the blood from body tissues to the lungs by one of the three methods: dissolution directly into the blood, binding to hemoglobin, or carried as a bicarbonate ion.

Blood carbon dioxide gas analyses conducted are:
- Partial pressure of carbon dioxide (pCO_2)
- The bicarbonate (HCO_3) and total CO_2

Partial Pressure of Carbon Dioxide (pCO_2)

These measures the pressure of carbon dioxide dissolved in the blood and how well carbon dioxide is able to move out of the body.

Partial pressure refers to the pressure exerted by a specific gas in a mixture of other gases. Partial pressure of carbon dioxide reflects amount of carbon dioxide passing from blood into pulmonary alveoli. These are those carbon dioxide molecules which are dissolved in plasma. Indirectly, the pCO_2 reflects the exchange of this gas through the lungs to the outside air. Two factors each have a significant impact on the pCO_2:

i. **How rapidly and deeply the individual is breathing:** Someone who is hyperventilating will "blow off" more CO_2, leading to lower

pCO_2 levels. Whereas, someone who is holding their breath will retain CO_2, leading to increased pCO_2 levels.

ii. **Lungs capacity for freely exchanging CO_2 across the alveolar membrane:** With pulmonary edema, there is an extra layer of fluid in the alveoli that interferes with the lungs' ability to get rid of CO_2. This leads to a rise in pCO_2. In case of acute asthmatic attack, even though the alveoli are functioning normally, there may be enough upper and middle airway obstruction to block alveolar ventilation, leading to CO_2 retention.

Determination of pCO_2:

pCO_2 can be measured using the formula:

$$pO_2 = \frac{(\text{Barometric pressure - Water vapor pressure})}{100} \times \% \, O_2$$

Normal range of pCO_2
- Adult/child = 35-45 mm Hg
- Child <2 years = 26-41 mm Hg
- Venous blood = 40-50 mm Hg

Increased pCO_2 is caused by:
- Pulmonary edema
- Obstructive lung disease

Decreased pCO_2 is caused by:
- Hyperventilation
- Hypoxia
- Anxiety
- Pregnancy
- Pulmonary embolism

Determination of pCO_2:

Measurement of CO_2 tension can be done with a silver-silver chloride electrode also known as Severinghaus electrode. The Severinghaus or carbon dioxide electrode is a modified pH electrode in contact with sodium bicarbonate solution and separated from the blood specimen by a rubber or Teflon semipermeable membrane. Carbon dioxide, but not hydrogen ions, diffuses from the blood sample across the membrane into the sodium bicarbonate solution, producing hydrogen ions and a change in pH.

$$CO_2 + H_2O \leftrightarrow H_2CO_3 \leftrightarrow H^+ + HCO_3^-$$

Hydrogen ions are produced in proportion to the pCO_2 and are measured by the pH-sensitive glass electrode. As with the pH electrode, the Severinghaus electrode must be maintained at 37°C, be calibrated with gases of known pCO_2 and the integrity of the membrane is essential. Because diffusion of the CO_2 into the electrolyte solution is required the response time is slow at 2–3 minutes.

The Bicarbonate (HCO_3) and Total CO_2

More than 90% of carbon dioxide in blood exists in the form of bicarbonate (HCO_3). The rest of the carbon dioxide is either dissolved as carbon dioxide gas (CO_2) or carbonic acid (H_2CO_3).

$$\text{Total } CO_2 = HCO_3^- + \text{Dissolved } CO_2.$$

Bicarbonate is a chemical buffer that keeps the pH of blood from becoming too acidic or too basic. When an acid-base imbalance is identified, estimation of bicarbonate (as part of the electrolyte panel) and blood gases may be ordered to evaluate the severity of the imbalance, to determine whether it is primarily respiratory (due to an imbalance between the amount of oxygen coming in and CO_2 being released) or metabolic (due to increased or decreased amounts of bicarbonate in the blood) in nature, and monitor its treatment until the acid-base balance is restored.

Normal range of HCO_3:
- Adult/child = 21–28 mEq/L
- Newborn/infants = 16–24 mEq/L

H_2CO_3 can be calculated by the following equation:

$$[H_2CO_3] = k_{H\,CO_2} \times pCO_2$$

where:
- $[H_2CO_3]$ is the concentration of carbonic acid in the blood
- $k_{H\,CO_2}$ is a constant including the solubility of carbon dioxide in blood. $k_{H\,CO_2}$ is approximately 0.03 (mmol/L)/mm Hg
- pCO_2 is the partial pressure of carbon dioxide in the blood

HCO_3^- (Bicarbonate) is calculated as—

$$HCO_3^- = \text{Total } CO_2 - H_2CO_3$$

or

$$HCO_3^- = 0.03 \times pCO_2 \times 10^{(pH-6.1)}$$

Low bicarbonate level include found in:
- Addison's disease
- Chronic diarrhea
- Diabetic ketoacidosis
- Metabolic acidosis
- Kidney disease
- Ethylene glycol or methanol poisoning
- Salicylate (aspirin) overdose

Increased levels may be due to:
- Severe vomiting
- Lung diseases, including Chronic obstructive pulmonary disease (COPD)
- Cushing syndrome
- Conn syndrome
- Metabolic alkalosis

Base Excess

The metabolic component of the acid–base balance is reflected in the base excess. This is a calculated value derived from blood pH and $PaCO_2$. It is defined as the amount of acid required to restore a liter of blood to its normal pH at a $PaCO_2$ of 40 mm Hg.

Base excess measures all bases, not just bicarbonate. However, because bicarbonate is the greater part of the base buffer, for most practical interpretations, BE provides essentially the same information as bicarbonate. Therefore, a tight range around zero (−3 to +3) is normal. In simple terms, a high BE excess is the same as a high HCO_3.

The calculation for the BE = $[HCO_3^-] - 24.8 + 16.2 \times (pH - 7.4)$.

Normal Range BE = >2 mEq/L (>2 mmol/L)

Positive BE occurs when there is surplus of HCO_3 and negative BE occurs when there is deficit of HCO_3.

pH

It is a measure of the balance of acids and bases in the blood. Decreased carbon dioxide or increased amounts of bases, like bicarbonate (HCO_3^-), can cause blood pH to increase (become alkaline).

pH Measurement

pH meter is used to measure pH. It is measured with a glass electrode suspended in the blood sample. The blood sample acts a conducting electrolyte. The potential difference across the electrode is proportional to the pH difference, and this can be measured. (see Chapter 26 for details)

Alternatively, it can be measured by Henderson-Hasselbalch equation:

$$[H^+] = \frac{24(PaCO_2)}{[HCO_3^-]}$$

Normal range of blood pH:
- Adult/child = 7.35–7.45
- Newborn = 7.32–7.49
- 2 months to 2 years = 7.34–7.46
- pH venous blood = 7.31–7.41

■ BLOOD GAS ANALYZER

It measures pH and blood gas, i.e., concentration of hydrogen ions (pH), partial pressure of carbon dioxide (pCO_2) and partial pressure of oxygen (pO_2), in whole blood. It may also measure electrolytes and metabolites. For example:

Electrolytes: cK^+ (potassium ion concentration), cNa^+, cCa^2, cCl^-

Metabolites: cGlu (glucose), cLac (lactate), ctBil (total bilirubin).

Working

Blood is collected from the patient and introduced into the analyzer **(Fig. 27.3)**. The analyzer aspirates the blood into a measuring chamber which has Ion Selective Electrodes (IE electrodes that are sensitive only to the measurement of interest).

The pH electrode compares a potential developed at the electrode tip with a reference potential, the resulting voltage is proportional to the concentration of hydrogen ions, $[H^+]$.

The pCO_2 electrode is a pH electrode with a Teflon or silicone rubber CO_2 semipermeable membrane covering the tip. CO_2 combines with H_2O in the space between the membrane and the electrode tip to

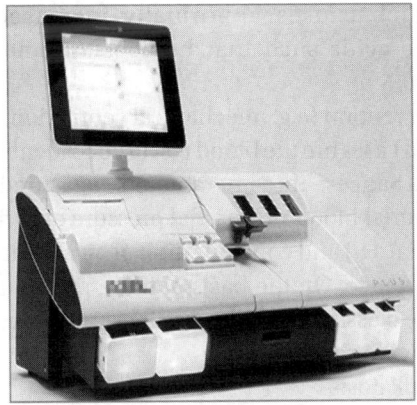

Fig. 27.3: Blood gas analyzer.
(For color version, see Plate 11)

produce free hydrogen ions in proportion to the partial pressure of CO_2. The voltmeter, although actually measuring $[H^+]$, is calibrated in pCO_2.

For pO_2, oxygen permeates a polypropylene membrane and reacts chemically with a phosphate buffer. The O_2 combines with water in the buffer, producing current in proportion to the number of oxygen molecules. The current is measured and expressed as partial pressure of oxygen.

After measurement the blood is automatically expelled into a waste container and the sample path is cleaned, and ready for the next sample. Results may be printed, displayed, and sent to the Laboratory Information System.

■ ACID-BASE BALANCE

The pH value of blood, serum or plasma is an indicator of the acid-base balance between the blood, renal (kidney), and lung (respiratory) systems, and is one of the most tightly controlled parameters in the body.

Disturbances of Acid-Base Balance

Most acid-base disturbances result from:
- Disease or damage to organs (kidney, lungs, brain) whose normal function is necessary for acid-base homeostasis.

- Disease which causes abnormally increased production of metabolic acids such that homeostatic mechanisms are overwhelmed.
- Medical intervention (e.g., mechanical ventilation, some drugs).

Arterial blood gases are the blood test used to identify and monitor acid-base disturbances. Three parameters measured during blood gas analysis, arterial blood pH, partial pressure of carbon dioxide in arterial blood ($PaCO_2$) and concentration of bicarbonate (HCO_3^-) are of crucial importance. On the basis of these parameters, acid-base disturbances are classified in following four categories:

1. Respiratory acidosis
2. Respiratory alkalosis
3. Metabolic acidosis
4. Metabolic alkalosis.

Respiratory Acidosis (Raised $PaCO_2$, Reduced pH)

Respiratory acidosis is characterized by increased $PaCO_2$ due to inadequate alveolar ventilation (hypoventilation) and consequent reduced elimination of CO_2 from the blood. Respiratory disease, such as bronchopneumonia, emphysema, asthma and chronic obstructive airways disease, all are associated with hypoventilation resulting in respiratory acidosis.

Some drugs (e.g., morphine and barbiturates) can cause respiratory acidosis by depressing the respiratory center in the brain. Damage or trauma to the chest wall and the musculature involved in the mechanics of respiration may reduce ventilation rate. This explains the respiratory acidosis that can complicate the course of diseases such as poliomyelitis, Guillain-Barré syndrome, and recovery from severe chest trauma.

Symptoms of respiratory acidosis include—headache, anxiety, blurred vision, restlessness, drowsiness, tremors, delirium and it may lead to coma.

Metabolic acidosis (Decreased HCO_3^-, Decreased pH)

Reduced bicarbonate is always a feature of metabolic acidosis. This occurs for one of two reasons—increased use of bicarbonate in buffering an abnormal acid load or increased losses of bicarbonate from the body. Diabetic ketoacidosis (due to insulin deficiency) and lactic acidosis(less oxygen to tissues) are two conditions characterized by overproduction of metabolic acids and consequent exhaustion of bicarbonate.

Examples include cardiac arrest and any condition associated with hypovolemic shock (e.g., massive fluid loss). The liver plays a major role in removing the small amount of lactic acid that is produced during normal cell metabolism, so that lactic acidosis can be a feature of liver failure.

Abnormal loss of bicarbonate from the body can occur during severe diarrhea. If unchecked, this can lead to metabolic acidosis. Failure to regenerate bicarbonate and excrete hydrogen ions explains the metabolic acidosis that occurs in renal failure.

Other causes for metabolic acidosis include—prolonged lack of oxygen, shock, poisoning, medications, dehydration and diarrhea.

Symptoms of metabolic acidosis: Symptoms of metabolic acidosis include—rapid breathing, confusion, lethargy, cold, clammy skin, tachycardia and arrhythmia.

If left untreated, acidosis can lead to acidemia. Acidemia occurs when the bloods pH is low (<7.35) due to an increased production of hydrogen ions by the body or its inability to form bicarbonate (HCO_3) in the kidneys.

If body is not maintained in a state of pH balance, its ability to eliminate the waste products slows down. To protect itself, the body converts acidic waste into solid waste and stores it in less critical areas of the body. The accumulation of solid waste can contribute to many health problems including excess weight, clogged arteries, arthritis, kidney stones, and various other chronic illnesses.

General causes for acidosis are:
- Eating food which include meat, fish, poultry, dairy, grains, refined or processed foods, fast food
- Drinks such as coffee, soft drinks, alcohol, many types of water (distilled, bottled)
- Stress, worries, anxiety, negative thoughts
- Pollution and toxins
- Intense physical exercise that produces lactic acid
- Dehydration which slows down the body's ability to cleanse itself through the kidneys.

Metabolic Alkalosis (Increased HCO_3^-, Increased pH)

Bicarbonate is always raised in metabolic alkalosis. This can occur if, excessive dose of $NaHCO_3$ is given in the treatment of metabolic acidosis or with massive blood transfusion with blood containing sodium citrate.

Rarely, excessive administration of bicarbonate or ingestion of bicarbonate in antacid preparation can cause metabolic alkalosis, but this is usually transient. Abnormal loss of hydrogen ions from the body can be the primary problem. Bicarbonate which would otherwise be consumed in buffering these lost hydrogen ions consequently accumulates in blood. Gastric juice is acidic and gastric aspiration or any disease process in which gastric contents are lost from the body represents a loss of hydrogen ions. In this situation, pH may increase upto 7.45.

Respiratory Alkalosis (Increased pH, Decreased PCO_2)

The primary decrease in PCO_2 is due to excessive ventilation. This occurs physiologically at high altitude. The stimulus is oxygen lack but it can be produced by excessively rapid and deep respiration in normal persons. Clinically seen in patients with encephalitis, hysterical attacks, fevers with septicemia, cerebral tumors, salicylate poisoning and tetany may also develop in alkalosis and when there is reduced ionized Ca^{3+} proportion of ionized Ca^{2+} falls as pH rises.

Other types of alkalosis are: Combined respiratory and Metabolic acidosis

Salicylates may cause vomiting and sufficient acid may be lost from stomach to produce alkalosis which has both respiratory and metabolic component. It may develop during treatment of primary respiratory acidosis.

This may leads to—confusion (can progress to stupor or coma), hand tremor, light-headedness, muscle twitching, nausea, vomiting, numbness or tingling in the face, hands, or feet and Prolonged muscle spasms (tetany)

Hypochloremic alkalosis

It is caused by an extreme lack or loss of chloride, such as from prolonged vomiting.

Hypokalemic alkalosis

It is caused by the kidneys' response to an extreme lack or loss of potassium. This can occur from taking certain water pills (diuretics).

Compensated alkalosis

It occurs when the body returns the acid-base balance to normal in cases of alkalosis, but bicarbonate and carbon dioxide levels remain abnormal.

SUMMARY

- For determination of blood gases, arterial blood is needed because arterial blood is a good mixture of blood from all parts of body and it gives information of how well oxygenation has taken place in the lungs.
- Blood is collected from radial or ulnar artery.
- The Allen test is a first-line standard test used to assess the arterial blood supply of the hand.
- The percentage of all the available heme binding sites saturated with oxygen is the hemoglobin oxygen saturation.
- Oximeters work by the principles of spectrophotometry—the relative absorption of red (absorbed by deoxygenated blood) and infrared (absorbed by oxygenated blood) light of the systolic component of the absorption waveform correlates to arterial blood oxygen saturations.
- Hemoreflector is based on the principle that intensity of light reflected by a layer of blood is determined. Light is more reflected by oxyhemoglobin than hemoglobin. Logarithm of reflected quantity of light is linear function of oxygen saturation.
- Oxygen capacity is the maximum quantity of oxygen that will combine chemically with the hemoglobin in a unit volume of blood.
- The oxygen content of blood is the volume of oxygen carried in each 100 mL blood.
- Partial pressure refers to the pressure exerted by a specific gas in a mixture of other gases.
- The partial pressure of oxygen in the plasma phase of arterial blood (PaO_2), is measured by an electrode that senses randomly-moving, dissolved oxygen molecules.
- Partial pressure of carbon dioxide (pCO_2) measures the pressure of carbon dioxide dissolved in the blood and how well carbon dioxide is able to move out of the body.
- Measurement of CO_2 tension can be done with a silver-silver chloride electrode also known as Severinghaus electrode.
- Bicarbonate is a chemical buffer that keeps the pH of blood from becoming too acidic or too basic.
- Base excess is defined as the amount of acid required to restore a liter of blood to its normal pH at a $PaCO_2$ of 40 mm Hg.

Section 3: Clinical Biochemistry

- Increased amounts of carbon dioxide and other acids can cause blood pH to decrease.
- Blood gas analyzer uses electrodes to determine pH and all blood gas parameters.
- Respiratory acidosis is characterized by raised $PaCO_2$, reduced pH.
- Metabolic acidosis is characterized by decreased HCO_3^-, decreased pH.
- Metabolic alkalosis is characterized by increased HCO_3^-, increased pH.
- Respiratory alkalosis is characterized by increased pH, decreased PCO_2.

PRACTICE QUESTIONS

1. Why arterial blood is preferred for determination of blood gases?
2. Why and how Allen test is performed?
3. Write a note on:
   i. Pulse oximetry
   ii. Kipp Hemoreflector
   iii. Oxygen saturation
   iv. Oxygen capacity
   v. Oxygen content
   vi. Partial pressure of O_2 (PO_2)
   vii. The partial pressure of oxygen in arterial blood (PaO_2)
   viii. Partial pressure of carbon dioxide (pCO_2)
   ix. Determination of pCO_2
   x. The bicarbonate (HCO_3)
   xi. Total CO_2
   xii. Base excess
4. What is measured by blood gas analyzer? Discuss its working.
5. What are causes of acid base disturbances in the body?
6. Differentiate between:
   i. Respiratory acidosis and metabolic acidosis
   ii. Metabolic alkalosis and respiratory alkalosis
7. Discuss the types of alkalosis.
8. What are causes of acidosis?
9. Discuss condition associated with—
   i. Decreased oxygen saturation
   ii. Decreased partial pressure of oxygen
   iii. Low bicarbonate level
10. Write formula for:
    i. Arterial oxygen content (CaO_2)
    ii. pO_2
    iii. pCO_2
    iv. Total CO_2
    v. HCO_3
    vi. Base excess
    vii. Henderson-Hasselbalch equation
11. Enlist the different parameters of arterial blood gases and respective normal values.

CHAPTER 28

Vitamin Assay

> **Keywords**
>
> Thiamine, riboflavin, niacin, pantothenic acid, biotin, pyridoxine, cyanocobalamin, folate, scurvy, pellagra, rickets, β-carotene, ergocalciferol, cholecalciferol, calcitriol, β-galactosidase, chemiluminescent immunoassay, tocopherols, phylloquinone, pyruvate dehydrogenase, beriberi, glossitis, competitive protein binding (CPB), Schilling test, ascorbic acid

■ INTRODUCTION

Vitamins are organic compounds that are essential in very small amounts for supporting normal physiologic function, growth, and development.

The characteristics of vitamins are follows:
- They are natural components of foods; usually present in very small amounts.
- They are essential for normal physiologic function (e.g., growth, reproduction, etc.).
- When absent from the diet, they will cause a specific deficiency.

There are 13 essential vitamins. This means that these vitamins are required for the body to work properly. They are are follows:
- Vitamin A
- Vitamin C
- Vitamin D
- Vitamin E
- Vitamin K
- Vitamin B1 (thiamine)
- Vitamin B2 (riboflavin)
- Vitamin B3 (niacin)

- Vitamin B5 (pantothenic acid)
- Vitamin B7 (biotin)
- Vitamin B6 (pyridoxine)
- Vitamin B12 (cyanocobalamin)
- Folate (folic acid and B9)

The eight types of vitamins are collectively known as vitamin B complex.

Vitamins are categorized as either fat soluble or water soluble depending on whether they dissolve best in either lipids or water.

A. **Fat soluble vitamins (Table 28.1):**
   - The four fat-soluble vitamins are vitamins A, D, E, and K. These vitamins are absorbed and transported passively by the body in the presence of dietary fat.
   - Fat soluble vitamins are excreted via feces, but it can also be stored in fatty tissues.
   - Deficiencies of fat-soluble vitamins can occur if it is not present in enough quantity in diet, if these vitamins are not absorbed properly in the body or a very low-fat diet.

B. **Water soluble vitamins (Table 28.2):**
   - There are nine water-soluble vitamins. These are vitamin B1 (thiamine), vitamin B2 (riboflavin), vitamin B3 (niacin), vitamin B5 (pantothenic acid), biotin (B7), vitamin B6 (pyridoxine), vitamin B12 (cyanocobalamin) and folate (folic acid and B9). Water soluble vitamins are absorbed and transported by both passive and active mechanisms. Their transport in the body relies on molecular "carriers".
   - Absorbed and transported more easily by the body in the presence of water.
   - The body must use water-soluble vitamins right away. Any leftover water-soluble vitamins are excreted in urine along with their breakdown products. Vitamin B12 is the only water-soluble vitamin that can be stored in the liver for many years.
   - Deficiencies of water-soluble vitamins can occur if it is not present in enough quantity in diet, or if these vitamins are not absorbed properly in the body.
   - Vitamins and their derivatives often serve a variety of roles in the body.

Table 28.1: Fat-soluble vitamins.

Nutrient	Functions	Sources	Deficiency diseases
Vitamin A (and its precursor,* beta-carotene)	Needed for vision, healthy skin and mucous membranes, bone and tooth growth, immune system health	Vitamin A from animal sources (retinol): Fortified milk, cheese, cream, butter, fortified margarine, eggs, liver Beta-carotene (from plant sources): Leafy, dark green vegetables; dark orange fruits (apricots, cantaloupe) and vegetables (carrots, winter squash, sweet potatoes, pumpkin)	Xerophthalmia, hyperkeratosis or dry, scaly skin
Vitamin D	Needed for proper absorption of calcium; stored in bones	Egg yolks, liver, fatty fish, fortified milk, fortified margarine. When exposed to sunlight, the skin can make vitamin D	Rickets, deformed bones Osteomalacia
Vitamin E	Antioxidant protects cell walls	Polyunsaturated plant oils (soybean, corn, cottonseed, safflower); leafy green vegetables; wheat germ; whole-grain products; liver; egg yolks; nuts and seeds	Ataxia, lack of reflexes
Vitamin K	Needed for proper blood clotting	Leafy green vegetables such as kale, collard greens, and spinach; green vegetables such as broccoli, Brussels sprouts, and asparagus; also produced in intestinal tract by bacteria	Bleeding problems, biliary obstruction

*A precursor is converted by the body to the vitamin.

Table 28.2: Water soluble vitamins.

Nutrient	Functions	Sources	Deficiency diseases
Thiamine (vitamin B1)	Part of an enzyme needed for energy metabolism; important to nerve function	Found in all nutritious foods in moderate amounts: pork, whole-grain or enriched breads and cereals, legumes, nuts and seeds	Beriberi, anorexia, weight loss
Riboflavin (vitamin B2)	Part of an enzyme needed for energy metabolism; important for normal vision and skin health	Milk and milk products; leafy green vegetables; whole-grain, enriched breads and cereals	Ariboflavinosis, glossitis of tongue, anxiety, loss of appetite
Niacin (vitamin B3)	Part of an enzyme needed for energy metabolism; important for nervous system, digestive system, and skin health	Meat, poultry, fish, whole-grain or enriched breads and cereals, vegetables (especially mushrooms, asparagus, and leafy green vegetables), peanut butter	Pellagra, dermatitis, stomatitis
Pantothenic acid (vitamin B5)	Part of an enzyme needed for energy metabolism	Widespread in foods	Tingling of feet, headache, fatigue, impaired muscle coordination.
Pyridoxine (vitamin B6)	Part of an enzyme needed for protein metabolism; helps make red blood cells	Meat, fish, poultry, vegetables, fruits	Cheilosis, glossitis, stomatitis, dermatitis

Contd...

Contd...

Nutrient	Functions	Sources	Deficiency diseases
Biotin (vitamin B7)	Part of an enzyme needed for energy metabolism	Widespread in foods; also produced in intestinal tract by bacteria	Hair loss (alopecia), neurological disorders, impaired growth
Folic acid	Part of an enzyme needed for making DNA and new cells, especially red blood cells	Leafy green vegetables and legumes, seeds, orange juice, and liver; now added to most refined grains	Macrocytic anemia, spina bifida in pregnancy, loss of appetite
Cobalamin (vitamin B12)	Part of an enzyme needed for making new cells; important to nerve function	Meat, poultry, fish, seafood, eggs, milk and milk products; not found in plant foods	Anemia and pernicious anemia, nerve degeneration
Ascorbic acid (vitamin C)	Antioxidant; part of an enzyme needed for protein metabolism; important for immune system health; aids in iron absorption	Found only in fruits and vegetables, especially citrus fruits, vegetables in the cabbage family, cantaloupe, strawberries, peppers, tomatoes, potatoes, lettuce, papayas, mangoes, kiwifruit	Scurvy, dry hair and skin, gum infections

■ PURPOSE OF VITAMIN DEFICIENCY TESTING

They are present in traces in different food content. Vitamins are required in the diet in only tiny amounts. Vitamins are essential to life. They contribute to good health by aiding in the metabolism and helping the biochemical processes that provide energy from digested food. Vitamins work with enzymes, helping the body perform all of its necessary activities.

Our body does not produce enough vitamins and hence, our body is prone to its deficiencies. There are different types of vitamins and each of them is important for the body. Deficiency of any vitamin will affect the daily functions of the body.

A vitamin may be present in the body, but it may not be properly activated, appropriately localized or have sufficient cofactors to function at a normal level of activity. No matter what the cause, the result will be a defect in the biochemical pathways that depend upon that nutrient for optimal function. A deficient or defective pathway may operate at a suboptimal level for many months, or even years, before a symptom appears. Even people with healthy dietary and life habits can have vitamin and mineral deficiencies. Biochemical individuality, absorption, chronic conditions, age, and lifestyle influence individual micronutrient requirements. Even a healthy-looking person can have vitamin, mineral or antioxidant deficiencies that may only be revealed through micronutrient testing.

Deficiencies suppress the function of the immune system and contribute to degenerative processes and diseases such as scurvy, pellagra, or rickets. Conversely, consuming too much of a certain vitamin can be toxic to a person's system. Vitamin tests are used to assess the level of certain vitamins in an individual's blood so that doctors can more accurately diagnose vitamin deficiency diseases or vitamin overdoses and advise effective therapy. The vitamins that are most commonly measured are folate, vitamin B12, vitamin K, vitamin D, and vitamin A.

■ ESSENTIAL VITAMINS

There are 13 essential vitamins. This means that these vitamins are required for the body to work properly. They are described in detail here.

Vitamin A

It is also known as retinol because it produces the pigments in the retina of the eye.

Biochemistry

Vitamin A is a generic term for retinol, retinal and retinoic acid, all of which are found in animals. Retinal and retinoic acid are the active forms of vitamin A. The provitamin of vitamin A is a plant pigment β-carotene and other carotenoids. β-carotene is converted in the small intestine to retinal and retinoic acid by the action of the β-carotene dioxygenase. Further metabolism in the enterocytes produces retinol and retinoic acid, which are transported to the liver for storage. It is excreted via bile and urine.

Function

- Vitamin A helps form and maintains healthy skin, teeth, skeletal and soft tissue, and mucus membranes.
- Vitamin A also helps regulate immune system and helps lymphocytes function more effectively in fighting infections.
- It is essential to the retina to form retinal, a light absorbing molecule which allows for low-light and color vision.
- It may also be needed for reproduction and breastfeeding.

Food Sources

There are two types of vitamin A that are found in the diet.
- Preformed vitamin A (retinyl acetate or retinyl palmitate) is found in animal products, such as meat, fish, poultry, and dairy foods.
- Provitamin A (carotenoids) is found in plant-based foods such as fruits and vegetables. The most common type of provitamin A is beta-carotene.
- Sources are orange and yellow vegetables and fruits, others such as broccoli, spinach, and most dark green, leafy vegetables. The more intense the color of a fruit or vegetable, the higher the beta-carotene content. Vegetable sources of beta-carotene are fat- and cholesterol free.
- Besides these natural sources, vitamin A is also present in fortified breakfast cereals and fortified skim milk and milk products.

Normal Value

28–94 μg/dL.

Recommended dietary allowance (RDA)

- Males age 14 and older: 900 μg/day
- Females age 14 and older: 700 μg/day (770 during pregnancy and 1,300 μg during lactation)

Deficiency

Deficiency of vitamin A has following effects:
- These include reversible night blindness and then non-reversible corneal damage known as xerophthalmia.
- Lack of vitamin A can lead to hyperkeratosis or dry, scaly skin.

Toxicity

Hypervitaminosis (high level of vitamin) A is caused by consuming excessive amounts of preformed vitamin A, (not the plant carotenoids) because, preformed vitamin A is rapidly absorbed and slowly cleared from the body.

It can cause nausea, headache, fatigue, loss of appetite, dizziness, and dry skin. Excess intake while pregnant can cause birth defects.

Laboratory Determination

High performance liquid chromatography (HPLC) method is very reliable method for diagnosis of vitamin A, mainly because of its ability to effect rapid separation and the high resolution achieved. Spectrophotometric method and colorimetric methods are also in practice.

Vitamin D

It is also known as the "sunshine vitamin," since it is made by the body after being in the sun.

Biochemistry

Vitamin D is a fat-soluble vitamin that also acts as a hormone. The animal form (obtained from animal source/ sunlight) is vitamin D3 (cholecalciferol) and the plant form (obtained from plant source) is vitamin D2 (ergocalciferol). Vitamin D2 and D3 are not biologically active; they must be modified in the body to have any effect.

The active form of vitamin D is a hormone and is known as 1,25-dihydroxyvitamin D3 [1,25(OH)$_2$D3] or calcitriol.

Following are the steps of vitamin D metabolism **(Fig. 28.1)**:

Step 1: Cholesterol is converted to 7-dehydrocholesterol, which is a precursor of vitamin D3. From there it begins two hydroxylation processes.

Step 2: After exposure to UVB radiation from sun, 7-dehydrocholesterol in the skin is converted to vitamin D3. It is 25-hydroxyvitamin D3/calcidiol, which is the primary circulating form of vitamin D and the most commonly measured form in serum.

Step 3: Vitamin D3 must then be hydroxylated and transformed into 1,25-dihydroxyvitamin D (calcitriol), which is the biologically

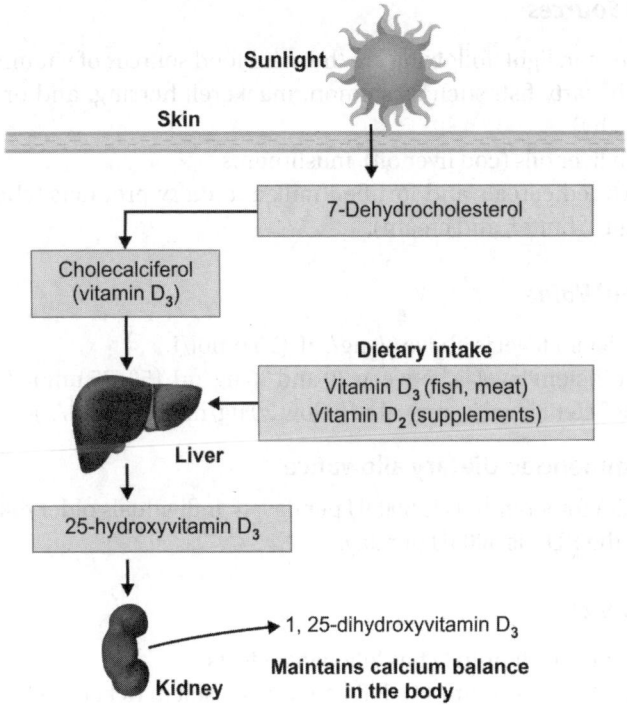

Fig. 28.1: Vitamin D metabolism.

active form of vitamin D. This happens in the liver and the kidneys to become active. At this point, it can exert its endocrine effect.

Function

Vitamin D has following multiple roles in the body:
- The active form of vitamin D helps to control the body's levels of calcium and phosphate. This maintains the health of bones and teeth. It also aids in preventing osteoporosis.
- Support the health of the immune system, brain and nervous system.
- It regulates insulin levels and aid diabetes management.
- It supports lung function and cardiovascular health.
- It influences the expression of genes involved in cancer development and helps to prevent chronic fatigue and certain cancers.

Food Sources

Besides sun light, following are the main food sources of vitamin D:
- Fish (fatty fish such as salmon, mackerel, herring, and orange roughy)
- Fish liver oils (cod liver oil), mushrooms
- Fortified cereals and fortified milk and dairy products (cheese, yogurt, butter, and cream).

Normal Value

- Sufficient level is above 30 ng/mL (75 nmol/L)
- Insufficient level is between 20 and 30 ng/mL (50–75 nmol/L)
- A deficient level is any value below 20 ng/mL (50 nmol/L)

Recommended dietary allowance

The RDA for vitamin D is 600 IU per day. In individuals older than 70 years, the RDA is 800 IU per day.

Deficiency

Deficiency of vitamin D has following effects:
- In children, a vitamin D deficiency can result in rickets, deformed bones, retarded growth, and soft teeth.

- In adults, a vitamin D deficiency can result in osteomalacia, softened bones, spontaneous fractures, and tooth decay.

Toxicity

- Hypervitaminosis D is not a result of sun exposure but from chronic supplementation.
- Excessive consumption of vitamin D can lead to the over calcification of bone and the hardening of blood vessels, kidney, lungs and heart.
- The most common symptoms of hypervitaminosis D are headache and nausea but can also include loss of appetite, dry mouth, a metallic taste, vomiting, constipation, and diarrhea.
- Excessive supplement use will result in excessive thirst, excessive urination, itching, muscle weakness, joint pain and disorientation.
- Calcification of soft tissues can also occur due to excess of vitamin D consumption.

Groups at Higher Risk for Vitamin D Deficiency

There are several groups at higher risk of vitamin D deficiency including—breastfed infants, older adults, dark skinned people (as melanin in darker skin reduces the ability to produce vitamin D from sunlight exposure), limited sun exposure, obesity (as vitamin D is fat soluble, which does not allow it to circulate as freely), gastric bypass patients have less small intestine available to absorb vitamin D.

Laboratory Determination

Earlier, vitamin D was measured by competitive binding methods, HPLC, and radioimmunoassay (RIA).

A commonly used RIA method is considered the gold standard. It is based on the principle of α-complementation of the enzyme β-galactosidase and competition between an enzyme donor 25-(OH)D in serum sample, and an anti-vitamin D antibody. Samples with higher 25-(OH)D concentrations produce higher β-galactosidase activities. A nitrophenyl-beta-galactoside analogue (NPGA) is used as the enzyme substrate and the accumulation of the reaction product has a maximum absorbance at 415 nm. The 25-(OH)D concentration of a patient sample is proportional to the measured beta-galactosidase activity.

High-performance liquid chromatography methods quantitate 25-hydroxy vitamin D_2 and D_3. HPLC methods are available in kit form in an effort to standardize test quality and to make the assays more cost-effective and less labor intensive. The Hitachi HPLC method uses a reverse phase column and diode array detection, which allow for highly sensitive simultaneous analysis at optimal wavelengths. This method can be used to analyze food and biological samples.

Newer chromatography methods have been developed to improve sensitivity, to simplify steps, and to measure all forms of vitamin D. One example is an LC-MS/MS method that was developed to analyze all forms and metabolites of vitamin D simultaneously, including D_2, D_3, and 25-hydroxy vitamin D in serum. The process uses an ionization detector technique known as atmospheric pressure photo ionization (APPI) to provide additional sensitivity for analysis. The method is less difficult compared with other LC methods because it does not require preconcentration steps.

Quantitative chemiluminescent immunoassay (CLIA) method measures total 25-hydroxy vitamin D and other hydroxylated vitamin D metabolites in human serum. During the first step, 25-hydroxy vitamin D is dissociated from its binding protein and binds to the specific solid phase antibody, followed by the addition of vitamin D-isoluminol tracer; unbound material is removed with a wash cycle. In the next step, the reagents are added to initiate the chemiluminescent reaction. The light signal is detected by a photomultiplier as relative light units; this measurement is inversely proportional to the concentration of 25-hydroxy vitamin D.

Vitamin E

Biochemistry

Vitamin E is the collective name for a group of fat-soluble compounds with antioxidant properties. These are called tocopherols. 90% of vitamin E present in human tissues is in the form of the natural isomer, α-tocopherol. Vitamin E occurs in eight forms, including alpha (α)-tocopherol and gamma (γ)-tocopherol. Chemically, it is chromane with isoprenoid side chain. It is transported by alpha-tocopherol transfer protein. It is stored in adipose tissue and parenchymal cells of the liver. It is excreted via bile.

Function

- It helps the body to form red blood cells and uses vitamin K.
- These vitamins have antioxidant properties and work to fight the damage of free radicals including oxidative stress which has been shown to cause certain types of cancer as well as heart disease.
- In addition vitamin E is also involved in immune function and supports healthy skin.
- It protects skin from ultraviolet light.
- It protects against prostate cancer and Alzheimer's disease.
- It maintains the integrity of cell membranes.
- Vitamin E is essential for the maintenance of the heart function, for functioning of sex organs and for cell protection.

Food Sources

- Avocado, tomatoes
- Dark green vegetables (spinach, broccoli, asparagus, and turnip greens)
- Margarine (made from safflower, corn, and sunflower oil)
- Oils (safflower, corn, and sunflower)
- Papaya, blueberries and mango
- Seeds and nuts (almonds, sunflower seeds, olives)
- Wheat germ and wheat germ oil

Normal Value

The reference range of vitamin E in adults is 5.5–17 µg/mL. In children, it is 3–18.4 µg/mL.

Recommended dietary allowance

The RDA for vitamin E is 10 mg/day for the adult man and woman.

Deficiency

Vitamin E deficiency occurs as a result of malnutrition, genetic defects or fat malabsorption syndromes.

Vitamin E deficiency in humans results in—ataxia, (poor muscle coordination with shaky movements), decreased sensation to vibration, lack of reflexes, and paralysis of eye muscles. One particular severe symptom of vitamin E deficiency is the inability to walk because of impaired balance. It is a very rare problem that results in damage to nerves.

Toxicity

People on blood thinners should not take vitamin E, because it increases the risk of hemorrhaging. Excess of Vitamin E can affect insulin requirements, so it may also be a risk for diabetics.

Minimal side effects have been noted in adults taking supplements in doses less than 2,000 mg/day. There is a potential for impaired blood clotting. Infants are more vulnerable.

Laboratory Determination

Vitamin E levels can be determined spectrophotometrically, although the HPLC method with fluorescence detection is preferred, as it permits the measurement of different forms of vitamin E; thus, total vitamin E activity. However, it is a sophisticated technique and requires trained personnel to execute the analysis.

Vitamin K

Biochemistry

Vitamin K refers to a group of vitamins which includes vitamin K1 and vitamin K2. Vitamin K1 is synthesized by plants. Vitamin K2 is mainly produced by both humans, animals, and also by bacteria found in the large intestine. These are varying in the number of isoprenoid units in their side chain. Vitamin K circulates as phylloquinone (vitamin K_1) and it is stored in liver in the form of menaquinones (vitamin K_2). It is transported via lipoproteins. Absorption of vitamin K depends on the ability to absorb fat. It is excreted by bile and urine. It is transported via lipoproteins, stored in liver and excreted via bile and urine.

Function

- Vitamin K facilitates the function of several proteins, including those that are responsible for blood clot formation.
- It plays a vital role in cell growth and in the metabolism of bone and other tissues.

- It is also involved in the prevention of bone loss. Vitamin K modifies the protein osteocalcin. This gives osteocalcin the ability to bind to calcium.
- It also prevents cardiovascular disease by preventing deposition of calcium in arteries.

Food Sources

- Cabbage, cauliflower, green beans, green peas, carrots
- Cereals and sprouts
- Dark green vegetables (broccoli, Brussels sprouts, and asparagus)
- Dark leafy vegetables (spinach, kale, collards, and turnip greens)
- Fish, liver, beef, and eggs

Normal Value

Vitamin K—0.13– 1.19 ng/mL.

Recommended dietary allowance

The RDA for vitamin K in individuals less than 6 months is 2 µg per day. The RDA in adult males and females is 120 µg per day and 90 µg per day, respectively.

Deficiency

- Among the most common signs and symptoms of vitamin K deficiency are heavy menstrual bleeding, gum bleeding, nose bleeding, and easy bruising. Vitamin K deficiency further includes bleeding within the digestive tract and blood in the urine.
- A deficiency of vitamin K can affect a newborn baby or fetus as well. Vitamin K deficiency may result in internal bleeding (in the skull), malformed fingers, and under-developed facial features such as ears, nose, and chin. Vitamin K helps in the overall development of the fetus. This explains why a pregnant woman is usually given vitamin K in the form of food supplements.
- Deficiency of vitamin K leads to a reduction in the prothrombin content of blood. Deficiency of vitamin K can also lead to Alzheimer's disease.
- Other prominent signs and symptoms of vitamin K deficiency are prolonged clotting times, hemorrhaging, and anemia.

- Vitamin K deficiency-related symptoms lead to excessive deposition of calcium in soft tissues. Hardening of the arteries or calcium-related problems, biliary obstruction, malabsorption, cystic fibrosis, and resection of the small intestine.

Toxicity

Vitamin K may interfere with glutathione. Although allergic reaction is possible, there is no known toxicity associated with high doses.

Laboratory Determination

Determination of serum vitamin K is performed by serum protein precipitation, followed by lipid extraction and HPLC with electrochemical or fluorometric detection.

Vitamin K status is generally determined indirectly by measuring the function of vitamin K-dependent proteins. Plasma prothrombin time (PT) and the international normalized ratio (INR, an expression of the PT as a fraction of control time) are the most commonly used tests. PT and INR increase in the case of vitamin K deficiency, reflecting clinically significant reduced clotting ability.

Vitamin B1 (Thiamine)

Biochemistry

Thiamine is important for carbohydrate metabolism. In its active form, thiamine pyrophosphate (TPP), it is a coenzyme of pyruvate dehydrogenase. It participates in a similar reaction of oxidative decarboxylation of α-ketoglutarate and also in the metabolism of branched chain amino acids. It is also a coenzyme for transketolase in the pentose phosphate pathway, and it is important in the production of hydrochloric acid in the stomach. It is stored mainly in kidneys, skeletal muscle, liver and brain. Thiamin and its metabolites are excreted mainly in urine.

Function

Thiamin functions as the coenzyme thiamin pyrophosphate (TPP) in the metabolism of carbohydrate that allows oxygen to convert carbohydrate into usable energy. The vitamin also provides nervous system support and aids in the process of creating the neurotransmitter acetylcholine used to relay messages between nerves and the muscles. Thiamin is involved in many body functions including the muscle function, metabolism, digestion and other biochemical processes.

Food Sources

- Dried milk, egg
- Enriched bread and flour
- Lean meats, pork/pork products, beef, liver
- Legumes (dried beans)
- Nuts and seeds
- Organ meats
- Peas, spinach, tomatoes, asparagus, lettuce, mushrooms
- Whole grains, soybeans

Normal Value

Blood thiamine—9-44 nmol/L.

Recommended daily intake

Men—1.2 mg, women—1.1 mg, pregnant/lactating women—1.4 mg.

Deficiency

- Symptoms include burning feet, weakness in extremities, rapid heart rate, swelling, nausea, fatigue, and gastrointestinal problems.
- Thiamine deficiency causes beriberi with swelling due to fluid retention (edema) in the lower limbs that spreads to the upper body, affecting the heart and leading to heart failure.
- Anorexia, weight loss, weakness, peripheral neuropathy—staggered gait, cross eyes, dementia, disorientation, and memory loss.
- Wernicke-Korsakoff syndrome is caused by poor food intake and by decreased absorption and increased excretion caused by alcohol consumption.

Toxicity

Not known. Because thiamine is water soluble and very little is stored in the body, depletion can occur rapidly.

Laboratory Determination

Whole blood is used to determine concentration of thiamin in blood. Erythrocytes contain about 80% of the total thiamine of whole blood. Determination of blood TTP is performed by a whole protein precipitation step, followed by formation of a fluorophore in alkaline condition with potassium ferricyanide and fluorometric measurement. For erythrocyte TTP determination, washed cells are used.

Vitamin B2 (Riboflavin)

Biochemistry

Riboflavin (vitamin B2) works with the other B vitamins. Riboflavin is attached to the sugar alcohol ribitol. The molecule is colored, fluorescent and decomposes in visible light but is heat stable. To prevent riboflavin breakdown, riboflavin-rich foods such as milk, milk products, and cereals are packaged in opaque containers.

It is found in the oxidoreductases such as the flavin mononucleotide (FMN) and the flavin adenine dinucleotide (FAD), and is required for the energy metabolism of both carbohydrates and lipids.

Function

- Riboflavin is a component of two coenzymes—FMN and FAD—that act as hydrogen carriers when carbohydrates and fats are used to produce energy.
- It is helpful in maintaining good vision and healthy hair, skin and nails, and it is necessary for normal cell growth.
- It is important for body growth and the production of red blood cells.

Sources

- Almonds, soybeans/tempeh, mushrooms
- Spinach, whole wheat, yogurt
- Mackerel, eggs, liver
- Fortified grain products such as cereal, and enriched products like bread, pasta, rice, and tortillas.

Normal Value

Blood riboflavin: 6.2–39 nmol/L.

Recommended daily intake

Men—1.3 mg, women—1.1 mg, pregnant women—1.4 mg, lactating women: 1.6 mg.

Deficiency

- A deficiency of this nutrient is usually a part of multinutrient deficiency and does not occur in isolation.
- Symptoms include glossitis of tongue, anxiety, loss of appetite, and fatigue, growth retardation, conjunctivitis, and nerve damage.
- Riboflavin deficiency causes a condition known as ariboflavinosis, which is marked by cheilosis (cracks at the corners of the mouth), oily scaling of the skin, and a red, sore tongue.
- In addition, cataracts may occur more frequently with riboflavin deficiency.

Toxicity

Excess riboflavin may increase the risk of DNA strand breaks in the presence of chromium. High-dose riboflavin therapy will intensify urine color to a bright yellow (flavinuria) but this is harmless.

Laboratory Determination

After protein precipitation, HPLC technique is used for the separation of coenzyme form (FMN, FAD), followed by measurement of intensity of fluorescence by a fluorometer.

Vitamin B3 (Niacin)

Biochemistry

Niacin exists in two forms—nicotinic acid and nicotinamide. Niacin is active as part of the coenzyme nicotinamide adenine dinucleotide (NAD^+) and nicotinamide adenine dinucleotide phosphate ($NADP^+$), both of which participate in oxidoreductase-catalyzed reactions. Both forms are readily absorbed from the stomach and the small intestine.

Niacin is stored in small amounts in the liver and transported to tissues, where it is converted to coenzyme forms. Any excess is excreted in urine. Niacin is one of the most stable of the B vitamins. It is resistant to heat and light, and to both acid and alkali environments. The human body is capable of converting the amino acid tryptophan to niacin when needed. However, when both tryptophan and niacin are deficient, tryptophan is used for protein synthesis.

Function

- Niacin helps the digestive system, skin, and nerves to function. It is also important for converting food to energy.
- Niacin helps to break down all three macronutrients—proteins, carbohydrates and fats.
- Vitamin B3 also helps regulate blood pressure and plays a role in cardiovascular health. Niacin acts as a blood vessel dilator as it helps blood vessels relax and widen to increase blood flow.

Sources

- Mushrooms, asparagus, peanuts
- Brown rice, corn, green leafy vegetables
- Sweet potato, potato, lentil, barley, carrots, almonds
- Chicken, meat, salmon, meat, poultry, fish
- Yeast, enriched and whole grain breads and cereals
- Milk and eggs.

Deficiency

A deficiency of niacin causes pellagra. The symptoms include—digestive problems, inflamed skin, and mental impairment.

Other deficiency symptoms include dermatitis, diarrhea, dementia, and stomatitis.

Normal Value

Blood niacin: 0.50–8.45 µg/mL.

Recommended daily intake

Men—16 mg, women—14 mg, pregnant women—18 mg, lactating women—17 mg.

Toxicity

Niacin from foods is not known to cause adverse effects. Supplemental nicotinic acid may cause flushing of skin, itching, impaired glucose tolerance, peptic ulcer and gastrointestinal upset. Intake of 750 mg per day for less than 3 months can cause liver cell damage. High dose nicotinamide can cause nausea and liver toxicity.

Laboratory Determination

Niacin is assayed semiquantitatively with sulfanilic acid to yield a yellow color. The intensity of the yellow color correlates with the amount of niacin present, which is measured against a set of standards.

HPLC methods are used to determine urinary metabolites. Determination of ratio NAD/NADH in erythrocytes can be useful to determine niacin deficiency. A ratio of NAD/NADH below 1.0 indicates niacin deficiency.

Pantothenic Acid (Vitamin B5)

The name is derived from Greek word pantothen meaning from everywhere. Small quantities of pantothenic acid are found nearly in every food.

Biochemistry

It is commonly found in the form of alcohol panthenol and calcium pantothenate. It is transported to blood via proteins. It is excreted in urine. Pantothenic acid is stable in moist heat. It is destroyed by vinegar (acid), baking soda (alkali), and dry heat. Significant losses occur during the processing and refining of foods.

Function

Pantothenic acid is released from coenzyme A in food in the small intestine. After absorption, it is transported to tissues, where coenzyme A is resynthesized. Coenzyme A is essential for the formation of energy as adenosine triphosphate (ATP) from carbohydrate, protein, alcohol, and fat. Coenzyme A is also important in the synthesis of fatty acids, cholesterol, steroids, and the neurotransmitter acetylcholine, which is essential for transmission of nerve impulses to muscles.

Sources

- Broccoli, lentils, split peas, avocado
- Whole wheat, mushrooms, sweet potato
- Sunflower seeds, cauliflower, green leafy vegetables
- Eggs, squash, strawberries, liver

Deficiency

Very unlikely dietary deficiency occurs in conjunction with other B-vitamin deficiencies. In severe malnutrition one may notice tingling of feet, headache, fatigue, impaired muscle coordination, abdominal cramps, and vomiting.

Normal Value

Blood pantothenic acid—37–147 µg/L.

Recommended daily intake

Men and women: 5 mg, pregnant women: 6 mg, lactating women: 7 mg.

Toxicity

Large doses of pantothenic acid do not cause symptoms, nausea, heartburn and diarrhea may be noticed with high dose supplements.

Laboratory Determination

Methods used for the determination of pantothenic acid are RIA and gas chromatography.

Vitamin B6

Biochemistry

Vitamin B6 is present in three forms—pyridoxal, pyridoxine, and pyridoxamine. All forms can be converted to the active vitamin-B6 coenzyme in the body. Pyridoxal phosphate (PLP) is the predominant biologically active form. Vitamin B6 is not stable in heat or in alkaline conditions, so cooking and food processing reduce its content in food. Both coenzyme and free forms are absorbed in the small intestine and transported to the liver, where they are phosphorylated and released into circulation, bound to albumin for transport to tissues. Vitamin B6 is stored in the muscle and only excreted in urine when intake is excessive.

Function

- PLP participates in amino acid synthesis and the interconversion of some amino acids.
- It catalyzes a step in the synthesis of hemoglobin, which is needed to transport oxygen in blood.
- PLP helps maintain blood glucose levels by facilitating the release of glucose from liver and muscle glycogen.
- It also plays a role in the synthesis of many neurotransmitters important for brain function.
- PLP participates in the conversion of the amino acid tryptophan to niacin and helps avoid niacin deficiency.
- Pyridoxine affects immune function, as it is essential for the formation of a type of white blood cell.

Sources

- Whole wheat, brown rice, green leafy vegetables
- Sunflower seeds, potato, garbanzo beans, banana
- Spinach, tomatoes, avocado, walnuts, peanut butter
- Salmon, lima beans, bell peppers, chicken meat, fish

Deficiency

Symptoms include—cheilosis, glossitis, stomatitis, dermatitis (all similar to vitamin B2 deficiency), nervous system disorders, sleeplessness, confusion, nervousness, depression, irritability, decline in immune function, interference with nerves that supply muscles and difficulties in movement of these muscles, and anemia. Prenatal deprivation results in mental retardation and blood disorders for the newborn.

Normal Value

Blood vitamin B6—5-50 µg/L.

Recommended daily intake

- Males age 14 to 50 years—1.3 mg/day
- Males over 50 years—1.7 mg/day
- Females age 14 to 50 years—1.3 mg/day
- Females over 50 years—1.5 mg/day
- Females of all ages 1.9 mg/day during pregnancy and 2.0 mg/day during lactation.

Toxicity

High doses of supplemental vitamin B6 may result in painful neurological symptoms (nerve destruction) and skin lesions.

Laboratory Determination

Plasma pyridoxal phosphate is considered to be one of the best indicators of vitamin B6 status in the body. Determination of serum PLP can be performed by HPLC techniques for separation of PLP, followed by fluorometric determination.

Biotin (Vitamin B7 or Vitamin H)

Biochemistry

Biotin is the most stable of B vitamins. It is composed of an uredio (tetrahydroimidizalone) ring fused with tetrahydrothiophene ring. It is commonly found in two forms—the free vitamin and the protein-bound coenzyme form called biocytin. Biotin is absorbed in the small intestine, and it requires digestion by enzyme biotinidase, which is present in the small intestine. Biotin is synthesized by bacteria in the large intestine.

Function

- Biotin containing coenzymes participate in key reactions that produce energy from carbohydrate and synthesize fatty acids and protein.
- It helps the body to process glucose.

- It also contributes toward healthy nails, skin and hair. It is, therefore, found in many cosmetic and health products for the skin and hair. It also helps to transfer CO_2.

Sources

- Chocolate, nuts and seeds, raspberries
- Cereal, whole grains
- Egg yolk, organ meats (liver, kidney), pork
- Legumes, green leafy vegetables
- Milk, yeast, salmon
- Avocado, cauliflower, carrots, papaya, banana

Deficiency

Deficiency is very rare in humans. Consuming raw egg whites over a long period of time can cause biotin deficiency. Egg whites contain the protein avidin, which binds to biotin and prevents its absorption.

Infants: Dermatitis, convulsions, hair loss (alopecia), neurological disorders, impaired growth.

Normal Value

Blood biotin: 221.0–3004.0 pg/mL

Recommended daily intake

Men and women—30 µg, pregnant women—30 µg, lactating women—35 µg.

Toxicity

Not known to be toxic.

Laboratory Determination

After separation by HPLC methods, ELISA techniques are used for the determination of serum biotin. In the methods based on ELISA, biotinylated primary antibodies are used against serum biotin (as an antigen). It is followed by detection step using streptavidin conjugated to horseradish peroxidase, followed by the color reaction with chromogen.

Vitamin B9 (Folic Acid, Folate, Folacin)

Folacin or folate, as it is usually called, is the form of vitamin B9 naturally present in foods, whereas folic acid is the synthetic form added to fortified foods and supplements. Both forms are absorbed in the small intestine and stored in the liver. The folic acid form, however, is more efficiently absorbed and available to the body. When consumed in excess of needs, both forms are excreted in urine and easily destroyed by heat, oxidation, and light.

Biochemistry

Folic acid (pteroyl-L-glutamic acid) exists in a number of derivatives collectively known as folates. Folic acid is physiologically inactive until reduced to dihydrofolic acid. Its main forms are tetrahydrofolate, 5-methyl tetrahydrofolate (N^5MeTHF), and N^{10}-formyltetrahydrofolate-polyglutamate derived from N^5MeTHF predominant in fresh food. Before polyglutamates can be absorbed, they must be hydrolyzed by glutamyl hydrolase in the small intestine. The main circulating form of folate is the monoglutamate-N^5-THF.

Function

- All forms of this vitamin are readily converted to the coenzyme form called tetrahydrofolate (THFA), which plays a key role in transferring single-carbon methyl units during the synthesis of DNA and RNA, and in interconversions of amino acids.
- Folate also plays an important role in the synthesis of neurotransmitters.
- Folate works with vitamin B12 to help form red blood cells.
- It is extremely important during pregnancy and helps to prevent conditions such as colon cancer, birth defects such as spina bifida and adult acute lymphocytic leukemia.

Sources

- Asparagus and broccoli, sprouts
- Beets, banana, papaya, citrus fruits
- Brewer's yeast
- Dried beans (cooked pinto, navy, kidney, and lima)
- Fortified cereals

- Green, leafy vegetables (spinach and romaine lettuce)
- Lentils, peanut butter, green peas
- Oranges and orange juice
- Wheat germ, whole grains

Deficiency

- Folate deficiency is one of the most common vitamin deficiencies. Early symptoms are nonspecific and include tiredness, irritability, and loss of appetite.
- One may notice sprue, leukopenia, thrombocytopenia, weight loss, cracking and redness of tongue and mouth, and diarrhea. In pregnancy, there is a risk of low birth weight and preterm delivery.
- Severe folate deficiency leads to macrocytic anemia, a condition in which cells in the bone marrow cannot divide normally and red blood cells remain in a large immature form called macrocytes.
- Large immature cells also appear along the length of the gastrointestinal tract, resulting in abdominal pain and diarrhea.
- Folate deficiency may lead to neural tube defects such as spina bifida (failure of the spine to close properly during the first month of pregnancy) and anencephaly (closure of the neural tube during fetal development, resulting in part of the cranium not being formed).
- Inadequate folate status is associated with some cancers.

Normal Value

Blood vitamin B9—2–20 ng/mL, or 4.5–45.3 nmol/L.

Recommended daily intake

Men and women—400 µg/day, pregnant women—600 µg, lactating women—500 µg.

Toxicity

No toxic effect.

Laboratory Determination

Competitive protein binding (CPB) assays are used for this determination of serum or erythrocyte folic acid, followed by RIA or fluorometric techniques. The protein used for binding folate is β-lactoglobulin together with radioactive ^{125}I-folate label or enzyme linked fluorescent compound.

Vitamin B12 (Cyanocobalamin)

Vitamin B12 is found in its free-vitamin form, called cyanocobalamin, and in two active coenzyme forms. Absorption of vitamin B12 requires the presence of *intrinsic factor,* a protein synthesized by acid-producing cells of the stomach. The vitamin is absorbed in the terminal portion of the small intestine called the ileum. Most of body's supply of vitamin B12 is stored in the liver.

Vitamin B12 is efficiently conserved in the body, since most of it is secreted into bile and reabsorbed. Vitamin B_{12} is stable when heated and slowly loses its activity when exposed to light, oxygen, and acid or alkaline environments.

Biochemistry

- Vitamin B12 is the largest of the B complex vitamins, with a molecular weight of over 1000. Vitamin B12 is commonly called cyanocobalamin.
- Vitamin B12 consists of six parts:
    - *(i to iv) Cobalt-corrin ring complex:* It is made up of cobalt as a central ion, and corrin ring. There are four parts of corrin ring (synthesized by bacteria). This cobalt-corrin ring complex gives vitamin B12 its red coloration.
    - *(v) A dimethylbenzimidazole group:* Different forms of vitamin B12 are similar in the the four parts and a dimethylbenzimidazole group, but differ in the sixth site.
    - *(vi)* Sixth site may contain cyano group (CN), hydroxyl group (OH), methyl group (CH3) and/or 5'- deoxyadenosyl group (C-CO).

Function

- Vitamin B12 coenzymes help recycle folate coenzymes involved in the synthesis of DNA and RNA, and in the normal formation of red blood cells.

- Vitamin B12 prevents degeneration of the myelin sheaths that cover nerves and help maintain normal electrical conductivity through the nerves.
- Vitamin B12, like the other B vitamins, is important for metabolism.
- The vitamin B12 is also needed for the synthesis of the red blood cells.
- It has been found to be very much needed for the growth and development of children.

Sources

B12 is a product of bacterial fermentation present in colon that is why it is not present in plant products.
- Meat, fish, poultry, eggs
- Fortified foods such as soymilk, fortified cereals
- Milk and milk products
- Organ meats (liver and kidney)
- Shellfish
- For vegetarian people and infants, fortified dairy products are important sources

Deficiency

Since vitamin B12 is well conserved in the body, it is difficult to become deficient from dietary factors alone. Deficiency is usually observed when B12 absorption is hampered by disease or surgery to the stomach or ileum, damage to gastric mucosa by alcoholism, or prolonged use of anti-ulcer medications that affect secretion of intrinsic factor. Elders are at a higher risk of developing a deficiency mainly due to decreasing absorption along with dietary changes or decreased food intake. Other causes include undergoing certain types of bariatric surgery that remove part of the stomach; bacterial overgrowth, which competes for vitamin B12; and alcohol consumption.
- Vitamin B12 deficiency results in macrocytic anemia and pernicious anemia, later is caused by a genetic problem in the production of intrinsic factor.
- The anemia caused by vitamin-B12 deficiency is accompanied by symptoms of nerve degeneration, which if left untreated can result in paralysis and death.

- Paresthesia (tingling and numbness in limbs), difficulty walking, loss of bowel and bladder control, dementia.

Normal Value

- Blood vitamin B12—200–900 pg/mL

Recommended daily intake

Men and women—2.4 µg, pregnant women—2.6 µg, lactating women—2.8 µg.

Toxicity

Not known from supplements or food. Only a small amount is absorbed via the oral route, thus the potential for toxicity is low.

Laboratory Determination

There are several approaches to diagnosing vitamin B12 deficiency. These include:

Indirect approach

Indirect tests to detect physiological correlates of vitamin B12 deficiency are:

i. **Blood film examination:** Hypersegmented neutrophils, oval macrocytes and circulating megaloblasts are typical features of vitamin B12 deficiency.
ii. **Mean cell volume (MCV):** MCV levels are increased up to 25% in vitamin B12 deficiency.

Other indirect tests for biochemical abnormalities associated with vitamin B12 deficiency, include—methylmalonic acid (MMA) or total homocysteine (Hcy) levels.

Two enzymatic reactions are known to be dependent on vitamin B12—

a. Methylmalonic acid is converted to succinyl-CoA using vitamin B12 as a cofactor. Vitamin B12 **deficiency**, therefore, can lead to increased levels of serum methylmalonic acid.
b. Total serum Hcy is an indicator of vitamin B12 deficiency because vitamin B12 is needed for the synthesis of methionine from Hcy. In case of vitamin B12 deficiency, methionine will not be produced, and the level of Hcy will be high.

However, for these indirect tests levels may not accurately indicate a deficiency as results can be altered by many other things.

Direct tests

Direct test for vitamin B12 include a wide range of tests with different advantages and drawbacks.

i. **Microbiological assay:** It has been the most commonly used assay technique. It relies on the specific requirement for vitamin B12 by certain bacterial organisms (e.g., *Lactobacillus delbrueckii*) to enable their growth in a supporting medium. Under appropriate conditions, the amount of bacterial growth obtained is proportional to the amount of vitamin B12 in the test extract.

ii. **Other assays:** Competitive protein binding and immunometric assays have been used for the quantitative determination of vitamin B12. In CPB methods serum vitamin B12 competes with radiolabeled cobalamin for a limited number of binding sites on intrinsic factor (IF). RIA methodology used to determine free and bound fractions of vitamin B12 to determine serum concentrations of vitamin B12. Most immunometric methods use solid phase separation by immobilizing the IF binder on beads or magnetic particles. In that case free vitamin B12 remains in the supernatant and bound vitamin B12 becomes a part of solid phase suspension. By determining ratio of bound to free fraction and calibrators, serum vitamin B12 concentration can be determined.

iii. **Schilling test:** Schilling test is performed to check for the efficiency of vitamin B12 absorption.

Intrinsic factor is produced in the stomach and is required for vitamin B12 absorption. Without the production of intrinsic factor, the body cannot absorb vitamin B12 and excreted in the urine.

The lack of intrinsic factor can be due to the damage of the stomach or its linings. Examples are pernicious anemia, partial removal of the stomach (gastrectomy), autoimmunity against gastric parietal cells and atrophic gastric mucosa.

Sample: Urine sample.

Stage 1: Oral vitamin B12 plus intramuscular vitamin B12 (without IF)

In the first part of the test, the patient is given oral dose of radiolabeled vitamin B12. The most commonly used radiolabels are ^{57}Co and ^{58}Co.

An intramuscular injection of unlabeled vitamin B12 is given an hour later. The purpose of the single injection is to temporarily saturate B12 receptors in the liver with enough normal vitamin B12 to prevent radioactive vitamin B12 binding in body tissues. So if radiolabeled B12 is absorbed from the GI tract, it will pass into the urine. The patient's urine is then collected over the next 24 hours to assess the absorption.

The normal test will result in a higher amount of the radiolabeled cobalamin in the urine because it would have been absorbed by the intestinal epithelium, but passed into the urine because all hepatic B12 receptors were occupied. An abnormal result is caused by less of the labeled cobalamin to appear in the urine because it was not absorbed and remain in the intestine and ultimately passed into the feces.

A normal result shows at least 10% of the radiolabeled vitamin B12 in the urine over the first 24 hours. In patients with deficiency due to impaired absorption, less than 10% of the radiolabeled vitamin B12 is detected.

Stage 2: Vitamin B12 and intrinsic factor
If an abnormality is found, i.e., the B12 in the urine is only present in low levels, the test is repeated, this time with additional oral intrinsic factor.

If this second urine collection is normal, this shows a lack of intrinsic factor production. This indicates pernicious anemia.

A low result on the second test implies an absorption defect in the terminal ileum, and further tests should be done to investigate.

Vitamin C (Ascorbic Acid)

Vitamin C is essential to the activity of many enzymes.

Biochemistry

Vitamin C serves as a reducing agent. Its active form is ascorbic acid, which is oxidized during the transfer of reducing equivalents, yielding dehydroascorbic acid. It is an antioxidant, also participates in the regeneration of another antioxidant vitamin—α-tocopherol.

Function

- By neutralizing free radicals, vitamin C may reduce the risk of heart disease, certain forms of cancer, and cataracts.

- It improves absorption of non-heme iron, and participates in bone mineral metabolism.
- Vitamin C is needed to form and maintain collagen, a fibrous protein that gives strength to connective tissues in skin, cartilage, bones, teeth, and joints. Collagen is also needed for the healing of wounds.
- When added to meals, vitamin C increases intestinal absorption of iron from plant-based foods. High concentration of vitamin C in white blood cells enables the immune system to function properly
- Vitamin C also recycles oxidized vitamin E for reuse in cells, and it helps folic acid convert to its active form, tetrahydrofolate (THF).
- Vitamin C helps synthesize carnitine, adrenaline, epinephrine, the neurotransmitter serotonin, the thyroid hormone thyroxin, bile acids, and steroid hormones.

Sources

- Broccoli, sprouts
- Cabbage, cauliflower
- Citrus fruits, strawberries, guava, kiwi, pineapple
- Potatoes, sweet potato
- Spinach, tomato

Deficiency

- Bruising, gum infections, lethargy, dental cavities
- Tissue swelling, dry hair and skin, bleeding gums
- Dry eyes, hair loss, joint paint, pitting edema, anemia
- Delayed wound healing, and bone fragility
- Long-term deficiency results in scurvy

Normal Value

Blood vitamin C: 0.6–2 mg/dL.

Recommended daily intake

Men—90 mg, women—75 mg, pregnant women—80–85 mg, lactating women—115–120 mg.

Toxicity

Possible problems with very large vitamin C doses including kidney stones, rebound scurvy, increased oxidative stress, excess iron absorption, vitamin B12 deficiency, and erosion of dental enamel. The 2 g or more per day can cause diarrhea, nausea, and abdominal cramps.

Laboratory Determination

Vitamin C can be quantitatively analyzed by either titrimetric or fluorometric methods. The titrimetric method involves the measurement of decolorization of 2,6-dichloroindophenol dye by ascorbic acid. The fluorometric method involves oxidation of ascorbic acid to dehydroascorbic acid, which reacts with phenylenediamine to produce a fluorescent compound whose intensity is proportional to the vitamin C concentration.

SUMMARY

- Vitamins are organic compounds that are essential in very small amounts for supporting normal physiologic function, growth, and development.
- Vitamin tests are used to assess the level of certain vitamins in an individual's blood so that doctors can more accurately diagnose vitamin deficiency diseases or vitamin overdoses and advise effective therapy.

PRACTICE QUESTIONS

1. What are vitamins? Write their characteristics.
2. What is vitamin B complex?
3. Differentiate between fat soluble and water soluble vitamins.
4. Justify, "vitamin deficiency testing is need of time".
5. Write any two functions sources and deficiency diseases for vitamin A.
6. Write any two functions sources and deficiency diseases for vitamin C.
7. Write any two functions sources and deficiency diseases for vitamin D.
8. Write any two functions sources and deficiency diseases for vitamin E.
9. Write any two functions sources and deficiency diseases for vitamin K.
10. Write any two functions sources and deficiency diseases for vitamin B1.
11. Write any two functions sources and deficiency diseases for vitamin B2.
12. Write any two functions sources and deficiency diseases for vitamin B3.
13. Write any two functions sources and deficiency diseases for vitamin B5.
14. Write any two functions sources and deficiency diseases for vitamin B7.

15. Write any two functions sources and deficiency diseases for vitamin B6.
16. Write any two functions sources and deficiency diseases for vitamin B12.
17. Write any two functions sources and deficiency diseases for folic acid.
18. With the help of vitamin D metabolism explain why it is called as sunshine vitamin?
19. Discuss methods for the laboratory determination of vitamin D.
20. What is mean by toxicity of vitamins? Write toxicity of all fat soluble vitamins.
21. Which is the largest of Vitamin B complex? Discuss its biochemistry.
22. What are indirect approaches to test vitamin B12?
23. Explain Schilling test.
24. Make a list of normal values for all vitamins.

CHAPTER 29

Tumor Markers

> **Keywords**
> Anaplastic lymphoma kinase (ALK), alpha-fetoprotein (AFP), beta-2-microglobulin (B2M), beta-human chorionic gonadotropin (beta-hCG), BRCA1 and BRCA2 gene, Philadelphia chromosome, B-RAF protein, stem cell factor (SCF), cancer antigen 15-3, cancer antigen 19-9, cancer antigen 125, calcitonin carcinoembryonic antigen (CEA), chromogranin A (CgA), cytokeratin epidermal growth factor, estrogen receptor (ER), lactate dehydrogenase, neuron-specific enolase (NSE), nuclear matrix protein 22, programmed death ligand 1 (PD-L1), prostatespecific antigen (PSA), chemiluminescent magnetic immunoassay (CMIA)

■ INTRODUCTION

Tumor markers are substances that are produced by cancer or by other cells of the body in response to cancer or certain benign (noncancerous) conditions. Most tumor markers are made by normal cells as well as by cancer cells; however, they are produced at much higher levels in cancerous conditions. These substances can be found in the blood, urine, stool, tumor tissue, or other tissues or bodily fluids of some patients with cancer. Most tumor markers are proteins. However, more recently, patterns of gene expression and in genetic material (DNA, RNA), have also begun to be used as tumor markers.

Many different tumor markers have been characterized and are in clinical use. Some are associated with only one type of cancer, whereas others are associated with two or more cancer types. No "universal" tumor marker that can detect any type of cancer has been found.

■ TYPES OF TUMOR MARKERS

Tumor markers are usually normal cellular constituents that are present at normal or very low levels in the blood of healthy persons.

There are five basic types of tumor markers. These are products that are over-expressed (produced in higher than normal amounts) by malignant cells. There are five basic types of tumor markers.

1. **Enzymes:** Many enzymes that occur in certain tissues are found in blood plasma at higher levels when the cancer involves that tissue. Enzymes are usually measured by determining the rate at which they convert a substrate to an end product, while most tumor markers of other types are measured by a test called an immunoassay. Some examples of enzymes whose levels rise in cases of malignant diseases are acid phosphatase, alkaline phosphatase, amylase, creatine kinase, gamma glutamyl transferase, lactate dehydrogenase, and terminal deoxynucleotidyl transferase.

2. **Tissue receptors:** Tissue receptors, which are proteins associated with the cell membrane, are another type of tumor marker. These substances bind to hormones and growth factors, and therefore affect the rate of tumor growth. Some tissue receptors must be measured in tissue samples removed for a biopsy, while others are secreted into the extracellular fluid (fluid outside the cells) and may be measured in the blood. Some important receptor tumor markers are estrogen receptor, progesterone receptor, interleukin-2 receptor, and epidermal growth factor receptor.

3. **Antigens:** Oncofetal antigens are proteins made by genes that are very active during fetal development but function at a very low level after birth. The genes become activated when a malignant tumor arises and produce large amounts of protein. Antigens comprise the largest class of tumor marker and include the tumor-associated glycoprotein antigens. Important tumor markers in this class are alpha-fetoprotein (AFP), carcinoembryonic antigen (CEA), prostate specific antigen (PSA), cathespin-D, HER-2/neu, CA-125, CA-19-9, CA-15-3, nuclear matrix protein, and bladder tumor-associated antigen.

4. **Oncogenes:** Some tumor markers are the product of oncogenes, which are genes that are active in fetal development and trigger the growth of tumors when they are activated in mature cells. Some important oncogenes are BRAC-1, myc, p53, RB (retinoblastoma) gene (RB), and Ph^1 (Philadelphia chromosome).

5. **Hormones:** The fifth type of tumor marker consists of hormones. This group includes hormones that are normally secreted by the

tissue in which the malignancy arises as well as those produced by tissues that do not normally make the hormone (ectopic production). Some hormones associated with malignancy are adrenal corticotropic hormone (ACTH), calcitonin, catecholamines, gastrin, human chorionic gonadotropin (hCG), and prolactin.

■ USES OF TUMOR MARKERS

High tumor marker levels can be a sign of cancer. Along with other tests, tumor marker tests can help doctors diagnose cancer and plan treatment. Tumor markers are most commonly used to do the following:
- **Screen:** Some of the tumor marker may be used to screen people who are at high-risk because they have a strong family history or specific risk factors for a particular cancer.
- **Diagnose:** In a person who has symptoms, tumor markers may be used to help detect the presence of cancer and help differentiate it from other conditions with similar symptoms.
- **Stage:** If a person does have cancer, tumor marker elevations can be used to help determine whether the cancer has spread (metastasized) to other tissues and organs and to what extent.
- **Determine prognosis:** Some tumor markers can be used to help determine how aggressive a cancer is likely to be.
- **Guide choice of treatment:** A few tumor markers provide information about which treatments might be effective against a person's cancer. A decrease in the level of a tumor marker or a return to the marker's normal level may indicate that the cancer is responding to treatment, whereas no change or an increase may indicate that the cancer is not responding.
- **Monitor success of treatment and detect recurrence:** Tumor markers can be used to monitor the effectiveness of treatment, especially in advanced cancers. If the marker level drops, the treatment is working; if it stays elevated, adjustments are needed. (The information must be used with care, however, since other conditions can sometimes cause tumor markers to rise or fall.) One of the most important uses for tumor markers, along with guiding treatment, is to monitor for cancer recurrence. If a tumor marker is elevated before treatment, low after treatment, and then

begins to rise over time, then it is likely that the cancer is returning. (if it remains elevated after surgery, then chances are that not all of the cancer was removed).

■ LIST OF TUMOR MARKERS

Tumor markers that are currently in common use are described here.
1. ***ALK* gene rearrangements and over-expression:** It is a gene that makes a protein called anaplastic lymphoma kinase (ALK), which may be involved in cell growth. Mutated (changed) forms of the *ALK* gene and protein have been found in some types of cancer, including neuroblastoma, non-small cell lung cancer, and anaplastic large cell lymphoma. These changes may increase the growth of cancer cells. Checking for changes in the *ALK* gene in tumor tissue may help to plan cancer treatment. It is also called *anaplastic lymphoma kinase* gene.
    - *Cancer types*: Non-small cell lung cancer and anaplastic large cell lymphoma.
    - *Tissue analyzed*: Tumor.
    - *How used*: To help determine treatment and prognosis.
2. **Alpha-fetoprotein (AFP):** It is a protein normally produced by a fetus. Alpha-fetoprotein levels are usually undetectable in the blood of healthy adult men or women (who are not pregnant). False elevated levels may be seen in pregnancy and liver disease (hepatitis, cirrhosis, toxic liver injury).
    - *Cancer types:* Liver cancer and germ cell tumors.
    - *Tissue analyzed:* Blood.
    - *How used:* To help diagnose liver cancer and follow response to treatment; to assess stage, prognosis, and response to treatment of germ cell tumors.
    - *Low levels present in both men and non-pregnant women (0–15 IU/mL);* generally results >400 are caused by cancer (half-life 4–6 days).
3. **Beta-2-microglobulin (B2M):** It is a small protein normally found on the surface of many cells, including lymphocytes, and in small amounts in the blood and urine. An increased amount in the blood or urine may be a sign of certain diseases, including some types of cancer. False elevated level may be seen in kidney disease and hepatitis.

- *Cancer types*: Multiple myeloma, chronic lymphocytic leukemia, and some lymphomas.
- *Tissue analyzed*: Blood, urine, or cerebrospinal fluid.
- *How used*: To determine prognosis and follow response to treatment.
- *Normal value*: < 2.5 mg/L.

4. **Beta-human chorionic gonadotropin (Beta-hCG):** It is a hormone found in the blood and urine during pregnancy. It may also be found in higher than normal amounts in patients with some types of cancer, including testicular, ovarian, liver, stomach, and lung cancers, and in other disorders. Measuring the amount of beta-hCG in the blood or urine of cancer patients may help to diagnose cancer and find out how well cancer treatment is working. It is also called beta-hCG. Beta-hCG is a type of tumor marker. False elevated levels are seen in pregnancy, hypogonadism (testicular failure) and cirrhosis.
    - *Cancer types*: Choriocarcinoma and germ cell tumors.
    - *Tissue analyzed*: Urine or blood.
    - *How used*: To assess stage, prognosis, and response to treatment.
    - *Normal value*: In men: < 2.5 U/mL, in non-pregnant women: < 5.0 U/mL.

5. ***BRCA1* and *BRCA2* gene mutations:** *BRCA1* is a gene on chromosome 17 and *BRCA2* is a gene on chromosome 13 that normally helps to suppress cell growth. A person who inherits certain mutations (changes) in these genes has a higher risk of getting breast, ovarian, prostate, and other types of cancer.
    - *Cancer type*: Ovarian cancer.
    - *Tissue analyzed*: Blood.
    - *How used*: To determine whether treatment with a particular type of targeted therapy is appropriate

6. **BCR-ABL fusion gene (Philadelphia chromosome):** It is a gene formed when pieces of chromosomes 9 and 22 break off and trade places. The *ABL* gene from chromosome 9 joins to the *BCR* gene on chromosome 22, to form the BCR-ABL fusion gene. The changed chromosome 22 with the fusion gene on it is called the Philadelphia chromosome. The *BCR-ABL* fusion gene is found in most patients with cancer.

- *Cancer type:* Chronic myeloid leukemia, acute lymphoblastic leukemia, and acute myelogenous leukemia.
- *Tissue analyzed:* Blood and/or bone marrow.
- *How used:* To confirm diagnosis, predict response to targeted therapy, and monitor disease status.

7. **BRAF V600 mutations:** It is a gene that makes a protein called B-RAF, which is involved in sending signals in cells and in cell growth. This gene may be mutated (changed) in many types of cancer, which causes a change in the B-RAF protein. This can increase the growth and spread of cancer cells.
   - *Cancer types:* Cutaneous melanoma and colorectal cancer,
   - *Tissue analyzed:* Tumor,
   - *How used:* To select patients who are most likely to benefit from treatment with certain targeted therapies.

8. **C-kit/CD117:** It is a protein found on the surface of many different types of cells. It binds to a substance called stem cell factor (SCF), which causes certain types of blood cells to grow. C-kit may also be found in higher than normal amounts, or in a changed form, on some types of cancer cells, including gastrointestinal stromal tumors and melanoma. Measuring the amount of c-kit in tumor tissue may help diagnose cancer and plan treatment. C-kit is a type of receptor tyrosine kinase and a type of tumor marker. It is also called CD117 and stem cell factor receptor.
   - *Cancer types:* Gastrointestinal stromal tumor and mucosal melanoma.
   - *Tissue analyzed:* Tumor.
   - *How used:* To help in diagnosing and determining treatment.

9. **CA15-3/CA27.29:** Cancer antigen 15-3 (CA 15-3) is a protein that is produced by normal breast cells. In many people with cancerous breast tumors, there is an increased production of CA 15-3 and the related cancer antigen 27.29. CA 15-3 is shed by the tumor cells and enters the bloodstream, making it useful as a tumor marker to follow the course of the cancer. False elevated values are seen in healthy people with certain conditions such as cirrhosis, hepatitis, and benign breast disease.
   - *Cancer type:* Breast cancer.
   - *Tissue analyzed:* Blood.
   - *How used:* To assess whether treatment is working or disease has recurred.

- *Normal value:* CA 15-3 ≤31 units/mL or <31 k units/L, CA 27-29 ≤38 units/mL or <38 k units/L.
10. **CA19-9:** Cancer antigen 19-9 (CA 19-9) is a protein that exists on the surface of certain cancer cells. It is shed by the tumor cells. Small amounts of CA 19-9 are present in the blood of healthy people. False elevated levels are seen in pancreatitis, ulcerative colitis and inflammatory bowel disease.
    - *Cancer types:* Pancreatic cancer, gallbladder cancer, bile duct cancer, and gastric cancer.
    - *Tissue analyzed:* Blood.
    - *How used:* To assess whether treatment is working.
    - *Normal value:* < 37 U/mL is normal and > 120 U/mL is generally caused by tumor.
11. **CA-125:** Cancer antigen 125 is a substance that may be found in high amounts in the blood of patients with certain types of cancer, including ovarian cancer. False elevation is seen in pregnancy, menstruation, endometriosis, ovarian cysts and fibroids.
    - *Cancer type:* Ovarian cancer.
    - *Tissue analyzed:* Blood.
    - *How used:* To help in diagnosis, assessment of response to treatment, and evaluation of recurrence.
    - *Normal value:* 0–35 U/mL.
12. **Calcitonin:** It is a hormone formed by the C cells of the thyroid gland. It helps maintain a healthy level of calcium in the blood. When the calcium level is too high, calcitonin lowers it. False elevation is found in chronic renal insufficiency.
    Cancer type: Medullary thyroid cancer.
    Tissue analyzed: Blood.
    How used: To aid in diagnosis, check whether treatment is working and assess recurrence.
    Normal value: <8.5 pg/mL for men and < 5.0 pg/mL for women.
13. **Carcinoembryonic antigen (CEA):** It is a substance that may be found in the blood of people who have colon cancer, other types of cancer or diseases, or who smoke tobacco. Carcinoembryonic antigen levels may help keep track of how well cancer treatments are working or if cancer has come back. It is a type of tumor marker. False elevation is found in cigarette smoking, pancreatitis, hepatitis and inflammatory bowel disease

- *Cancer types*: Colorectal cancer and some other cancers.
- *Tissue analyzed:* Blood.
- *How used:* To keep track of how well cancer treatments are working or check if cancer has come back.
- *Normal value:* <2.5 ng/mL in non-smokers <5 ng/mL in smokers; generally, > 100 signifies metastatic cancer.

14. **CD20:** It is a protein found on B cells (a type of white blood cell). It may be found in higher than normal amounts in patients with certain types of B-cell lymphomas and leukemias. Measuring the amount of CD20 on blood cells may help to diagnose cancer or plan cancer treatment.
    - *Cancer type:* Non-Hodgkin lymphoma.
    - *Tissue analyzed:* Blood.
    - *How used:* To determine whether treatment with a targeted therapy is appropriate.

15. **Chromogranin A (CgA):** It is a protein found inside neuroendocrine cells, which release chromogranin A and certain hormones into the blood. Chromogranin A may be found in higher than normal amounts in patients with certain tumor. False elevation is found in proton-pump inhibitors (medications given to reduce stomach acid).
    - *Cancer type:* Neuroendocrine tumors, small cell lung cancer, prostate cancer.
    - *Tissue analyzed:* Blood.
    - *How used:* To help in diagnosis, assessment of treatment response, and evaluation of recurrence.
    - Normal varies on how tested, but typically < 39 ng/L is normal.

16. Chromosomes 3, 7, 17, and 9p21:
    - *Cancer type:* Bladder cancer.
    - *Tissue analyzed:* Urine.
    - *How used:* To help in monitoring for tumor recurrence.

17. Circulating tumor cells of epithelial origin
    - *Cancer types:* Metastatic breast, prostate, and colorectal cancers
    - *Tissue analyzed:* Blood
    - *How used:* To inform clinical decision making, and to assess prognosis

18. **Cytokeratin fragment 21-1:** It is a type of protein found on epithelial cells, which line the inside and outside surfaces of the body.

Cytokeratins help form the tissues of the hair, nails, and the outer layer of the skin. They are also found on cells in the lining of organs, glands, and other parts of the body. Certain cytokeratins may be found in higher than normal amounts in patients with different types of epithelial cell cancers. False elevation is found in other lung disease.
- *Cancer type:* Lung cancer, breast, colorectal, bladder, and head and neck cancers.
- *Tissue analyzed:* Blood.
- *How used:* To help in monitoring for recurrence.
- *Normal value:* 0.05–2.90 ng/mL.

19. **EGFR gene mutation analysis:** It is the protein found on the surface of some cells and to which epidermal growth factor binds, causing the cells to divide. It is found at abnormally high levels on the surface of many types of cancer cells, so these cells may divide excessively in the presence of epidermal growth factor. It is also called epidermal growth factor receptor, ErbB1, and HER1.
    - *Cancer type:* Non-small cell lung cancer.
    - *Tissue analyzed:* Tumor.
    - *How used:* To help determine treatment and prognosis.

20. **Estrogen receptor (ER)/progesterone receptor (PR):** These are hormones found inside the cells of the female reproductive tissue, some other types of tissue, and some cancer cells. The hormone estrogen will bind to the receptors inside the cells and may cause the cells to grow.
    - *Cancer type*: Breast cancer.
    - *Tissue analyzed:* Tumor.
    - *How used:* To determine whether treatment with hormone therapy and some targeted therapies is appropriate.

21. **Fibrin/fibrinogen:** These are proteins found in blood.
    - *Cancer type:* Bladder cancer.
    - *Tissue analyzed:* Urine.
    - *How used:* To monitor progression and response to treatment

22. **HE4:** It is a protein found on cells that line the lungs and reproductive organs, such as the ovaries. HE4 may be found in higher than normal amounts in patients with some types of cancer, including ovarian epithelial cancer.
    - *Cancer type:* Ovarian cancer.
    - *Tissue analyzed:* Blood.

- *How used:* To plan cancer treatment, assess disease progression, and monitor for recurrence.
23. **HER2/neu gene amplification or protein overexpression:** It is a protein involved in normal cell growth. It is found on some types of cancer cells, including breast and ovary. Cancer cells removed from the body may be tested for the presence of HER2/neu to help decide the best type of treatment. HER2/neu is a type of receptor tyrosine kinase. It is also called c-erbB-2, human EGF receptor 2, and human epidermal growth factor receptor 2.
    - *Cancer types*: Breast cancer, gastric cancer, and gastroesophageal junction, adenocarcinoma.
    - *Tissue analyzed*: Tumor.
    - *How used:* To determine whether treatment with certain targeted therapies is appropriate.
24. Immunoglobulins:
    - *Cancer types*: Multiple myeloma and Waldenström macroglobulinemia (lymphoplasmacytic lymphoma).
    - *Tissue analyzed:* Blood and urine.
    - *How used:* To help diagnose disease, assess response to treatment, and look for recurrence.
25. ***KRAS*** gene mutation analysis:
    - *Cancer types:* Colorectal cancer and non-small cell lung cancer.
    - *Tissue analyzed:* Tumor.
    - *How used:* To determine whether treatment with a particular type of targeted therapy is appropriate.
26. **Lactate dehydrogenase:** This is one of a group of enzymes found in the blood and other body tissues and involved in energy production in cells. An increased amount of lactate dehydrogenase in the blood may be a sign of tissue damage and some types of cancer or other diseases. False elevated levels are seen in Hepatitis, MI (heart attack), stroke and anemia (pernicious and thalassemia).
    - *Cancer types:* Germ cell tumors, lymphoma, leukemia, melanoma, and neuroblastoma.
    - *Tissue analyzed:* Blood.
    - *How used:* To assess stage, prognosis, and response to treatment.
    - Normal values are 100–333 µg/L.

27. **Neuron-specific enolase (NSE):** False elevated levels are seen in proton pump inhibitor treatment, hemolytic anemia and hepatic failure.
    - *Cancer types:* Small cell lung cancer and neuroblastoma.
    - *Tissue analyzed:* Blood.
    - *How used:* To help in diagnosis and to assess response to treatment.
    - Normal < 9 µg/L.
28. **Nuclear matrix protein 22:** False elevated levels are seen in benign prostatic hypertrophy (BPH) and prostatitis.
    - *Cancer type:* Bladder cancer.
    - *Tissue analyzed:* Urine.
    - *How used:* To monitor response to treatment.
    - Normal < 10 U/mL.
29. Programmed death ligand 1 (PD-L1):
    - *Cancer type:* Non-small cell lung cancer
    - *Tissue analyzed:* Tumor.
    - *How used:* To determine whether treatment with a particular type of targeted therapy is appropriate.
30. **Prostate-specific antigen (PSA):** This is a protein made by the prostate gland and found in the blood. Prostate-specific antigen blood levels may be higher than normal in men who have prostate cancer, benign prostatic hyperplasia, or infection or inflammation of the prostate gland. False elevated levels are seen in BPH, nodular prostatic hyperplasia and prostatitis.
    - *Cancer type:* Prostate cancer.
    - *Tissue analyzed:* Blood.
    - *How used:* To help in diagnosis, assess response to treatment, and look for recurrence.
    - Normal < 4 ng/mL (half-life 2–3 days)
31. **Thyroglobulin:** It is the form that thyroid hormone takes when stored in the cells of the thyroid. If the thyroid has been removed, thyroglobulin should not show up on a blood test. Doctors measure thyroglobulin level in blood to detect thyroid cancer cells that remain in the body after treatment.
    - *Cancer type:* Thyroid cancer.
    - *Tissue analyzed:* Blood.
    - *How used:* To evaluate response to treatment and look for recurrence.

32. **Urokinase plasminogen activator (uPA) and plasminogen activator inhibitor (PAI-1):** These enzymes are produced in the kidney and found in urine. A form of this enzyme is made in the laboratory and used to dissolve blood clots or to prevent them from forming.
    - *Cancer type*: Breast cancer.
    - *Tissue analyzed:* Tumor.
    - *How used:* To determine aggressiveness of cancer and guide treatment.
33. **5-Protein signature (OVA1):**
    - *Cancer type:* Ovarian cancer.
    - *Tissue analyzed:* Blood.
    - *How used:* To preoperatively assess pelvic mass for suspected ovarian cancer.
34. **21-Gene signature (Oncotype DX):**
    - *Cancer type:* Breast cancer.
    - *Tissue analyzed:* Tumor.
    - *How used:* To evaluate risk of recurrence.
35. **70-Gene signature (MammaPrint):**
    - *Cancer type:* Breast cancer.
    - *Tissue analyzed:* Tumor.

■ TESTING OF TUMOR MARKERS

Testing of tumor markers is performed by a variety of method which includes:

Serology	*Enzyme assays*
Immunological	Immunohistochemistry
	Radioimmunoassay
	Enzyme-linked immunosorbent assay
Flow cytometry	
Cytogenetic analysis	Fluorescent in-situ hybridization
	Spectral karyotyping
	Comparative genomic hybridization
Genetic analysis	Sequencing (automated)
	Reverse transcription

Contd...

Contd...

Serology	Enzyme assays
	Gel electrophoresis
	DNA microarray analysis
Proteomics	Surface-enhanced laser desorption/ionization

Immunological detection usually relies on monoclonal antibodies that specifically bind to epitopes on tumor markers and are in turn tagged for identification with dyes in immunohistochemistry (IHC), radioactive tags in radioimmunoassay (RIA), or enzymes in enzyme-linked immunosorbent assay (ELISA). Alternatively, in a suspension, flow cytometry can analyze the presence and percentage of antibody-tagged cells. These methods are highly sensitive and can detect quantities in the nanogram to picogram range (10^{-6} to 10^{-9} g). Of these, the most commonly used technique today is IHC. Uses of IHC in oncology include categorization of undifferentiated malignant tumors, categorization of leukemias and lymphomas, determination of site of origin of metastatic tumors and detection of molecules of prognostic or therapeutic significance (e.g., estrogen/progesterone receptors (ER/PR) in breast cancer).

Meanwhile, the emergence of nanotechnology is opening new horizons for highly sensitive detection of tumor markers. Due to their excellent properties, many kinds of nanomaterials have been employed in colorimetric assays for detecting tumor markers.

Tumor markers are intended primarily for monitoring patients with cancer, i.e., the test is usually indicated by the oncologist. The dynamics of change is important. First, the individual level should be determined, i.e., the concentration in the stabilized condition following surgery, i.e., removal the tumor mass. The next step is repeated follow-up monitoring, frequent at the beginning, and later at intervals of about 3–6 months. A rise in three consecutive samples and a rise in the marker by more than 25% are considered significant. Such increased marker level, although in the reference range, may provide an earlier warning of relapse than imaging methods, and suggests the indication of additional diagnostic and therapeutic procedures. Several markers should be monitored at the same time because this increases the chance that a relapse is detected (usually the two markers most suitable for the region are chosen).

■ LIMITATIONS OF TUMOR MARKERS

Ideally, markers could be used as a screening tool for the general public. The goal of a screening test is to diagnose cancer early, when it is the most treatable and before it has had a chance to grow and spread. For a screening test to be useful, it should have very high sensitivity (ability to correctly identify people who have the disease) and specificity (ability to correctly identify people who do not have the disease). But no tumor marker identified to date is sufficiently sensitive or specific to be used on its own to screen for cancer. Other tests are usually needed to learn more about a possible cancer or recurrence. Some of the limitations of tumor markers are listed here.

- A condition or disease other than cancer can elevate tumor marker levels.
- Some tumor marker levels may be high in people without cancer (benign conditions).
- Tumor marker levels may vary over time, making it hard to get consistent results.
- The level of a tumor marker may not rise until a person's cancer worsens. This is not helpful for early detection, screening, or watching for recurrence.
- Some cancers do not make tumor markers that are found in the blood. This includes cancers with no known tumor markers. Also, some patients do not have higher tumor marker levels even if the type of cancer they have usually makes tumor markers.

A positive finding of tumor markers has a diagnostic value; a negative finding does not necessarily mean the absence of cancer. Thus we can conclude that, tumor markers can be very helpful in following response to treatment and recurrence, but they cannot replace physical examination, evaluation of symptoms, and radiologic studies (CT scan, MRI, PET, etc.). Histopathological examination complemented by tumor marker demonstration is always decisive for the diagnosis. An increase in a tumor marker does not always necessarily mean cancer, it may be caused by inflammation, benign lesion, trauma, use of effective therapy or liver or kidney injury in the case of markers eliminated by these organs.

SUMMARY

- Tumor markers are substances that are produced by cancer or by other cells of the body in response to cancer or certain benign (noncancerous) conditions.
- Tumor markers are enzymes, tissue receptors, antigens, oncogenes, or hormones.
- Tumor markers are used to screen, diagnose, prognosis, to guide choice of treatment and to monitor success of treatment.
- ALK gene rearrangements and overexpression is useful in nonsmall cell lung cancer and anaplastic large cell lymphoma.
- Alpha-fetoprotein (AFP) is useful in liver cancer and germ cell tumors.
- Beta-2-microglobulin (B2M) is useful in multiple myeloma, chronic lymphocytic leukemia, and some lymphomas.
- Beta-human chorionic gonadotropin (beta-hCG) is useful in choriocarcinoma and germ cell tumors.
- *BRCA1* and *BRCA2* gene mutations are useful in ovarian and breast cancers.
- BCR-ABL fusion gene (Philadelphia chromosome) is useful in chronic myeloid leukemia, acute lymphoblastic leukemia, and acute myelogenous leukemia
- BRAF V600 mutations are useful in cutaneous melanoma, Erdheim–Chester disease, colorectal cancer, and nonsmall cell lung cancer.
- C-kit/CD117 is useful in gastrointestinal stromal tumor, mucosal melanoma, acute myeloid and leukemia
- CA15-3/CA27.29 is useful in breast cancer.
- CA19-9 is useful in pancreatic, gallbladder, bile duct, and gastric cancers.
- CA-125 is useful in ovarian cancer.
- Calcitonin is useful in medullary thyroid cancer.
- Carcinoembryonic antigen (CEA) is useful in colorectal cancer and some other cancers.
- CD20 is useful in non-Hodgkin lymphoma.
- Chromogranin A (CgA) is useful in neuroendocrine tumors.
- Chromosomes 3, 7, 17, and 9p21 are useful in bladder cancer.
- Cytokeratin fragment 21-1 is useful in lung cancer.
- *EGFR* gene mutation is useful in non-small cell lung cancer.
- Estrogen receptor (ER)/progesterone receptor (PR) is useful in breast cancer.
- Fibrin and fibrinogen are useful in bladder cancer.
- HE4 is useful in ovarian cancer.
- *HER2/neu* gene amplification or protein overexpression is useful in breast, ovarian, bladder, pancreatic, and stomach cancers.
- Immunoglobulins are useful in multiple myeloma and Waldenström macroglobulinemia.

- *KRAS* gene mutation is useful in colorectal cancer and non-small cell lung cancer.
- Lactate dehydrogenase is useful in germ cell tumors, lymphoma, leukemia, melanoma, and neuroblastoma.
- Nuclear matrix protein 22 is useful in bladder cancer. Programmed death ligand 1 (PD-L1) is useful in non-small cell lung cancer, liver cancer, stomach cancer.
- Prostate-specific antigen (PSA) is useful in prostate cancer.
- Thyroglobulin is useful in thyroid cancer.
- Urokinase plasminogen activator (uPA) and plasminogen activator inhibitor (PAI-1) is useful in breast cancer.
- 70-gene signature (MammaPrint) is useful in breast cancer.
- There are different serological as well as enzymatic assays to detect tumor markers such as ELISA, RIA, genetic analysis and flow cytometry.
- Tumor markers can be very helpful in following response to treatment and recurrence, but they cannot replace physical examination, evaluation of symptoms, and radiologic studies.

PRACTICE QUESTIONS

1. Define tumor markers.
2. Explain the types of tumor markers with example.
3. Discuss the use of tumor markers.
4. Enlist all the tumor markers, their biochemical structure and use.
5. Discuss the different methods to test tumor marker.
6. What are the limitations of tumor markers?

CHAPTER 30

Therapeutic Drug Monitoring

Keywords
Therapeutic range, therapeutic index, half-lives antibiotics, bronchodilatants, antiepileptics, cytostatics, psychoactive ELISA, pharmacokinetics, pharmacodynamics

■ INTRODUCTION

Therapeutic drug monitoring (TDM) is a branch of clinical chemistry and clinical pharmacology that specializes in the measurement of medication levels in blood. Its main focus is on drugs with a narrow therapeutic range, i.e., drugs that can easily be under- or overdosed.

Generally, a person must be given a drug dose at regular intervals to ensure that the effective or the therapeutic concentration of the drug is maintained in the body. For some drugs, maintaining this steady state is not as simple as giving a standard dose of medication. Each person will absorb, metabolize, utilize and eliminate drugs at different rates based upon their age, general state of health and genetic makeup. The determining factor of pharmacological action is drug concentration at the site of action. The aim is to create an objective basis for rational drug dosing and also for individual treatment, taking the individual differences of patients into account. Making an effort to adjust doses to individual needs is very important in ensuring effective treatment and reducing the rate of adverse drug effects.

The drug concentration in the body may be enhanced or decreased by the interference of other medications that a patient may be taking along with the drug which has to be monitored. This is also known as drug-drug interaction.

Therapeutic drug monitoring is the measurement of specific drugs and/or their breakdown products (metabolites) at timed intervals to maintain a relatively constant concentration of the medication in the blood. Some of the monitored drugs tend to have a narrow "therapeutic index," which is a ratio between the toxic and therapeutic (effective) dose of medication.

As soon as a drug enters the body, different processes start removing the drug from the body. The amount of time it takes for the body to reduce the drug concentration to half from the initial value is called a half-life of the drug. It generally takes around five half-lives to remove a drug completely from the body. The concentration of drugs, the level of which changes quickly (drugs with a short elimination half-life), is determined.

INDICATIONS FOR DRUG LEVEL DETERMINATION

The following properties are drug characteristics suitable for monitoring:
- Narrow therapeutic width
- Risk of toxicity
- High interindividual variability
- Steep dependence between the dose and the effect
- Concentration-effect relationship is closer than the dose-effect relationship
- Nonlinear pharmacokinetics TDM is beneficial for the patient in the following cases:
  - Elimination of patient non-compliance (failure of drug therapy)
  - Changes during physiological conditions (pregnancy, childhood, old age)
  - Changes during pathological conditions (fever, renal, hepatic or cardiac failure)
  - Drug interactions.

DRUGS FOR THERAPEUTIC DRUG MONITORING

Therapeutic drug monitoring is currently used for the following groups of drugs:
- **Antibiotics:** Aminoglycosides (gentamicin, amikacin), vancomycin.
- **Bronchodilatants:** Theophylline, caffeine.

- **Antiepileptics:** Phenobarbital, primidone, phenytoin, ethosuximide, carbamazepine, valproic acid, clonazepam, lamotrigine, topiramate, levetiracetam.
- **Cytostatics/anticancer:** Methotrexate, busulfan.
- **Cardiac:** Amiodarone, digoxin.
- **Immunosuppressive drugs:** Cyclosporine A, tacrolimus, sirolimus, everolimus, mycophenolate.
- **Psychoactive drugs:** Lithium, diazepam, antidepressants, antipsychotics.

In certain cases, it is advisable to determine the basic metabolite of the parent active substance:
- **Carbamazepine:** 10,11 epoxycarbamazepine.
- **Primidone:** Phenobarbital.
- **Amiodarone:** Desethylamiodarone.
- **Diazepam:** Desmethyldiazepam.
- **Metoprolol:** Hydroxy metoprolol.

INFORMATION REQUIRED FOR THERAPEUTIC DRUG MONITORING

Detailed information about drug, patient and medical history is needed before going for TDM.

The route of administering the drug is important—maximum concentration in the blood following IV application is reached within 30 minutes, following IM application in an hour. Following oral administration even after a longer time depending on the pharmaceutical form of the drug administered (tablets, capsules, matrix tablets, film-coated tablets with extended release, etc.). The entire dose is absorbed after IV application, while different portions are absorbed after oral administration, and depend on the type of the drug, galenical form of the drug and condition of the GIT.

Correct interpretation in terms of the concentration of the drug thus requires filling in a lot of information on the request for laboratory analysis.

Information about the drug type and form:
- Dose history, current dose, compliance, length of therapy
- Patient's condition (age, weight, height, organ functions)
- Time of administering the dose and time of blood sampling

- Type of biological material (blood, plasma, serum)
- Medication history (concurrently administered drugs)

■ COLLECTION OF SAMPLE

The timing of the collection of the sample is important as the drug concentration changes during the dosing interval. The least variable point in the dosing interval is just before the next dose is due. This predose or trough concentration is what is usually measured. For drugs with long half-lives such as phenobarbitone and amiodarone, samples can be collected at any point in the dosage interval.

Correct sample timing should also take into account absorption and distribution. For example, digoxin monitoring should not be performed within 6 hours of a dose, because it will still be undergoing distribution and so plasma concentrations will be erroneously high.

Blood Testing

Blood testing methods, normally involves an initial screen test using enzyme-linked immunosorbent assay (ELISA) technology, which combines the specificity of antibodies with the sensitivity of simple enzyme assays by coupling antibodies or antigens to an easily-assayed enzyme. This makes it possible to measure extremely low levels of drugs in solutions as whole blood, serum, urine, and tissues. ELISA results are confirmed and quantified through gas chromatography/mass spectrometry (GC/MS), regarded as the "gold standard" in drug testing for its unique combination of chromatography for separation of drugs and mass spectrometry for identification and quantization.

The biggest advantage to testing blood is its slim margin for error. It cannot be adulterated, in addition, the drug levels found in a person's blood sample directly correlate to the dosage currently present in his or her system. Therefore, the quantization level found on the report can be used to accurately calculate the amount of the drug.

However, the window of detection is short; it takes only a few hours for a drug to filter through the blood, which can cause a false negative result. This type of testing is also time-consuming and intrusive. For these reasons that urine drug testing is the method of choice most preferred by physicians.

Urine Testing

Method of testing is same, using immunoassay or ELISA, and then quantified through GC/MS. It commonly screens for eleven different substances, including alcohol, amphetamines, barbiturates, benzodiazepines, cannabinoids, cocaine, fentanyl, methadone, opiates, phencyclidine, and propoxyphene. The sample's creatinine level is also checked to determine if any adulteration has taken place. In the case of a positive barbiturate, benzodiazepine, or opiate, it will also list the specific substance present.

A urine test can detect if a drug is present, but cannot determine the quantity of it. There is also a higher risk of manipulation. The dilution and concentrations factors associated with the consumption of fluid can cause drug concentrations in urine to exhibit an additional tenfold variation. However, the test's popularity suggests that its benefits far outweigh the shortcomings.

■ PHARMACOKINETIC ANALYSIS

Pharmacokinetics is the study of the fate of drugs in the body including drug absorption, distribution, biotransformation (metabolism) and elimination. These processes can be described by mathematical methods and a pharmacokinetic analysis can be used to determine the pharmacokinetic parameters. Pharmacokinetic information acquired when registering the drug registration and further information gained at subsequent stages of clinical testing form the basis to understand the parameters of the population pharmacokinetic curve for the relevant drug and its pharmaceutical form. It is possible to compare this information to even just one measured drug concentration for the examined patient. Together with the drug type, the measured drug concentration, dose, time of administration, and time of biological sample collection, patient's weight and age and other data are entered onto a special computer program, which evaluates whether the measured concentration complies with the average population pharmacokinetics.

In case if unexpected concentrations are found, it is necessary to consider whether the wrong dose has been taken, drugs have interacted with one another, the drug has been used inappropriately, whether absorption disorders are present, collection took place at the wrong time, kidney and liver disease are present, there has been a change in the strength of the bond to serum proteins or the possibility of patient non-compliance (use of a higher or lower dose).

Pharmacodynamics describes the intensity of a drug effect in relation to its concentration in a body fluid, usually at the site of drug action.

■ TARGET DRUG CONCENTRATION RANGE

If the measured values do not range within certain therapeutic limits and there is no doubt that all the entered data is correct, then there should be a change of dose to be simulated or for the dosing interval to comply with requirements for optimum method of treatment. The drug concentration should be within the target range. The concept of the target drug concentration range (replaces the older term "therapeutic range") is based on two concepts: (1) the minimum effective concentration and (2) maximum safe concentration for the relevant medicine. Values between these concentrations represent the maximum therapeutic effect and at the same time a minimum risk of toxicity and side effects for most patients.

The target range has to be always connected with, not replaced by, a clinical assessment of the patient's condition. The objective is not to reach the "target range" but to treat patient's health problems.

Advanced Therapeutic Drug Monitoring

Further development in this area leads to advanced therapeutic drug monitoring (ADTM), which introduces the determination of free (pharmacologically effective) drug fraction, metabolites of the drug, determination of drug concentration in target tissues (e.g., immunosuppressive drugs in lymphocytes), and each patient is tested while taking into account genetic and phenotype predispositions for the metabolism of each drug group.

SUMMARY

- Therapeutic drug monitoring is the measurement of specific drugs and/or their breakdown products (metabolites) at timed intervals to maintain a relatively constant concentration of the medication in the blood.

- TDM is performed for the drugs with narrow therapeutic width, or failure of drug therapy.
- There are different categories of drugs used for TDM, such as antibiotics bronchodilatants, antiepileptics, cytostatics, psychoactive drugs.
- Lots of information such as dose history, current dose, compliance, length of therapy is needed for correct interpretation.
- Time of sample collection is important. Generally, it is just before the next dose is due.
- Blood or urine samples are tested by ELISA and then GC/MS.
- Pharmacokinetics is the study of the fate of drugs in the body including drug absorption, distribution, biotransformation (metabolism) and elimination.
- Pharmacodynamics describes the intensity of a drug effect in relation to its concentration in a body fluid, usually at the site of drug action.
- The drug concentration should be within the target range, which is the minimum effective concentration and maximum safe concentration for the relevant medicine.
- Advanced therapeutic drug monitoring introduces the determination of free (pharmacologically effective) drug fraction, metabolites of the drug, determination of drug concentration in target tissues.

PRACTICE QUESTIONS

1. Define therapeutic drug monitoring.
2. In which case therapeutic drug monitoring is needed?
3. What are the characteristics of drugs for which TDM is done?
4. Name different categories of drugs with example for which TDM is used?
5. What are different information required before going for TDM?
6. While collecting samples for TDM what are the points to be taken care of?
7. Why it is said that urine testing for TDM is beneficial over blood testing?
8. Define pharmacokinetics and pharmacodynamics.
9. If unexpected concentrations of drugs are found in the sample what are the other possibilities to be ruled out before entering the drug dose? Define therapeutic range.
10. What is advanced therapeutic drug monitoring?

Automation in Clinical Biochemistry

CHAPTER 31

> **Keywords**
> Signal processing, data handling, quality control, continuous flow analyzers, centrifugal analyzer, discrete analyzers, batch analyzers, Stat analyzers, dry chemical analyzers, dispensing system, Technicon autoanalyzer, Hitachi 917, Cobas Mira, VITROS DT60 II, BioMeriex VIDAS, ELISA reader, total laboratory automation (TLA), biosensors, nanotechnology

■ INTRODUCTION

During the past few years, in Clinical Biochemistry there has been a considerable increase in clinical demand for laboratory investigations. When the volume of work increased, there arose a need for work simplification. Monostep methods are introduced to replace multistep cumbersome and inaccurate methods such as Folin-Wu's blood sugar determination. The efficiency of monostep methods was further increased by the introduction of automatic dispensers and diluters. For the common test such as blood glucose, blood urea, etc., however, most large laboratories found this approach still inadequate to deal with workload and instruments designed to handle the whole analytical process in mechanized fashion have become common place in last decade. This procedure is called *automation*.

Automation refers to machines with intelligence and adaptability which reduces our workload and need for nonstop supervision. It is a self-regulating process, where the specimen is accurately pipetted by a mechanical probe and mixed with a particular volume of the reagent and results are displayed in digital forms and also printed by a printer. There is an element of feedback which detects any tendency to malfunction. The function of autoanalyzer in clinical biochemistry is to replace with automated devices the steps of pipetting, preparation of protein free filtrated, heating the color forming reagents in a waterbath and increase the accuracy and precision of the methods.

Advantages of automation: It has a lot of benefits for the laboratory personnel, which can be summarized as:
1. Reduces the workload.
2. Increases turnaround time (saves time used per analysis).
3. Increases total number of tests done in less time.
4. Eliminates repetition and monotony from human life so decreases human error, improves accuracy.
5. Improves reproducibility (repeatability).
6. Work economically by using smaller quantities of samples and reagents.

■ STEPS IN AUTOMATED ANALYSIS

There are several individual steps in the analysis process as a whole in a laboratory such as:
1. Sample collection
2. Identification of patient
3. Specimen measurement and delivery
4. Sample preparation
5. Reagent system and delivery
6. Chemical reaction phase
7. Measurement phase
8. Signal processing and data handling

1. **Sample collection:** Blood collection using the evacuated tube provides blood samples for analysis. Here the phlebotomist need not pull the syringe, blood gets sucked in due to negative pressure filling the vacuum. The blood goes directly from the patient's vein into the appropriate test tube. The vacuum system consists of a double-pointed needle, a tube holder, and a series of vacuum tubes with rubber stoppers of various colors. The tube stopper color indicates the type of additive present.
2. **Identification of patient:** Automation in identification of patient consists of using computer generated bar coding technology for labeling samples. It has the advantage that it can be scanned and read by bar code reader accurately so transcriptional error (mistake in writing manually) is avoided. It has all information

about patient, tests to be done, time of sample collection, and other necessary information. Bar coding of the patient, unique sample identity is attached to his/her wrist. Even when patient is sleeping or unconscious, nurse can read the code for patient identification.

3. **Specimen measurement and delivery:** Most of the laboratories rely on human pick up system or conveyer belt system. Though cheaper, it may lead to human error, delays, etc.

   Pneumatic tube systems (use of pressurized gas to move the tubes containing samples) are used in some laboratories. However, care has to be taken that acceleration and deceleration should not damage any sample. In very advanced laboratory mobile robots are used.

4. **Sample preparation:** Most of the laboratories depend on technicians for sample processing (such as serum separation) as soon as sample arrives. However introduction of automation can reduce the workload on technicians and save their time and expertise for analysis purpose. Therefore, nowadays many semiautomated devices are developed which can analyze whole blood itself. For example, automated ion selective electrode, use of dry chemistry, etc.

   These automated sample processors can do the following tasks: sorting of samples, removing caps, separating samples, bar coding, etc., having an automated sample processor solves the task of bar coding and sample delivery via conveyer belt system.

5. **Reagent system and delivery:** Reagents could be dry or liquid. Dry reagents could arrive as lyophilized powder or in a tablet form (some instruments have a tablet crusher on board). Delivery of reagents is analyzer type dependent (refer to the Types of Analyzers for more details later).

6. **Chemical reaction phase:** This phase mainly consists of mixing, separation, incubation, and reaction time.

7. **Measurement phase:** Ultraviolet (UV) light, fluorescent, flame photometry, ion-selective electrodes (ISE), gamma counters and luminometers are various methods for measuring product formed. Most common methods are still visible and UV spectrophotometer. Analyzers that measure light need monochromators to produce specific wavelength, classically filter wheels have been used to separate light, which are usually computer controlled.

Electrochemical techniques are the latest one:
- *Direct potentiometry:* The use of ISEs is widespread and mainly used for assaying ions in samples. This method is used to measure ions such as Na^+, K^+, Cl^- and Li^+. ISEs are sensors capable of determining the concentration of ions in a solution by measuring the current flow through an ion-selective membrane.
- *Indirect potentiometry:* This method also uses ISEs. It allows high throughput and is most commonly used in centralized laboratories. It requires prior dilution, unlike direct potentiometry, and the results are expressed in molarity.

A biochemistry analyzer can offer several measurement principles.

8. **Signal processing and data handling:** Accurate calibration is essential to obtain reliable results. This requires proper use of standards, which then reflect the data on standard curve according to which the sample results are interpreted. After the calibration has been performed and the chemical or electrical analysis of the specimen is either in progress or completed, the instruments computer goes into data acquisition and calculation mode. This process may involve signal averaging which may involve hundreds of data pulses per second.

Points to consider while buying analyzer:
There is hundreds of variety of analyzers available in market and so are types of laboratories. Each laboratory can have different requirements to meet. To find an analyzer perfectly suitable for respective laboratory, following points are to be considered:
- What is the maintenance cost?
- What does the software do?
- How will it interact with the lab's laboratory information system (LIS)?
- What quality control (QC) package is included?
- How easy is the QC to review for technicians?
- What is the full test menu?
- What is in development?
- Will this instrument meet a lab's needs for the next 5 years?
- Does a lab still need an analyzer to cover one or two very important tests?

■ CLASSIFICATION OF ANALYZERS

- According to the number of simultaneously measurable items, it is divided into—single channel and multichannel.
- According to the degree of automation of the instrument, it is divided into—fully automated and semiautomatic biochemical analyzers.
- According to the function and complexity of the instrument, it is divided into—small, medium, large and super large automatic biochemical analyzers.
- According to the structure of the instrument reaction device, it is divided into—continuous flow type, discrete type, centrifugal type and dry chemical type.

Following are the different types of autoanalyzers used in clinical chemistry laboratories.

1. **Continuous flow analyzers:** The early form of automation was introduced by Technicon Instrument Corporation. It was based on continuous flow analysis. Liquids (reagents, diluents and samples) are pumped through a system of continuous tubing. Samples are introduced in a sequential manner, following each other through the same network. Series of air bubbles at regular intervals serve as separating and media. The internal diameter of the tubing and the rate of flow determine the volumes of sample prior to mixing with the reagents and the turnaround time of the result. An oil heating bath is used to promote color development or the completion of enzymatic reaction.

    Principle of detection: Detection is by measuring absorbance by spectrophotometer through a continuous flow cuvet (cell).

    When there is no sample, the sampler probe is placed in distilled water to avoid blockages and precipitation. More sophisticated continuous flow analyzers use parallel single channels to run multiple tests on each sample. For single channel machines, results are plotted on a chart recorder. For multichannel machines, computer and printers are used to report the results in the appropriate units.

    Uses: Major use for certain test profiles (e.g., liver function, lipid function).

    Single channel machines may be used for frequently requested independent analysis (e.g., blood glucose, blood total protein).

Disadvantages:
- The machine does not allow test selection; all tests must be performed even if not requested.
- The machine must run continuously even when there are no tests. Because of the continuous flow, reagents must be drawn at all times even when there are no tests to perform, which results in wastage of reagent. Therefore a good stock of reagents must be available to avoid system malfunction due to reagent depletion.
- The instrument must be closely monitored all the time for air bubbles uniformity; tubing integrity and most important of all carry over problems.
- Multichannel machines are usually large in size and occupy large space.

2. **Centrifugal analyzer:** Samples and reagents are added in an especially designed centrifugal type cuvet that has three main compartments. The sample and the reagent are placed in the rotor position of the centrifuge. When the centrifuge is started, the sample and the reagent in the rotor mix and react by the centrifugal force, after incubation, the reaction liquid finally flows into the colorimetric groove of the outer ring of the shaped reactor, the colorimetric result is obtained. In the analysis process, each step of mixing, reacting and detecting the sample and the reagent is completed at the same time, which belongs to "synchronous analysis".

Advantages:
- Rapid test performance by analyzing multiple samples.
- Batch analysis is a major advantage because reactions in all cuvets are read virtually simultaneously.
- Use less sample and less reagent. It can be programmed to carry out many different assay methods.

Disadvantages:
- Only one test type can be performed each time.
- Each cuvet must be uniformly matched to each other to maintain quality handling of each sample.

3. **Discrete analyzers:** Discrete analyzers have the capability to run multiple tests one sample at a time or multiple samples one test

at a time. They are the most versatile analyzers. Discrete analysis is a separation of each sample and accompanying reagents in a separate container. Each sample is treated differently according to the tests requested and programmed by the operator.

For example, sample 1 glucose, urea, creatinine and electrolytes, sample 2 total protein, albumin, calcium, sample 3 triglycerides, cholesterol, sample 4 bilirubin, ALT, AST, ALP.

These instruments are heavily dependent on electronic control. Sample is aspirated by the autosampler from the sample cup and placed in the reaction cuvet. Mixing of sample and reagents may be achieved by several methods such as:

a. Spinning of the cuvet at high speed followed by sudden stop.
b. Introducing the reagent into the cuvet by jet action.
c. Introducing air bubbles into the cuvet.

The reaction chamber temperature is controlled for color development or enzyme assay to proceed. The absorbency of the reaction in the reaction cuvet is read by a spectrophotometer, which is housed in the reaction chamber. Computer then calculates the results and produces it in printed format. Many of these machines have a QC system built in and automatically checks on the results of the QC samples to determine whether to accept or reject the results of the run. Deproteinization is not performed to save time. Kinetic rather than endpoint methodologies are used (minimize protein error and give more accurate results). Some of these machines have the ability to store or file patient results. Some can be connected to laboratory or mainframe computers.

These work on the principle that non-continuous flow using random access fluid which is a hydrofluorocarbon liquid to reduce surface tension between samples/reagents and their tubing and therefore reduce carry over.

Uses: Analytes that can be measured by reflectance photometry include glucose, BUN, ammonia, bilirubin, uric acid, cholesterol, triglycerides, total calcium, total protein, albumin, creatinine, phosphorus, and serum enzymes.

Advantages: Assay by reflectance photometry offers advantages:
- The storage requirements for reagents are minimal since no wet reagents are required.

- No pipetting steps are needed as the manufacturing company prepares the slides.
- No sample dilution is required and 10 or 11 µL of sample per test is used.

Disadvantages: Since each sample is in a separate reaction container, uniformity of quality must be maintained in each cuvet so that a particular sample quality is not affected by the cuvet it is placed in.

The various types of discrete autoanalyzers used in the clinical chemistry laboratories are—

A. Batch analyzers and
B. "Stat" (means immediate reporting or emergency determination analyzers).

A. **Batch analyzers:** These are convenient to analyze specimen in batches such as of sugar, urea creatinine, etc., state testing may not be conveniently carried out on these analyzers. The batch analyzers can be further differentiated as: (I) semiautomated and (II) fully automated.

(I) *Semiautomated (batch) discrete analyzers:* In case of these analyzers, the initial part of the procedure, i.e., pipetting of reagent and specimen, mixing and incubation is carried out by the technician. Rest of the procedure, i.e., setting of incubation temperature (for kinetic determinations), zero setting, photometric readings, result display, automatic printing and data management and processing is carried out by the analyzer.

Advantage of semiautoanalyzers:
- The semiautoanalyzers are cheap and compact, compared to other fully automated alyzers.
- Specimen analysis is cheap, since volume of reagent used is 0.5–1.0 mL.
- Enzyme determinations by kinetic methods are performed accurately in 1–3 minutes.
- The enzymatic reagents are not corrosive and involve monostep testing.

(II) **Fully automated batch analyzers:** These analyzers carry out all the function of a semiautomated analyzer, in addition to the pipetting of specimen and reagents and also the mixing

of the reaction mixtures. The basic working stages of these analyzers, after selecting general system parameters are as follows:
  a. The specimen cups are placed on the sampler.
  b. The required quantity of reagent is dispensed by a reagent probe, in the reaction cups.
  c. The respective specimens from the sampler are pipetted into the appropriate reaction cups by another sample probe.
  d. The reaction cups are shaken mechanically to mix the contents.
  e. After observing the required incubation time (for delay time in the case of kinetic determinations) the reaction mixture is aspirated by a probe for photometric readings.
  f. The resulted values are printed and displayed in appropriate units by digital display.
B. **Stat analyzers (random access analyzers):** In the case of these analyzers many reagents (8-20 or more) can be pipetted one after another, so that various biochemical determinations can be performed on one specimen, according to the number of tests ordered for the patient. Hence, these are patient (or specimen) orientated autoanalyzers.

The advantages of a fully automatic "stat" (or random access) analyzer are as follows:
- It performs a single test, a profile, an organ panel or a "stat" determination.
- It reduces the cost per test by utilization of microvolumes of a reagent.
- It performs automatic monitoring of specimen and reagent volumes.
- It can perform various methodologies such as end point, kinetic, initial rate and bichromatic (readings at two different wavelengths) to eliminate errors which may arise due to hemolytic, icteric or lipemic sera.
- The analyzer can perform repetition of tests with or without automatic dilution.

4. **Dry chemical analyzers:** Dry chemical methods utilize reagent slides that are composed of several layers which may include: 1—spreading layer; 2—scavenger layer; 3—reagent layer(s); 4—plastic or support layer.

The reagent layer(s) contains enzymes, dye precursor, and buffers necessary for the analysis of a specific component.

Sample, control, or standard is deposited on the spreading layer. Selected components are allowed to penetrate to the reaction layer(s), which in turn activate the dehydrated reagents. A chemical reaction is initiated to produce a color. Light is passed from beneath the support or plastic layer and is directed through the reagent layer(s). As the light hits the white spreading layer, some of the light reflects back through the reagent layer(s) to a photocell. The amount of reflected light, which is in proportion to color intensity, is used to determine the concentration of the analyte.

A dry chemical method is utilized to determine sodium, potassium, chloride, and carbon dioxide (electrolytes) which employs ISEs that are joined by a paper bridge.

A drop of reference sample and a drop of patient sample are deposited, each on its respective electrode. The samples interact with coated reagent layers to create a pair of electrochemical half-cells. The drops spread toward one another across the paper bridge, meeting at the center and forming a stable liquid junction. A voltmeter measures the potential difference of the two half-cells, which is then used to determine the concentration values.

Uses:
Widely used in many clinical laboratories. Many offer the ability for the operator to include his own test procedures (open system). For examples, The Hitachi group of analyzers (Hitachi 717, Hitachi 917), The Technicon RA 1000.

Advantages:
- Uses dry chemistry hence incurring minimum storage costs.
- ISE has a major advantage which allows a sample to be analyzed for electrolytes separately even when the analyzer is analyzing a batch of other samples for various other tests.

Disadvantages: Samples with abnormal high protein may introduce significant errors (sample dilution may be necessary).

■ CARE AND MAINTENANCE OF ANALYZERS

- On ending the working day, once the analyzer has been switched off, always empty the waste container.

- Never use detergents or abrasive products for cleaning the surface of the analyzer. Use only a damp cloth with water and pH-neutral soap.
- If a reagent or corrosive product spills or splashes onto the apparatus, clean it with a damp cloth and soap immediately.
- All the elements of the analyzer have drainage conduits leading to the exterior to enable the elimination of any liquid spilled and to prevent the apparatus from flooding. If the spillage is significant, the liquid spilled onto the table through the drainage conduits and the analyzer must be adequately cleaned.
- When not in use, close the main cover of the analyzer to protect it from dust.
- Time to time calibration is needed as guided by manufacturer.

Cleaning the Dispensing System

The dispensing system should be cleaned with washing solution at the start and end of each working day to ensure that it is completely free from air bubbles and is perfectly clean.

Once the wash has been performed, the analyzer asks the user to replace the container with system liquid and it automatically performs a wash and rinse of the dispensing system with system liquid. With the initial wash, the system is ready for working in optimum conditions during the entire working day, offering maximum performance. With the final wash, the analyzer cleans the needle at the end of the working day, keeping it in optimum condition for future working days. The user can also wash the dispensing system whenever he wishes by means of the Dispensing System Wash tool on the user program, while the analyzer is in standby mode. It is also appropriate to clean and check the filters of the system liquid container at least once every 3 months. If the needle is obstructed by solid residue and needs cleaning with the metal cleaning rod supplied with the analyzer, it can be disassembled for cleaning out of the analyzer. For this, disassemble dispensing needle utility on the user program must be used. It is also recommendable to periodically clean the outside surface of the needle with a piece of cotton or a soft cloth dampened with alcohol. The needle must be replaced if it noticeably deteriorates.

Cleaning the semidisposable reactions rotor: When the reactions rotor is completely full, the user must change it for one that is empty, clean and dry. The reactions rotors can be reused if they are carefully cleaned immediately after use. The procedure is as follows:
- Remove the reagents from the rotor wells and rinse abundantly with running water.
- Immerse the material in a 5% wash solution (Extrán® Merck) for 30 minutes.
- Rinse thoroughly with running water.
- Deproteinize the rotor by adding a 3% nitric acid solution for 5 minutes.
- Rinse thoroughly with distilled water.
- Immerse in distilled water for 30 minutes and allow to dry at room temperature.
- Only deproteinize the rotor when tests for ions such as magnesium, calcium, etc., are required. Organic solvents (alcohol, benzene) or alkaline solutions must not be used.
- They must be left to dry completely before being reused. High temperatures must not be used during drying.
- The rotors must be rejected if they are noticeably deteriorated.

The optical status of a rotor must be verified by means of the reactions rotor verification utility on the user program. The useful lifetime of each rotor depends drastically on its use and care.

■ ROUTINE BIOCHEMISTRY ANALYZERS

These are machines that process the bulk of the samples going into a hospital or private medical laboratory. And the results should be out as quickly as possible. There will often be a method that can get urgent specimens moved more quickly through.

The type of tests required are often enzyme levels (such as many of the liver function tests), ion levels (e.g. sodium and potassium), and other chemicals (such as albumin or creatine).

Simple ions are done with ion selective electrodes that let one type of ion through and measure voltage differences. Enzymes are measured by the rate they change one colored substance to another; the results for enzymes are given as an activity, not a concentration of enzyme. Other tests use colorimetric changes to determine the concentration.

Turbidity (as created when an antibody reacts with a test compound) can also be measured with these machines. Examples of these types of machines are:

Technicon Autoanalyzer

Autoanalyzer is an automated analyzer using a special flow technique named "continuous flow analysis" (CFA) first made by the Technicon corporation. The instrument was invented in 1957 by Leonard Skeggs and commercialized by Jack Whitehead's Technicon Corporation. The first applications were for clinical analysis, but methods for industrial analysis soon followed.

Instruments

The best known of Technicon's CFA machines are the autoanalyzer II (introduced 1970), the sequential multiple analyzer (SMA, 1969), and the sequential multiple analyzer with computer (SMAC, 1974). Bran+Luebbe continued to manufacture the autoanalyzer II and TRAACS, a micro-flow analyzer for environmental and other samples, and went on to develop the autoanalyzer 3 in 1997 and the QuAAtro in 2004.

Today, there are other manufacturers of CFA instruments. Astoria-Pacific International, for example, was founded in 1990 by Raymond Pavitt. Its products include the Astoria Analyzer lines for environmental and industrial applications; the SPOTCHECK analyzer for neonatal screening; and FASPac (flow analysis software package) for data acquisition and computer interface.

Clinical Analysis

Autoanalyzers were used mainly for routine repetitive medical laboratory analyses, but they had been replaced during the last years more and more by discrete working systems which allow lower reagent consumption. These machines typically determine levels of albumin, alkaline phosphatase, serum glutamic oxaloacetic transaminase (SGOT), blood urea nitrogen, bilirubin, calcium, cholesterol, creatinine, glucose, inorganic phosphorus, proteins and uric acid in blood serum or other bodily samples. Autoanalyzers automate repetitive sample analysis steps which would otherwise be done manually by a technician, for such medical tests as the ones mentioned previously. This way, an autoanalyzer can analyze hundreds of samples every day with one operating technician. Early autoanalyzer instruments each tested multiple samples sequentially for individual analytes. Later, model autoanalyzers such as the SMAC tested for multiple analytes simultaneously in the samples.

Operating Principle

In a continuous flow analyzer, a peristaltic pump contains several tubes including one for the sample, one or more for various reagents and one or more to generate air bubbles. The pump tubes deliver into the "manifold" of junctions, coils and tubing where the reactions take place. In segmented flow analyzers (SFA), the sample is mixed with small reproducible volumes of the required reagents and air bubbles are introduced into the flow, creating about 20–100 segments of liquid for each sample, keeping them separated as they flow sequentially through the tubing. The inlet side of the sample pump tube is connected to the sample probe in an autosampler. The sample probe moves between the small cups holding liquid samples and a reservoir of wash solution, normally pure water, which also serves to generate a baseline response. The sample/reagent mixture flows through mixing coils and depending on the method a heated coil for elevated reaction temperature or other modules to develop a color proportional to the amount of analyte in each sample. The samples with developed color flow through a colorimeter to measure the color. Other detectors such as a flame photometer, a fluorometer or an ISE module are used for some applications.

Flow injection analyzers (FIA) operate similar to SFA, but without the air segmentation. A FIA introduces sample into a flowing stream of reagents using an injection valve. The reagents and sample are mixed together while passing through tightly coiled narrow bore teflon tubing and other modules to develop a product that is measurable by a detector. Normally, the same chemistries possible by SFA are possible by FIA. SFA methods have a clear advantage at obtaining lower detection limits, and the ability to bring all chemical reactions to completion prior to measurement.

Previously a chart recorder and more recently a PC records the detector output as a function of time so that each sample output appears as a peak whose height depends on the analyte level in the sample. In medical testing applications and industrial samples with high concentrations or interfering material, there is often a dialyzer module in the instrument in which the analyte permeates through the diaphragm into a separate flow path going on to further analysis. The purpose of a dialyzer is to separate the analyte from interfering substances such as protein, whose large molecules do not go through the dialysis membrane but go to a separate waste stream. The reagents, sample and reagent volumes, flow rates, and other aspects of the instrument analysis depend on which analyte is being measured.

Hitachi 917

The *Hitachi 917* (**Fig. 31.1**) is an automated biochemistry analyzer used by medical laboratories to process biological fluid specimens, such as urine, cerebrospinal fluid, but most commonly blood.

Manufactured by Boehringer Mannheim, the Hitachi 917 is a commonly used routine chemical bichromatic analyzer. Capable of doing 1200 test/hour with ion selective electrode (ISE), it is a popular choice among small to medium size laboratories.

Appearance and Use

The 917 has two trays for racks, plus a stat rack. Racks that hold five test tubes slide in on the left side of the machine. There are two reagents

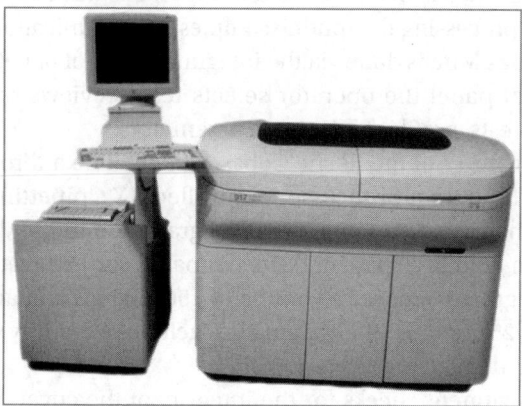

Fig. 31.1: Hitachi 917.

carousels on the right side of the 917. In the center, towards the back, are the reaction vessels, where the chemical reactions take place. ISE reagents and components are in front of the reaction carousel.

Tests Available

- Ion-selective electrode—Na, K, Cl
- Rate—CK
- End point
- Immunoturbidity

Cobas Mira

The Roche Cobas Mira is a bench top, random access biochemistry analyzer. This system allows for the selective analysis of chemistries in either a routine or STAT mode. Testing sequence is by patient rather than test (batch). The optional ISE module for sodium, potassium and chloride determinations expand the capabilities of the instrument.

The Roche Cobas Mira is ideal in the laboratory situation where patient samples arrive throughout the day and night. With random access instrumentation, these samples may be placed on the analyzer and results will be available within minutes. With random access, samples do not have to be saved for a major run as with batch analyzers. STAT samples may be placed on the instrument at any time. Once the STAT has been completed, the Cobas Mira automatically returns to processing the routine samples. Communication with the Roche Cobas Mira is done via the integrated control panel. Through the control panel the operator selects tests, reviews results and programs tests, profiles and system parameters.

Other features of the Roche Cobas Mira include a throughput of 140 tests/hour, microprocessor controlled XYZ pipetting system, 104 test channels including 23 preprogrammed methods and the capacity to hold 2100 patient results, capacity for 72 cuvettes (six 12 cuvette segments), cuvette volume of 150–600 µL and an analysis interval of 25 seconds. The system also includes a security system for laboratory-defined parameters.

The instrument checks for the integrity of the cuvette, the rack reader, temperature, the monitor and printer.

The other important examples include:
- Hitachi 912
- Abbott Aeroset
- Dade Dimension
- Beckman-Coulter LX
- Berkman Astra
- Dupont Automated Clinical Analyzer
- Kodak Ektachem 700

The VITROS DT60 II random access dry chemistry analyzer can perform a broad chemistry menu, including basic chemistries, electrolytes, enzymes, full lipid profile, and special chemistry tests. Wide ranges allow for fewer dilutions and repeats. We can obtain results in 2–5 minutes, with hard copy printout of results and patient ID. Fast throughput delivers up to 10 tests in 5 minutes, over 100 tests per hour. It facilitates quicker diagnosis so treatment can commence earlier—enhancing patient care, satisfaction, and outcomes. VITROS dry-slide technology minimizes the effects of common interferences to provide precise, accurate results while yielding cost and convenience benefits—no mixing of wet reagents, no waste, no need for special plumbing.

BioMeriex VIDAS is a fully automated immunoassay analyzer, which offers flexible and convenient operation with STAT capability, multiparametric testing, single sample testing, and batch testing (up to 100 tests/2 hour) BioMerieux VIDAS's test menu includes tumor markers, thyroid hormones, therapeutic drug monitoring, serology, infectious disease, reproductive hormones, and coagulation. The BioMerieux VIDAS instrument provides results for serology and immunochemistry assays in 20–60 minutes. At the same time, the antigen assay results can be obtained in 30–150 minutes. Also the analyzer is featured with five independent testing areas with 6 positions, LIS and barcode patient demographic interface capabilities, calibration every 14 days, automated barcode identification, single-dose and ready-to-use reagents.

ELISA Reader

ELISA reader is a strip reader used for microwell. ELISA determinations which can store 100 different parameters with their calibration curves and can perform immunoassays for proteins, enzymes, autoimmune diseases, and hormones. An ELISA reader measures and quantitates the color differences in the 12 wells of the plate. ELISA readers are based on spectrophotometry; additionally, ELISA plate readers can also measure fluorescence and luminescence. Chemical dyes fluoresce or emit one color or wavelength when exposed to light. The amount of reflection, absorption and the color identify, and measure the amount of a substance.

Advantages of ELISA Reader

Spectrophotometers require more sample per measurement. To use a spectrophotometer or ELISA plate reader, the molecule must be dissolved in solution. A spectrophotometer requires between 400 µL and 4 mL, depending on the manufacturer and model. An ELISA plate reader needs about 2–100 µL; ELISA plate readers use much less of a sample to get a result.

ELISA plate readers measure more samples in a shorter period of time. A spectrophotometer measures one to six samples at a time. Typically, an ELISA plate measures 96 wells in an equivalent amount of time.

■ TOTAL LABORATORY AUTOMATION

Rapid changes in the diagnostic sector coupled with parallel advances in technology have stimulated the evolution of approaches for total laboratory automation (TLA) and artificial intelligence (AI) and robotic elements in the routine laboratory process flow. These measures offer promise in streamlining the clinical laboratory process flow.

The implementation of AI, cloud computing, machine learning, adoption of paperless workflows is instrumental in the transformation of the laboratory, more specifically, influencing clinical validation, procedure efficiency, data handling, data analysis, and much more. AI helps in computing the risk stratification score of laboratory data and clinical data using an expert system and evidence based guidelines. Increasing cost containment pressures make the application of this technology highly approachable.

Total laboratory automation, where most analyzers performing different types of tests (i.e., clinical chemistry, immunochemistry, hematology, hemostasis and so forth) on different sample matrices (e.g., whole blood, serum, heparinized or citrated plasma) are physically integrated as modular systems or connected by assembly lines (e.g., tracks, belts and other types of conveyers). In the broader models of TLA, many preanalytical and postanalytical steps (e.g., sample input, check-in, sorting, decapping, centrifugation, separation, aliquoting, sealing and storage) are automatically performed in workstations physically connected with the analyzers and efficiently managed by software programs.

On the other hand, developing a model of TLA presents some potential problems, mainly represented by higher costs on the short-term, enhanced expenditure for supplies, space requirement, and infrastructure constraints. Advantages and limitations of TLA are summarized in **Table 31.1**.

Table 31.1: Potential advantages and limitations of TLA.

Advantages	Limitations
• Lower costs in the long-term	• Higher costs in the short-term
• Reduction of manual workforce	• Project accommodation
• Lower number of blood tubes	• Installation
• Decreased congestion	• Larger equipment
• Improved efficiency	• Increased costs for supplies
• Shorter TAT	• Maintenance
• Higher throughput	• Energy
• Enhanced complexity	• Water
• Possibility to manage different tubes types and sizes	• Tips for aliquotters and caps for sealers
• Lower need of urgent testing	• Space requirement and infrastructure constraints
• Improved sample management	• Overcrowding of personnel
• More efficient management of rerun	• Increased generation of noise, heat and vibration
• More efficient management of reflex testing	• Higher risk of downtime
• Easier add-on	• Higher risk of system failures
• Enhanced traceability	• Shortage of personnel for response to emergency situations

Contd...

Contd...

Advantages	Limitations
• Improved process standardization for certification/accreditation	• Psychological dependence on automation
• Improved quality of testing	• Differential requirements for sample management
• Enhanced standardization	• Generation of potential bottlenecks
• Lower risk of errors	• Disruption of staff trained in specific technologies
• Lower sample volume	• Risk of transition toward a manufacturer's-driven laboratory
• More efficient integration of tests results	
• Lower biological risk for operators	
• Staff requalification and job satisfaction	

■ BIOSENSORS

In recent years, the demand has grown in the field of medical diagnostics for simple and disposable devices that also demonstrate fast response times, are user-friendly, cost-efficient, and are suitable for mass production. Biosensor technologies offer the potential to fulfill these criteria through an interdisciplinary combination of approaches from nanotechnology, chemistry and medical science.

Analytical devices that consists a combination of biological detecting elements like sensor system and a transducer is termed as biosensor.

Biosensors can be defined as self-sufficient integrated devices that have capacity to provide specific qualitative or semiquantitative analytical information using a biological recognition element which is in direct-spatial contact with a transductional element.

In simple words, biosensors are analytical devices that detect changes in biological processes and transform the biological data into electrical signal.

Components of Biosensor

The biosensor consists of three segments namely, sensor, transducer, and electrical circuit.

1. **Sensor or detector:** The first segment is the sensor or detector which is a biological component. It is a biochemical receptor. It interacts with the analyte and signals the change in its composition as electrical signal.
2. **Transducer:** The second segment is the transducer and it is a physical component which amplifies the biochemical signal received from detector, alters the resulting signal into electrical and displays in an attainable way.
3. **Electrical circuit:** It is the associated part which consists of signal conditioning unit, a processor or microcontroller and a display unit.

Principles of Biosensors

- Biosensors works on the principle of signal transduction and biorecognition of element.
- All the biological materials including enzyme, antibody, nucleic acid, hormone, organelle or whole cell can be used as sensor or detector in a device. But the desired bioreceptor is usually a specific deactivated enzyme.
- The deactivated enzyme is placed in proximity to the transducer.
- The tested analyte links to the specific enzyme (bioreceptor) and inducing a change in biochemical property of enzyme. The change in turn gives an electronic response through an electroenzymatic approach.
- Electroenzymatic process is the chemical process of converting the enzymes into corresponding electrical signals with the aid of transducer.
- Now, the outcome from transducer, i.e., electrical signal is a direct representation of the biological material (i.e., analyte and enzyme in this case) being measured.

The electrical signal is usually converted into physical display for its proper analysis and representation.

Biosensors are ideally suited for caregivers or patients in non-hospital settings, and by patients at home.

■ NANOTECHNOLOGY

Biotechnology and nanotechnology are two of the 21st century's most promising technologies. Nanotechnology is defined as the design, development and application of materials and devices whose least functional make up is on a nanometer scale. Generally, nanotechnology deals with developing materials, devices, or other structures possessing at least one dimension sized from 1 to 100 nanometers. Meanwhile, biotechnology deals with metabolic and other physiological processes of biological subjects including microorganisms. Association of these two technologies, i.e., nanobiotechnology can play a vital role in developing and implementing many useful tools in the study of life.

A number of clinical applications of nanobiotechnology, such as disease diagnosis, target-specific drug delivery, and molecular imaging are being laboriously investigated at present. Some new promising products are also undergoing clinical trials. Such advanced applications of this approach to biological systems will undoubtedly transform the foundations of diagnosis, treatment, and prevention of disease in future. Diagnostic applications are discussed here.

Current diagnostic methods for most diseases depend on the manifestation of visible symptoms before medical professionals can recognize that the patient suffers from a specific illness. But by the time those symptoms have appeared, treatment may have a decreased chance of being effective. Therefore, the earlier a disease can be detected, the better the chance for a cure is. Optimally, diseases should be diagnosed and cured before symptoms even manifest themselves. Nucleic acid diagnostics will play a crucial role in that process, as they allow the detection of pathogens and diseases/diseased cells at such an early symptomless stage of disease progression that effective treatment is more feasible. Current technology, such as polymerase chain reaction (PCR) leads toward such tests and devices, but nanotechnology is expanding the options currently available, which will result in greater sensitivity and far better efficiency and economy.

Future Trends in Automation

Automation and technology will continue to evolve, and laboratories need to position themselves for such changes as demand for pathology services and consumer expectations will continue to rise.

System integration and miniaturization with more technologically advanced computer power will persist to accommodate more portable analyzers for more precise testing. Automated analyzers will have AI where by the computer will "think" or make decisions if sufficiently programmed with infinite scenarios of data. Spectral mapping or multiple wavelength monitoring, with high-resolution photometers and polychromators will become standard.

SUMMARY

- Automation refers to machines with intelligence and adaptability which reduces our workload and need for nonstop supervision.
- Analyzers save time and reduce cost as well.
- The steps in analysis process as a whole in a laboratory are—sample collection, identification of patient, specimen measurement and delivery, sample preparation, reagent system and delivery, chemical reaction phase, measurement phase and signal processing and data handling.
- To find out most suitable analyzer as per one's need, the points to consider are—cost, quality control, menu, software, and dimensions.
- Analyzers are classified on the basis of measurable items, degree of automation, complexity of instrument and instrument reaction.
- In continuous flow analyzers, detection is by measuring absorbency by spectrophotometer through a continuous flow cuvet.
- In centrifugal analyzer, the sample and the reagent in the rotor mix and react by the centrifugal force, after incubation, the reaction liquid finally flows into the colorimetric groove.
- Discrete analyzers have the capability to run multiple tests one sample at a time or multiple samples one test at a time. It works on the principle that non-continuous flow using random access fluid which is a hydrofluorocarbon liquid to reduce surface tension between samples/reagents and their tubing.
- Batch analyzers are convenient to analyze specimen in batches such as of sugar, urea creatinine, etc.
- In case of Stat analyzers (random access analyzers), many reagents (8–20 or more) can be pipetted one after another, so that various biochemical determinations can be performed on one specimen.
- Dry chemical methods utilize reagent slides that are composed of several layers, the amount of reflected light, which is in proportion to color intensity, is used to determine the concentration of the analyte.
- Care, maintenance proper cleaning, and calibration of analyzer is needed.

- An ELISA reader measures and quantitates the color differences in the 12 wells of the plate. ELISA readers are based on spectrophotometry; additionally, ELISA plate readers can also measure fluorescence and luminescence.
- Analyzers consume much less time and cost as compared to ELISA reader.
- Total laboratory automation (TLA) includes use of combinations of analyzers connected physically to perform all steps efficiently.
- TLA has some limitations such as higher short term cost, space requirement, etc.
- Biosensors can be defined as self-sufficient integrated devices that have capacity to provide specific qualitative or semiquantitative analytical information using a biological recognition element which is in direct-spatial contact with a transductional element.
- Nanotechnology deals with developing materials, devices, or other structures possessing at least one dimension sized from 1 to 100 nanometers.
- System integration and miniaturization with more technologically advanced computer power will persist to accommodate more portable analyzers for more precise testing.

PRACTICE QUESTIONS

1. Define automation.
2. Justify that "automation is a need of time".
3. Enlist the advantages of automation.
4. What are individual steps in analysis and how they are automized? Explain it with at least one example for each step.
5. What are the points to be considered while buying an auto autoanalyzer?
6. Discuss the classification of analyzers on different basis.
7. Write principle, uses, and advantages for continuous flow analyzer.
8. Explain working of centrifugal analyzer and its disadvantages.
9. Explain discrete analyzer and its advantages.
10. Differentiate between batch analyzer and stat analyzer.
11. How semiautoanalyzer are useful?
12. What are the advantages of fully automatic analyzer?
13. What is dry chemical analyzer? Explain its working.
14. How to clean semidisposable reaction rotors.
15. Explain working and advantages of any two latest models of analyzers.
16. What is ELISA reader and how it is beneficial?
17. Write a note on:
    i. Total laboratory automation
    ii. Biosensors
    iii. Nanotechnology
18. Compare the advantages and limitations of total laboratory analyses automation.

Index

Page numbers followed by *f* refer to figure, *fc* refer to flowchart, and *t* refer to table

A

Abetalipoproteinemia 479
Acetoacetyl-coenzyme A 170
Acid 3, 7
  base
    Arrhenius theory of 7
    Lowry and Brønsted concept of 8
    status, assessment of 541
  base balance 420, 555
    disturbances of 555
    renal regulation of 538
    respiratory regulation of 536
  maltase 327
  phosphates 299
  sphingomyelinase 337
Acidic solution 72
Acidosis 15
  acute 491
  causes of 13
  metabolic 553, 556, 557
  mild 13
  respiratory 556
Acidurias, organic 341
Acinar cells 290
Acne 369
Acrolein, formation of 180
Acrosome 505
Addison's disease 318, 365, 409, 491, 553
Adenine 197, 249
Adenocarcinoma 605
Adenohypophysis 355
  hormone of 356
Adenosine
  deaminase 518
  diphosphate 302, 305
  triphosphate 133, 180, 285, 305, 317, 581
Adipocytes 137
Adipose tissue 137, 372
  cells 294
Adrenal corticotropic hormone 598
Adrenal failure 359
Adrenal gland 363, 364*f*
  hormone 364
  disorders of 365
Adrenal hyperplasia, congenital 370, 371
Adrenal medulla, hormone of 366
Adrenaline 366
Adrenocorticotropic hormone 318, 359
  disorders of 359
Advanced therapeutic drug monitoring 617
Agarose 89, 269
Alanine 165

aminotransferase 426
transaminase 166
Albumin 159
  serum 159
Alcohol 43, 307, 401
Alconox 225
Aldehydes 43
Alditols 141
Aldolase B 330
Aldosterone 313, 366
Alkaline
  phosphatase 277, 420, 434, 519, 521
  picrate method 453
  urine 15
Alkalosis 559
  causes of 14
  development of 15
  hypochloremic 14, 558
  hypokalemic 559
  metabolic 14, 491, 553, 558
  respiratory 558
Alkane 45
Alkapton 332
Alkaptonuria 332
Alkenes 46
Allopurinol 288
Alpha-fetoprotein 597, 599
Alpha-glucosidase 506
Alpha-ketoglutarate 148
Alumina 251
Aluminum oxide 251
Amines 44
Amino acid 163, 166, 171, 173, 258, 312, 334, 507
  carbon skeletons of 170*f*
  dehydrases 167
  desulfhydrases 168
  glucogenic 170
  lysine 335
  metabolism 185
  oxidase 167
  oxidative deamination of 168*f*
  phenylalanine 172
  types of 166
Amino group, removal of 167
Amiodarone 614
Ammonia 12, 141, 465, 519
Amniocentesis 206
Amniotic fluid 507, 508
  findings, abnormal 509
Amputation 391
Amylase 142, 290, 291, 516, 519, 521
  pancreatic 290

Index

Amylopectin 142, 327
Amylopectinosis 327
Anabolism 142, 311
Anaplastic lymphoma kinase 599
Andersen's disease 153
Androgen 369
Angiokeratomas 188, 338
Aniline 141
Animal cell 130, 135f
    functional units of 134
Anion 5
    exchange chromatography 245, 246, 246f
        applications of 247
        principles of 246
Antibiotics 613
Antibody 261, 263, 266, 269
    monoclonal 412
    secondary 277
    staining 277
Anticancer 614
Anti-C-peptide antibody, sandwich of 407
Antidepressants 614
Antidiuretic hormone 313, 347, 362, 396
    disorders of 363
Antiepileptics 614
Antigen 261, 264, 597
    carcinoembryonic 516, 519, 597, 602
Anti-nuclear antibodies 269
Antipsychotics 359, 614
Antithyroid therapy 386
Anuria 491
Anxiety 551
Apolipoproteins 279
Arginine, hydrolysis of 169
Arterial blood 541
    collection 227
    gas 541, 543
        analysis 543
    specimen, collection of 542
Arthritis 13
    types of 526
Artificial intelligence 636
Aryl halides 43
Ascites
    biliary 522
    cardiac 522
    mixed 522
    pancreatic 522
Ascitic fluids 234
Ascorbic acid 565, 592
Asparagine 165
Aspartate transaminase 166
Asthma, bronchial 57
Atmospheric pressure
    ionization-mass spectrometer 258
    photo ionization 572
Atomic number 5

Atomic weight 6
Atoms 4
    structure of 3, 4, 4f
Autoantibodies, multiple 411
Autoimmune
    disease 379
    disorder 358
    endocrine disorders 411
    thyroid disease 387
Automation 619, 620
Avogadro number 217
Axillary hairs 369
Axons 349
Azoospermia 505

B

Bacteria 519
Basal metabolic rate 143, 378
Basal metabolism 143
Batch analyzer 235, 626
Beam balance 62f
Beer's law 73
Benedict's quantitative reagent 414
Benedict's test 141, 413, 413f
Benzene 244
Berthelot reaction method 448
Beta-2-microglobulin 599
Beta-cells 409
Beta-human chorionic gonadotropin 600
Beta-oxidation
    cyclic representation of 183f
    steps of 182
Bicarbonate 19, 552
    carbonic acid buffer 535
Bile pigments 437, 440
    detection of 438
    metabolism of 438
Bile salts 437, 440
    detection of 437
    metabolism of 437
Biliary tract disease 293
Bilirubin
    conjugation 421
    creation of 421
    estimation of 422
    excretion 422
    formation of 421
    metabolism of 421, 421f
    serum 420
Biochemical tests 212f, 505, 511, 516, 524
    use of 211
Biochemistry 31, 125, 126, 567, 568, 572, 574, 576, 578, 581, 582, 584, 586, 588, 592
    fundamentals of 123
    scope of 126
Biometry 92
Biomolecules 128

Index

Biosensors 638
    components of 639
    principles of 639
Biostatistics 92
Biotin 562, 565, 584
Biuret method 431
Biuret test 162
Bladder 604
    cancer 603, 604, 606
Blindness 391
Blood 227, 447, 599-606
    biotin 585
    carbon dioxide analysis 543, 550
    cell 136, 138
    collection of 227, 228, 542f
    film examination 590
    gas
        analyzer 554, 555f
        determination of 541
    glucose 369, 396, 397
        high 395
        level 401, 446
    oxygen analysis 543
    pH 13, 529
        normal range of 554
        respiratory regulation of 537fc
    plasma 534
    pressure 92
        diastolic 103
        high 379, 395
        systolic 103
    sampling technique 230
    sugar
        fasting 103, 396
        low 330, 395
        random 397
    test 453, 457, 615
    urea nitrogen, estimation of 447
Blotting techniques 271
Body
    fluids 502
    temperature 288
Bone
    abnormalities 331
    cell 136, 138
    marrow 601
Bovine serum albumin 277
Bowel obstruction 522
Bowman's capsule 446
Bradford assay 276
Brain
    cancer 303
    injury 303
    maturity of 378
Branched-chain
    alpha-keto acid dehydrogenase complex 334
    ketoaciduria 334

Breast 604
    cancer 601, 604, 605, 607
    metastatic 603
Brewer's yeast 321
Bromine 39
Brownian movement 53
Budd-Chiari syndrome 522
Buffer solution 19, 498
Buffer system 529, 534
    need of 533
Bulbourethral glands 503
Busulfan 614

C

Calcitonin 598, 602
Calcitriol 446
Calcium 316, 324, 462, 465, 498
    absorption 27
    oxalate 462
    phosphate 462
    serum 498
    standard 498
Cancer
    bile duct 602
    colorectal 601, 603, 605
    ovarian 600, 602, 604, 607
    pancreatic 602
Capillary blood collection 227
Carbamazepine 614
Carbamoyl phosphate 169
Carbohydrate
    biochemical importance of 155
    classifications of 139, 140fc
    detective tests of 141
    metabolism 144, 185f, 326
        disorders of 151
    study of 139
Carbon 39
    atoms 46
    dioxide 168
        partial pressure of 550
        pressure of 551
    skeleton, fate of 170
Carbonate 465
Carboxylic acids 43
Carcinoma, prostatic 301
Carcinomatosis, peritoneal 522
Cardiac function tests 469, 471
Cardiomyopathy 327
Cardiovascular disease 370
Carnitine 506
Catabolism 143, 166, 311
Catalase 315
Catalysis, reaction of 284, 306
Catecholamines 598
Cation exchange chromatography 247, 247f
    steps of 248

Celiac disease 205
Cell 534
   membrane 131, 138, 347
      functional units of 347
   organelles 131, 138
   structure of 130
   tadpole-shaped 136
   types of 136
Cellular
   components 313
   metabolism reactions 282
   respiration 134
Cellulose 155, 254, 263
   acetate 89
Central nervous system, abnormality of 303
Centrifuge 67
Centrosome 133, 138
Ceramide 337
Cerebrospinal fluid 211, 233, 234, 312, 510, 600
Cerebrotendinous xanthomatosis 189
Charcoal 263
Chemical
   buffer system 534, 539
   method, limitations of 466
   reaction 125, 621
Chemiluminescent microparticle immunoassay 386
Chemistry
   extracellular 125
   inorganic 3, 34, 312
   organic 39
Chickenpox 267
Chi-Square
   distribution 118
   test 118
Chloride
   reagent 493
   serum 492
   standard 493
Chlorine 39
Chloroform 244
Cholecystitis, acute 293
Cholecystokinin 372
Cholesterol 179, 237, 396, 469, 471, 472, 475, 517
   high levels of 472
   lower 307
   reagent 473, 476
   standard 473, 476
   total 473
Choriocarcinoma 600
Chorionic villi sampling 206
Chromatographic procedures 243
Chromatography 242, 243f, 263
   thin layer 251, 252f
Chromic acid 225
Chromium 321, 324

Chromogranin A 603
Chromosomal mutations 206
Chromosome 136
Chronic obstructive pulmonary disease 553
Circulation
   pulmonary 471
   types of 470
Cirrhosis 522, 600
   hepatic 515
Citrate 147
   formation of 147
Citric acid
   cycle 144, 170
   total 506
Clonazepam 614
Cobalamin 565
Cobalt-corrin ring complex 588
Cobas mira 634
Cocaine 307
Codon 165
Coenzymes 282
Colloid 52, 376, 377
   biological significance of 54
   properties of 53
   solution 53
Colorimeter 73, 75f, 81, 81t
   parts of 75
Column chromatography 243, 245f
   principles of 244
   steps of 244
Complete blood count 464
Compound 5
Confusion 14
Conjunctiva 313
Conn syndrome 553
Connective tissue disease 522
Constipation 379
Continuous flow analyzers 623
Copper 319, 324
Corpus luteum 371
Corticosteroids, hypersecretion of 365
Corticotropin 359
   releasing hormone 354
Covalent bond 40
C-peptide 407, 408
   amount of 407
   low 408
   test 407, 408
Cramps, abdominal 317
Creatine kinase 305
   isoenzymes, diagnosis of 304
Creatine phosphokinase 283
   isoenzymes test 302
   types of 302
Creatinine 453
   clearance test 456
Cretinism 358
Critical value method 116

Index

Cushing's disease 359
Cushing's syndrome 365, 409, 412, 491, 553
Cyanocobalamin 562, 588
Cyclic adenosine monophosphate 347
Cyclosporine A 614
Cyst, ovarian 294
Cystic fibrosis 205
Cystine 463, 465
Cytochrome
    oxidase 315
    system 316, 322
Cytogenetic analysis 607
Cytokeratin fragment 603
Cytology 519
Cytoplasm 131
    cells 165
Cytosine 164, 197, 249
Cytoskeleton 134, 138

D

Decarboxylases 282
Dehydration 15, 141, 365, 416, 490
Dementia 338
Dendrites 349
Dengue virus 267
Densitometer 89
Deoxyribonucleic acid 192, 348
    replication 198f
    structure of 193, 195f
Deoxyribose 194, 197
Depression 379
Desethylamiodarone 614
Desmethyldiazepam 614
Dextrin 142
Deydrogenases 284
Diabetes
    insipidus 490
    mellitus 391, 396, 401, 414
        complications 393, 395
        diagnosis of 394, 396, 417
        gestational 394, 396
        juvenile 392
        mild 405
        noninsulin-dependent 392
        signs 393
        symptoms 393
        type 1 392, 408, 409, 411, 412
        type 2 392, 394, 408, 409, 412
Diabetic ketoacidosis 294, 296, 414, 416, 553
Diacetylmonoxime method 449
Diarrhea 15, 153, 318
    chronic 553
    severe prolonged 491
Diazepam 614
Dieresis 363
Dietary iodine deficiency 379
Digestion 130, 281
Digoxin 614

Dihydroxyacetone phosphate 294
Diluted test serum 401
Dilution 22, 23
Dimethylbenzimidazole group 588
Dinitrophenyl hydrazine 297
Diploid cell 136
Direct immunofluorescence 268, 268f
Distal convoluted capsule 446
Dopamine 366
Double-beam spectrophotometer 79f
Down syndrome 204, 206
Dry chemical analyzers 627
Duchenne muscular dystrophy 205
    symptoms of 205

E

Ebola 255
Edema, pulmonary 551
Egg
    albumin 159
    cell 138
Ehrlich's test 439
Eicosanoids 346
Electric
    centrifuge 68f
    circuit 639
    current 215
    injuries 303
Electrochemical techniques 622
Electrode 17
    internal 71
Electrolytes 484, 554
    classifications of 484
Electromagnetic spectrum 81
Electromotive force 17
Electromyography 304
Electron
    capture 30
    microscopy 466
Electrophoresis 269, 271, 275, 277, 306
    bands of 271f
    capillary 258
Electrophoretogram 307
Encephalopathy 175
Endocrine
    disorders 401
    system 353
    glands of 346
Endoplasmic reticulum 131, 132
Energy
    metabolism 143
    unit of 143
Enzymatic
    method 473, 474
    reaction 56, 282
Enzyme 78, 126, 134, 261, 288, 300, 360, 597
    activity of 288
    assay 281

catalytic activity 282
classifications of 284
concentration of 287
deficiency 326-329, 332-334, 336-339
denaturation of 288
diseases 401
inhibition, types of 287
inhibitor 288, 308
   complex 287
linked immunosorbent assay 263, 269, 340, 411, 412, 607, 608
   direct 265f
   indirect 266f
   method, principles of 412
   reader 635, 636
   sandwich 266f
   technique 382, 615
   test 264f
lysosomal 378
mechanism of 285
phenylalanine hydroxylase 333
properties of 281
replacement therapy 187
residual 341
substrate complex 285, 287
unit of 282
use of 289
Epididymis marker 506
Epinephrine 366, 401
Epoxycarbamazepine 614
Erythrocyte sedimentation rate 105
Erythropoietin 372, 446
Esters 43
Estrogen 370
   receptor 604
Ethers 44
Ethosuximide 614
Ethyl acetate 244
Ethylene glycol 553
Ethylenediaminetetraacetic acid 229, 230
Ethyne 46
Evelyn method 422
Everolimus 614
Excretory function 420
Exercise, strenuous 304
Eye 312
   disease 406
   sockets 379

F

Fabry disease 188, 338, 339
Fasting glucose
   impaired 396
   test 396
Fat 186
   cells 137, 138
Fatty acid 179, 184
   beta-oxidation of 181

biosynthesis of 181, 185
metabolism 180
oxidation disorders 181, 188
synthetase 181
Fatty acyl-coenzyme A 182
Fecal collection 233
Fehling's test 141
Ferrocyanide 403
Fetal death 371
Fibrin 604
Fibrinogen 604
Flagellum 136
Flame photometer 85, 87, 621
   components of 86
   use of 88
Flavin
   adenine dinucleotide 283, 578
   mononucleotide 578
Flavoproteins 161
Flow cytometry 607
Fluid
   analysis 525
   cholesterol 514
   classifications of 519
Fluorescent in situ hybridization 607
Fluorimeter 82, 85f
   components of 84
Fluorine 39
Fluorochromes 267
Fluorophores 84, 267
Folacin 586
Folate 562, 586
Folic acid 562, 565, 586
Folin blood sugar test 398
Folin uric acid reagent 465
Folin-Wu
   blood sugar tube 398, 398f
   method 397
   procedure 399
Follicle
   cell 378
   membrane 378
   stimulating hormone 382
Food
   contamination 255
   sources 567, 570, 573
Forbes' disease 153
Formaldehyde agarose gel 275
Fouchet's test 438
Fourier transform infrared spectroscopy
   analysis 466
Free thyroxine 381
Free triiodothyronine 381
Fructose
   intolerance, hereditary 154, 330
   total 506
Fungi 519
Furan 42

Index

G

G proteins 347
Galactorrhea 360
Galactose 152
   1-phosphate uridyltransferase 329
Galactosemia 152
Galactosuria 329
Gallbladder cancer 602
Galvanometer 76, 80
Gamma rays 30
Gas chromatography 252, 253f
   principles of 252
   steps of 253
Gastric
   aspirate 211
   cancer 602, 605
   inhibitory peptide 372
Gastrin 372, 598
Gastrointestinal stromal tumor 601
Gastrointestinal tract 290, 353, 372
Gaucher's disease 186, 187, 338
Gel
   chromatography 248, 249f
   electrophoresis 272, 608
Gene signature 607
Genetic
   analysis 607
   code 162
   disorders 204
      detection of 206
      types of 204
   engineering 126
   material 130
Genomic hybridization 607
Germ cell tumors 599, 600, 605
Ghrelin 372
Gigantism 357
Gland 346, 503
   endocrine 344, 345, 353
   pineal 367
   pituitary 353-355, 388
   suprarenal 363
Glass
   bulb 71
   cleaners 225
   instruments, types of 221
   membrane 72
   types of 220
Glasswares, types of 221
Globulin 159
   serum 434
Glomerular filtration rate 456, 461
Glucagon 368
Glucocerebroside 338
Glucocorticoid hormone 351
Glucometer 402
Gluconeogenesis 144
Gluconic acid 403
Glucosazone 141
Glucose 413, 414, 511, 515, 517, 519, 521, 524
   6-phosphate dehydrogenase 305
      deficiency of 174
   amount of 391
   concentration 397
   meters 403
   oxidase 400, 401, 416
      method 397, 400
   peroxidase 78, 289
   procedure 401
   phenylhydrazone 141
   quantity of 404
   standard 401
   tolerance 396
   test 394, 397, 404, 405, 405f, 416
Glucosuria 401
Glucosylceramide 338
Glutamate
   dehydrogenase 167
      role of 167
   pyruvate transaminase 426
Glutamic acid 410
Glutamine 511
Glutaric
   acid 335
   acidemia 334
   aciduria 334
Glutaryl-coenzyme A 335
Glutelins 159
Glutenin 159
Glyburide 409
Glycerol 179
   kinase 294
Glycine reagent 297
Glycogen 142
   accumulation 326
   hydrolysis of 327
   storage disease 152, 326
      characteristics of 153t
      types of 152, 153t, 328, 329
Glycogenesis 144, 368
Glycogenosis 326, 328
Glycolipid 155, 179
Glycolysis 144, 145fc, 151
   oxidative phase of 146
   preparatory phase of 145
   stages of 144
Glycoproteins 155, 161, 279
Glycosuria
   causes of 414
   nondiabetic 414
Glyoxal agarose gel 275
Gmelin's test 439
Golgi apparatus 131
Golgi bodies 133, 138
Gomori's method 495, 497

Index

Gonadotropin 361
  releasing
    factor 361
    hormone 354
Gradient elution technique 244
Gram's stain 511, 525
Graves' disease 379
Growth 135
  hormone 356
    deficiency 357
    inhibiting hormone 354
    releasing hormone 349
    noncancerous 408
Guanine 197, 249
Guanosine
  diphosphate 148
  triphosphate 148
Guillain-Barré syndrome 556
Gum infections 391

H

Hashimoto's disease 358, 379
Hay's test 437, 438f
Head and neck cancers 604
Hearing loss 338
Heart 372
  defibrillation 303
  disease 391, 396, 406
    coronary 237, 477
  external view of 470f
  failure, congestive 299
  function of 469
  injury 303
  muscle 303
  structure of 469
Heartbeat, slow 379
Heinz bodies 174
Hematuria 340
Hemoglobin 406, 534
  amount of 92, 406
  glycosylated 406
Hemolysis, intravascular 491
Hemophilia 205
Hemoreflector, construction of 546
Henderson-Hasselbalch equation 10
Henle loop 446
Henry-Caraway method 458
Heparin 155
Hepatic disease 401
Hepatitis, alcoholic 522
Herrings bodies 356
Hers' disease 153, 328
Hexosaminidase A 337
Hexoses 139
High-density lipoprotein 396, 472, 476
  estimation of 476

High-performance liquid chromatography 254, 254f, 568
  methods 572
Hirsutism 369
Histidine, deamination of 168
Histogram 98
Histones 195
Holoenzyme 282, 308
  structure of 283f
Homeostasis 344
Homeostatic systems 13
Homocysteine 335
Homocystinuria 172, 173, 335
Homogentisate oxidase 332
Hormone 126, 262, 344, 347, 597
  action, mechanism of 346
  chemical nature of 345
  classes of 345
  fat-soluble 347
  functional units of 344
  gonadotropic 361
  hydrophilic 346, 347f, 348f
  hypercalcemic 380
  hyperglycemic 368
  hypothalamic 353
  lactogenic 360
  lipophilic 347
  parathyroid 380
  peptides 346, 379, 380
  placental 394
  producing cells 346
  prolactin
    inhibiting 354
    releasing 354
  receptor complex 348
  secretion, control of 348
  somatotropic 356
  test 412
  thyroid 377, 384
  thyrotrophic 358
  tropic 349
  water-soluble 346
Horseradish peroxidase 277, 386, 412
Huble's reagen 180
Huble's test 180
Human chorionic gonadotropin 382, 598
Huntington's disease 205
Hybridization 274, 275
Hydration 149, 182
Hydride ions 284
Hydrocarbons 44
  characteristics of 45t
Hydrogen 39
  bonding 285
  ions 72, 529
    concentration 72

Index

Hydrolases 284
Hydrolysis test 162
Hydronium, formation of 10
Hydroxy metoprolol 614
Hypercalcemia, idiopathic 317
Hypercalciuria 500
Hypercholesterolemia 475
Hyperglycemia 368, 391, 395
Hyperlipidemia 186, 326
Hyperthyroid pregnancies 389
Hyperthyroidism 379
Hypertonic solution 51
Hypertrophy, benign prostatic 606
Hyperuricemia 326, 329, 339
Hyperventilation 551
Hypervitaminosis 568, 571
Hypocholesterolemia 475
Hypoglycemia 154, 326, 365, 394, 395, 402, 408, 409
    fasting 328
Hypogonadism 360
Hyponatremia 491
Hypopituitarism 412
Hypotension 365
Hypothalamus 314, 353
Hypothesis test 114, 115
    form of 116
Hypothyroid pregnancy 388
Hypotonia 327
Hypotonic solution 51
Hypoxia 551

I

Immune system 387
    development of 380
Immunoassay 261
    types of 263
Immunoenzymometric assay 307
Immunofluorescence
    immunoassay 267
    indirect 268, 268f
    types of 268
Immunoglobulins 605
Immunohistochemistry 607, 608
Immunoradiometric assay 381
Immunosuppressive drugs 614
Infarction, pulmonary 303
Infection, parasitic 515
Infundibulum 353, 354
Inhibitors, effect of 288
Inorganic phosphorus excretion 497
Insomnia 316
Insulin 368, 394, 409, 412, 491
    absence of 414
    autoantibodies 410
    concentration of 412
    dependent diabetes mellitus 392
    resistance 395, 409
    secretion of 349
Insulinoma 408, 409
Interferon gamma release assays 518
International enzyme commission 284
Interstitial cell stimulating hormone 361
Intestinal infarction 296
Iodide ions 377
Iodine 39, 319, 324
    test 142, 180
Iodometric method 291
Ion 5
    beam 257
    exchange chromatography 245
    selective electrode 88, 621, 633, 634
Ionization 256
    chamber 257
Iron 315, 324
    deficiency of 316
    serum 316
Islet cell
    antibody 409
    cytoplasmic autoantibodies 410
Isocitrate, formation of 148
Isocratic elution technique 244
Isoenzyme 283, 303, 307
    sources of 283
Isoleucine 173
Isomerases 285
Isotonic solution 51
Isotope 3, 25, 26
Isthmus 376

J

Jaffe reaction 453
Jaundice 154, 330
Jendrassik-Grof method 424
Joints 313
Juxtaglomerular cells 372

K

Ketone 43, 326, 414
    bodies 413
Kidney 353, 372
    collecting duct 362
    disease 391, 406, 553
    functional units of 444, 446
    stones 13
    structure of 444, 445f
    transplant 339
Kipp hemoreflector 546
Krebs cycle 151
    significance of 149
Kwashiorkor 171

Index

L

Laboratory information system 622
Lactate dehydrogenase 283, 297, 514, 516, 519, 525
   serum 297, 299
Lactic acidosis 326
Lactobacillus delbrueckii 591
Lambert's law 74
Lamotrigine 614
Langerhans islets 368
Lesch-Nyhan syndrome 339
Leucine 173
Leukemia 605
   acute
      lymphoblastic 601
      myelogenous 601
   chronic
      lymphocytic 600
      myeloid 601
Leukocytes 294
Levetiracetam 614
Leydig cells 369
Ligases 285
Light's criteria 514t
Linoleic acid 179
Lipase
   activator 295
   determination of 289
   serum 294
   substrate buffer 295
   tests 296
Lipidosis 186
Lipids 57, 186, 469
   biochemical importance of 189
   classifications 178
   compound 179
   derived 179
   detective tests of 180
   metabolism 180, 185, 336
      disorders of 186
      hereditary disorders of 189
   simple 178
   study of 178
Lipogenesis 181
   reactions 181
Lipoproteins 161, 179
   high-density 396, 472, 476
   low-density 471, 472, 478, 479
   very low-density 471, 478
Lithium 87, 614
Liver 353, 418
   cancer 186, 599
   diseases 294, 299
   dysfunction 206
   function tests 418, 420
   metastasis, massive 522
   morphology 419f
   regeneration 418
Lock and key model 285, 286
Low-density lipoproteins 471, 472, 478, 479
Lung
   cancer 604
   diseases 553
Luteinizing hormone 382
Luteotropin 360
Lyases 284
Lymphatic leak, postoperative 522
Lymphocyte 338
Lymphoma 515, 605
   lymphoplasmacytic 605
Lysosome 131, 132, 326

M

Macroamylasemia 294
Macrominerals 315
Magnesium 318, 324
   ammonium phosphate 463
   chloride reagent 476
Malaria 112
Malloy method 422
Malnutrition 491
Mammalian cells 195
Mammotropin 360
Manganese 319, 324
Maple syrup urine disease 172, 173, 334
Marasmus 171
Maruna and Trinder's method, modified 486
Mass
   number 5
   spectrometer 257
      parts of 256
   spectroscopy 255, 256f, 258
Master gland 353
McArdle disease 153, 328
Melanoma 605
   cutaneous 601
   mucosal 601
Melatonin 368
Meniscus 223
Menstrual cycle 371
Mental deterioration 154, 330
Metabolic function 419
Metabolism 135, 142, 311, 318, 322, 344, 471
   inborn errors of 325, 340
Metabolites 554
Metallic pointer 61
Metalloproteins 161
Methanol poisoning 553
Methionine 163, 165
Methotrexate 614
Methyl methanoate 43
Methylmalonic acid 590
Metoprolol 614

Index

Microfilaments 131
Microminerals 315
Microtubules 131
Milk
  carbohydrate of 360
  protein of 360
Millon's test 162
Minerals 314
  metabolism 311
Miscarriage 371
Mitochondria 131, 133, 181, 190
Mitosis 135
Moilsch test 141
Molar solution 20
Molybdate reagent 495
Molybdenum 320, 324
Monochromators 86
Monoglyceride lipase 294
Monohydroxy 179
Monosaccharides 139
Monostep methods 619
Motilin 372
Mucic acid test 142
Mucopolysaccharidoses 154, 330
  types of 331
Muscle
  cells 136, 138, 328
  injury 304
  stress 304
  weakness 328
Muscular dystrophy 304
Mutants, bacterial 127
Myalgia 328
Mycophenolate 614
Myeloma, multiple 600, 605
Myocarditis 303
Myophosphorylase 328
Myxedema 522

N

Nanotechnology 640
Nebulizer 86
Necrozoospermia 505
Nephrocalcinosis 317
Nephrons 445
  structure of 445f
Nephrotic syndrome 522
Nernst filament 79
Nerve
  cells 137, 138
  damage 406
  problems 391
Nervous system 349
  autonomic 143
  sympathetic 349
Neuroblastoma 605, 606

Neurohypophysis 356, 362
  hormone of 362
Neuron-specific enolase 606
Neutron radiation 31
Niacin 561, 562, 564, 579
Nicotinamide adenine dinucleotide
  phosphate 90, 283
Niemann-Pick disease 187, 188, 336, 337
Nitric oxide 347
Nitrophenyl-beta-galactoside analogue 571
Non-Hodgkin lymphoma 603
Non-oxidative deamination 167
Non-protein nitrogen 447
Non-small cell lung cancer 599, 604, 606
Noradrenaline 366
Norepinephrine 366
Northern blot 274, 278t
  procedure 275
Nuclear
  matrix protein 606
  membrane 165
Nucleic acid 192
  biological importance of 207
  components of 192
  metabolism 339
  molecule 192
  study of 192
Nucleoproteins 161
Nucleoside 193
Nucleotides 193, 194, 317
  interconversion of 203
  synthesis of 322
Nucleus 4, 131
Nuclide 26
Nutrition 130

O

Obesity 370, 412
Obstruction, pyloric 15
Obstructive lung disease 551
Ochronosis 332
O-cresolphthalein complexone
  method 498
  reagent 498
Oligo-amenorrhea 369
Oligosaccharide 139
Oligospermia
  mild 505
  severe 505
Oliguria 491
Oncogenes 597
Optical density 78
Oral estrogen use 479
Oral glucose tolerance test 396
Organic compounds 39, 312
  classifications of 41t, 42

Organic phosphates 317
  synthesis of 322
Oryzenin 159
  formation of 141
Osmosis 50
Osmotic pressure 51, 362
Osteoporosis 335, 370
O-toluidine method 397, 399, 416
Ovary 370
Oxalate 465
Oxaloacetate 148
Oxidation 142, 148, 182, 183, 312
Oxidative deamination 167, 168f
Oxidize alcohol 183
Oxidoreductases 284
Oxygen 39
  capacity 548
    determination of 543
  content 548
    determination of 544
  partial pressure of 544, 548
  saturation 544
    determination of 543, 545
Oxygenation, adequacy of 541
Oxytocin 313, 354, 363
  disorders of 363

P

Palmitic acid, energy yield of 184
Pancreas 368, 394, 408
Pancreatectomy 409
Pancreatic beta cells inhibits insulin secretion 349
Pancreatitis 293, 296, 401
Pantothenic acid 562, 564, 581
Paper chromatography 250
  principles of 250
  steps of 250
Paracentesis 520
  biochemistry 521
Paralysis, familial hyperkalemic 491
Parametric test 94
Parathyroid gland 377f, 379
  pairs of 379
Peal plasma blood sugar, post- 397
Penicillin acylase 288
Pentoses 139
Pentosuria 329, 341
Pericardial fluid 512
  tests 513
  types of 512
Pericardial interferon-gamma 515
Pericardiocentesis 513
  biochemistry 514
Peritoneal fluid 518
  normal values of 519
  tests 520

Peritoneum 313
Peritonitis, tuberculous 522
Peroxidase 315, 416
Peroxide hydrogen peroxidase 400
Peroxisomes 131, 134
pH 3, 10, 72, 517, 553
  effect of 288
  indicators 15
  measurement of 530, 554
  meter 16, 69, 88, 530
    calibration 18f
    parts of 531f
    working principle 530
    scale 69, 70f, 71f
Phenobarbital 614
Phenol reagent 401
Phenyl phosphate 300
Phenylacetic acid 333
Phenylalanine hydroxylase 333
Phenylketonuria 172, 333
  pathway of 334fc
Phenytoin 401, 614
Philadelphia chromosome 597, 600
Phlebotomy 227
Phosphate 299, 315, 465
  buffer system 19, 535
Phosphocreatine 302
  kinase 302
Phosphoenolpyruvate 146
Phosphofructokinase 328, 329
Phosphokinase isoenzymes 303
Phospholipids 179, 317
  synthesis of 322
Phosphoproteins 161, 317
  synthesis of 322
Phosphorescence 83
Phosphoric acid monoesters 299
Phosphorus 317, 324
  serum 495, 496
  standard 495
Phosphotungstic acid reagent 476
Photodetector 87
  system 76
Photometric analysis 84
Photometry, fundamental laws of 73
Photomultiplier tubes 84, 85
Pie chart 98
Pinguecula 338
Pituitary disease 388
Pituitary gland 353-355, 388
  hormone of 356
  morphology of 355f
Plant cells 130
Plasma 51, 386
  enzyme 290
  heparinized 365, 474
  membrane 131

Index

preparation 397
protein 19, 420
tension of 57
urea 212
Plasminogen activator inhibitor 607
Pleural fluid 234, 515
analysis 516
Pneumonia 57
P-nitrophenol 292
Pollution, control of 127
Polyacrylamide 89
gel 275
Polycystic ovary syndrome 395
Polymerase chain reaction 126
Polynucleotides 200
hydrolysis of 200
Polysaccharide 141
types of 142
Polystyrene tube 381
Polyuria 363
Polyvinylidene difluoride 276
Pompe's disease 153, 326
Porphyrinoproteins 161
Portal vein thrombosis 522
Potassium 318, 324, 489
ferricyanide 300
imbalance 365
reagent 488
serum 485, 487
Potentiometry, direct 622
Preeclampsia 395
Pregnancy 551
ectopic 371
fatty liver of 522
Prehybridization 273, 275
Primidone 614
Progesterone 371
receptor 604
Prokaryotes 192
Prolactin 359, 360, 598
disorders of 360
stimulates 360
Prolamins 161
Propyne 46
Prostate 503, 603
cancer 603, 606
carcinoma of 301
marker 506
specific antigen 597, 606
Prostatitis 606
Protein 57, 175, 264, 269, 279, 312, 511, 519, 521, 525
buffers 534
catabolism of 166
classifications of 160fc
conjugated 161
deficiency diseases of 171

derived 161
energy malnutrition 171
free filtrate, preparation of 398, 454
kinases 347
metabolism 162, 171, 332
serum 420, 431
study of 159
synthesis 162, 163f, 281
tests for 162
Proximal convoluted tubule 446
Psychoactive drugs 614
Pulmonary disease, chronic 479
Pulse
oximetry 545
rate 92, 97
Purine 199, 201
catabolism 201
nucleotides, de novo synthesis of 201
salvage pathway 202
P-value 115, 116, 118
method 118
Pyridoxal phosphate 582
Pyridoxine 562, 564
Pyrimidine 200
anabolism 201
catabolism 201
metabolism 199
nucleotides, de novo synthesis of 202
Pyruvate
carboxylase, absence of 155, 332
dehydrogenase complex deficiency 155, 331
metabolism 331
disorders of 155

Q

Quantitative chemiluminescent immunoassay 572

R

Radiation
hazard 32
safety measures 33
types of 29
Radioactivity 29, 35
Radioimmunoassay 31, 262, 359, 571, 607, 608
principles of 263f
Radioisotope 3, 25, 29, 261
use of 31, 32t
Rathke's pouch 355
Red blood cell 51, 93, 365, 516, 522
Refsum's disease 189
Renal buffer system 534
Renal function tests 444, 447
Renal glomerular disease 491
Renal tubular

acidosis 15
  damage 491
Renin 372
  angiotensin-aldosterone system 446
Respiration 130, 135, 281
Respiratory buffer system 534
Respiratory distress syndrome 57, 395
Retinoblastoma 597
Reye's syndrome 479
Rhabdomyolysis 304
Riboflavin 561, 562, 564, 578
Ribonucleic acid 192
  messenger 196
  ribosomal 196
  structure of 195
Ribosome 131, 132, 165
Rotavirus 267
Rothera's test 340, 415, 415f

S

Salicylate
  intoxication 15
  overdose 553
  poisoning 14
Saliva, secretion of 313
Salts
  poisoning 491
  types of 9
Schilling test 591
Schoenfeld and Lewellen's method, modified 493
Scleroproteins 161
Secretin 372
Seizure 154, 303, 330, 338
Selenium 321, 324
Sella turcica 354
Semen 234, 502
  analysis, biochemical variables of 506t
  sample, preparation of 506
Seminal fluid 502
Seminal vesicle 503
  marker 506
Serositis 522
Serum albumin 159
  estimation of 432
Serum ascites albumin gradient 522
Serum glutamic oxaloacetic transaminase 289, 420, 631
  estimation of 428
Serum glutamic pyruvic transaminase 289, 420
  estimation of 426
Serum uric acid 458
  estimation of 458
Sheehan syndrome 359
Shock 416
Sickle cell anemia 204
Silica gel 251

Sirolimus 614
Sitosterolemia 189
Skeletal muscle 327
  inflammation 304
Skin 372
  growths 188
Sleep 360
Small cell lung cancer 603, 606
Sodium 317, 324, 365, 489
  carbonate 458
  serum 485
Solid-liquid chromatography technique 244
Somatostatin 356
Southern blot 272, 273f, 278t
  procedure 272
Spectrophotometer 78, 81, 81t
Sperm
  cells 136, 138
  concentration 505
  morphology, normal 505
  nucleus 505
Sphingomyelin 187, 337
Sphingomyelinase 336
Sphingosine 179
Spinal tap 233
Splenic rupture 294
Sputum 234
Squamous cell carcinoma 267
Stable isotope 26
  use of 27
Starch 142, 291
Starvation 15
Steatorrhea 185
Stem cells 136, 138
Steroid 179, 307, 365
  androgenic 365
  hormone 347
Stone analysis 465
Stress 360
Stroke 391, 406
Strontium 87
Sucrose 154
Sudan III test procedure 180
Sugar determination, quantitative test for 414
Sulfhydryl 288
Sulfonamides 288
Sulfuric acid 382, 473, 476
Sweating, excessive 318
Synovial fluid 234, 523
  characteristics of 526
  normal constituents of 524
Syphilis 267

T

Tacrolimus 614
Tandem mass spectrometry 340
Tarui's disease 153, 329

Index

Tay-Sachs disease 187, 337, 338
Test tube 75
Testicular failure 600
Testis 369, 503
Testosterone 369, 370
Tetrahydrofolate 586
Tetramethyl rhodamine isothiocyanate 268
Tetramethylbenzidine 382, 412
Tetroses 139
Thalassemias 206
Therapeutic drug monitoring 612, 614
Thiamine 561, 562, 564, 576
    deficiency 175
    pyrophosphate 283, 576
Thoracentesis 515
Thymus 380
    gland, location of 376, 380f
Thyrocalcitonin 379
Thyroglobulin 377, 378, 606
Thyroid
    cancer 606
        medullary 602
    follicles 376
    function
        diagnosis of 386
        tests 376, 380, 381t, 387, 388t
    gland 376, 377f, 379
        functional units of 376
        hormone of 378
        morphology of 376
        regulation of 352f
    hormone 377, 384
        level of 381
        release of 377
        synthesis of 377
        thyroxine 380
    stimulating hormone 349, 358, 377, 380, 381, 388
        determination of 382
        disorders of 358
        receptor 358
        test 380
Thyrotropin
    releasing hormone 380
    serum 381
Thyroxine 384
    binding globulin 378, 381
    deficiency of 379
    index 386
    serum 381
Tissue
    receptors 597
    samples 304
Topiramate 614
Toxic multinodular goiter 386
Toxicity 317, 318, 568, 571, 574, 576, 577, 581, 582, 584, 585, 590, 594

Toxicology 84
Toxoplasmosis 267
Trabeculae 376
Trace minerals 322
Trachea 376
Transaminases 426
Transcellular fluids 312
Trauma, pancreatic 293
Tricarboxylic acid cycle 147
Trichloroacetic acid 162, 495
Triglyceride 182, 515, 517, 521
    serum 471, 480
Triiodothyronine 384
    serum 381
Trypsin 289
T-test 117
Tubular necrosis, acute 492
Tumor 408, 599, 601, 604-607
    extrapancreatic 401
    malignant 515
    markers 517, 596, 608
        limitations of 609
        testing of 607
        types of 596
        use of 598
    neuroendocrine 603
    ovarian 370
Turbidometric method 488
Turkish saddle 354
Turner's syndrome 205
Tyndall phenomenon 53
Tyrosine, abnormal metabolism of 333fc
Tyrosinemia 172, 174, 336

U

Ultraviolet
    light 621
    radiation 273
Uracil 249
Uranyl magnesium acetate solution 487
Urea 447
    clearance 452
    cycle 168, 169f
    metabolism 447
Uric acid 339, 340, 457, 462, 465, 525
    metabolism 457
    serum 458
Urinary calculi 462
Urinary tract
    infection 464
    obstruction 15
Urine 340, 600, 603, 605, 606
    analysis 437
    calcium 498-500
    chloride 492, 494
    collection 231, 232
    cortisol 366

Index

creatinine 455
inorganic phosphorus 496, 497
ketone test 414
normal value 415
output 401
pH 14
phosphorus 495
potassium 491, 492
sample 232, 291, 407
types of 232
sodium 491, 492
sugar test 413
test 413, 447, 453, 457, 616
urea 451
uric acid 460
Urinometer 88, 88f
Urobilinogen 437, 440
detection of 439
Urokinase plasminogen activator 607
Uterine tissue 303

V

Vacuoles 133
Valine 173
Valproic acid 614
Varicella zoster virus 267
Vasopressin 313, 362
Veno-occlusive disease 522
Venous blood collection 227
Ventilation, adequacy of 541
Very low-density lipoprotein 471, 478
Vitamin 561
 A 463, 561, 567
 assay 561
 B1 561, 562, 564, 576
 B12 562, 565, 588, 589, 592
 deficiency 589, 590
 test 231
 B2 561, 562, 564, 578
 B3 561, 562, 564, 579
 B5 562, 564, 581
 B6 166, 562, 564, 582
 B7 562, 565, 584
 B9 562, 586
 C 319, 561, 565, 592, 593
 characteristics of 561
 D 561, 563, 568, 570
 deficiency of 570, 571
 metabolism 569f
 deficiency testing, purpose of 566

E 561, 563, 572
 essential 566
 fat-soluble 562, 563t
 H 584
 high level of 568
 K 561, 563, 574
 water-soluble 282, 562, 564t
Vomiting 154, 318, 330
 severe 491, 553
von Gierke's disease 153, 326

W

Waldenström macroglobulinemia 605
Water
 balance 312
 intake 312
 output 312
 passage of 314
 physiological functions of 313, 322
 quality 255
 self-ionization of 10
Watson method 473
Waxes 179
Weakness 379
Weight gain 379
Wernicke-Korsakoff syndrome 175
Western blot 275, 278t
 procedure 276
Whatman paper 250f
White blood cell 516
 count 514, 522, 525
Wolman's disease 189

X

Xanthine dehydrogenase 339
Xanthinuria, hereditary 339
Xanthomas 189
Xanthoproteic test 162
Xylitol dehydrogenase 329

Z

Z data 116
Z test 114, 116
Zinc 320, 324
 test 506
Zona
 fasciculata 364
 glomerulosa 364